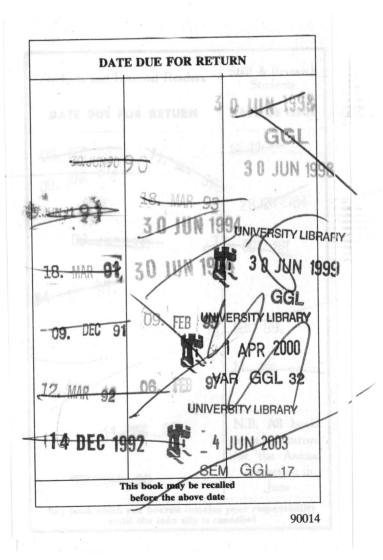

ALFRED BENZON SYMPOSIUM 20

Natural Products and Drug Development

NATURAL PRODUCTS AND DRUG DEVELOPMENT

Proceedings of the Alfred Benzon Symposium 20 held at the premises of the Royal Danish Academy of Sciences and Letters, Copenhagen 7–11 August 1983

EDITED BY

P. KROGSGAARD-LARSEN

S. BRØGGER CHRISTENSEN

HELMER KOFOD

Published by
Munksgaard, Copenhagen

Distributed in Japan by
Nankodo, Tokyo

Printed in Denmark by P. J. Schmidts Bogtrykkeri, Vojens
ISBN 87-16-09563-4
ISSN 0105-3639

Distributed in Japan by
Nankodo Company Ltd.

Contents

List of Participants

E. X. ALBUQUERQUE
Department of Pharmacology &
Experimental Therapeutics
University of Maryland
660 West Redwood Street
Baltimore, Maryland 21201
U.S.A.

NITYA ANAND
Central Drug Research Institute
Chattar Manzil
P. O. Box 173
Lucknow
226001 India

P. S. ANDERSON
Merck Sharp & Dohme
Research Laboratories
West Point, Pennsylvania 19486
U.S.A.

F. ARCAMONE
Ricerca & Sviluppo Chimico
Farmitalia Carlo Erba
Viale Bezzi 24
20146 Milan
Italy

ATTA-UR-RAHMAN
H.E.J. Research Institute of Chemistry
University of Karachi
Karachi-32
Pakistan

J. T. BAKER
Sir George Fischer Centre for Tropical
Marine Studies
James Cook University of North Queensland
Townsville, Qld. 4811
Australia

G. BLUNDEN
School of Pharmacy
Park Building
King Henry I Street
Portsmouth PO1 2DZ
England

PER M. BOLL
Department of Chemistry
Odense University
DK-5230 Odense M
Denmark

J. M. CASSADY
Department of Medicinal Chemistry and
    Pharmacognosy
Purdue University
Pharmacy Building
West Lafayette, Indiana 47907
U.S.A

S. B. CHRISTENSEN
Department of Chemistry BC
Royal Danish School of Pharmacy
2 Universitetsparken
DK-2100 Copenhagen Ø
Denmark

C. Christophersen
University of Copenhagen
H. C. Ørsted Institute
5 Universitetsparken
DK-2100 Copenhagen Ø
Denmark

J. E. Davies
Biogen, S. A.
3, Route de Troinex
1227 Carouge/Geneva
Switzerland

C. Djerassi
Department of Chemistry
Stanford University
Stanford, California 94305
U.S.A.

E. Falch
Department of Chemistry BC
Royal Danish School of Pharmacy
2 Universitetsparken
DK-2100 Copenhagen Ø
Denmark

N. R. Farnsworth
College of Pharmacy
University of Illinois at Chicago
P. O. Box 6998
Chicago, Illinois 60612
U.S.A.

H. H. S. Fong
W. H. O. Collaborating Centre for
Traditional Medicine
University of Illinois at Chicago
Chicago, Illinois 60612
U.S.A.

R. K. A. Giger
Pharmaceutical Division
Preclinical Research
Sandoz AG
CH-4002 Basle
Switzerland

H. Hikino
Pharmaceutical Institute
Tohoku University
Aoba-Yama
Sendai 980
Japan

Huang Liang
Institute of Materia Medica
Chinese Academy of Medical Sciences
Beijing
People's Republic of China

J. Jaroszewski
Department of Chemistry BC
Royal Danish School of Pharmacy
2 Universitetsparken
DK-2100 Copenhagen Ø
Denmark

W. Keller-Schierlein
Laboratorium für organische Chemie
ETH-Zentrum
CH-8092 Zürich
Switzerland

H. Kofod
Department of Chemistry BC
Royal Danish School of Pharmacy
2 Universitetsparken
DK-2100 Copenhagen Ø
Denmark

P. Krogsgaard-Larsen
Department of Chemistry BC
Royal Danish School of Pharmacy
2 Universitetsparken
DK-2100 Copenhagen Ø
Denmark

J. P. Kutney
Department of Chemistry
University of British Columbia
2036 Main Mall
Vancouver, British Columbia V6T 1Y6
Canada

M. LAZDUNSKI
Centre de Biochimie du CNRS
Université de Nice
Parc Valrose
F-06034 Nice Cedex
France

C. LUND-JENSEN
Department of Chemistry BC
Royal Danish School of Pharmacy
2 Universitetsparken
DK-2100 Copenhagen Ø
Denmark

L. A. MITSCHER
Department of Medicinal Chemistry
University of Kansas, School of Pharmacy
Lawrence, Kansas 66045
U.S.A.

K. NAKANISHI
Department of Chemistry
Columbia University
New York, N.Y. 10027
U.S.A.

P. S. PORTOGHESE
Department of Medicinal Chemistry
University of Minnesota
308 Harvard Street, S.E.
Minneapolis, Minnesota 55455
U.S.A.

H. RAPOPORT
Department of Chemistry
University of California at Berkeley
Berkeley, California 94720
U.S.A.

R. K. RAZDAN
Sisa Incorporated
763D Concord Avenue
Cambridge, Massachusetts 02138
U.S.A.

VICHAI REUTRAKUL
Department of Chemistry
Mahidol University
Rama VI Road
Bangkok 10400
Thailand

T. TAKITA
Microbial Chemistry Research Foundation
Institute of Microbial Chemistry
14–23 Kamiosaki 3-chome
Shinagawa-ku
Tokyo 141
Japan

H. WAGNER
Institute für Pharmaceutische Biologie und
    Phytochemie der Universität München
Karlstrasse 29
D-8000 München 2
Federal Republic of Germany

M. E. WALL
Chemistry and Life Sciences
Research Triangle Institute
P. O. Box 12194
Research Triangle Park, North Carolina 27709
U.S.A.

T. R. WATSON
Pharmacy Department
The University of Sydney
Sydney, New South Wales 2006
Australia

B. WITKOP
National Institute of Health
National Institute of Arthritis, Diabetes and
    Digestive and Kidney Diseases
Bethesda, Maryland 20205
U.S.A.

Preface

It is a historic fact that a considerable number of efficient drugs have originated from natural products, principally plant products. Even in the industrialized countries today, a fair percentage (estimated 25) of prescribed, registered medicine contain active pharmaca derived from the plant kingdom (extracts, pure compounds, modifications or analogues).

A different approach to drug development is rational design of (synthetic) drugs, ideally based on detailed insight into the detrimental biochemical mechanisms underlying the pathogenesis of diseases and disorders. It has to be admitted that so far this ambitious approach has been successful only to a limited extent, because the available basic knowledge of the biochemical defects in diseases normally is incomplete and, frequently, negligible. The synthetic approach of the medicinal chemist, therefore, is still largely based on the principle of trial and error. These facts and the limitations of human inventiveness prompt the medicinal chemist also to find inspiration from other sources, primarily biologically active natural products.

An increasing amount of computerized data, scientific documentation, as well as ethnomedical reports indicate that the abundant plant resources, especially in developing countries, are far from being exhausted with respect to potentially bioactive substances, which may act as lead structures in future drug development. It is our opinion that contrary to what is often advocated by believers in herbal medicine and traditional medical systems, natural products and isolates are rarely optimal for therapeutic purposes. By structural modification, it is nearly always possible to optimize the desired effect and, if necessary, to minimize adverse effects. Thus, drug development on a sound scientific basis will always involve an element of rational drug design, even when inspiration is derived from nature.

The "toxic" actions of naturally occurring compounds frequently reflect selective or specific interactions with physiological processes in humans and animals. Screening for biological activities and analysis of the toxic mechanism may reveal compounds with biological effects pertinent to severe human diseases. There are many examples of successful utilization of this approach, but the potential of biologically active natural products as lead structures in drug design has, so far, only been explored to a limited extent.

The aim of this symposium was to focus on examples of successful conversion of natural products into therapeutic agents and on areas in this research field, which at present are under development. Furthermore, the symposium was dealing with general aspects relating to the selection of biologically active material from plants or animals for more detailed pharmacological and medicinal chemical investigations.

Due to the dimensions of the scientific field it has been necessary to be selective with respect to the choice of topics. As hoped, the symposium did form the frame of fruitful and stimulating exchange and development of ideas in this research in the borderlands between chemistry and biology.

Povl Krogsgaard-Larsen, Søren Brøgger Christensen and Helmer Kofod

I. Terrestrial Sources for Active Constituents and Lead Structures

The Role of Medicinal Plants in Drug Development

Norman R. Farnsworth

Why is it that many scientists, especially during the last two decades have been intrigued with the chemistry of natural products and, especially, in the chemistry of secondary metabolites from plants? Undoubtedly a majority of scientific investigation directed toward the chemistry of plants has been motivated by an inherent curiosity by these scientists to solve the structure of complex secondary metabolites and then to duplicate them through synthetic procedures. Others have been fascinated by the biosynthetic routes through which plants form these secondary metabolites. Hence, the pure drive of scientific exploration of the unknown has probably been the primary factor responsible for the considerable body of knowledge currently available on the chemistry of plants. As this knowledge began to accumulate, other scientists directed their attention to the phylogenetic relationships that seemed to be connected with the often obvious, orderly occurrence of secondary metabolites within plant taxa. This led to the birth of chemotaxonomy, a developing art that someday may present a suffcient basis for its application to the general classification of plants. It is also obvious from an overview of the scientific literature that a motivating force for some chemists in the field of natural products, is a desire to publish.

In more recent times, a great deal of attention has been directed toward developing a better understanding of the interrelationhips that are apparent between plants, insects and man, with an obvious focus on their chemistry (Jacobson 1982). Why do some insects thrive on certain plants and clearly avoid others as a source of food and energy? Conversely, why do a few selected plants have an affinity for insects, sufficient enough to attract, capture and destroy

Program for Collaborative Research in the Pharmaceutical Sciences, College of Pharmacy, Health Sciences Center, University of Illinois at Chicago, Chicago, Illinois 60612, U.S.A.

NATURAL PRODUCTS AND DRUG DEVELOPMENT, Alfred Benzon Symposium 20.
Editors: P. Krogsgaard-Larsen, S. Brøgger Christensen, H. Kofod, Munksgaard, Copenhagen 1984.

them? Why are some plants susceptible to insect, fungal or bacterial infestation, while others apparently are able to withstand this type of attack from the environment? As the chemistry of these types of relationships unravel, can this knowledge be applied somehow to explain man's ability to select those plants useful to him for nutrition, recreation and medicine? Or must we continue to believe in the "trial and error" theory of discovery?

Since we know that plants are an important, in some cases indispensible, source of drugs for human use, will it be necessary to further develop useful drugs from the abundant and renewable flora of the earth through an evolution of the imagination, interests and energies of chemists, or will a revolution be required?

Up to recent times, scientists have more-or-less been free to identify their research interests in an undirected manner. Perhaps for a selected few scientists, this Utopian option will continue. However, most likely the vast majority of scientists active today, will find difficulty acquiring the support necessary to conduct their research, if some aspects of it are not directed toward solving some of the problems facing the world. The chemist interested in natural products surely will not be exempt from this type of pressure.

Based on the title of this presentation, it seems that a major goal for me is to identify the role, if any, that medicinal plants play in drug development. However, the term "medicinal" seems to imply that plants to be used in answering this question, should have proven therapeutic efficacy. It is not my intent to follow this definition.

MAJOR HISTORICAL ROLES OF PLANTS IN DRUG DEVELOPMENT
Other than for purposes of pure scientific inquiry, plants historically seem to have served as models in drug development for 3 reasons. First, at least in the industrialized countries, about 25% of all prescription drugs contain active principles that are still extracted from higher plants and this situation has persisted for at least the last 25 years (Farnsworth & Morris 1976, Farnsworth 1982b). Further, it is generally accepted that as many as two-thirds of the people in developing countries rely on plants as sources of drugs. Suffice it to say that plants continue to provide useful drugs for man.

Second, very often, interesting biologically active substances derived from plants may have a poor pharmacological/toxicological profile, at least for the purposes of using them as drugs in humans per se. Such compounds can often serve as templates for synthetic modification and structure-function studies with the anticipation that useful drugs for humans will result.

Third, many highly active secondary plant constituents have unequivocal value as pharmacologic tools that are often found to be useful in studying biological systems and disease processes. A look at the topics being presented at this symposium clearly points out the importance being paid to a study of natural toxins as pharmacologic tools.

Thus, any of these models can be documented as useful approaches applicable to initiating plant-derived drug development programs. The interests and training, as well as the facilities available to a scientist, will determine to a great degree, the direction that a drug development program might take.

Even though the first chemical substance to be isolated from plants was benzoic acid, discovered in the year 1560, the search for useful drugs of known structure from the plant kingdom did not really begin until about 1804, when morphine was separated from the dried latex of *Papaver somniferum L.* (Opium). Since this important event, many useful drugs from higher plants have been discovered. However, less than 100 plant-derived drugs of defined structure are in common use today throughout the world. Less than half of these are accepted as useful drugs in the industrialized countries (Table I). It is interesting that less

Table I
Plant-Derived Drugs Widely Employed in Western Medicine

Acetyldigoxin	*Ephedrine	*Pseudoephedrine
Aescin	Hyoscyamine	Quinidine
Ajmalicine	Khellin	Quinine
*Allantoin	Lanatoside C	Rescinnamine
Atropine	Leurocristine	Reserpine
Bromelain	α-Lobeline	Scillarens A & B
*Caffeine	Morphine	Scopolamine
Codeine	Narcotine	Sennosides A & B
Colchicine	Ouabain	Sparteine
*Danthron	Papain	Strychnine
Deserpidine	*Papaverine	Tetrahydrocannabinol
Digitoxin	Physostigmine	*Theobromine
Digoxin	Picrotoxin	*Theophylline
*L-Dopa	Pilocarpine	Tubocurarine
Emetine	Protoveratrines A & B	Vincaleukoblastine
		Xanthotoxin

* Produced industrially by synthesis.

Table II

Plant-Derived Drugs Used Widely But Not Generally in Western Medicine

Adoniside	Curcumin	Palmatine
Anabasine	Galanthamine	Peonol
Andrographolide	Glycyrrhizin	Quercetin
Anisodamine	Hemsleyadin	Rorifone
Arecoline	Hesperidin	Rotundine
Berberine	Hesperidin methyl chalcone	Rutin
Brucine	Hydrastine	Saligenin
Cephaeline	Kawain	α-Santonin
Cissampeline	Neoandrographolide	Silybin
Cocaine	Nicotine	Tetrandrine
Convallatoxin	Pachycarpine	Vincamine
		Yohimbine

than 10 of these well-established drugs are produced commercially by synthesis, even though laboratory syntheses have been described for most of them.

In the United States, the consumer paid about $ 8.0 billion for prescription drugs during 1980 in which the active principles are still obtained from plants (Farnsworth & Morris 1976, Farnsworth 1982b). In spite of this, not a single pharmaceutical manufacturer in the United States has a serious research program designed to discover new drugs from the plant kingdom. With the exception of Japan, there does not appear to be much intensity of interest in plant-derived drug development programs in other developed countries of the world. The idea of developing drugs with plants as a starting point has always been high in the developing countries since most of them have abundant starting material in their natural flora and scientific expertise is usually available to implement this type of program. Organizational capability, modern equipment and administrative encouragement, however, appear to be less than sufficient to expect programs to be productive.

Table II lists additional plant-derived drugs that are either widely used in developed countries, perhaps without medical acceptance as to efficacy, or are medically accepted, but less widely used, and/or are included in the pharmacopoeias of many developing countries, for example, the People's Republic of China. That a drug is unknown to western medicine and has pharmacopoeial status in a country with more than 1 billion people, should provide reasonable evidence of utility. Naturally, there are many other minor plant-derived substances of known structure that are used as drugs, such as camphor, menthol, eucalyptol, capsaicin, several minor cardiotonic glycosides, etc., which have not been included in Tables I and II.

ATTITUDES TOWARD INITIATION OF PLANT-DERIVED DRUG
DEVELOPMENT PROGRAMS

Several recent papers addressing the topic of support/non-support for plant-derived drug development programs have been published. In these, specific examples have been cited that have most likely contributed to the negative attitudes that seem to have developed in the minds of decision makers in government, industry, and in private foundations and this has resulted in a lack of attention to this promising area of drug discovery (Djerassi 1979, Farnsworth 1982a, Farnsworth & Bingel 1977, Schneider 1964, Tyler 1979). It would serve no useful purpose to reiterate the details of these arguments at this time. However, a summary of this problem might be useful.

1. Industry, especially in developed countries, generally feels that patent protection for plant-derived drugs is weak. Process patent usually offer little protection and difficulties arise when active principles are found whose chemical structures are known (Schneider 1964, Tyler 1979).

In developed countries, the cost of taking a drug from the discovery stage to the market place can exceed $50 million and span a period of several years (Djerassi 1979, Pillow 1979). Thus, industry is reluctant to invest in the development of any drug when its investment cannot be recovered. Patent protection is mandatory for this reason. However, this does not constitute a problem in most developing countries, where a major thrust behind drug development programs is to conserve hard currency. Approval for use of a new drug in many of the developing countries is not as complicated a procedure as in most developed countries of the world.

2. For a drug being marketed in developed countries, the manufacturer must have assurance of a continued supply of starting material for its synthesis or extraction. Starting material for synthetic drugs can usually be obtained from several sources so that dependence on a single supplier minimizes this problem. Generally speaking, it is felt that if the plant source for a useful drug is geographically restricted to a country where there is instability in the government, that source of supply could be disrupted with predictable consequences, especially since the vast majority of plant-derived drugs are not amenable to commercial synthesis. A look at this problem shows that virtually every plant-

derived drug of importance can be obtained from several different geographic regions, or the plant can be cultivated. Thus, a well-planned drug development program requiring plants as starting material, should include advanced planning to assure availability.

3. How often does one hear or read that "biological variation" is a major frustration when studying plants for pharmacologic activity. This occurs when there is a failure to be able to duplicate an initial interesting biological activity in a second collection of plant material. It has been the experience of our research group that perhaps about one-quarter of the plants that we have found to present an interesting biological activity, based on test results from an initial collection, failed to show the activity when recollections of the "same" plant were similarly evaluated. However, it has never been clearly demonstrated that failure to confirm activity in a second collection is due exclusively to biological and/or chemical variation of a sample. In other words, unless one has complete control over the botanical, chemical and biological aspects of a plant-derived drug development program, it is difficult to identify where problems of this type reside. Further, it is a rare instance when a pharmaceutical firm would employ a full-time botanist - reliance is usually made for plant collections through a commercial botanical importer. We have rarely been able to acquire adequate voucher specimens from commercial importers who have provided plant samples for our programs. This makes it difficult to verify the identification of recollections, especially when they are small, to determine whether we were actually working with the same plant.

4. It is also known that a major complaint of biologists or pharmacologists who are involved in attempting to make a biological assessment of plants, is that crude extracts are most frequently water-insoluble and/or they are difficult to place into a suitable homogeneous suspension for administration to an animal. If the route of administration of an extract to a test animal has to be intravenous, particulate matter cannot be administered. As a consequence, such extracts are often left on the shelf and forgotten. For the most part, problems of this type are not insurmountable, based on advances in pharmaceutical technology, i.e. preparation of co-precipitates that solubilize plant extracts.

Most of the pharmacologists that we have worked with often indicate that assessment of the pharmacologic effects of crude plant extracts is something that they are totally unprepared for, based on their classical training. Clear cut results are rare, good dose-response curves are infrequently seen and effects elicited following the administration of extracts under experimental conditions are often ambiguous. When fractionation of a promising extract is carried out, the pharmacological effects usually become more distinct and exciting. Work of this type is often delegated to a technical assistant, who cannot, in most cases, be expected to identify subtle and perhaps unanticipated effects produced by plant extracts.

Finally, the failure of many major programs to produce useful drugs after several years of intensive effort and millions of dollars, signals to many that plants are an uninteresting source of useful drugs. For example, the recent decision to eliminate the National Cancer Institute (NCI) contract program involving a search for tumor inhibitors in plants, will most likely produce a negative effect on support for plant-derived drug development programs of all types throughout the world for a long period. Could it be possible that leurocristine and vincaleukoblastine, indole alkaloids from the Madagascan Periwinkle, are the only two clinically useful antitumor agents, present in the plant kingdom, when more than 250,000 species of higher plants are thought to exist on this planet?

APPROACHES TO PLANT-DERIVED DRUG DEVELOPMENT
As there are currently no scientific methods applicable for the selection of plants that can be expected to contain novel biologically active substances, the planning for plant-based drug development programs must utilize approaches that are considered to be "non-scientific" by some. Historically, scientists claiming to have an interest in drug discovery from natural products have used the following approaches.

1.0 Phytochemical screening
The literature is abundant with papers in which thousands of plants, randomly selected, have been subjected to a series of spot tests or color reactions to identify those containing one or more broad classes of chemical constituents, i.e., alkaloids, sterols, triterpenes, flavonoids, saponins, tannins, lactones, quinones, cyanogenics, glycosides, essential oils and others (Farnsworth 1968). Justification for this approach is usually made on the basis that biologically active and/or useful drugs can be identified within each of the chemical groups for which tests are being made and, hence, related chemical compounds might be found that will have a drug potential. For the most part, the results from these types of screening procedures are unreliable and in many instances do not reflect

the presence of the substance for which the test was devised. To the best of my knowledge, useful drugs for humans have not been found based on data derived from phytochemical screening programs.

2.0 Selection of plants having a specified class of chemical compound, followed by bioassay

Several years ago the Smith Kline & French Co. in the U.S.A. supported for more than a decade a program involving the selection of alkaloid-containing plants on a random basis throughout the world. This was followed by pharmacological screening of the alkaloid-containing fractions from those plants. The program has never been described in the literature and, thus, the problems and potentials of this approach are unknown. Suffice it to say that the program was terminated and it did not produce useful drugs during its existence.

3.0 Selection of plants based on folkloric use

Virtually all of the currently useful drugs derived from plants were discovered through scientific investigation of folkloric claims of human efficacy. The discovery of reserpine and related useful alkaloids is perhaps the most recent success story that was based on a pursuit of folklore. However, quinine, digoxin, digitoxin, tubocurarine, morphine, codeine and a majority of other useful drugs were also derived from plants in a similar fashion. On the other hand, there are those who believe that all important medicinal folklore has been tapped relative to its value in discovering useful drugs (Tyler 1979).

4.0 Selection of plants based on pharmacological screening

As indicated previously, the most intensive program of this type was recently terminated. The National Cancer Institute in the United States no longer supports a so-called random-selection screening program of plant, animal and marine extracts selected from the flora and fauna of the world. However, at least during the past 15–20 years, this program has not been based on a selection of plants randomly collected. It was also not an especially expensive program relative to the total cost of developing all types of useful antitumor agents. While some active and promising plant-derived compounds remain to be fully evaluated from the NCI program, such as taxol, indicine-N-oxide, harringtonine, phyllanthoside and others, the program over the past 25 or more years did not identify a single agent for general use in the treatment of human cancer. On the other hand, the number of cytotoxic and/or experimental antitumor agents identified by the program was enormous. Follow-up studies of many of these active compounds by biologists have contributed immensely to a better understanding of the cancer process and mechanisms of action of antitumor agents. Structure-activity studies made possible through synthetic work by chemists has also contributed significantly to a better understanding of the types of molecules required to elicit antitumor effects. These represent spin-off benefits of any drug development program.

As mentioned previously, there has been success in the development of useful antitumor agents from plants as evidenced by the discovery of leurocristine and vincaleukoblastine from *Catharanthus roseus* (L.) G.Don. The latter alkaloid was discovered almost simultaneously in 2 different laboratories, i.e., at the Eli Lilly Company, U.S.A. by the team of Svoboda, Gorman and Neuss, and in Canada by Noble, Beer and Cutts. The paper published by the latter group, interestingly enough, was titled "Chance Observations in Chemotherapy-*Vinca rosea*", which contained the following statement ... " ... The results of our research, which are presented here in detail for the first time, should not be considered in terms of a new chemotherapeutic agent, but rather in terms of a chance observation that has led to the isolation of a substance with potential chemotherapeutic possibilities" (Noble *et al.* 1958).

In Svoboda's laboratory at the Eli Lilly Company, *Catharanthus roseus (Vinca rosea* L.) was selected for inclusion in a broad biological screening program by Svoboda because of its reputation as a folkloric hypoglycemic agent. However, extracts of the plant did not show hypoglycemic activity. Instead, a remarkable prolongation of life in mice infected with the P1534 leukemia was noted. *Catharanthus roseus* was the 40th of 200 plants selected by Svoboda to be screened for a broad spectrum of biological activities. Extracts prepared from this plant were submitted for antitumor testing on December 23, 1957, and the antitumor effect was identified in January of 1958. Vincaleukoblastine was isolated shortly thereafter and was approved by FDA and marketed in the United States for the treatment of Hodgkin's disease and choriocarcinoma in March of 1961. Leurocristine was discovered during this period of time and was approved by FDA for use as an antitumor agent in July of 1963. Leurocristine is considered worldwide to be the drug-of-choice for the treatment of childhood leukemias (Farnsworth & Bingel 1982).

Thus, it is important to point out that in the NCI plant screening program for antitumor agents, no useful drug arose from the program after testing perhaps

40,000 species of plants and the Lilly screening program yielded two useful and marketed antitumor agents after screening only 40 species.

ELEMENTS OF AN IDEAL PLANT-BASED DRUG DEVELOPMENT PROGRAM
It is obvious from the approaches just mentioned that others are possible and variations of these have been used as well. However, with the exception of the approach involving a follow-up of folkloric information, all have been unsuccessful except in a few cases where the actual discovery of a useful drug involved an element of serendipity. Based on a general knowledge of industrial viewpoints and some personal experience and associations with groups desirous of setting up plant-derived drug development programs, together with a reasonable feel for the approaches used by academic scientists, it has become very clear that definite elements must be included in a plant-based drug development program in order to anticipate success. These are as follows.

1. Effective and successful programs can only be anticipated in which a multidisciplinary group of scientists, working harmoniously in a collaborative way, and being situated in proximity, is put together. Minimally, the group must consist of scientists having expertise in botany, chemistry and biology. Real collaboration involves agreement to work together toward a common goal with input by all parties from the beginning. To me, meaningful collaboration does not exist between a botanist and a chemist or between a chemist and a biologist, when one of the pair only provides a service to the other. Too many so-called collaborative efforts in the field of natural products involve the latter situation.

2. A well-thought-out strategy must be developed, taking into account (a) the scientific expertise available to the program (b) the local or national drug priorities, (c) available physical facilities and equipment required to attain the goals of the program, (d) the extent of funding (e) a mechanism to insure that a significant discovery can be taken to the market place or be introduced into the medical system of the country and finally, (f) effective leadership.

3. Since, in most cases, development of a drug requires a long and complex procedure before it can be used in humans, any research group embarking on a drug development program must enlist an industrial partner. Such a partner should be involved at the planning stage of the program and not only when a potentially useful drug has been discovered.

4. Even under the best of circumstances, a drug development program requires time. There are no shortcuts without predictable consequences, and organizational or institutional commitment for this must be assured.

It would be an interesting experiment if we could arrange for everyone present at this Symposium to work together under one roof, augmented with a few other experts in specialized areas of biology and botany, with a resolve to develop new drugs from natural sources. There is little doubt in my own mind that such an experiment would pay off handsomely in less than five years, providing the previously mentioned guidelines were followed. On the other hand, working singly or restricting our own work to self-directed scientific interests, we most likely will go into retirement knowing that our contributions may be of value to science or to other scientists somewhere and sometime, but the likelihood that new and useful drugs will arise from our individual laboratories would be remote.

CONCLUSION

Plants remain as an untapped reservoir of potentially useful chemical compounds (a) as drugs, (b) as unique templates that could serve as a starting point for analog preparation by chemists primarily interested in synthetic work, or (c) as interesting tools that can be applied to a better understanding of biological processes. The last two possibilities are strongly tied to the former. It is my personal opinion that the discovery of useful drugs from plants will best be carried out through a concentrated multidisciplinary attack on the plant kingdom by means of collaboration, good planning, imaginative and creative thinking, dedication, a touch of luck, and a great deal of serendipity.

REFERENCES

Djerassi, C. (1979) *The Politics of Contraception,* pp. 68–69, W. W. Norton & Company, New York.
Farnsworth, N. R. (1968) Biological and phytochemical screening of plants. *J. Pharm. Sci.* 55, 255–276.
Farnsworth, N. R. (1982a) Rational approaches applicable to the search for and discovery of new drugs from plants. In: *1er Symposium Latinoamericano y del Caribe de Farmacos Naturales, Havana, Cuba, 21–28 June, 1980. Acad. Cienc. Cuba and Comision Nacl. Cuba ante la UNESCO,* Montevideo, Uruguay, pp. 27–59.
Farnsworth, N. R. (1982b) The potential consequences of plant extinction in the United States on the current and future availability of prescription drugs. Unpublished invited paper at a symposium on Estimating the Value of Endangered Species: Responsibilities and Role of the Scientific Community, American Association for the Advancement of Science annual meeting, Washington, D. C., January 4, 1982.

Farnsworth, N. R. & Bingel, A. S. (1977) Problems and prospects of discovering new drugs from higher plants by pharmacological screening. In: *New Natural Products and Plant Drugs with Pharmacological, Biological or Therapeutical Activity,* eds. Wagner, H. & Wolff, P., pp. 1–22, Springer-Verlag, New York.

Farnsworth, N. R. & Morris, R. W. (1976) Higher plants-the sleeping giant of drug development. *Amer. J. Pharmacy* 147, 46–52.

Jacobson, M. (1982) Plants, insects and man – their interrelationships. *Econ. Botany* 36, 346–354.

Noble, R. L., Beer, C. T. & Cutts, J. H. (1958) Role of chance observations in chemotherapy: *Vinca rosea. Ann. N. Y. Acad. Sci.* 76, 882–894.

Pillow, W. F., Jr. (1978–1979) Editorial, *Tile & Till 64,* 13.

Schneider, J. H. (1964) Patentability of natural products, plant isolates and microbiological products. In: *Patents for Chemical Inventions.* ed. Gould, R. F., pp. 99–106. American Chemical Society, Washington, D. C.

Tyler, V. E. (1979) Plight of plant-drug research in the United States today. *Econ. Botany* 33, 377–383.

DISCUSSION

WALL: Why were so few useful, active plants developed by the formal National Cancer Institute Program? Could it be that no true collaboration between physicians, chemists, and botanists existed?

FARNSWORTH: It is my opinion based on more than 20 years experience in the NCI program that a major weakness could be an almost total lack of interaction between chemists, botanists, biologists, and physicians.

ARCAMONE: We have never found correspondence between reported fold-use and test for anti-inflammatory, anti-cancer, or anti-virus activities. Could this discrepancy be explained by the necessary differences between the preparation of folk medicines and extracts for pharmacological tests?

FARNSWORTH: To the best of my knowledge no definitive studies have been published suggesting that the inability to correlate folkloric claims with experimental pharmacological test results in many cases is due to differences in the type of extract employed for testing. Perhaps of greater importance is that medicinal folkloric information found in the literature is incomplete and poorly described. It is difficult to understand how primitive man could document the etiology of a disease such as poliomyelitis or cancer. In his treatment of such diseases he could only describe a series of symptoms treated with plant products. It is therefore difficult to envision how reliable correlations of cause-effect situations for certain diseases can be made that would allow one to select an appropriate bioassay. On the other hand, for example, treatment of intestinal parasitic diseases with plant extracts represents more believable information, since the observation of expulsion of parasites from the body in the feces, following treatment, is a more reliable indicator of efficacy.

DJERASSI: You have not explained of what the 25% prescribed drugs derived from plant sources really consist. Neither did you mention if and how the use of plant-derived drugs has changed during the last decade.

FARNSWORTH: We have documented in detail the breakdown of types of plant products comprising the 25% of prescriptions over the period 1967 to 1973 in several publications (1, 2, 3, 4). We have not analyzed the raw data on prescription frequency that has accumulated due to lack of time. However, we do know that the percentage of prescriptions containing plant-derived active compounds has remained at ca. 25% up through the year 1980. Since relatively few new plantderived drugs were introduced to the market place during this period of time, it is quite possible that the relative percentage of each plant-derived type of prescription has remained constant as described in our previous cited publications.

(1) Farnsworth, N. R. (1969) Drugs from higher plants. *Tile & Till 55,* 33–36.

(2) Farnsworth, N. R. (1977) The current importance of plants as a source of drugs. In: *Crop Resources.* ed. Seigler, D. S., pp. 61–73. Academic Press, New York.

(3) Farnsworth, N. R. & Bingel, A. S. (1977) Problems and prospects of discovering new drugs from higher plants by pharmacological screening. In: *New Natural Products and Plant Drugs with Pharmacological, Biological or Therapeutical Activity.* Springer-Verlag, New York, eds. Wagner, H. & Wolff, P., pp. 1–22.

(4) Farnsworth, N. R. & Morris, R. W. (1976) Higher plants – the sleeping giant of drug development. *Am. J. Pharm. 147,* 46–52.

Bioactive Compounds from Nature

Koji Nakanishi

Most natural products exist in nature for specific purposes and, thus, it is not surprising that they would exhibit some interesting bioactivities. In most cases, however, they are not sufficiently active or are too toxic to be of immediate practical use. In such cases, the structures have to be chemically modified for activity enhancement or toxicity reduction, either empirically, or more logically, if the mode of action is known. In any event, it is the structural uniqueness of natural products that is so valuable and indispensable in acquiring new leads for bioactive molecules. In the following, we present some results from our recent and current research in the general area of bioactive natural products.

GENERAL STRATEGY

In the past we have carried out systematic extraction studies of plants, mostly East African medicinal herbs, in order to isolate and identify the active constituents. The air-dried 40% aqueous methanol extract of the plant is extracted successively with hexane, ether, methanol, and the residue is taken up in water. Each extract is then bioassayed separately to monitor the isolation and characterization of the active principle(s). The in-house assays carried out are insect antifeedant tests using the army-worm (*Spodoptera exempta, S. litoralis* or *S. eridania*), Mexican bean beetle (*Epilachnia varivestes*), or spruce bud-worm, helicocidal tests with *Biomphalaria pfeifferei* (a South American snail which is a host for schistosomes, parasitic trematodes responsible for the widespread occurrence of schistosomiasis), and plant growth regulatory tests using lettuce seeds.

Department of Chemistry, Columbia University, New York, N. Y. 10027, U.S.A. and Suntory Institute for Bio-organic Research, Osaka 618, Japan.

NATURAL PRODUCTS AND DRUG DEVELOPMENT, Alfred Benzon Symposium 20.
Editors: P. Krogsgaard-Larsen, S. Brøgger Christensen, H. Kofod, Munksgaard, Copenhagen 1984.

Once an active factor has been characterized, it is subjected to other biological activity tests such as antibiotic, antifungal, antiyeast assays, and other pharmacological tests, provided there is sufficient material. Past experience has shown that practically all insect antifeedants isolated exhibit other activities; therefore, insect antifeedant tests could be used as a relatively simple guide for isolating active factors from plants. It should also be mentioned that tropical flora have given a much higher probability of yielding antifeedants (or bioactive compounds), a finding which is not surprising because they are exposed to a greater variety of predators as compared to their temperate-zone counterparts (Kubo & Nakanishi 1977a, 1979). Plants which are resistant to insects are a good source; folk-medicinal herbs are also good sources for antifeedants as well as pharmacologically active principles.

An alternative scheme for isolating bioactive factors is, of course, to follow specific intrinsic attributes such as hormonal and pheromonal; this frequently involves interdisciplinary collaboration between organic chemists and biologists, biochemists, etc.

INSECT ANTIFEEDANTS

a. *Specionin* (Chang & Nakanishi 1983) (Fig. 1)

This is a case in which the compound is synthesizable and, thus, can be subjected

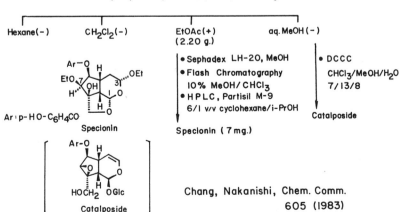

Fig. 1. Isolation of specionin from *Catalpa* leaves following the spruce bud-worm antifeedant assay.

more readily to structural modifications. The isolation scheme is a slight variant of the general procedure described above. Furthermore, since the search for antifeedants against the Eastern spruce bud-worm was the specific purpose of this project, the isolation was monitored with the worm raised on an artificial diet or on natural spruce.

The spruce bud-worm infests North American fir and spruce forests and inflicts enormous damage on the lumber industry. Leaves of 40 tree species that are not attacked by the worms were collected and extracted with ethanol. The active principle, specionin, isolated from *Catalpa speciosa* Warder (Bignoniaceae), 7 mg from 9 g of dried leaves, had an activity level of 50–100 ppm in a choice test. Although this activity is rather moderate, it should be noted that the spruce bud-worm larvae are voracious animals difficult to control.

b. *Azadirachtin* (Zanno *et al.* 1975) and *warburganal* (Kubo *et al.* 1976) (Fig. 2) Of the close to 30 antifeedants that we have isolated to date from East African plants, these 2 are the most potent. Azadirachtin was first isolated by Butterworth and Morgan (1968) from the seeds of *Azadirachta indica* A. Juss (Indian neem tree), and the closely related *M. azedarach* using feeding inhibition tests with the desert locust (*Shistocerca gregaria*) (Morgan & Thornton 1973); 100% inhibition is caused by 40 μg/l or when impregnated on filter paper by 1 ng/cm^2. Besides being a systemic growth disruptor (Gill & Lewis 1971, Ruscose 1972) it is an effective antifeedant against a wide variety of insects. Its liminoid structure (Zanno *et al.* 1975) is too complex to be synthesized, but on the other

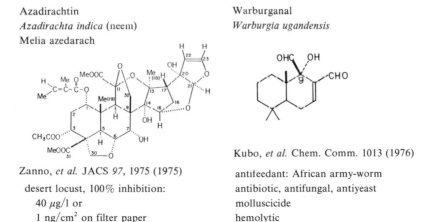

Azadirachtin
Azadirachta indica (neem)
Melia azedarach

Zanno, *et al.* JACS 97, 1975 (1975)

   desert locust, 100% inhibition:
     40 μg/l or
     1 ng/cm^2 on filter paper

Warburganal
Warburgia ugandensis

Kubo, *et al.* Chem. Comm. 1013 (1976)

   antifeedant: African army-worm
   antibiotic, antifungal, antiyeast
   molluscicide
   hemolytic

Fig. 2. Azadirachtin, a potent antifeedant and warburganal, a strongly bioactive principle.

hand, the tree is common in India and Africa and the yield of azadirachtin is quite high (800 mg from 300 g of seeds under favorable conditions, i.e., season, etc.), and being a traditional herb used as a toothbrush (twigs), or orally for malaria treatment, etc., it has no acute toxicity. Field tests with the leaf sap have been carried out in Nigeria with positive results. The tree is, thus, attracting considerable attention throughout the world. International Conferences on the Neem Tree have been held in Europe since 1980.

Warburgia stuhlmannii and *W. ugandensis,* from which warburganal was isolated (leaves), are also widely used in folk medicine and food spices (bark) in East Africa. Warburganal is a very potent antifeedant against the African army-worm (*Spodoptera exempta,* oligophagous, 0.1 ppm), but is less active against *S. littoralis* (polyphagous, 10 ppm), and non-active against the Southern army-worm (*S. eridania,* polyphagous), a pest in the Texas and Florida regions. Electrophysiological studies show that warburganal irreversibly blocks the taste buds of *S. exempta* (Ma 1977) so that when the worm is placed on a corn leaf treated with warburganal for 1 h and then transferred onto an untreated leaf, it starves to death. Warburganal is active against a host of micro-organisms, e.g., *Candida utilis* 3.1 μg/ml (Kubo & Nakanishi 1979, Nakanishi 1980), and is also a potent molluscicide (LD_{100} 5 ppm in 2 h against *B. pfeifferi*) (Kubo & Nakanishi 1977b). Although when taken orally warburganal is non-toxic (it is contained in "ta-de", a spicy plant traditionally accompanying sashimi, the Japanese raw fish dish), upon injection it exhibits strong, acute toxicity (LD_{50} 20.4 mg/kg with mice) and cytotoxicity (KB test 0.01 μg/ml). Warburganal has been synthesized by many groups.

c. *Trichilins* (Nakatani *et al.* 1981) (Fig. 3)
These complex antifeedants against the spruce bud-worm and other insects were isolated from the root bark of the East African plant *Trichila roka* (Meliaceae). Tests with the Southern army-worm have shown that substituents at C-1, -2 and -3 do not exert a great effect but C-12 is crucial: i.e., trichilin B 200 ppm, A 300 ppm, B 12-acetate and 12-desoxy-A (or -B) 400 ppm, C inactive (unpublished). The trichilin structures were found to be very closely related to aphanastatin (Polonsky *et al.* 1978), the isolation of which was directed by lymphocytic leukemia P388 bioassay. Exchange of samples showed aphanastatin and trichilins to be potent antifeedants and cytotoxic agents, respectively. The coincidence of antifeedant activity and cytotoxicity has been encountered in other cases (Kubo & Nakanishi 1977a, 1978) in addition to warburganal (see

Fig. 3. The insect antifeedant trichilins and antileukemic factor aphanastatin.

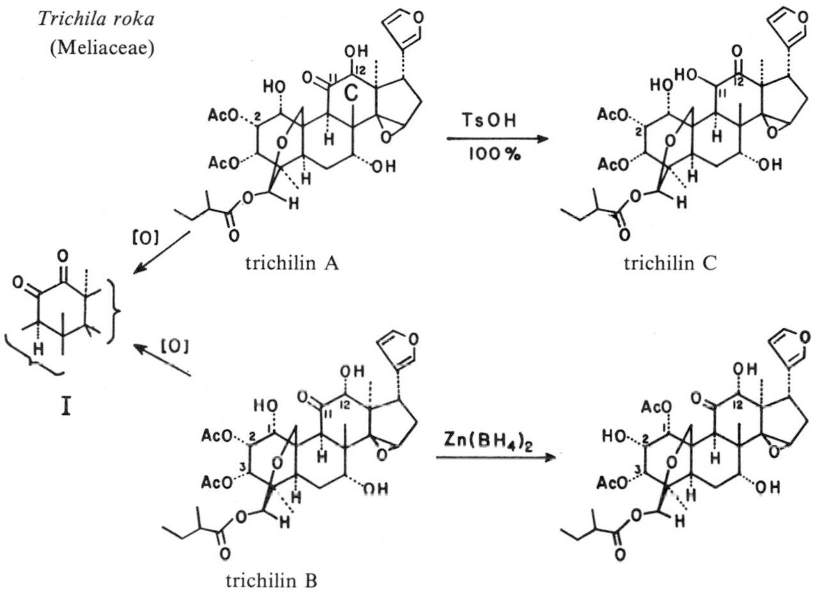

above). The coincidence is probably due to the fact that the majority of insect antifeedants isolated have an electrophilic moiety.

MOLLUSCICIDE FROM *ACACIA NILOTICA*
(Chang 1982)

Schistosomiasis, a serious tropical disease affecting several million people every year, is one of the major problems for which WHO is actively seeking an inexpensive remedy. Since the snails *Biomphalaria pfeifferei* and *B. glabratus* serve as hosts for the miracidium, a stage in the life cycle of the flukes responsible for schistosomiasis, we are looking for principles which cause hemolysis of these snails (which are very readily raised in a plain-water tank with lettuce leaves). *Acacia nilotica* is widely used in Sudan to kill the snails which proliferate in swamps and puddles after rain storms. The lyophilized fruits were extracted with ether and then with ethyl acetate, the latter giving 5 g of crude tannin, which was fractionated by a tedious procedure involving rotation locular counter-current chromatography (RLCC, Snyder *et al.* 1983) and tlc to give 50 mg of an extremely unstable powder; the snail assay was employed for monitoring the isolation. Structural studies carried out on the deca-acetate elucidated the molluscicidal factor as a compound containing 2 gallates (Structure I). The isolated compound is too unstable to be of practical use, but it is apparently protected from oxidation in the fruit and the crude tannin.

PHYTOALEXINS PRODUCED BY THE SWEET POTATO
(Schneider & Nakanishi 1983, Schneider *et al.* 1983a, b) (Fig. 4)

The furanosesquiterpene (+)ipomeamarone, which is produced in large quantities by the sweet potato (*Ipomea batata*) upon infection by black rot fungus *Ceratocystis fimbriata,* is one of the first phytoalexins to be isolated (1943). The conflict in its absolute configuration has now been settled (Schneider *et al.* 1983). Careful isolation studies have yielded 6 new related compounds, thus, bringing the total to ca. 30 (Schneider *et al.* 1983b); many of these exhibit antifungal activity.

The more polar fraction of the extract which had not been investigated before has given the new selinene 7-hydroxycostal which has a stronger germination inhibitory activity against *C. fimbriata* (Schneider & Nakanishi 1983). Since costal is devoid of antifungal properites, the activity of the 7-hydroxy derivative is attributed to the generation of acrolein as shown in Fig. 4 (a conversion which has been verified upon incubation for 1 week).

Sweet potato (*Ipomea batatas*) infected with
black rot fungus (*Ceratocystis fimbriata*)
PHYTOALEXINS

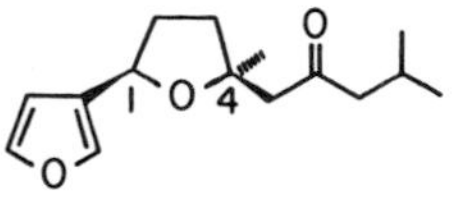

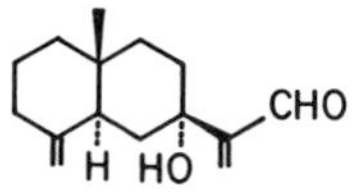

Ipomeamarone
(Kubota, 1953)

Schneider, *et al.*
Chem. Comm. 352 (1983)

7-Hydroxycostal
0.45 g from 15 g CHCl₃ extract

Schneider, Nakanishi
Chem. Comm. 353 (1983)

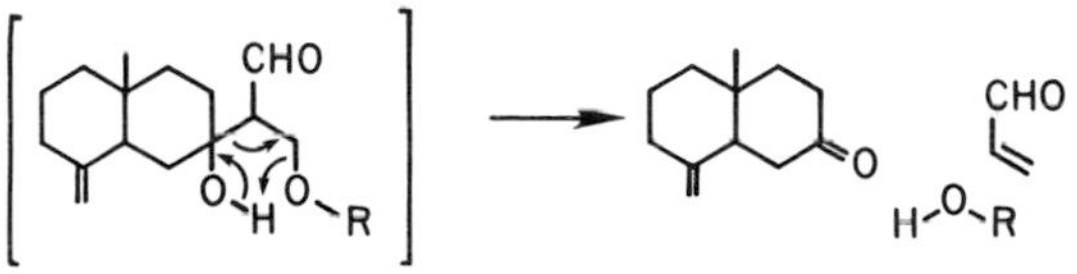

Fig. 4. Sweet potato phytoalexins ipomeamarone and 7-hydroxycostal.

A SESTERTERPENOID KAIROMONE
(Tempesta *et al.* 1983) (Fig. 5)

The scale insect *Ceroplastes rubens*, which attaches to citrus and other trees as
deep red hemispheres about 3 mm in diameter, are widespread orchid pests in
Japan. The insect bodies have given 5 sesterterpenes which represent a new class
as exemplified by cerorubenic acid-I (Fig. 5). Interestingly, some of these
compounds act as a kairomone responsible for the ovipositional behavior of the
parasitic wasp Anicetus beneficus; the eggs of this wasp hatch inside the host
insect and destroy it. Kairomones with a simpler structure could potentially be
used to control pest insects by attracting their natural enemies.

Ceroplastes rubens Maskell (scale insect)
cerorubenic acid-I

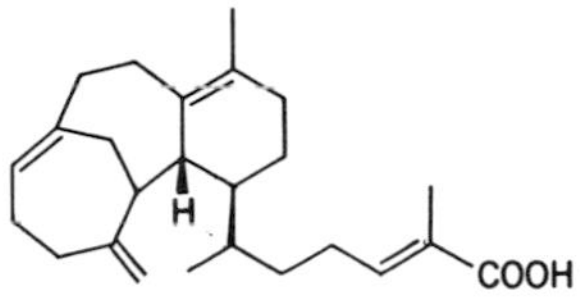

kairomone: *Anicetus beneficus*
(parasitic wasps)

Tempesta, *et al.* Chem. Comm.

Fig. 5. A sesterterpene with kairomone activity isolated from the scale insect.

Relative activities in receptor binding

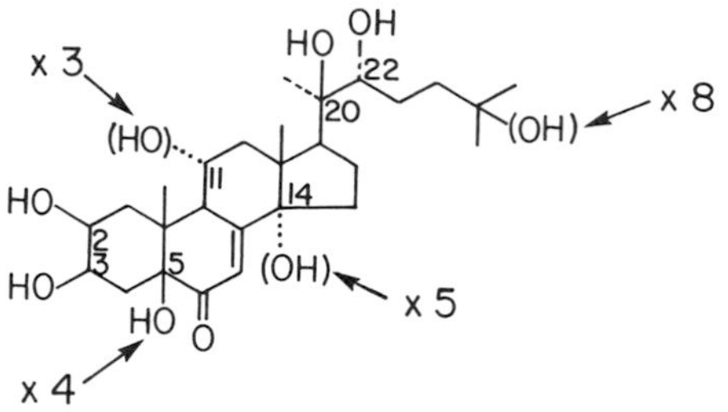

Fig. 6. Relative affinities for ecdysteroid receptor. Number n by parenthesized OH indicates n-fold increase in affinity upon removal of OH; number n by non-parenthesized OH indicates n-fold increase with introduction of OH.

14-DEOXYMURISTERONE
(Cherbas *et al.* 1982) (Fig. 6)

Treatment of the phytoecdysteroid muristerone (Canonica *et al.* 1972) with $Me_3SiCl/NaI/CH_3CN$ under Ar for 3 h at room temperature gave the 14-desoxy compound in 25% yield (the reaction was initially carried out in an attempt to introduce radioactive iodine in the ecdysteroid). Although the molting-inducing activity was diminished it was found that the 14-deoxy compound was ca. 50 times more active than the natural molting hormone 20-hydroxyecdysone when assayed by the morphological response of *Drosophila* Kc-H cells in culture; this assay roughly parallels the affinity for the ecdysteroid receptor.

Removal of the 14-hydroxyl from other ecdysteroids with Zn/AcOH gave an unusually clear-cut structure/activity relation in terms of receptor affinity assay as shown in Fig. 6 (Stonard *et al.* 1983). Namely, removal of OH groups in parentheses led to an increase in activity, 8-fold for 25-OH, 5-fold for 14-OH and 3-fold for 11-OH, whereas presence of 5-OH results in a 4-fold increase. We have prepared 14-deoxyponasterone A with ^{3}H in the side-chain and are planning to utilize its strong receptor affinity (120-fold that of 20-hydroxyecdysone) to clarify the mode of action of insect molting, i.e., what is the series of molecular events which activate the genes involved in molting? The 14-OH is required for molting by probably being metabolized to a more active hormone *in vivo*. The 14-deoxy compound, which is weak in terms of its molting activity, binds strongly to the natural ecdysteroid receptor. In this sense it is similar to a suicide enzyme and this should have adverse effect on insects, an aspect under investigation.

CABENEGRINS, ANTI-SNAKE VENOM FACTORS
(Nakagawa *et al.* 1982) (Figs. 7, 8)

An aqueous alcoholic extract "especificio pesara" of the root of an as yet unidentified Amazonian plant "Cabeca de negra" is available to plantation workers in the jungle as an oral antidote against snake venom (*Fer de lance* or *Bothrops atorax*) and spider venom. A tedious extraction procedure using mice

anti-snake venom factors from *Cabeca de negra*

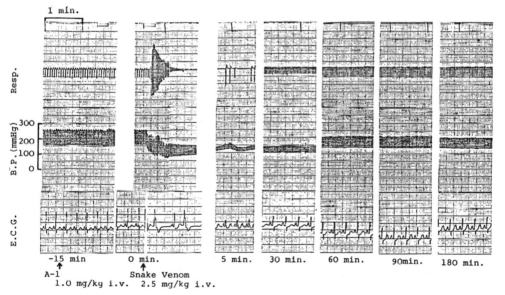

cabenegrin A-I   cabenegrin A-II

M. Nakagawa, *et al.* Tet. Lett. 3855 (1982)

Fig. 7. Two anti-snake venom factors isolated from a South American plant extract.

anesthetized beagle dog, 9 kg
Bothrops atorox

Fig. 8. Effect of cabenegrin A-I on respiratory and cardiovascular responses to the snake venom (*Fer de lance* or *Bothrops atorox*) in anesthetized dog (sodium pentobarbital 35 mg/kg, i.v.). Resp: respiration, B.P.: blood pressure, E.C.G.: electrocardiograph.

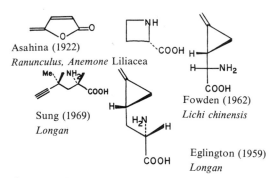

Fig. 9. Procaryote antimutagens from plants.

as the monitoring animal (2.5-fold lethal dose of *Fr de lance* venom was intraperitonially injected, the fractions were injected immediately after envenomation and mice were checked for survival after 24 h) led to the isolation of cabenegrins A-I and -II. Both pterocarpans were subsequently synthesized (Ishiguro *et al.* 1982). Injection of 2.5 mg/kg i.v. (lethal dose) of the snake venom to a male beagle dog (9 kg weight) led to immediate respiratory and cardiac arrest and hypotension; however, pre- (15 min) or post- (several min) injection of cabenegrins restores the respiratory and cardiovascular responses (Fig. 8).

ANTIMUTAGENS FOR PROCARYOTES ISOLATED FROM PLANTS
(Minakata *et al.* 1983, Komura *et al.* 1983) (Fig. 9)
The screening of over 500 plants for the presence of antimutagens according to a bioassay system using *E. coli* B/r WP2 *trp* (UV, MNNG-induced mutation), *S. tryphimirium* TA 100 *his* (spontaneous mutation) or *B. subtilis* NIG 1125 *his* (spontaneous mutation) has led to the characterization of protoanemonine from *Ranunculus* and *Anemone* plants (Minakata *et al.* 1983), L-azetidine-2-carboxylic acid from Lilliaceae and Clavariaceae plants, L-α-(methylenecyclopropyl) glycine from *Litchi chinensis* (Sapindaceae), and 2-amino-4-methylhex-5-ynoic acid and hypoglycine from *longan* (Komura *et al.* 1983). All compounds had been isolated from various plants earlier. The antimutagenic tests with eucaryotes should be performed.

THE RED TIDE TOXINS BREVETOXINS
(Lin *et al.* 1981) (Fig. 10)
The dinoflagellate toxins responsible for the massive fish kills, mollusc poisoning and human food-poisoning along the Florida coast and Gulf of

Toxins from *Ptychodiscus brevis*

BTX-A[1] T^2_{46} – CHO

BTX-B[1]   GB-2[3,4] T^5_2 T^6_{34} T^2_{47} – CHO

BTX-C[7,1]   ↓   ↓   – CH$_2$Cl

         GB-3[3] T^8_{17} – CH$_2$OH

1. Lin, *et al., JACS,* 6773 (81)
2. Risk, *et al., "Toxic Din. Blooms,"* 351 (79)
3. Chou, Shimizu, *TL,* 5521 (82)
4. Shimizu, *"Marine Nat. Prod.,"* I, 1 (78)

5. Alam, *et al., J. Pham. Sci.,* 865 (75)
6. Baden, *et al. Toxicon,* 455 (81)
7. Golik, *et al., TL,* 2535 (82)
8. Baden, Mende, *Toxicon,* 452 (82)

brevetoxin-B

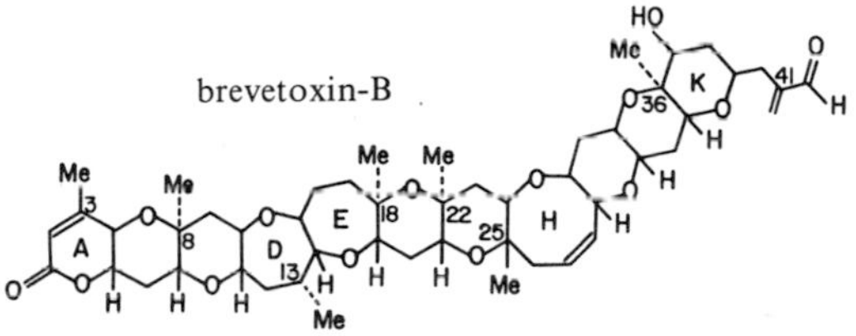

Fig. 10. Neurotoxins from the red-tide dinoflagellate *Ptychodiscus brevis* and structure of the main component brevetoxin-B. The chart summarizes the various notations assigned to the toxins in the past; those on the same horizontal line denote the same toxin, e.g., BTX-A and T$_{46}$ are the same and the terminal group is -CHO (the structure of this still remains to be elucidated). Superscripts in the chart denote the references.

Mexico are produced by blooms of *Ptychodiscus brevis.* Davis. The major toxin (BTX-B) was first purified and characterized in 1981 by Lin *et al.* Because of the attempts by different groups to isolate the toxins for 20 years, the nomenclature has been quite confusing as summarized in Fig. 10. The structure of BTX-B (C$_{50}$H$_{70}$O$_{14}$) is unprecedented. It is made up of a single carbon chain locked into a ladder comprising trans-fused ene-lactone and 10 ether rings. The structures of BTX-C (Golik *et al.* 1982) and GB-3 (Chou & Shimizu 1982) have also been determined; the terminal enal is a chloroketone in BTX-C and an allylic alcohol in GB-3.

It has recently been shown that the brevetoxins are potent neurotoxins which open the sodium channel and that they have a receptor site different from other neurotoxins. The ca. 30 Å length of the brevetoxins makes it relatively easy to modify one end and still retain the toxicity, although at a diminished level; such modifications should be suited for isolating the receptor site and will enable us to gain some insight into the mechanisms of sodium transport.

ACKNOWLEDGEMENTS

I am most indebted to all colleagues who carried out the studies described. The work has been supported by NIH grants AI 10187, CA 11572, and the Suntory Company.

REFERENCES

Butterworth, J. E. & Morgan, E. D. (1968) Isolation of a substance that supresses feeding in locusts. *J. C. S. Chem. Commun.* 23–24.

Butterworth, J. H. & Morgan, E. D. (1971). Title of paper *J. Insect Physiol. 17,* 969.

Canonica, L. Danieli, B., Weisz-Vincze, I. & Ferrari, G. (1972)Title of paper *J. C. S. Chem. Commun.* 1060–1061.

Chang, C. C. (1982) title of paper Ph. D. Thesis, Columbia University.

Chang, C. C. & Nakanishi, K. (1983) Specionin, an iridoid insect antifeedant from *Catalpa speciosa. J. C. S. Chem. Commun.* 605–606.

Cherbas, P., Trainor, D. A., Stonard, R. & Nakanishi, K. (1982) 14-Deoxymuristerone, a compound exhibiting exception moulting hormone activity. *J. C. S. Chem. Commun.* 1307–1308.

Chou, H.-N. & Shimizu, Y. (1982) A new polyether antibiotic from *Gymnodinium breve* Davis. *Tetrahedron Lett.* 5521–5524.

Gill, J. S. & Lewis, C. T. (1971) Systemic action of an insect feeding deterrent. *Nature 232,* 402–403.

Golik, J., James, J. C., Nakanishi, K. & Lin, Y.-Y. (1982) The structure of brevetoxin C. *Tetrahedron Lett.* 2535–2538.

Ishiguro, M. Tatsuoka, T. & Nakatsuka, N. (1982) Synthesis of (I)-cabenegrins A-I and A-II. *Tetrahedron Lett.* 3859–3862.

Kada, T. (1982) Mechanisms and genetic implications of environmental antimutagens. In: *Environmental Mutagens and Carcinogens,* ed. Sugimura, T., Kondo, S. & Takabe, H., pp. 355–359. Univ. Tokyo Press, Tokyo.

Komura, H., Minakata, H., Nakanishi, K. & Kada, T. (1983). Unpublished.

Kubo, I., Lee, Y.-W., Pettei, M., Pilkiewicz, F. & Nakanishi, K. (1976) Potent army-worm antifeedants from the East African *Warburgia* plants. *J. C. S. Chem. Commun.* 1013–1014.

Kubo, I. & Nakanishi, K. (1977a) Insect Antifeedants and Repellents from African Plants. In: ACS Symposium Series No. 62 *Host Plant Resistance to Pests,* ed. Hedin, P. A., pp. 165–178. Am. Chem. Soc.

Kubo, I. & Nakanishi, K. (1979) Some Terpenoid Insect Antifeedants from Tropical Plants. In: *Advances in Pesticide Science,* Part 2, ed. Geissbuhler, H., pp. 284–294. Pergamon Press, New York.

Lin, Y.-Y., Risk, M., Ray, S. M., Van Engen, D., Clardy, J., Golik, J., James, J. C. & Nakanishi, K. (1981) Isolation and structure of Brevetoxin B from the "red tide" dinoflagellate *Ptychodiscus brevis (Gymnodinium breve). J. Am. Chem. Soc. 103,* 6773–6775.

Ma, W.-C. (1977) Alterations of chemoreceptor function in army-worm larvae (*Spodoptera exempta*) by a plant-derived sesquiterpenoid and by sulfhydryl reagents. *Physiol. Entomol. 2,* 199–207.

Minakata, H., Komura, H. Nakanishi, K. & Kada, T. (1983) Protoanemonin, an antimutagen isolated from plants. *Mutation Res. 116,* 317–322.

Morgan, E. D. & Thornton, M. D. (1973). Azadirachtin in the fruit of *Melia azadarach. Phytochem.* *12,* 391–392.

Nakagawa, M., Nakanishi, K., Darko, L. & Vick, J. A. (1982) Structures of cabenegrins A-I and A-II, potent anti-snake venoms. *Tetrahedron Lett.* 3855–3858.

Nakanishi, K. (1980) Insect Antifeedants from Plants. In: *Insect Biology in the Future* "VBW80", ed. Locke, M. and Smith, D. S., pp. 603–611. Academic Press, New York.

Nakatani, M., James, J. C. & Nakanishi, K. (1981) Isolation and structures of trichilins, antifeedants against the Southern army-worm. *J. Am. Chem. Soc. 103,* 1228–1230.

Polonsky, J. Varon, Z., Arnoux, B., Pascard, C., Pettit, G. R., Schmidt, J. H. & Lange, L. M. (1978) Isolation and structure of aphanastatin. *J. Am. Chem. Soc. 100,* 2575–2576.

Ruscose,, C. N. E. (1972) Growth disruption effect of an insect antifeedant. *Nature New Biol. 236,* 159–160.

Schneider, J. A. & Nakanishi, K. (1983) A new class of sweet potato phytoalexins. *J. C. S. Chem. Commun.* 353–355.

Schneider, J. A., Yoshihara, K. & Nakanishi, K. (1983a) The absolute configuration of (+)-ipomeamarone. *J. C. S. Chem. Commun.* 352–353.

Schneider, J. A., Lee, J., Naya, Y., Nakanishi, K., Oba, K. & Uritani, I. (1983b) The fate of the phytoalexin ipomeamarone: new furanoterpenes and butenolides from *Ceratocystic fimbriata*-infected sweet potatoes, Submitted to *Phytochem.*

Stonard, R. Trainor, D. A., Nakanishi, K. & Cherbas, P. (1983) Unpublished.

Tempesta, M. S., Iwashita, T., Miyamoto, F., Yoshihara, K. & Naya, Y. (1983) A new class of sesterterpenoids from the secretion of *Ceroplastes rubens* (Coccidae). *J. C. S. Chem. Commun.,* in press.

Zanno, P. R., Miura, I., Nakanishi, K. & Elder, D. L. (1975) Structure of the insect phagorepellent azadirachtin. *J. Am. Chem. Soc. 97,* 1975–1977.

DISCUSSION

ANDERSON: The importance of the hydroxy groups for the molting activity of 14-deoxymuristerone makes me ask, if there is a reason to believe that cAMP has anything to do with the molting.

NAKANISHI: I don't know.

ANDERSON: Is anything known about the mechanism inside the *Acacia nilotica* that protects molluscicide from oxidation?

NAKANISHI: Probably some anti-oxidant is present.

KROGSGAARD-LARSEN: Is there a physiological receptor for the ecdysteroids or is the binding site the active site of an enzyme?

NAKANISHI: There is a physiological receptor. We plan to do 2 things with Dr. Peter Chebas, one is to isolate the protein which carries the binding site, and the other is to localize the binding site in the living cell using tritium-labelled ecdysteroids.

ALBUQUERQUE: Can you explain why you are able to protect the animals against fer-de-lance venom by pretreatment with, or by administration of, cabenegrins to poisoned animals?

NAKANISHI: I think it is a fascinating pharmacological problem, but it is not known. The cabenegrins are also active against poisoning from rotten food, botulism, and this may suggest a common mechanism.

LAZDUNSKI: Do the cabenegrins protect against the toxicity of the other types of toxins present in snake venoms, especially the cytotoxins?

NAKANISHI: Professor Ching, China, recently tested the cabenegrins against venom from the Southeast Asian Habu snake and found no activity.

BAKER: A great challenge to the organic chemist is to protect labile groups in potential drugs, and still ensure bio-activity in human administration. Also we should try to simplify complex substances by identifying the important functional groups and synthesizing analogues. In one compound given, cerorubenic acid, there is a complex cyclic structure. Were any tests conducted to determine if the α,β-unsaturated carboxylic acid is the functional group and if the hydrocarbon portion can be simplified?

NAKANISHI: I believe that it is the general sesterpene that is scattered in itself.

Plant Products Produced in Cell Culture

James P. Kutney

It is well known that plants provide a fertile source of natural products many of which are clinically important medicinal agents. In numerous instances, the present source of the medicinal drugs still derives from large plantations propagated in appropriate areas of the world where climatic conditions, etc., are optimum for growth. In such cases, the supply and cost of the active agent is dependent upon the complexity of the plant extract from which it is isolated, the concentration which, in turn, may vary depending upon the season of plant collection, etc. Within certain areas of medicinal applications, for example, cancer chemotherapy, lack of the target compound may be associated with difficulties of plant collections due to geographical locations or even political problems. In order to alleviate such situations, various laboratories have recently addressed themselves to studies with tissue cultures derived from such plants in the hope that this technique would afford methodology for laboratory controlled production of selected medicinal agents.

In addition, plant tissue cultures also provide excellent media for detailed biosynthetic investigations and, via cell-free extracts derived from such systems, potentially important sources of enzymes for various studies of interest to the scientific community. Various books (Street 1977, Reinert & Bajaj 1977), and recent review articles (Kurz & Constabel 1979, Kurz & Constabel 1979a) provide an excellent background to the methods involved and summaries of earlier studies in the tissue culture area. The present lecture will summarize the recent experiments which have been obtained in our tissue-culture program directed specifically to cultures propagated from plant species known to produce clinically important anticancer drugs. The specific experiments which we have conducted concern the following plant species: 1) *Catharanthus roseus* L. G. Don; 2) *Maytenus buchananii;* 3) *Tripterygium wilfordii;* 4) *Cephalotaxus*

Department of Chemistry, University of British Columbia, Vancouver, B. C., Canada V6T 1Y6.

NATURAL PRODUCTS AND DRUG DEVELOPMENT, Alfred Benzon Symposium 20.
Editors: P. Krogsgaard-Larsen, S. Brøgger Christensen, H. Kofod, Munksgaard, Copenhagen 1984.

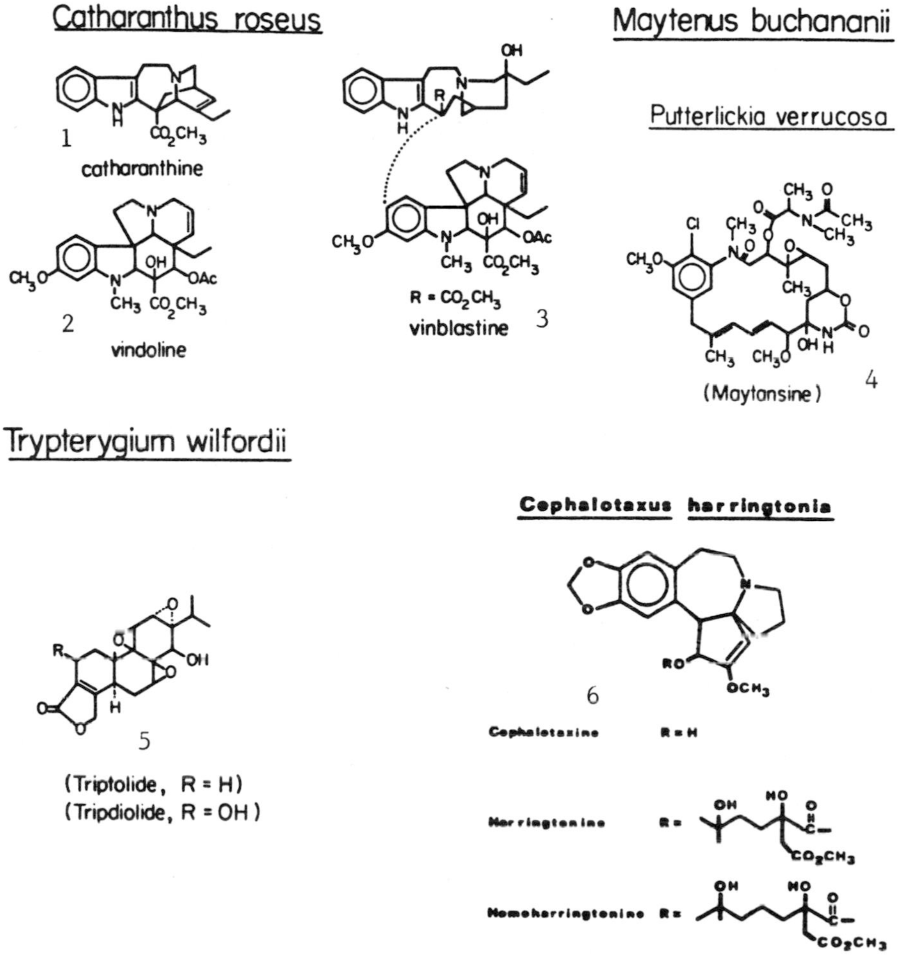

Catharanthus roseus

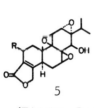

1
catharanthine

2
vindoline

R = CO₂CH₃
vinblastine 3

Maytenus buchananii

Putterlickia verrucosa

(Maytansine) 4

Trypterygium wilfordii

5

(Triptolide, R = H)
(Tripdiolide, R = OH)

Cephalotaxus harringtonia

6

Cephalotaxine R = H

Harringtonine R =

Homoharringtonine R =

Fig. 1. Plant species under study and the target compounds involved.

harringtonia, and Figure 1 summarizes the target compounds which are involved in our program. Due to lack of time the discussion will focus largely on *C. roseus* and *T. wilfordii.*

STUDIES WITH *CATHARANTHUS ROSEUS*

Our studies concerning the various avenues of research within this aspect of our program involve a collaborative effort between our group at the University of British Columbia and the National Research Council of Canada, Prairie

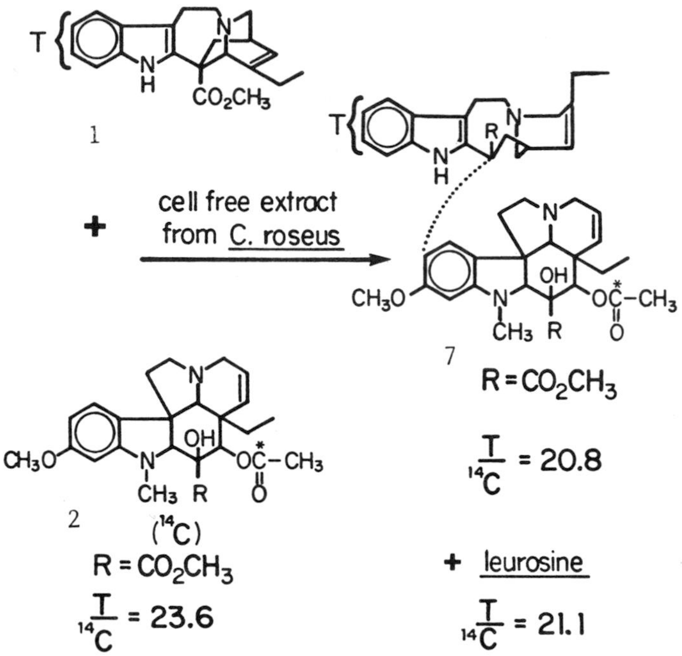

Fig. 2. The biosynthesis of 3′,4′-anhydrovinblastine (7) and leurosine (8) from catharanthine (1) and vindoline (2) employing cell free extracts.

Regional Laboratory, Saskatoon. The direction of this program was influenced considerably by our earlier studies on the synthesis and biosynthesis of bisindole alkaloids within the vinblastine family. Vinblastine (3), one of the clinically important anti-tumor agents isolated from *C. roseus,* represents an important member of these complex natural products and synthetic routes to (3) from more readily available starting materials have been under study for some years. The development of the "biogenetic" approach in our (Kutney *et al.* 1976, Kutney 1978, Kutney *et al.* 1980), and other (Potier *et al.* 1976, Potier *et al.* 1979) laboratories and involving the coupling of catharanthine N-oxide with vindoline provide an important route to the bisindole alkaloid system. Furthermore, in a parallel study in our laboratory and utilizing cell-free extracts from *C. roseus* (Kutney *et al.* 1978a, b, c), we were able to demonstrate that 3′, 4′-anhydrovinblastine (7) is also formed in the enzymatic process via the coupling of catharanthine (1) and vindoline (2) (Fig. 2). Subsequent enzymatic transformation of this bisindole system (7) to the clinical drug vinblastine (10, R = CH₃) and the bisindole alkaloids leurosine (8) and catharine (9) (Fig. 3) is also

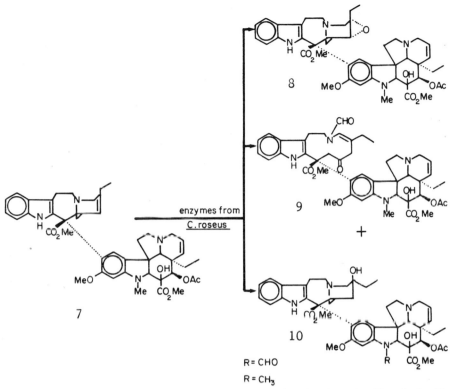

Fig. 3. Enzyme catalyzed conversion of 3′,4′-anhydrovinblastine (7) to leurosine (8), catharine (9) and vinblastine (10, R=CH₃) employing cell free extracts.

achieved with the enzymes obtained in the cell-free extract. A simultaneous independent study by Scott (Scott *et al.* 1978) provided results analogous to those summarized in Fig. 2. These various studies clearly demonstrated the overall importance of the 2 monomeric alkaloids vindoline and catharanthine and consequently the production of these compounds via the tissue culture methodology became of primary concern. Details of these studies are available in various recent publications (Kutney *et al.* 1980a–d, 1981, 1981a–e, 1982) so the following discussion provides only an overall summary of our experiments.

Callus grown from anthers generally originated at the cut of the filament and in the anther walls, i.e., diploid tissue. When grown to a size of 1–2 g freshweight, about 2 cm in diameter, the callus was cut into small pieces and serially subcultured on fresh agar medium or transferred to liquid medium (Gamborg's

B5 medium) giving rise to a cell suspension. For large scale production Zenk's alkaloid production medium was employed.

The alkaloid production varied with the cell line and age of the subculture and ranged from 0.1–1.5% of cell dryweight. The relative amounts of alkaloids produced was fairly constant under conditions given and appeared cell-line-specific. Monitoring of alkaloid production is achieved by HPLC so that not only relative concentrations of total alkaloids produced can be ascertained but comparative concentrations of specific alkaloids, for example structures 11–24, with time, etc., can be accurately determined.

All subcultures of cell lines grown in 7.5 liter *Microferm* bioreactors followed essentially the pattern shown in Fig. 4. After incubation with actively growing cell-suspension, the mitotic index (MI) dropped to zero within 24 h and remained there for 2–3 days. Thereafter, the index rose sharply and reached its maximum (MI 1.8–3.0) within 2 days and declined again gradually over the

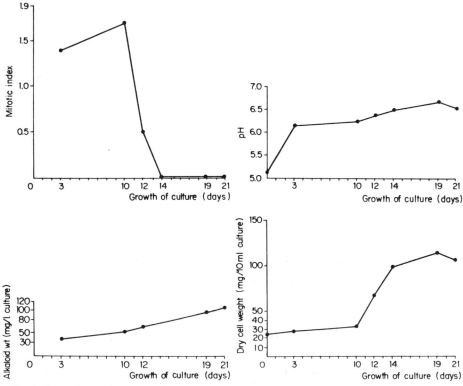

Fig. 4. General growth pattern of *C. roseus* tissue culture in bioreactor.

following 10–15 days to zero. The cell dryweight over the culture period increased by a factor of 8 to 10 while the variation in pH stayed within half a unit.

During an 8 week culture period alkaloids have been found as soon as 2 weeks after inoculation. Most cell lines showed a maximum accumulation of alkaloids in the 3rd-5th week of culture. Having established a large number of cell lines capable of alkaloid production, we proceeded to a more detailed study with several of the more promising lines. The results from 2 such lines coded as "953" and "200GW" are summarized below.

a. *The 953 line*
Studies with this selected line were performed both in shake flasks and bioreactors employing the 1B5 medium for inoculum growth and then Zenk's alkaloid production medium. Detailed accounts of these experiments are published (Kutney *et al.* 1980d, 1981b) so only a brief summary is provided. On harvesting the culture, the water is removed by freeze drying and the alkaloids are extracted in the conventional manner to provide the data summarized in Table I. The crude alkaloid mixtures were fractionated by intermediate-scale reverse-phase high-performance liquid chromatography (HPLC). Final purification by analytical reverse-phase HPLC allowed the isolation of the following alkaloids, characterized by their physical and spectral data and by comparison with authentic materials: ajmalicine (11), yohimbine (12), isositsirikine (13), vallesiachotamine (14), strictosidine lactam (15), lochnericine (16), hörhammericine (17), hörhammerinine (18), vindolinine (19), 19-epivindolinine (20), 19-acetoxy-11-methoxytabersonine (21), 19-hydroxy-11-methoxytabersonine (22), and dimethyltryptamine (23).

As general alkaloid formation was not observed during the initial periods of rapid cell growth, it was decided to examine whether the appearance, disappearance or build-up of particular components could be observed over different time periods. The results are given in Tables I and II. These show that the percentage of alkaloid per gram of cell weight increases with time, with optimum production at 3–4 weeks. It is also observed that maximum cell dry weight occurs during the same period and coincides with a zero value of the mitotic index. With respect to the earlier periods of culture growth, it is noted that there is a more rapid increase in the biosynthesis of ajmalicine (11) and yohimbine (12) (Corynanthé family) than in the biosynthesis of vindolinine (19) (Aspidosperma family). That is, the simple Corynanthé alkaloids ajmalicine (11)

Table I

Alkaloid yields from batches of 953 line C. roseus *cell cultures*

Sample	Culture method	Weight of freeze dried cells (g)	Weight of basic fraction (g)	% Alkaloid
1	Bioreactor (10 days)	90.5	0.168	0.185
2	Bioreactor (11 days)	110.0	0.178	0.16
3	Bioreactor (22 days)	26.9	0.058	0.21
4	Shake flask (14 days)	40.6	0.065	0.16
5	Shake flask (21 days)	49.66	0.182	0.37

Table II

Alkaloid yields from 953 line C. roseus *shake flask cultures*

Cultivation time	Weight of freeze dried cells (g)	Weight of basic fraction (g)	% Alkaloid
3 Weeks	65.9	0.15	0.23
4 Weeks	51	0.15	0.29
5 Weeks	87.6	0.24	0.28
6 Weeks	19.8	0.125	0.63
7 Weeks	19.7	0.1	0.51

and yohimbine (12) reach maximum concentration at a much earlier period in culture growth than the biosynthetically more complex vindolinine (19).

b. *The 200GW line*

Another particularly interesting cell line under recent investigation is coded as "200GW". The general procedures concerning tissue propagation, HPLC analyses, etc., are very similar to those discussed above. However, this line is uniquely different from the 953 line and produces its own "spectrum" of alkaloids as summarized in Table III. Of particular interest is the alkaloid catharanthine (1, 0.005% dry cell wt) isolated for the first time in our studies. This line originally provided this alkaloid in amounts *ca.* three times that normally obtainable from *C. roseus* plant material. Indeed, recent optimization studies with this line have shown even a further improvement.

c. *Biotransformation studies*

The above discussion has demonstrated the capabilities of different tissue-culture cell lines from *C. roseus* to produce various types of alkaloids. Another area of potential importance for the purpose of increasing cell yield of desired products, as well as for biosynthetic investigations, concerns the use of selected cell lines for biotransformation of appropriate substrates introduced into the culture medium at variuos stages of culture growth. Studies involving the transformation of various functional groups within organic compounds by plant tissue culture techniques have been reported (Kurz & Constabel 1979a), but compared to the extensively studied area of microbial transformation, much research is still required with such cultures before a proper understanding of this method can be attained. To this end we have initiated some studies (Kutney *et al.* 1982) with selected *C. roseus* cell lines and appropriate substrates available from our earlier investigations.

The substrate 3', 4'-anhydrovinblastine (7) available from the synthetic route outlined in Fig. 1, was selected for our initial experiments. Several serially cultured cell lines have been propagated for the preliminary screening to determine their capability of biotransforming 7 into desirable products. From these studies we chose a line coded as '916' since this cell line was unique in that it exhibited satisfactory growth characteristics, etc., but did not produce any alkaloids. In the initial study with the 916 cell line, 3–5 mg of 3',4'-anhydrovin-blastine (7) was incubated with the cells in shake flasks for 2, 6, 12, 18, 24, 48 and 72 h. In the sample incubated for 2 h, mainly 7 was found; samples incubated for

Table III
Alkaloids isolated from the 200GW cell line

Alkaloid	% Yield from dry cell wt.	% of crude alkaloid mixture
1	0.005	1.35
20	0.015	4.05
epimer of 20	0.026	7.02
11	0.006	1.62
17	0.002	0.54
18	0.005	1.44
19	0.002	0.54
20	0.002	0.54
15	0.224	60.48

% figures refer to *isolated* yields.

6–72 h contained a new, less polar compound. However, the highest concentration of this new product was observed in 24- and 48-h incubation samples. In the 72 h incubation samples the concentration of the new product was decreasing and degradation products appeared. From these samples the new compound was subsequently isolated by TLC and HPLC methods and shown to be dimeric ($C_{46}H_{54}N_4O_{11}$) by mass spectrometry although no further studies were performed. Further large scale experiments (3', 4'-anhydrovinblastine, 300 mg added as the hydrogensulfate salt) involving an incubation time of 48 h were performed in a *Microferm* bioreactor (cell line 916, 5.5 l) and allowed a more detailed study of the biotransformation process. Based on the amount of recovered substrate, the transformation of 7 to leurosine (8) and catharine (9) was 25.5 and 16.3% respectively, or, approximately 42% of 7 had been utilized by the cells. It should be noted, however, that no attempts have yet been made to optimize the yields of specific products.

The results also indicate that these high-molecular-weight alkaloids have passed through the cell walls since bisindole alkaloids were present in both the cell material and the culture medium.

Finally, the short period of time required for such biotransformations (24–48 h) is interesting, particularly when compared to plant cell culture production of alkaloids from nutrients present in the growth medium (usually several weeks). The inoculation of suspension cultures with biosynthetically 'advanced' precursors which reduce time periods for the production of target compounds may provide an important avenue for the commercial production of such pharmaceutically important agents. Further studies are underway.

d. *Studies with cell-free systems*

Plant tissue cultures can provide excellent media for biosynthetic studies either directly with whole cells or with enzyme mixtures available from cell-free systems. We have initiated some investigations with such systems in the hope of understanding the biosynthetic pathways involved with the above-mentioned natural products and, in particular, to attempt an evaluation of the enzymes responsible for optimum production of such target compounds.

Brief mention has already been made (Figs. 2, 3) of earlier experiments with cell-free systems prepared from *C. roseus* leaves, but a more detailed discussion is now appropriate in order to relate the results of the most recent investigations.

The purification procedure employed in all our studies concerned with leaves and/or tissue cultures involve initially a homogenization of leaves and/or cells in 0.1 M potassium phosphate buffer (pH 6.3) and centrifugation at 30,000×g for 20 min to provide the supernatant which represents the cell-free extract (or crude enzyme extract) to be utilized in the various experiments. In more recent studies, we have refined the method in order to obtain more information concerning the late stages of the biosynthetic pathway. Of particular interest to us was the enzyme(s) involved in the coupling of catharanthine (1) and vindoline (2) to 3′, 4′-anhydrovinblastine (7) and its subsequent transformation to the other bisindole alkaloids (Fig. 2, 3). Thus, we have initiated a study directed at the recognition and purification of the relevant enzyme(s) involved in this coupling reaction.

The coupling enzyme activity was determined by monitoring the formation of 3′, 4′-anhydrovinblastine (7) and leurosine (8) using radiolabelled tracer techniques with $(Ar-^3H)$-catharanthine and vindoline as substrates. We also applied HPLC methodology to analyse the protein contents of the cell-free enzyme mixtures. The HPLC system employed 2 protein columns (Waters Associates I-250 and I-125) which were calibrated with a number of standard proteins and from the HPLC analysis it was clear that a mixture of proteins varying in molecular weight of 15,000–450,000 were present. In order to establish a relationship between the molecular size of the enzyme(s) involved in the coupling of catharanthine and vindoline to the bisindole system, we proceeded to further separate the cell-free extract (crude enzyme) by precipitation, dialysis and chromatographic techniques to a "partially purified" enzyme stage.

The crude enzyme extract was brought to 70% saturation with ammonium sulfate. The precipitate, thus formed, was dialysed against phosphate buffer (pH 6.8) and the dialysate was applied on a DEAE-cellulose column equilibrated

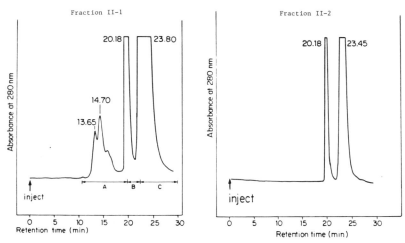

Fig. 5. HPLC. profiles of fractions II-1 and II-2 from Sephadex G-200 chromatography.

with potassium phosphate buffer (20 nM, pH 6.8) with a total of 50 fractions generally being collected. Fractions 21 to 30 found to possess the coupling enzyme activity were, therefore, combined and concentrated to a small volume by ultrafiltration. This concentrate was then subjected to Sephadex G-200 chromatography employing UV absorbance at 280 nm to monitor the separation. Fractions 9–22 were combined to form Fraction II-1 while fractions 23–29 were similarly combined to form Fraction II-2. Analyses of II-1 and II-2 by HPLC (Fig. 5) and assay for coupling activity by incubation with (Ar-^{3}H)-catharanthine and vindoline revealed that II-1 contains the necessary enzymes.

It is clear from these investigations that the enzyme system(s) involved in the biosynthesis of 7 and 8 from the appropriate monomeric alkaloids are present in the short HPLC retention-time region (11–20 min). From the standard protein calibrations this indicates proteins of molecular weight greater than 25,000. We intend to pursue these studies further employing the various cloned lines (953, 200GW, 916, etc.) of *C. roseus* tissue cultures as sources of the relevant enzymes. Clearly cell and/or enzyme immobilization studies will be highly interesting.

STUDIES WITH *TRIPTERGIUM WILFORDII*

Tripdiolide (5, R=OH) and triptolide (5, R=H) are interesting diterpene triepoxides with significant activity *in vivo* against L-1210 and P-388 leukemias in the mouse and *in vitro* against cells derived from human carcinoma of the

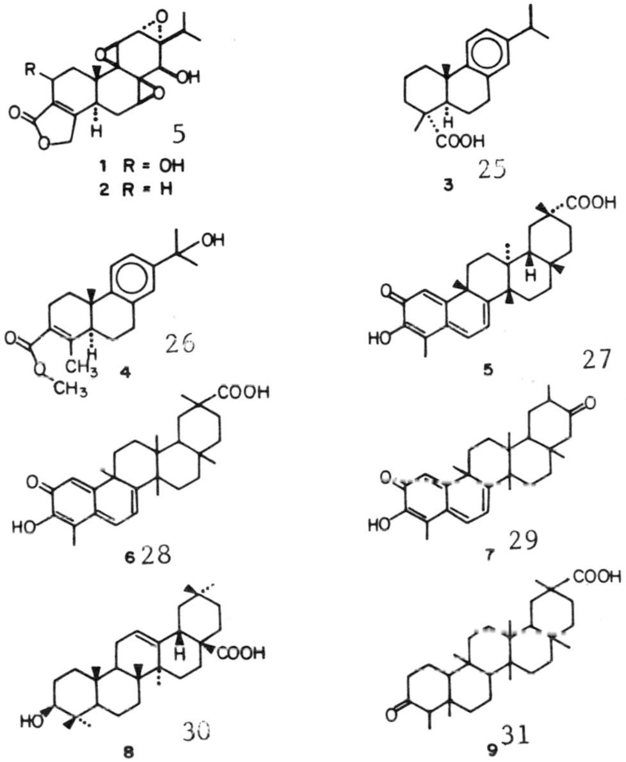

Fig. 6. Natural products isolated from *Tripterygium wilfordii* cultures.

nasopharynx (KB) (Kupchan *et al.* 1972). The plant, *Tripterygium wilfordii,* in which they occur in low concentration (0.001%), is not readily accessible and, thus, studies with tissue cultures were of interest in our program.

Plant tissue culture cells were grown in callus and in suspension employing modified B-5 and PRL-4 media. Experiments with shake flasks over varying times revealed upon subsequent analysis, the presence of tripdiolide and other components. An extensive study concerned with varying parameters (media, various additives, time of growth, etc.) for the culture growth has been undertaken and will be published elsewhere. It is sufficient to mention here that, in general, tripdiolide appears in the culture after several weeks (4–7 weeks), and its concentration depends on the media and other parameters. Large scale experiments both in shake flasks and in bioreactors have been completed and an extensive investigation of the natural products present has been undertaken. In addition to tripdiolide, 14 other compounds have been isolated and some of the

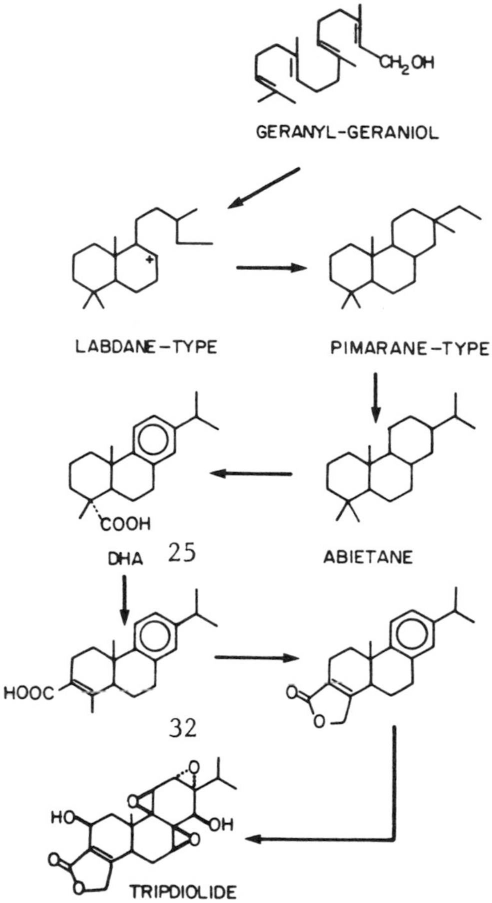

GERANYL-GERANIOL

LABDANE-TYPE   PIMARANE-TYPE

DHA 25   ABIETANE

32

TRIPDIOLIDE

Fig. 7. Proposed biosynthetic pathway leading to tripdiolide.

established structures are summarized in Fig. 6. Some of these are quinone methides similar to those encountered in the studies with *M. buchananii,* while others are di- and triterpenoid in nature. It is important to note that in the present tissue culture studies the concentration of tripdiolide is *significantly* higher than in the plant and recent optimization studies have provided levels *20* times that in the plant.

The isolation of dehydroabietic acid and the unsaturated ester provides interesting information about the possible biosynthetic pathway leading to the tripdiolide system (Fig. 7). It is suggested that 25 and the unsaturated carboxylic acid 32 are possible biosynthetic intermediates leading to tripdiolide.

Appropriate experiments are presently underway. Several publications concerning the above studies are available (Kutney *et al.* 1980e, 1981 f, g), and further details of these various experiments are presented.

In summary, it is hoped that the above discussion had demonstrated that plant tissue cultures can provide interesting alternatives for producing plant-derived natural products and also allow other avenues of research to be pursued within biosynthetic and enzyme related areas.

REFERENCES

Constabel, F., Rambold, S., Chatson, K. B., Kurz, W. G. W. & Kutney, J. P. (1981a) Alkaloid production in *Catharanthus roseus* (L.) G. Don VI. Variation in alkaloid spectra of cell lines derived from one single leaf. *Plant Cell Reports, 1.* 3–5.

Constabel, F., Rambold, S., Shyluk, J. P., Le Tourneau, D., Kurz, W. G. W. & Kutney, J. P. (1981e) Alkaloid production in *Catharanthus roseus* cell cultures. X. Mitotoxic effect of 3′,4′-dehydrovinblastine. *Z. Pflanzenphysiol. 105,* 53–58.

Kupchan, S. M., Court, W. A., Dailey, R. G., Gilmore, C. J. & Bryan, R. F. (1972) Triptolide and tripdiolide. Novel antileukemic diterpenoid triepoxides from *Tripterygium wilfordii. J. Amer. Chem. Soc. 94,* 7194–7195.

Kurz, W. G. W., Chatson, K. B., Constabel, F., Kutney, J. P., Choi, L. S. L., Kolodziejczyk, P., Sleigh, S. K., Stuart, K. L. & Worth, B. R. (1980a) Alkaloid production in *Catharanthus roseus* cell cultures: initial studies on cell lines and their alkaloid content. *Phytochemistry 19,* 2583–2587.

Kurz, W. G. W., Chatson, K. B., Constabel, F., Kutney, J. P., Choi, L. S. L., Kolodziejczyk, P., Sleigh, S. K., Stuart, K. L. & Worth, B. R. (1980d) Alkaloid production in *Catharanthus roseus* cell cultures. IV. Characterization of the 953 cell line. *Helv. Chim. Acta 63,* 1891–1896.

Kurz, W. G. W., Chatson, K. B., Constabel, F., Kutney, J. P., Choi, L. S. L., Kolodziejczyk, P., Sleigh, S. K., Stuart K. L. & Worth, B. R. (1981c) Alkaloid production in *Catharanthus roseus* cell cultures. VIII. Characterisation of the PRL-200 cell line. *Planta Medica 42,* 22–31.

Kurz, W. G. W. & Constabel, F. (1979) Plant cell suspension cultures and their biosynthetic potential. In: *Microbial Technology,* eds. Peppler, H. J. & Perlman, D., Vol 1, pp 389–415. Academic Press, New York.

Kurz, W. G. W. & Constabel, F. (1979a) Plant cell cultures, a potential source of pharmaceuticals. In: *Advances in Applied Microbiology,* ed. Perlman, D., Vol. 25, pp 209–240. Academic Press, New York.

Kutney, J. P. (1978) Synthetic studies in indole alkaloids. Biogenetic considerations. *Bioorganic Chem. 2,* 197–228.

Kutney, J. P., Aweryn, B., Choi, L. S. L., Kolodziejczyk, P., Kurz, W. G. W., Chatson, K. B. & Constabel, F. (1981d) Alkaloid production in *Catharanthus roseus* cell cultures. IX. Biotransformation studies with 3′,4′-dehydrovinblastine. *Heterocycles 16,* 1169–1171.

Kutney, J. P., Aweryn, B., Choi, L. S. L., Kolodziejczyk, P., Kurz, W. G. W., Chatson, K. B. & Constabel, F. (1982) Alkaloid production in *Catharanthus roseus* cell cultures. XI. Biotransformation of 3′,4′-anhydrovinblastine to other bisindole alkaloids. *Helv. Chim. Acta 65,* 1271–1278.

Kutney, J. P., Choi, L. S. L., Kolodziejczyk, P., Sleigh, S. K., Stuart, K. L., Worth, B. R., Kurz, W. G. W., Chatson, K. B. & Constabel, F. (1980b) Alkaloid production in *Catharanthus roseus* cell cultures: isolation and characterization of alkaloids from one cell line. *Phytochemistry 19,* 2589–2595.

Kutney, J. P., Choi, L. S. L., Kolodziejczyk, P., Sleigh, S. K., Stuart, K. L., Worth, B. R., Kurz, W. G. W., Chatson, K. B. & Constabel, F. (1980c) Alkaloid production in *Catharanthus roseus* cell cultures. III. Catharanthine and other alkaloids from the 200GW cell line. *Heterocycles 14,* 765–768.

Kutney, J. P., Choi, L. S. L., Kolodziejczyk, P., Sleigh, S. K., Stuart, K. L., Worth, B. R., Kurz, W. G. W., Chatson, K. B. & Constabel, F. (1981) Alkaloid production in *Catharanthus roseus* cell cultures. V. Alkaloids from the 176G, 299Y, 340Y and 951G cell lines. *J. Natural Prod. 44,* 536–540.

Kutney, J. P., Choi, L. S. L., Kolodziejczyk, P., Sleigh, S. K., Stuart, K. L., Worth, B. R., Kurz, W. G. W., Chatson, K. B. & Constabel, F. (1981b) Alkaloid production in *Catharanthus roseus* cell cultures. VII. Effect of parameter changes and catabolism studies on cell line PRL No. 953. *Helv. Chim. Acta 64,* 1837–1842.

Kutney, J. P., Hibino, T., Jahngen, E., Okutani, T., Ratcliffe, A. H., Treasurywala, A. M. & Wunderly, S. (1976) Total synthesis of indole and dihydroindole alkaloids. IX. Studies on the synthesis of bisindole alkaloids in the vinblastine-vincristine series. The biogenetic approach. *Helv. Chim. Acta, 59,* 2858–2882.

Kutney, J. P., Honda, T., Kazmaier, P. M., Lewis, N. J. & Worth, B. R. (1980) Total synthesis of indole and dihydroindole alkaloids. XVIII. Isomers and analogues of vinblastine. *Helv. Chim. Acta, 63,* 366–374.

Kutney, J. P., Beale, M. H., Salisbury, P. J., Sindelar, R. D., Stuart, K. L., Worth, B. R., Townsley, P. M., Chalmers, W. T., Donnelly, D. J., Nilsson, K. & Jacoli, G. G. (1980e) Tripdiolide from tissue culture of *Tripterygium wilfordii. Heterocycles, 14,* 1465–1467.

Kutney, J. P., Sindelar, R. D. & Stuart, K. L. (1981f) Rapid thin-layer chromatographic assay of tripdiolide using fluorimetric detection. *J. of Chromatography, 214,* 152–155.

Kutney, J. P., Hewitt, G. M., Kurihara, T., Salisbury, P. J., Sindelar, R. D., Stuart, K. L., Townsley P. M., Chalmers, W. T. & Jacoli, G. G. (1981g) Cytotoxic diterpenes triptolide, tripdiolide and cytotoxic triterpenes from tissue cultures of *Tripterygium wilfordii. Can. J. Chem. 59,* 2677–2683.

Langlois, N., Guéritte, F., Langlois, Y. & Potier, P. (1976) Application of a modification of the Polonovski reaction to the synthesis of vinblastine-type alkaloids. *J. Amer. Chem. Soc. 98,* 7017–7024.

Mangeney, P., Andriamialisoa, R. Z., Langlois, N., Langlois, Y. & Potier, P. (1979) Preparation of vinblastine, vincristine, and leurosidine, antitumor alkaloids from *Catharanthus spp.* (Apocynaceae). *J. Amer. Chem. Soc. 10,* 2243–2245.

Reinert, J. & Bajaj, Y. P. S. (1977) *Plant Cell, Tissue and Organ Culture,* Springer-Verlag, New York.

Scott, A. I., Gueritte, F. & Lee, S.-L. (1978) Role of anhydrovinblastine in the biosynthesis of the antitumor dimeric indole alkaloids. *J. Amer. Chem. Soc. 100,* 6253–6255.

Street, H. E. (1977) *Plant Tissue and Cell Culture,* University of California Press, Berkeley.

Stuart, K. L., Kutney, J. P., Honda, T. & Worth, B. R. (1978b) Studies on the biosynthesis of bisindole alkaloids. The final stages in biosynthesis of vinblastine, leurosine and catharine. *Heterocycles, 9,* 1391–1395.

Stuart, K. L., Kutney, J. P., Honda, T. & Worth, B. R. (1978c) Intermediacy of 3′,4′-dehydrovinblastine in the biosynthesis of vinblastine type alkaloids. *Heterocycles, 9,* 1419–1427.

Stuart, K. L., Kutney, J. P. & Worth, B. R. (1978a) Studies on the synthesis of bisindole alkaloids. XIV. Enzyme catalyzed formation of leurosine. *Heterocycles, 9,* 1015–1022.

DISCUSSION

RAPOPORT: Did you isolate the enzyme preparations from the plant or tissue culture?

KUTNEY: The enzyme preparations are now isolated from tissue cultures, but we can show that the preparation isolated from, say, the 953-line, contains the same kind of enzymes as the *Catharanthus roseus* leaves.

RAPOPORT: Did you isolate pure enzymes from the cultures?

KUTNEY: No, we look at the appropriate mixtures and correlate the HPLC profile to the ability to convert tritium or carbon-14-labelled precursors into products. A major programme is to obtain enzyme preparations, which are able to convert established synthetic precursors into end products. In the use of enzyme preparations for synthetic purposes a great deal of time-consuming refining work and development of methodology has to be done.

DAVIES: Can you manipulate the cell lines genetically *in vitro* or by mutagenesis?

KUTNEY: This is still a frontier-breaking and very interesting area.

WATSON: How do changes in the medium and bio-regulators affect your enzyme systems?

KUTNEY: Bio-regulators do appear to influence production although our studies are still preliminary. On the other hand, changing of nutrients is a very complicated question, which requires months of research. We have observed that changes of, for example, calcium or magnesium concentrations in the medium induces changes in the appropriate appearance of enzymes as monitored by HPLC. These changes, in turn, tell what will relate to the concentration of end product.

ATTA-UR-RAHMAN: Having refined the isolation procedure for catharanthine, vindoline, and vinblastine we are now able to isolate 10 g of pure vinblastine from 40–50 kg of leaves, and the procedure can be further optimized.

KUTNEY: Tissue-culture methodology may not be able to oust plantation, but for people in the Western world it might be a safe source for a number of drugs.

NAKANISHI: Dr. Y. Ohta and collaborators at the Suntory Institute for Bio-organic Research have found streptomycin able to change the ratio of secondary metabolites in liverwort cultures. Do you find a parallel between the greeness of the material and the production of secondary metabolites?

KUTNEY: No, the most important relationship is the metabolic phase of the cell. Without exception, maximum production of secondary metabolites was obtained in the secondary metabolic phase.

ATTA-UR-RAHMAN: In plantations, a maximum content of vinblastine is found in 6-month-old plants.

ANAND: At our Institute we have successfully used plant tissue culture for producing an interferon-like antiviral factor by infecting *Cassia fistula* callus with Ranikhet disease virus (1).

KUTNEY: This is another important field, the triggering of appropriate enzymes in callus or liquid cell suspension by adding various substances.

ARCAMONE: Do the 3 states of your tissue cultures parallel changes in the medium? We have observed that for the ergotamine fermentation of *C. purpureæ* the first phase showed rapid uptake of inorganic phosphate from the medium, the second one lasted until nitrogen-source exhaustion, and the third "maintenance" phase is sustained by presence of less available carbon sources.

KUTNEY: We are studying that type of experiment at present. Perhaps more exciting information may be obtained by withdrawal of the nutrients of the medium after 14 days of production, and then resuspension in a buffer. That gives you a very good, clean system in which you can study the effects of different buffers and other parameters.

LAZDUNZKI: How stable are the cloned lines?

KUTNEY: By subculturing techniques we have maintained the stability of cultures for about 4 years. To safeguard we use 2 procedures to ensure cell line stability, one is slow freezing and slow thawing of the culture, the other is to stimulate root formation and, thereby, obtain cell-differentiated plants which can be stored in a greenhouse.

LAZDUNSKI: How much do you understand of the genetic control of alkaloid production?

KUTNEY: Nothing at present.

WAGNER: Will HPLC in future replace radioimmunoassays for monitoring tissue cultures?

KUTNEY: There are tremendous advantages in HPLC methodology. In one HPLC chromatogram you can monitor, let us say, the presence of 13–20 alkaloids in a cheap and quick way, whereas it would be necessary to perform many radioimmunoassays to achieve the same result. The sensitivity of UV-monitoring in the HPCL analysis is sufficiently high in our case, and we use this method almost exclusively in our present program.

(1) Babbar, O. P. & Madan, A. R. (1981) *Ind. J. Exp. Biol. 19,* 349–355.

Application of Genetic Engineering to the Production of Pharmaceuticals

Julian E. Davies

Pharmacologically active agents for use in human and animal therapy have been obtained traditionally from natural product sources, by chemical synthesis, or by a combination of the two (semi-synthesis). In the isolation of drugs from natural sources, such as micro-organisms (bacteria, moulds, plants) yields and products are dictated, in general, by the growth properties and the biochemical physiology of the producing organism. Yields are often poor, due to low levels of production or difficulties in extraction. Much experimental effort (most of it empirical) has been expended in attempts to improve yields of natural products by inducing genetic changes in the organism or in the environmental conditions necessary for its propagation. In those cases where genetic manipulations of the producing organism are feasible, yields of the natural product can be altered substantially. Such adjustments have been most dramatic in the case of antibiotics, vitamins and amino acids where successive strain improvement steps, usually carried out by random mutagenesis accompanied by changes in culture conditions such as medium, temperature, growth phase, etc., have been applied to produce large amounts of the required metabolite with substantial reductions in cost and in availability. These efforts have been remarkably successful in many cases, resulting in 1000-fold increases in yield, but have been almost completely empirical and there is virtually no genetic or biochemical pedigree for the successive improvements. The organisms (Elander 1982) now used to produce antibiotics such as tetracycline, penicillin, streptomycin, etc., on the commercial scale, although they are identified as the same species as the original producing isolate, are probably distantly related progeny as a result of

Biogen S. A., 3, Route de Troinex. 1227 Caroúge/Genève, Schweiz.

NATURAL PRODUCTS AND DRUG DEVELOPMENT, Alfred Benzon Symposium 20.
Editors: P. Krogsgaard-Larsen, S. Brøgger Christensen, H. Kofod, Munksgaard, Copenhagen 1984.

the many genetic manipulations that have been imposed in the process of strain improvement.

As a result, very little has been learned of the metabolic pathways leading to useful natural products, and the control of their expression. The large amount of specific, empirical information has, only in rare cases been translated into biochemical knowledge that can be used as the basis for rational organism manipulations (Vining 1983).

By contrast, plants and, especially, animals cannot be subjected to genetic and biochemical exploitation in the same empirical (albeit convenient) way and their rare products must remain rare (and expensive). As an example, one can quote human growth hormone for which, until recently, the only source was human cadavers. The situation is somewhat different for animal hormones, but even if large amounts of, say, bovine growth hormone are needed for animal growth promotion on a large scale, the natural source is limited and the product expensive. Insulin for diabetes treatment at present relies on the ready availability of bovine and porcine sources; this is a fortunate situation since the hormone (unlike many other physiologically active proteins) shows little or no species specificity and the small variations in protein structure are not antigenically important.

It is in the case of human and animal proteins that the most obvious applications of recombinant DNA technology come into play. The ability to remove a gene from any source, to engineer this gene so that it can be expressed and its product isolated from simple micro-organisms, is now a highly developed and efficient technology. Any given gene in an organism can be detected by several different methods; most conveniently if the sequence of the protein product is known and short oligonucleotide probes can be synthesized chemically and used to screen gene libraries or banks, by means of nucleic acid hybridization. Once all, or part, of the required gene is isolated it is introduced onto a suitable vector adjacent to an appropriate expression system (promotor plus ribosome binding site) (Lathe & Lecocq 1983). Introduction of the engineered vector into an appropriate host will then allow production of the necessary protein product (Fig. 1). Recent advances in genetic engineering permit the production of single foreign proteins in E. coli at levels of 10–20% of the total cellular protein, often providing something like 1 gram/litre of product from a dense bacterial culture. This means that large (almost unheard of!) amounts of human proteins such as interferons, growth hormones, etc., can be manufactured using normal fermentation/extraction processes with an E. coli

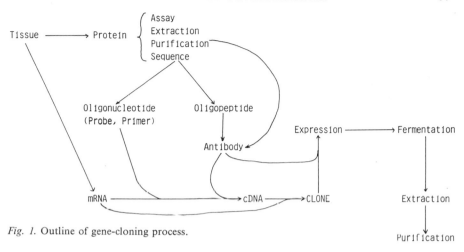

Fig. 1. Outline of gene-cloning process.

host that has been engineered to produce a particular protein. Table 1 lists some eukaryotic proteins that have been cloned and produced in micro-organisms; it is anticipated that other, even rarer, proteins will be produced in the same way in the near future. One result of this technological advance will be the development of new approaches to disease treatment: application of human proteins in the therapy of human diseases.

Recombinant DNA techniques have opened up another important pharmaceutical application: vaccines. In spite of the fact that conventional vaccines against many bacterial and viral diseases are available and provide acceptable degrees of protection, not all vaccines are foolproof and others cannot be made because of difficulties in cultivating the pathogenic virus or micro-organism under laboratory conditions. The production of many vaccines requires the manipulation of large amounts of infectious materials, creating a hazard for the workers involved in the collection of source material and in the preparation of the vaccine product. Rabies vaccine is not easy to produce because of the difficulty in growing the virus *in vitro;* hepatitis B virus cannot be grown in cell culture and the only present source of vaccine material is blood collected from infected humans. In addition, the safety and efficacy of conventional (killed or attenuated) vaccines has frequently been questioned, and outbreaks of disease have been initiated by the use of unstable or incompletely inactivated virus particles in a vaccine. Using recombinant DNA techniques viral genomes can be fragmented and the gene(s) for the appropriate viral antigens cloned and expressed in bacteria, thus providing a completely non-infectious source of the

Table I
Some eukaryotic genes cloned in micro-organisms

Human proteins, hormones etc.	Viral antigens
Interferons (α, β, γ)	Hepatitis B (surface and core)
Growth hormone	Polyoma
Growth-hormone releasing factor	Influenza
Insulin	Foot and Mouth disease
Somatostatin	Rabies
Interleukin-2	Herpes
Antitrypsin	
Plasminogen activator	
Blood factor IX	
Serum albumin	

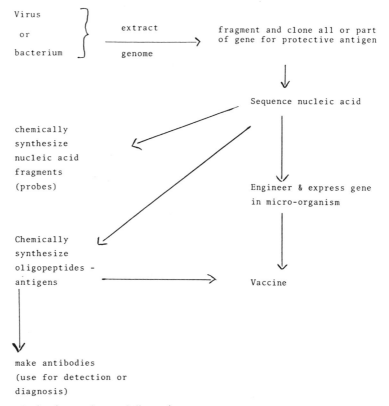

Fig. 2. Gene cloning for vaccines and diagnosis.

SIMPLE

SINGLE   EXPRESSION
 GENE   VECTOR   ⟶   (HOST MICRO-ORGANISM)

                                          │
                                          ↓
                                   PROTEIN PRODUCT

COMPLEX

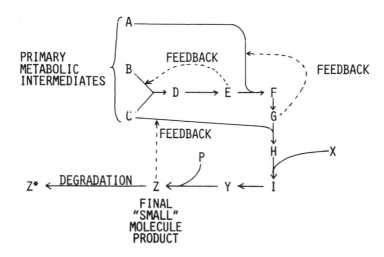

Fig. 3. Simple *versus* complex biosynthetic processes.

antigen for vaccine production (Küpper *et al.* 1981) (Fig. 2). This guarantees the safety of the vaccine since it contains no infectious nucleic acid.

In precisely the same way, the protective antigens of bacteria can be cloned and expressed in more convenient hosts for growth and production. Success has already been reported in the cloning and expression the antigens of virulent *E. coli* enteropathogenic for swine (Nature 1982), and a commercial vaccine has been developed. It can be anticipated that other vaccine materials will become available by this route in the near future. An additional benefit from the cloning of viral or bacterial antigens is their application for a variety of diagnostic purposes. Using either sensitive nucleic acid hybridisation or immunological methods, it will be possible to provide rapid identification systems for viruses and micro-organisms, disease-related antigens and antibodies, and target-directed drug applications.

The applications of genetic engineering discussed above all involve the manipulation of single genes and their resulting products; recombinant DNA technology has been and will continue to be, extremely successful in numerous applications in this area. However, an entirely different situation exists when more complex genetic and biochemical processes need to be manipulated, for example the production of antibiotics and alkaloids (Fig. 3). These usually involve multistep pathways with complex biosynthetic and regulatory circuits; the optimistic prediction that antibiotics would be made in *E. coli* has not been realised and this remains a daunting but also unnecessary (?) prospect. The many genes involved in the synthesis of a simple antibiotic are not necessarily present as a single genetic linkage group and cloning of the genes required would necessitate numerous operations, often without the advantage of selective methods to detect the presence of the cloned genes. The same technical problems associated with multicomponent antibiotic synthesis apply to the genetic engineering of improved yields of most secondary metabolites, for example, alkaloids in plants. The latter are further complicated by the fact that appropriate host-vector systems have yet to be developed for the application of recombinant DNA techniques to plants, although several promising approaches are being pursued (Barton & Brill 1983).

However, as an optimist (there is no point in being in science unless you are) I cannot leave this discussion on an entirely pessimistic note since there are a number of technical prospects (Table II). If in the biosynthesis of antibiotics, there is a single rate-limiting step in the pathway it might be possible to clone the

Table II
Improvement of antibiotic production

1. Fermentation conditions
2. Random mutation (regulation, excretion, resistance etc.)
3. Cloning and amplification of rate limiting step(s)
4. Cloning resistance genes – higher expression
5. Different host organism – transfer of production
6. Precursor feeding – mutasynthesis

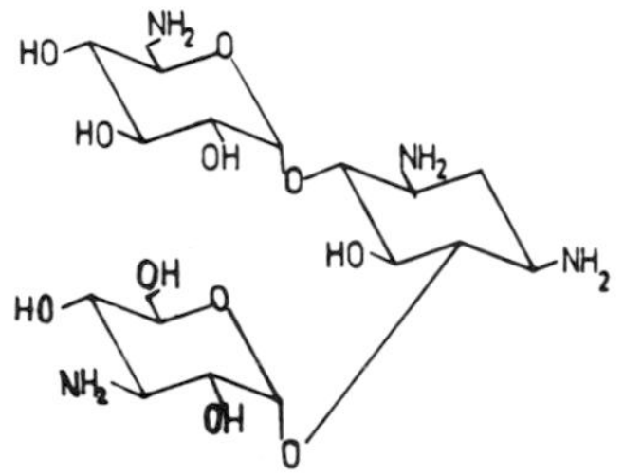

kanamycin A
Streptomyces kanamyceticus

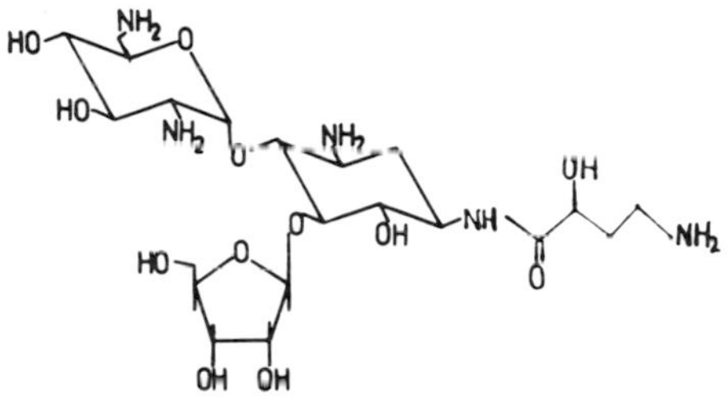

butirosin
Bacillus circulans

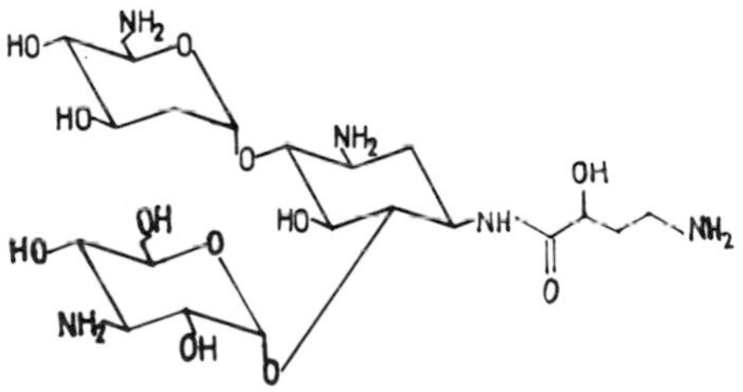

amikacin
(1-HABA-kanamycin A)

Fig. 4. Amikacin and its "parent" antibiotics.

Table III

Possible approaches to amikacin production in micro-organisms

1. Chemical modification of kanamycin A (current process)
2. Precursor feeding of appropriate *B. circulans* or *S. kanamyceticus* deriviative
3. Introduce *B. circulans* genes for HABA synthesis (plus acylase?) into *S. kanamyceticus*
4. Introduce *S. kanamyceticus* genes for 3-amino 3-deoxaglucose moiety into *B. circulans*
5. Fusion of *B. circulans* with *S. kanamyceticus*

Protoplast fusion

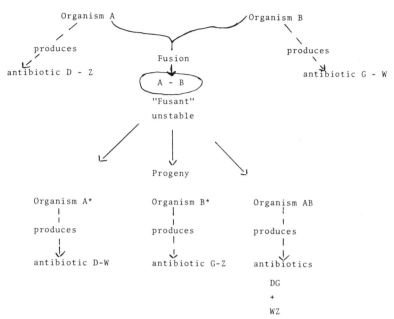

Fig. 5. Protoplast fusion for modified antibiotic production.

gene for this step by selecting for increased antibiotic production by shotgun cloning back into the producing organism. An alternative approach to achieve increased levels of antibiotic production might also be envisaged by cloning appropriate genes on multicopy or high expression vectors (Vournakis & Elander 1983). What do we mean by appropriate genes? Antibiotic resistance levels of the producing-organism may limit the extent to which an antibiotic can be produced and raising the resistance level by augmenting those pre-existing, or adding new resistance mechanisms would be useful. In addition it seems likely that antibiotic-producing organisms might be engineered to produce hybrid or specifically modified antibiotics. As an example, we can consider amikacin which is a chemically synthesized derivative of kanamycin and an important agent for the treatment of serious gram-negative infections in hospitals. Amikacin is currently the most effective aminoglycoside drug that is available to the physician. The structures of amikacin and its "parent" antibiotics are shown in Figure 4; in order to produce amikacin by microbiological methods it will be necessary to combine the genes for kanamycin biosynthesis and hydroxyamino-

Table IV

Recombinant DNA methods applicable to pharmaceuticals

1. Gene cloning
2. Gene manipulation – directed mutagenesis
3. Gene fusion – recombination
4. Organism fusion – changed cytoplasm
5. Gene synthesis (chemical)
6. Combinations of 1–5

butyric acid (HABA) biosynthesis. Several approaches are outlined in Table 3, the question that remains unanswered is whether or not the HABA adding enzyme will be capable of acting on the 1- position of a 4,6 disubstituted 2-deoxystreptamine (as in kanamycin) in place of the existing 4,5 disubstituted ribostamycin. There is recent evidence that kanamycin, when fed to kanamycin-resistant mutants of the butirosin-producing strain is converted to amikacin and this would that suggest that a shift in substrate would be possible for the HABA-adding enzyme (Cappelletti & Spagnoli 1983). This is an example of the production of a hybrid antibiotic of immediate commercial value; many other examples involving combinations of antibiotic-modifying enzymes in conjunction with a given antibiotic biosynthetic pathway can be envisaged. For the future, as antibiotic biosynthetic pathways become better defined and their corresponding genes identified, *in vitro* mutagenesis techniques should make it possible to produce "unnatural" enzymatic modifications of antibiotics and other therapeutically active agents.

The "ultimate shotgun" approach in recombinant DNA techniques is cell fusion, when protoplasts of 2 or more parental strains are allowed to fuse to produce, in principle, an infinite number of progeny that might contain all possible combinations of genetic recombinants as a result of the recombination of the activities of 2 distinct genomes (Baltz 1980) (Fig. 5). The progeny could then be screened for specific products using tests that would distinguish from the parental antibiotics. This shot-gun approach is likely to provide a rich new source of "new" antibiotic-producing organisms that would be screened in the same way that random soil isolates are screened at present. The advantage of this method would be that, starting with known producers with known biochemical functions, one could predict the nature of the hybrids and screen them. The problems associated with this approach are concerned with the stability of the products of fusion and limitations in gene function as a result of breakdown of "foreign" DNA by cytoplasmic nucleases. Nonetheless, proto-plast fusion of different antibiotic producing strains has been shown to lead to the production of hybrid molecules (Okami 1983) – the method works! In all biological production systems, the laws of chemistry must be obeyed and unnatural enzymatic transfers would be precluded. We have to rely on the organic chemist to produce truly unusual molecules, either by synthesis or site-directed mutagenesis (Lathe & Lecocq 1983) of the isolated genes of known enzymes.

In summary, recombinant DNA techniques are likely to be a powerful approach and rich source for producing large quantities of rare and novel pharmaceuticals both by simple gene cloning and expression techniques, and also by *in vitro* manipulation of gene sequences (Table 4). Some caution must be exercised in predicting success with the products of multistep biochemical pathways that may involve complex regulatory controls, as our knowledge of the controls if not non-existent, is quite primitive. In spite of optimism in the application of these new techniques to the production of pharmaceuticals it should be remembered that we cannot write down, with confidence, the complete biosynthetic pathway for any of the major antibiotic species known!

In addition to the recombinant approaches mentioned above, several other important tools are available that complement this methodology and will allow an increasing range of applications to useful pharmaceuticals. The ability to synthesize genes, peptides and proteins has enormous implications in genetic engineering for the production of proteins, antibodies, vaccines, etc. These, combined with monoclonal antibody techniques will provide a wealth of detection and diagnostic methods, plus the prospect of "targetting" drugs through specific cell receptor interactions (Gilliland *et al.* 1980).

REFERENCES

Baltz, R. H. (1980) Genetic recombination by protoplast fusion in *Streptomyces. Dev. Ind. Microbiol 21:* 43–54.

Barton, K. A. & Brill, W. J. (1983) Prospects in plant genetic engineering. *Science 219,* 617–676.

Cappelletti, L. M. & Spagnoli, R. (1983) Biological transformation of kanamycin A to amikacin (BBK-8). *J. Antibiotics 36,* 328–330.

Elander R. P. (1982) "Trends in the genetic improvement of antibiotic producing microorganisms" In: *"Trends in Antibiotic Research"* (eds. H. Umezawa, A. L. Demain, T. Hata, C. R. Hutchinson) *Japan Antibiotics Res. Assn. Tokyo* pp 16–31.

Gilliland, D. G., Steplewksi, Z., Collier, R. J., Mitchell, K. F., Chang, Th. & Koprowski, H. (1980) Antibody directed cytotoxic agents; use of monoclonal antibody to direct the action of toxin A chains to colorectal carcinoma cells. *Proc. Natl. Acad. Sci. U.S.A. 77,* 4539–4543.

Küpper, H., Keller, W., Kurz, C., Forss, S., Schaller, H., Franze, R., Strohmaier, K., Marquardt, O., Zaslavsky, V. G. & Hofschneider, P-H. (1981) Cloning of cDNA of major antigen of foot and mouth disease virus and expression in *E. coli Nature 289,* 550–559.

Lathe, R. F. & Lecocq, H. P. (1983) DNA engineering: the use of enzymes, chemicals and oligo nucleotides to restructure DNA sequences *in vitro.* In: "*Genetic Engineering*" (ed. R. Williamson) Academic Press. London Vol 4. pp 1–56.

New era Vaccine, see *Nature 296,* 792 (1982).

Okami, Y. (1983) unpublished observation – (see Vournakis & Elander 1983, ref. 31).

Vining, C. L. (1983) "*Biochemistry and genetic regulation of commercially important antibiotics*" Addison-Wesley Reading, Mass.

Vournakis, J. N. & Elander, R. P. (1983) Genetic manipulation of antibiotic producing micro-organisms. *Science 219,* 703–709.

DISCUSSION

WITKOP: I am very glad that proteins are recognized as important natural products, insulin being a clear-cut example. Eli Lilly now makes insulin added to the lactose operons of *E. coli* by genetic engineering, and taking advantage of the absence of methionine, they can liberate the insulin by cyanogen bromide.

DAVIES: You mention the very important problem that small proteins are often unstable, and in order to overcome this one has to make a hybrid protein. If the protein contains no methionine, a way of cleaving the hybrid protein is to use cyanogen bromide. Another way is to apply specific peptide "linkers", which can be cleaved by the right kind of proteinases. The "linker" has to be synthesized as an oligonucleotide and inserted between the gene and its "carrier" sequence.

DJERASSI: Which of the listed potential improvements will be the first one to show some real practical, commercial impact?

DAVIES: I think that the first application is obviously going to be high yields, as it has been utilized in the production of interferons. Schering-Plough expects to get FDA approval for the sale of a-2-interferon by the end of 1984 for a variety of specific anti-viral and anti-tumour indications.

DJERASSI: I do not believe that interferon prepared by this technique will be on the market in 1985.

LAZDUNSKI: Although there might be fewer contaminants in products obtained by these techniques, the contaminants will come from bacteria, so they might be immunogenic or even immunostimulants.

DAVIES: The human peptides prepared from bacteria such as insulin, interferons, interleukins, etc., can be prepareds free of bacterial contaminants and should not raise antibodies. There are a variety of analytical and immunological tests that can be applied to demonstrate the absence of bacterial antigens; these tests will be important before marketing.

LAZDUNSKI: How many of these compounds are secreted from the producing organism?

DAVIES: Everybody has chosen *E. coli* as their major tool for genetic engineering, and *E. coli* does not excrete proteins into the culture medium. In order to overcome this problem bacillus and yeast are being studied, as these organisms might produce proteins in the excreted form.

Integrated Approach to Development of New Drugs from Plants and Indigenous Remedies

Nitya Anand & Swarn Nityanand

INTRODUCTION

Drugs, from whatever source they may be derived, are a means to relieve suffering and to achieve and maintain good health. In the past five decades the development and introduction of new drugs has indeed been remarkable, these have been mainly synthetics and antibiotics and have led to miraculous successes in the control of many diseases. But still drugs derived from plants form the mainstay of medical treatment in the developing countries (Anand 1978). According to the June 1983 issue of "World Health", it is estimated that more than one-half of the world's population, most of them in the developing countries, relies mainly on traditional remedies. Even in industrialized countries a distinct trend is noticeable towards the use of plant drugs, perhaps as a sequel to the reports of occurrence of iatrogenic diseases caused by some synthetic drugs and antibiotics.

There are several factors for the continued popularity of traditional remedies. One is their ready availability, compared to modern drugs, in rural areas and less accessible regions in developing countries; another is the shortage of practitioners of modern medicine in such areas. But more important is the sociocultural reason. In some countries where reverence for tradition is a way of life, there exists a long tradition of the use of such remedies. People, particularly in the rural areas, have more faith in the traditional physician as he is a part of their community. The doctor speaks the same language as the village people, explains in the terms and concepts that are familiar to them and uses raw

Central Drug Research Institute, Lucknow, 226001, India

NATURAL PRODUCTS AND DRUG DEVELOPMENT, Alfred Benzon Symposium 20.
Editors: P. Krogsgaard-Larsen, S. Brøgger Christensen, H. Kofod, Munksgaard, Copenhagen 1984.

materials that are generally available in the neighbourhood for the preparation of his remedies. Both patient and physician are part of the same cultural milieu. Moreover, since modern medicine in these countries came in the wake of colonialism, it was considered as an alien system imposed on the people. With independence, there has been a renewal of interest in the past of developing countries, including in their traditional systems of healing. This almost emotional attachment to traditional medicine is, thus, a part of the national resurgence.

The traditional remedies and the traditional physicians cannot, therefore, be ignored and have to be integrated into one comprehensive system of health care which also includes the best from traditional systems. Because their objectives are the same, a conscious effort has to be made to narrow down the divergence between the traditional systems and modern medicine.

In this context it is also necessary to appreciate that traditional materia medica, as part of well-established systems of medicine, have evolved on a scientific basis. Thus, there is a need to differentiate between these remedies and folk medicines. The former are based on a corpus of organized knowledge, reduced to writing, while the latter consists merely of individual empirical observations without any theoretical basis. The major traditional systems of medicine in Asia are: the Chinese as practised in China and, with modifications, in Japan, Korea and Indo-China; the Ayurvedic, practised in India, Bangladesh, Nepal, Sri Lanka and to some extent Burma, and the Unani-Tibb (Graeco-Arab) limited also largely to the Indian sub-continent. These systems of medicine can by no means be considered empirical. They are based on a considerable amount of knowledge accumulated, by and large, through application of scientific method, individual observations, confirmation of these observations by others, formulation of hypotheses, followed by testing of the hypotheses by experimentation. Granted that some of the tools employed in ancient times when these systems were evolving were primitive by modern criteria, but the approach was undoubtedly scientific.

I shall try to illustrate my point by referring to *Charak Samhita,* one of the most important texts of the Ayurvedic system. According to Charak, knowledge is gained through: (i) "pratyaksha", that is direct observation, and (ii) "anumana", that is inference, induction, deduction and analogy, and the basis of "anumana" is "pratyaksha". He further states that although theoretical knowledge may be derived from authoritative instruction, this knowledge must then be investigated by observation and inference. While knowledge gained by direct visual perception is considered the most dependable, that gained by other senses is also valid.

"Anumana" based on "pratyaksha" enables one to draw conclusions in 3 ways having regard to the 3 aspects of time: past, present and future, a series of cause and effect. And "anumana" is again derived in 3 ways: a posteriori, a priori and commonly observed.

In addition to existing authoritative and valid knowledge, observation and inference, Charak also refers to "yukti" as a method for determining the truth. He has defined "yukti" as reasoning with a view to arrive at a correct judgement or conclusion. The faculty of reasoning is a function of "buddhi" or intellect, which evaluates the nature of several forces at work in a particular phenomenon having regard to the 3 aspects of time.

Thus, greater credence would have to be given to the materia medica of the traditional systems and a deeper study and understanding of the principles of these systems is required in order to make effective use of the knowledge enshrined in them. Only in this way can the full potential of traditional medicine be harnessed for the development of new drugs.

APPROACHES TO DRUG DEVELOPMENT

I would now like to discuss how best modern scientific methodology could be applied to investigate traditional remedies so that the results are acceptable to modern physicians and these drugs could be incorporated and integrated into one comprehensive armamentarium. Some of the approaches available are discussed below.

Standardisation of traditional remedies

A serious limitation of traditional medicines is the absence of standardisation in regard to: (i) raw materials, (ii) method of production, and (iii) quality control of the finished product. Traditional physicians, who are generally their own pharmacists, rely on their individual experience or descriptions contained in ancient texts or verbally handed down for the identification of plants, which can sometimes be erroneous. Advancements made in recent years in pharmacognosy, phytochemistry and physicochemical instrumentation techniques can be of immense value in removing this major shortcoming of traditional medicine. These techniques could be utilized for: (i) correct botanical identification of the plants used, (ii) standardisation of processing and compounding methods, (iii) development of quality control methods.

It is often argued that as traditional remedies are made from powdered plants or their whole extracts, whose active constituents may not have been identified or only partly identified, what should be the criteria for quality control of such preparations. The fact that such remedies are frequently compounded of more than one plant only adds to the complexity of the problem. Of course, chemical assay would be almost impossible in the case of such complex mixtures containing unknown substances. A practical solution would be to develop bioassay methods, which are now possible with the advances that have taken place in techniques of bioassay *in vitro* and *in vivo*. But, with the improvements in methods of isolation using GLC and HPLC it would not be difficult to finger print even complex preparations and obtain at least qualitative idea of the chemical composition. Thus, the criteria of bioassay and composition finger print could help to control batch to batch variation.

Safety criteria of largely used traditional drugs
A number of traditional remedies, particularly general tonics and those recommended for chronic conditions, are very popular and used for long periods in developing countries. As it is often difficult to clinically or experimentally evaluate the efficacy of such products in the absence of suitable parameters or animal models respectively, and as these are used by large numbers of people, at least the safety of these preparations should be ensured. This would be particularly necessary for those drugs which, in the light of modern knowledge, are known to contain ingredients that may have harmful effects after prolonged use. It is, therefore, essential to scientifically evaluate the safety of such traditional drugs by the well-established preclinical toxicological studies.

Evaluation of efficacy of traditional remedies
We have also to consider how to evaluate scientifically traditional remedies so as to sift out drugs that are therapeutically effective from the useless ones, and to compare the effective ones with other drugs having similar action available today. As already mentioned, traditional remedies are generally compounded of a number of plants. The usual approach to investigating the efficacy of these remedies is to prepare alcoholic extracts of the individual plants separately and to subject each crude extract, semi-purified fractions prepared from it and in some cases even isolated pure product(s) to a biological test corresponding to the reputed therapeutic efficacy. It is not inconceivable that the processing of the

plants according to traditional methods may modify the activity of the active ingredient(s), or that various chemical constituents present in the preparation may interact with each other resulting in alteration of the activity or toxicity of the individual constituents. Thus, good correlation between the results of biological testing of crude extracts, semi-purified fractions or pure constituents of individual plants and those of the compounded drug, may be lacking. It would, therefore, be more meaningful to carry out the initial screening for biological activity of the drug in the very form it is used in clinical practice. If the activity is confirmed, then each individual plant could be tested to pinpoint the activity.

In the context of development of drugs from plants, the drug-control regulations of various countries have to be taken into consideration. In many developing countries which have a system of drug regulation, traditional drugs, if prepared strictly according to the methods laid down in the texts of their systems, are allowed to be used without fulfilling the strict requirements of safety and efficacy evaluation, mandatory for new drugs. So, if the activity of a traditional drug is confirmed scientifically it could be promoted for use in modern medical practice without further evaluation. This would be particularly important in the areas of degenerative diseases and tropical parasitic diseases where there is a lack of effective drugs. In some cases, pure compounds isolated from these remedies may be more potent or have less side-effects than the remedies themselves. But prior to clinical use of such pure compounds, mandatory preclinical and clinical studies would have to be done, which normally take about 10 years. Thus, for diseases for which modern drugs are not available, but a traditional remedy is, it would be expedient to promote the use of the latter, even if it is not an ideal one according to modern criteria. Development of the ideal new drug from its pure constituent could continue side by side.

In this context, I would say that undue importance has been attached to the use of pure single ingredient from plants. In many cases this is not at all necessary from the standpoint of therapeutic efficacy and would certainly make the drug more expensive. This point is well illustrated by our work on the development of a hypolipidaemic product from *Commiphora mukul* resin, discussed later. Isolation of pure active constituents and elucidation of their structures is no doubt essential for study of structure-activity relationship and design of better synthetic drugs, but not necessarily for the use of these constituents in therapeutics.

Broad spectrum biological screening of plants

The number of plants used for preparing traditional remedies in various countries and those that have so far been investigated scientifically constitute only a small fraction of the plant resources of the world. A majority of the plants growing in developing countries, particularly of Africa and S. America, have not been investigated. Moreover, even in the case of plants that have been screened, one has to bear in mind the well-known possibility of variation in the chemical composition of the same plant growing in different geographical and climatic regions. It is, therefore, necessary for every country to undertake systematic biological screening of all the available plants from different climatic zones. It must be emphasized that the collection, storage and processing of plants must be done in such a manner that their chemical constituents are not affected. Bioassays, *in vitro* and *in vivo* have to be developed which can measure even weak activities due to minor constituents. The biological test systems employed should be particularly directed to the therapeutic conditions for which satisfactory drugs are not so far available. Here it should be pointed out that the above approach is quite different from the classical investigation of medicinal plants. The latter concentrates primarily on isolation of pure chemical constituents, their characterisation and structural elucidation, and the testing for biological activity of pure constituents comes later. In contrast, the former approach involves monitoring for biological activity at every step of chemical fractionation/purification.

I would now like to discuss a few examples of these approaches from our own work on the development of new drugs from plants/traditional remedies.

A HYPOLIPIDAEMIC AGENT FROM *COMMIPHORA MUKUL* RESIN

The resin (gum guggul) obtained from *Commiphora mukul* is an important drug in the Ayurvedic system for arthritis and inflammation. There is one reference regarding its anti-obesity activity also in *Charak Samhita*. This activity of the resin had been first reported by Satyavati (1966) on the basis of a limited clinical trial. As good hypolipidaemic drugs are not yet available, gum guggul was taken up for investigation for hypolipidaemic activity, based on this reference, by our Institute jointly with Dr. Sukh Dev, formerly of the National Chemical Laboratory, Pune, and now Director, Malti-Chem Research Centre, Baroda.

By treating the gum with ethyl acetate, soluble and insoluble fractions were obtained; activity was found only in the former fraction, a thick brownish yellow liquid (named as 'gugulipid'), while the insoluble fraction had no activity but showed some hepatotoxicity (Nityanand & Kapoor 1971, 1973, 1975). Such toxicity was subsequently observed in the total gum guggul. This was followed by further fractionation of gugulipid, monitored by the hypolipidaemic activity as tested in animal models of triton-induced acute hyperlipidaemia and alcohol-induced hypertriglyceridaemia. The fractionation procedure is given in Chart I and the biological activity of the different fractions as also of the isolated pure steroids (guggulsterones) (Patil *et al.* 1972) shown in Fig. 1, is given in Table I.

Surprisingly, the activity of gugulipid (total ethyl acetate extractive) and that of the mixture of guggulsterones was found to be almost the same, although the proportion of the latter in the extractive was only about 4.4%. As the other substances present in gugulipid besides guggulsterones do not have any significant hypolipidaemic activity, this would indicate that some of the inactive substances potentiate the activity of the guggulsterones, perhaps by increasing the bioavailability of the latter. This point is still under investigation. Because the order of activity of the gugulipid fraction and that of the pure guggulsterones

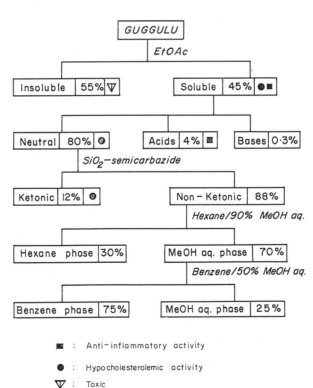

Chart 1

■ : Anti-inflammatory activity

● : Hypocholesterolemic activity

▽ : Toxic

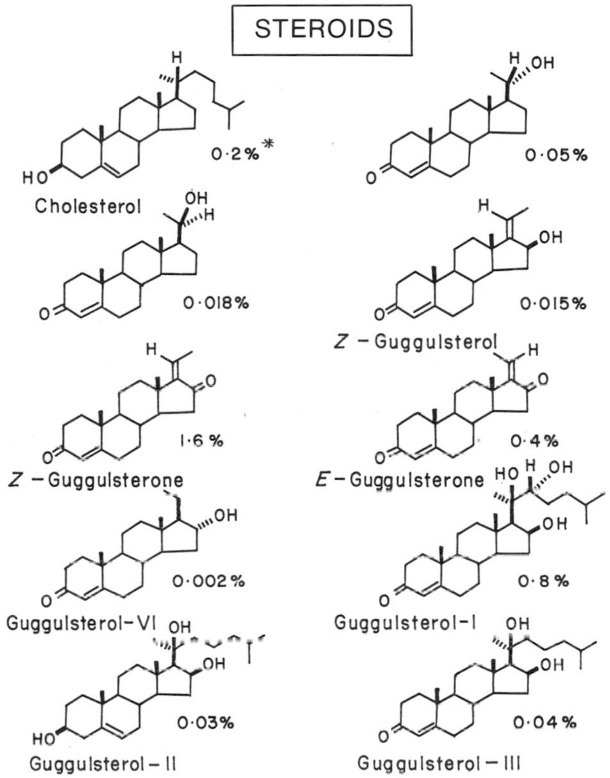

STEROIDS

Cholesterol   0·2% *

0·05%

0·018%

Z − Guggulsterol   0·015%

Z − Guggulsterone   1·6%

E − Guggulsterone   0·4%

Guggulsterol−VI   0·002%

Guggulsterol−I   0·8%

Guggulsterol−II   0·03%

Guggulsterol−III   0·04%

* Based on gum-resin

Fig. 1

was the same, it was decided to concentrate on developing gugulipid as a new drug.

The next problem was to standardise a suitable method for quality control of gugulipid. After considerable study, both a bioassay and a chemical assay method have been developed. The bioassay is based on testing the hypolipidaemic activity in triton-induced hyperlipidaemia and alcohol-induced hypertriglyceridaemia in rats, while the chemical assay is based on the absorption in UV of gugulipid, and on the finger-print TLC and the quantitative determination of the steroid fraction extracted from the TLC. We have investigated a large number of samples of gum guggul collected from different regions of the country and stored for varying periods and found a very satisfactory agreement between the bioassay and chemical assay results of gugulipid prepared from them.

Table I

Hypolipidaemic Effect of Guggul Fractions in Normal Rats

Fraction[1] Dose: 100 mg/kg per oral for 30 days	% Lowering of Serum		% Inhibition of Cholesterol Biosynthesis in rat liver homogenates
	Cholesterol	Triglycerides	
1. EtOAc soluble (GUGULIPID)	33.0	24.0	31.0
2. Insoluble	no effect	no effect	–
3. Neutral	35.0	26.0	32.0
4. Acid	no effect	no effect	no effect
5. Basic	no effect	no effect	no effect
6. Ketonic	30.5	26.0	27.5
7. Guggulsterone Z+E	35.0	28.0	35.0
8. Non-Ketonic	15.0	16.0	12.5
9. Clofibrate 100 mg/kg	43.0	30.0	40.0

[1] For methods see Nityanand and Kapoor, 1971, 1973, 1975

The biological activity results obtained so far, are given in Table II and show that gugulipid is effective in lowering serum cholesterol and triglycerides, and also raising the HDL/LDL ratio, in inhibiting cholesterol biosynthesis and platelet aggregation. This product has now undergone preclinical toxicology, including teratogenic and mutagenic studies, Phase I clinical trial for safety and Phase II trial for efficacy and is now in Phase III trial in seven hospitals in India (Nityanand *et al.* 1980, 1981).

In view of the marked hypolipidaemic activity shown by gugulipid, we have synthesized a number of steroids related to guggulsterones and some of them have shown good activity without any significant side-effects (Table III). One of these compounds is now in an advanced stage of development (Nityanand *et al.,* unpublished).

This example of development of a traditional remedy as a modern drug was chosen because it shows how an unexploited observation recorded in an old text of a traditional system of medicine can provide a useful lead. Thus, there is need for in-depth study of old texts. But the descriptions of the plants and their properties will have to be carefully interpreted in terms of modern scientific concepts and terminology.

Table II

Lipid Lowering Activity of Gugulipid

| Test System[1] | % Lowering of Serum | | % Change in Serum Lipoproteins | | |
	Cholesterol	Triglycerides	LDL	VLDL	HDL
1. Normal rats 100 mg/kg p.o. for 30 days	34	24	–	–	–
2. Triton treated rats, 200 mg/kg i.p. single dose	36	30	–	–	–
3. Ethanol treated rats, 200 mg/kg p.o. for 4 days	46	24	–	–	–
4. Hyperlipemic rabbits, 50 mg/kg p.o. for 90 days	40	30	-25	-27	$+29$
5. Normal Monkeys 60 mg/kg p.o. for 90 days	25	22.5	-50	-30	ns

[1] For methods see Nityanand and Kapoor, 1973, 1975.
LDL: Low density lipoproteins, VLDL: Very low density lipoproteins; HDL: High density lipoproteins; ns: no significant change; –: not done.

Table III

Lipid Lowering Activity of Some Steroids Related to Guggulsterones in Triton Treated Rats

Compound	Dose i.p. mg/kg	% lowering of serum cholesterol
80/429	50	43.0
80/430	50	38.5
80/574	50	37.5
80/575	50	39.0
80/613	50	30.5
80/550	50	32.5
Gugulipid	200	37.5
Clofibrate	200	not active

BROAD SPECTRUM BIOLOGICAL SCREENING

Apart from these investigations on plants and remedies used in traditional systems of medicine, Central Drug Research Institute has also been carrying out

Table IV

Distribution of Biological Activity in 2000 Plants Screened at C.D.R.I.

Screen	No. active	Screen	No. Active
Antiinfective		Pharmacological	
Antibacterial	} 14	Cardiovascular	27
Antifungal		-hypotensive	
Antiprotozoal	2	-hypertensive	
Antiviral	8	-cardiotonic	
Antihelminth	1	C.N.S. depressant	27
		Diuretic	10
Endocrinal		Antiinflammatory	24
Antifertility	15	Antiallergic	2
-antiimplantation		Hepatoprotector	2
-spermicidal			
-semen coagulant		Anticancer	72
Hypoglycemic	3		
Hypolipidaemic	2		

a broad biological screening of plants collected from different parts of India. The collection is done by our own botanists so that the authenticity of the plant material is ensured and the site and the season of collection is known. Collection is not restricted to those plants mentioned for therapeutic activity; rather, all plants available in a particular region which have so far not been investigated are included.

A methanolic or ethanolic extract of the plant, and in some cases after defatting, is subjected to biological screening. The various screens that are routinely used are given in Table IV. A total of 2800 plants have been collected so far, and an analysis of the activities observed in 2000 plants is included in the table. A part of this work has recently been reviewed (Rastogi & Dhawan 1982), wherein a classified list of the active plants with the parts of the plant used, is given. The order of activity in about 8% of these plants was such as to warrant secondary screening. These studies have led to the characterisation of the active constituents from a number of plants. A few of these which have reached an advanced stage of preclinical or clinical development are mentioned below.

A SPERMICIDE FROM *SAPINDUS MUKOROSSI* FRUITS

The saponins from a number of plants were shown to possess spermicidal activity, out of which the saponin mixture from the pericarp of *S. mukorossi*

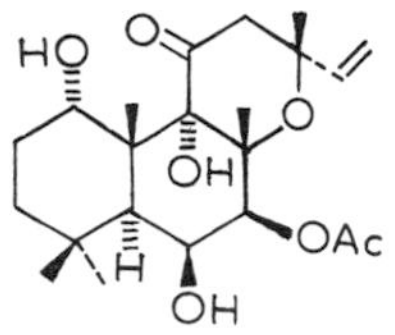

Fig. 2   Coleonol

fruits showed the most potent activity (Setty *et al.* 1976). The spermicidal activity in this plant is associated with olean-C-28-carboxylic acid type of sapogenins. A cream made from the saponins is at present under clinical trial as a local contraceptive, after extensive pharmacological and clinical studies.

AN ANTIHYPERTENSIVE FROM *COLEUS FORSKOHLII* ROOTS
From the roots of this plant, 2 groups of workers, one at the Central Drug Research Institute, and the other at the Hoechst Research Centre, Bombay, isolated a number of polyhydroxyditerpenoids (Bhatt *et al.* 1977, Tandon *et al.* 1977), some of which displayed significant antihypertensive and cardiotonic properties. The best of these, coleonol (Forskolin of Hoechst) (Fig. 2) is undergoing intensive preclinical evaluation at both the Centres (Lindner *et al.* 1978, Dubey *et al.* 1981).

CONCLUSION
The results, described above, of the chemo-pharmacological investigations of plants currently used in the traditional systems of medicine and of a broad biological screening programme of plants, collected at random or referred to in some texts, were interesting. While in the former category, the majority showed weak to strong activity, in the latter category the percentage showing activity was rather low (about 8–9 %); this percentage remained almost the same whether the plants were collected at random or were those mentioned in some compilations. However, in these investigations absolutely unexpected activities were discovered and many compounds of novel structure were isolated. Thus, both these approaches have their own place in the search for new drugs from plants and are complementary.

Only with this diversity of approach and provision of appropriate scientific inputs to the investigation of natural products and traditional remedies, would it be possible to fully utilise the materia medica of the traditional systems and exploit the abundant plant resources of the world.

ACKNOWLEDGEMENTS

I wish to express my appreciation to the colleagues at the Central Drug Research Institute who have made their results available; Dr. Sukh Dev, Director, Maltichem Research Center, Baroda, India who has collaborated in the work on Gugulipid; and to Alfred Benzon Foundation for their kind invitation to present this talk and to attend this symposium.

REFERENCES

Anand, N. (1978) An integrated approach to research on medicinal plants. *Symp. UNIDO Technical Consultation on Production of Drugs from Medicinal Plants in Developing Countries,* Lucknow, India, 13–20 March, 1978 UNIDO Doc. No. ID/WG. 271/3.

Bhat, S. V., Bajwa, B. S., Dornaur, H., de Souza, N. J. & Fehlhaber, H. W. (1977) Structure and stereochemistry of new labdane diterpenoids from *Coleus forskohlii* Briq. *Tetrahedron Lett 19,* 1669–1672.

Dubey, M. P., Srimal, R. C., Nityanand, S. & Dhawan, B. N. (1981) Pharmacological studies on coleonol, a hypotensive diterpene from *Coleus forskohlii. J. Ethanopharmacol. 3,* 1–13.

Lindner, E., Dohadwala, A. N. & Bhattacharya, B. K. (1978) Positive inotropic and blood pressure lowering activity of a diterpene derivative isolated from *Coleus forskohlii. Arzneimittel-Forschung 28,* 284–289.

Nityanand, S. & Kapoor, N. K. (1971) Hypocholesterolemic effect of *Commiphora mukul* resin (guggul). *Indian J. Exptl. Biol. 9,* 376–377.

Nityanand, S. & Kapoor, N. K. (1973) Cholesterol lowering activity of the various fractions of the guggul. *Indian J. Exptl. Biol. 11,* 395–396.

Nityanand, S. & Kapoor, N. K. (1975) Hypolipidaemic effect of ethyl acetate fraction of *Commiphora mukul* (guggul) in rats. *Indian J. Pharmacol. 7,* 106.

Nityanand, S., Asthana, O. P., Agarwal, S. S., Gupta, P. P., Tangri, A. N., Puri, V. & Dhawan, B. N. (1980) Tolerance and hypolipidaemic activity of gugulipid; the steroidal fraction of *Commiphora mukul. Abstr. World Conf. Clin. Pharmacol. Therapy,* London No. 0667.

Nityanand, S., Asthana, O. P., Gupta, P. P., Kapoor, N. K. & Dhawan, B. N. (1981) Clinical studies with gugulipid – a new hypolipidaemic agent. *Indian J. Pharmacol. 13,* 59.

Patil, V. D., Nayak, U. R. & Sukh Dev (1972) Chemistry of *Ayurvedic* Crude Drugs – I *Guggulu* (resin from *Commiphora mukul*)-1: Steroidal constituents. *Tetrahedron 28,* 2341–2352.

Rastogi, R. P. & Dhawan, B. N. (1982) Research on medicinal plants at the Central Drug Research Institute, Lucknow (India). *Indian J. Med. Res. 76 (Suppl),* 27–45.

Satyavati, G. V. (1966) Effect of an indigenous drug (*Commiphora mukul* Eng) on disorders of lipid metabolism with special reference to atherosclerosis and obesity. Thesis submitted for the degree of Doctor of Ayurvedic Medicine, Banaras Hindu University,

Setty, B. S., Kamboj, V. P., Garg, H. S. & Khanna, N. M. (1976) Spermicidal potential of saponins isolated from Indian medicinal plants. *Contraception 14,* 571–578.

Tandon, J. S., Dhar, M. M., Ram Kumar, S. & Venkatesan, K. (1977) Structure of coleonol, a biologically active diterpene from *Coleus forskohlii. Indian J. Chem. 15B,* 880–883.

DISCUSSION

RAZDAN: I would like to hear your comments on the CNS profile of coleonol.

ANAND: It had practically no CNS effects. It produced a fall in blood pressure, both in normotensive animals (cats, dogs and monkeys), and also in spontaneously hypertensive rats.

WALL: I noticed in one of your early slides that you have tested for anti-tumour activity and had positive tests for some hundred or more plants. What sort of extracts were used and how did you prepare them?

ANAND: This study is carried out under contract with the National Cancer Screening Programme, N.I.H., Bethesda, and we follow their protocols for extraction. In earlier studies it used to be 50% ethanolic extract, but more recently, we defat the plant material and then make ethanol and chloroform extracts, which are tested.

WALL: What are the results of these studies?

ANAND: Out of about 2400 plant extracts screened, activity was found in about 600 extracts in primary screening, confirmed in 126 extracts, and active constituents isolated from about 20 of them; most of them had a very low therapeutic ratio, and none of them could be taken up for a clinical study, and provided only new leads for molecular modifications.

ATTA-UR-RAHMAN: The World Health Organization published a resolution in 1977, in which they recommended direct clinical trials on some of these herbal extracts after preliminary toxicological studies. It seems to me that there is an over-obsession in Western medicine for single ingredients, and certainly Western laws would forbid such medical trials in the respective countries, but these could be undertaken in countries like Pakistan. I was wondering how you feel about this possibility?

ANAND: I agree there is an unnecessary obsession for single constituent drugs from plants; I feel a fraction or a mixture should be acceptable as a drug provided its method of production is properly standardised, and a suitable chemical or bio-assay method is available for quality control, and the product has definite therapeutic gain over known products; this view is exemplified by the development of gugulipid which has been discussed in my paper. I understand some Scandinavian and West European countries have somewhat relaxed regulations in this matter.

PORTOGHESE: Did you examine any compound for the ability to raise HDL relative to LDL?

ANAND: We have studied the effect of gugulipid on lipoproteins, both in experimental animals and in human subjects, and find that in most of the cases there was a distinct trend towards a relative rise of HDL over LDL.

Drug Research Based upon the Leads of the Chinese Traditional Medicine

Huang Liang (L. Huang)

The bewildering varieties of molecular structures accomplished by the nature's chemical architecture incite the chemists' enthusiasm and curiosity to explore the kingdom of nature, especially in searching for biologically active constituents. Traditional medicine and folklore are based on long periods of practical experience in treating human disease. Taking them as the leads for drug search may save one from drowning in costly random screening. The written document of Chinese traditional medicine can be traced back to *Shen Nong Ben Cao Jing* (A.D. 22–250). Since then, it has been refined and enriched continously, and more than 300 classical books have been published. *Ben Cao Gang Mu* written by the greatest physician and naturalist Li Shizhen has been regarded as a more comprehensive pharmacopoeia containing total of 1894 entries published in 1596. *Ben Cao Gang Mu,* as well as the other classics, still serve as the valuable references for teaching, practicing and guides for drug research in China. About 80% of the Chinese traditional medicine comes from the plant kingdom. The animal and marine products and minerals cover the remaining 20%. A recent survey of Chinese traditional drugs and folklore has identified that about 2000 plant species are concerned. Majority of the plant species have been more or less investigated chemically throughout the world, but few pharmacological studies have been undertaken until recent years. Not all traditional medicines including the folkloric are as useful as described, but we do treasure them as an invaluable heritage and have confidence in most of their practical values. They have left medicinal chemists a vast, fertile field to be

Institute of Materia Medica, Chinese Academy of Medical Sciences, Beijing, China

NATURAL PRODUCTS AND DRUG DEVELOPMENT, Alfred Benzon Symposium 20.
Editors: P. Krogsgaard-Larsen, S. Brøgger Christensen, H. Kofod, Munksgaard, Copenhagen 1984.

developed. To verify the clinical values of the traditional prescriptions and to bridge the gap between the traditional self-contained theories and the "modern aspects", and then to find the active principles and take them as the leads for drug design, is not easy. The meagre experience obtained indicates that it is a difficult and complicated task which demands not only great effort and endurance, but also more advanced scientific and medical knowledge and techniques, some of which have yet to be devised. The study of the famous tonic ginseng started in 1905 in Japan. Since then, its chemical constituents and biological properties have attracted the interests of the scientists in various parts of the world. Nearly 80 years have elapsed. Many constituents have been identified among which over 10 glycosides of triterpenes have been shown to have the biological activities somewhat related to those described in the classics for ginseng, such as antistress, cardiovascular, antiinflammatory, immuno-stimmulating and antitumor action. However, it still demands more elaborate study to understand the polychrestic biological activities described, and to assign each activity to the individual constituent to permit a basis for drug design. Therefore, it continues to be an active subject of investigation.

However, not all the studies on the traditional medicines are as perplexed and costly as the case of ginseng, some of the projects are quite rewarding. The following 4 examples are selected to illustrate the more or less successful results obtained in the drug development based on the leads of the traditional medicines. 1. Qinghao (*Artemisia annua* L.): The Chinese drug Changshan (roots of Dichroa febrifuga Lour.) the oldest remedy for malaria which has been known since 200 B.C. Febrifugine 1, the active principle was isolated in 1948. The toxicity of the alkloid, especially the adverse action on gastrointestinal system, hindered it from developing into an useful remedy. Derivatives were prepared to lower its toxicity but with only limited success.

Qinghao was first described as the remedy for malaria in "*Zhou Hou Bei Ji Fang*" in 340 A.D. It also has been collected in "*Ben Cao Gang Mu*". But its value had been somewhat ignored until recent years. Ruziska first reported the study of Artemisia in 1936. Since then, the chemical studies of about 60 species of Artemisia including *Artemisia annua* have been carried out by other chemists, nothing pertaining to the antimalarial activity had been noticed until the isolation of artemisinine 2 (qinghaosu) in 1972 which was reported by Chinese scientists (Anonymous 1977a). Along with artemisinine, 6 biologically inactive sesquiterpenes 3–8, the structures of which are closely related to artemisinine, have also been isolated (Tu 1981, 1982). They all have the basic skeleton of amorphane 9, cis-fused decalin ring with an isopropyl group trans to the angular hydrogen.

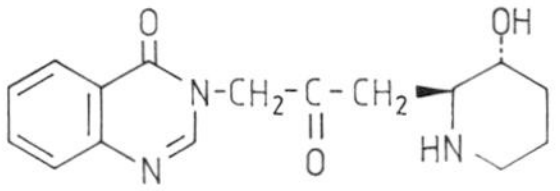

1

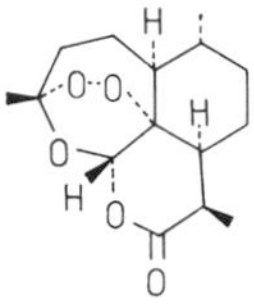

2 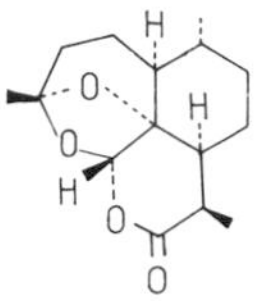   3 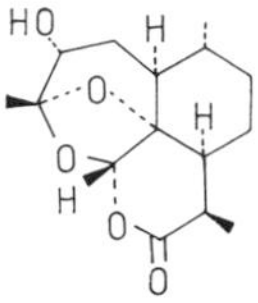   4

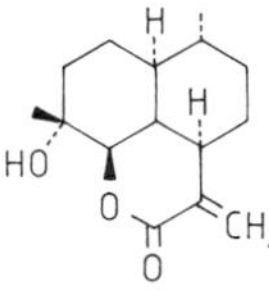

5 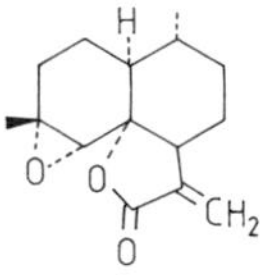   6 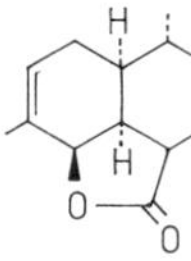   7

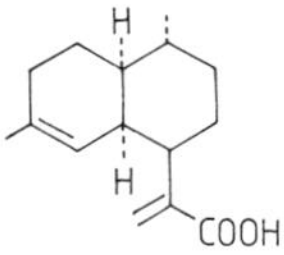

8 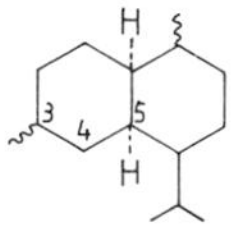   9

Compounds 2–4 biogenetically might be regarded as formed from amorphane through scission of C_3-C_4 bond by oxygen, then recyclization. Compounds 3 and 4 with all the structural features of artemisinine except the presence of an oxide ring in place of the peroxide bridge in the latter, are completely inactive. The importance of the presence of peroxide bridge for its biological activity is, thus, conceivable. In order to overcome the recrudescence after the treatment of artemisinine, preparation of derivatives has been undertaken. The hemilactol, hydroartemisinine 10 obtained as a mixture of $C_{12}\alpha$ and βOH in a ratio close to 1:1 by $NaBH_4$ reduction is twice as active as the parent compound. Furthermore, the hemilactol provides a functional group OH which makes the preparation of derivatives possible without touching the basic structure particularly the peroxide bridge. Nearly 100 derivatives in the form of ethers, carboxylates and carbonates were prepared (Anonymous 1982a). Most of the derivatives are more active than artemisinine and the esters are more potent than the ethers. The carbonates is the most active class.

10 R H
11 R CH_3
12 R $-C-CH_2CH_2COONa$
$\quad\quad\ ||$
$\quad\quad\ 0$

The quantitative structure-activity relationships were analyzed by Hansch's approach using various parameters. The following 2 parabolic equations for ethers and esters illustrated the close relationship between lipophilicity and antimalarial activity. The optimal values, $logP_0$ for ether and ester are 2.60 and 2.9 respectively. The electronic charater of the substituents also plays its role in ethers as introduction of Taft's σ^* gives better correlation coefficient. The indicator variable $I_{\alpha,\beta}$ equals to 1 for C_{12} β-substitution and 0 for the α-epimers.

Ester: $log_c^{\frac{1}{}} = 1.202 - 0.1983(logP)^2 + 1.549\ logP - 0.6125\ I_{\alpha,\beta}$
$\quad$ n=49, r=0.9111, s=0.153, $logP_0$=2.91
Ether: $log_c^{\frac{1}{}} = 0.9575 - 0.2231\ (logP)^2 + 1.1620\ logP - 0.837\ \sigma^* - 0.1451\ I_{\alpha,\beta}$
$\quad$ n=14, r=0.906, s=0.168, $logP_0$=2.60

The therapeutic index against chloroquine-sensitive strain of *P. berghei* in mice of artemisinine (oil suspension) and artemether 11 (oil solution) given by intramuscular injection (im), and sodium artesunate 12 (water solution) given by intravenous injection (iv) are 4987, 447 and 1733 respectively compared with the value of 95 for chloroquine (im) (Anonymous 1982b). This indicates that artemisinines are much less toxic than chloroquine. The artemisinines are also effective against chloroquine-resistant *P. berghei* strain and the artemether and sodium artesunate are more active (Anonymous 1982c). After i.v. and oral administration of artemisinine and artemether, the drug concentrations in the blood were of short duration, while i.m. gave a prolonged blood level. As sodium artesunate (iv) was also eliminated very rapidly from the body, intravenous drip was recommended (Anonymous 1982d). The artemisinines can pass through the blood-brain and blood-placenta barrier and, hence, adverse

effects on neuro and embryo systems should be taken into consideration. On the
other hand, it may be useful in the treatment of cerebral malaria. In the past 7
years, clinically 3368 cases of *plasmodium falciparum* and *Plasmodium vivax*
malaria were treated with artemisinine (2099 cases), artemether (1088 cases),
and sodium artesunate (181 cases, Anonymous 1982e). Artemisinine and
artemether gave the radical cure rates of ca. 90% in falciparum cases and sodium
artesunate showed a lower cure rate. They all are effective in the treatment of
chloroquine-resistent *P. falciparum,* therefore, they may be the drug of choice
for chloroquine-resistent falciparum malaria. No apparent toxic effect on heart,
liver or kidneys has been observed in the clinical trails. From the urine of
patients taking artemisinine, 3 inactive metabolites (3, 13, 14) have been
identified. It was suggested that the metabolism is a reductive deactivating
process. The preliminary studies suggested that the membrane system of the
parasites may be the main site of action exerted by artemisinine and this mode of
action may differ from the other known classical antimalarials. The importance
of the discovery of artemisinine not only provides an useful antimalarial agent,
but its greater significance lies more in the novel and unique structure with no
precedent in the antimalarias. Recently, the total synthesis of artemisinine from
isopulegal has been reported by Schmid (Schmid 1983).

13   14   15

In the early 70's, another antimalarial herb *Artabotrys uncinatus* L. Merr was
studied in our institute (Liang 1979). The antimalarial action of *yingzhaosu* A 15
was verified, preliminarily both in experimental malaria and in clinic. The
limited source of the plant interrupted further investigation. *Yingzhaosu A,* a
sesquiterpene with the basic skeleton differs from artemisinine but it is most
amazing that a peroxide bridge is also present in the molecule. The coincidence
is indisputable evidence of the significance of the peroxide bridge. The structural
differences between artemisinine and *yingzhaosu A* indicated the flexibility of the
basic structure required for the biological activity. In retrospect, it seems more
fruitful in researching parasiticides from traditional medicine, because the

simple therapeutic action is identical to the direct screening method. Besides the antimalarias mentioned above, the ascaricides quisqualic acid 16 from the nuts of *Quisqualis indica* L. and the triterpene *chuanliansu* 17 (Hsie *et al.* 1975) from the bark of *Melia toosendan* S. et Z. The latter is especially welcomed by the pedistricians due to its efficacy and low toxicity. Agrimophol 18 (Anonymous 1977b) a taeniafuga isolated from the winter root-sprout of *Agrimonia pilosa* Ledeb. showed an efficacy as high as 98% (Anonymous 1974). Agrimorphol is a biphloroglucinol with an unusual linkage between the 2 phloroglucinol moieties.

16   17   18

Qingdai

Correlating the theory behind the Chinese traditional medicine to the symptoms of patients with chronic myelocytic leukemia (CML), of which the term is missing in the old medical classics, led to the treatment of CML with a commercially available honey pill "*Dang Gu Lu Hui Wan*". 16 of the 22 treated cases showed positive reponse. The pill contains 11 ingredients. By subsequent combination and elimination of the ingredients based on the traditional medical theory and clinical results, "*Qingdai*" is found to be the active constituent. It is the floating solid formed after the indican-containing leaves of *Baphicacanthus custa* have been soaked in water for 2 days and then treated with lime. The solid contains indigo as its major organic component with a small amount of indirubin, indigo brown, etc. Further study showed that indirubin 19 is responsible for the antitumor activity exhibited by qingdai. Indirubin is active against transplantable leukemia L_{7212}, Lewis lung carcinoma in mice and Walker Ca 256 in rats (Ji *et al.* 1981). Of 314 CML patients treated with indirubin, 87% response rate was obtained. Abdominal pain and diarrhea are the side effects observed. Pharmacological studies revealed that indirubin has no effect on the hemopoietic system and immuno-system in normal rats and mice. The profiles of the content of uric acid (metabolite of purine), and of β-amino-isobutyric acid (metabolite of thymidine) eliminated in the urine of patients treated with indirubin, are different from those obtained with myleran, 6-MP and radiation therapy. Indirubin combined with DNA and inhibited the syntheses of DNA, RNA and protein in Walker 256 ascitic cells (Anonymous 1979). Indirubin has been known for 100 years and can easily be synthesized by condensation of indoxyl with insatin. In 1946 Friedman (Friedman 1946) reported the isolation of indirubin from urine of patients suffering from CML, and Landsheere (Landsheere 1951) found intramuscular administration of indirubin to guinea pigs caused the maximum reduction of the white blood cell count to 60%, eosinophils to 20%, granulocytes to 40% and no significant effect on lymphocytes and monocytes combined count compared with that of vehicle control. But no antitumor action was reported. However, their observations supported the therapeutic effect on CML found 2 decades later. Indirubin with its high m.p. is insoluble in water and its solubilities in most organic solvents are also exceedingly low. It was postulated that substitution on the nitrogen atom might increase the solubility and facilitate the absorption to improve the therapeutic effect (Huang *et al.* 1983). Among the derivatives prepared, compounds 20–23 with substution on the amino nitrogen exhibited higher inhibitory action on experimental tumors than indirubin, while substitution on the other nitrogen atom abolished the activity.

To our surprise, introduction of low alkyl group to one of the nitrogens of isoindigotin or indigo, rendered these inactive isomers of indirubin exhibiting antitumor action (Wu *et al.* to be published). It is then suggested that in this type of bisindole derivative, the positions linking the 2 moieties play a less crucial role for their antitumor activity.

19 R=H
20 R=C₂H₅
21 R=C₃H₇
22 R=COOH
23 R=COCH₃

Schizandra chinensis Baill

The dried kernal of *Schizandra chinensis* Baill (*Wuweizi*) is a herb described to have various physiological actions in the Chinese medical classics. It is a common ingredient in prescriptions and also can be used alone as a tonic, astringent, etc. Since the early 70's, Chinese traditional doctors have used the honey pills of the kernal to treat hepatitis based upon the theory of Chinese traditional medicine. The therapeutic effects obtained soon induced an impetus to the chemical and pharmacological studies of this herb in China.

Chemical studies of Schizandra was first reported by the Russian chemists in 1952. Later, 5 dibenzocyclooctadiene lignans, schizandrin, r-schizandrin, deoxyschizandrin, schizandrol and pseudo-r-schizandrin were isolated by Kochetkov. In our institute, study under the pharmacological and clinical guidlines, ascertained that the ethanol extract possessed a lowering effect on the serum glutamic pyruvic transaminase (SGPT). On further studies, 7 dibenzo-cyclooctadienes 24–30 were isolated from the alcoholic extracts (Chen & Li 1976a, b). Th structures were assigned by chemical degradation and spectra analysis. During 1979–1982 a series of papers published by Ikeya (Ikeya *et al.*

(Sin A) (R)	(Sin B) (dl)	(Sin C) (S)	(Sol A) (R)
24	25	26	27
Deoxyschizandrin	r-Schizandrin	Wuweizisu-C	Schizandrin

(Ser A) 29

R = -CO-

(Gomisin C)

R = -CO-C=C$\overset{CH_3}{\underset{CH_3}{\overset{|}{C}}}$H

(Sol B) (R)	(S)	(Ser B)	(DDB)
28	Schizandrer	(Gomisin B)	31
Schizandrol B			

1979–1982) reported the isolation of 34 dibenzocyclooctadienes and assignment of the absolute configurations based upon NOE of ^{1}HNMR, X-ray analysis and circular dichroism, but no pharmacological effects were mentioned. The 7 compounds 24–30 mentioned above, demonstrated various effects on the liver functions (Bao *et al.* 1979). They decreased the CCl$_4$ and thioacetamide-induced hepatotoxicity as indicated by the lowering of SGPT in the treated mice. The relative efficacies are in the order of Ser B>Sol B>Sin C>Sin B>Sin A≥Ser A≥Sol A. Sol B, Sol A, Sin B and Sin A increased the liver glycogenesis of the starved mice, but no significant activity was showed by the remaining 3. All 7 compounds affected the pentobarbitol sleeping time in mice. Some of their inhibitory actions pertinent to the liver microsomes (Liu *et al.* 1982) might explain their protective activity against hepatoxicity. Their biological activities varied with the slight change of structures. No structure-activity relationship can be drawn from the present data. However, the ability of increasing the liver glycogenesis seemed to be linked with R configuration of the biphenyl group. During the total synthesis of *Wuweizisu* C, one of the by-products of the intermediates, the substituted biphenyl ester 31 (Xie *et al.* 1982) also showed protective action against hepatoxicity caused by CCl_4 and thioacetamide in mice as the schizandrin series and in addition, it lowered the elevated SGPT level induced by prednisolone while the schizandrins are inactive (Liu *et al.* 1979). Since 1977, 500 patients with a virus chronic hepatitis have been treated with DDB. About 85% of these patients showed a reduction of SGPT level and relief of other symptoms through a course of treatment. No side effect was observed. DDB is more effective than the flavone-lignon (silymarin) in a parallel comparative clinical study. The effectness of DDB sheds light on the therapeutic value of the simple diphenyl compound.

Pueraria lobata Ohwi *(Wild)*
In an attempt to relieve the stiff neck of hypertensive patients which usually persisted even after the blood pressure returned to normal, the study of the root of *Pueraria lobata,* a Chinese medicine described in the classics, as a remedy for fever, thirst, eye pain and stiffness of the neck, was undertaken in early 70's. The decoction and also the ethanol extract of the root were introduced to the clinical trials and satisfactory results were obtained. From the alcoholic extract an isoflavone, daidzein 32 as well as its 3 glucosides, daidzin 33, puerarin 34 and daidzein 7,4'-diglucoside 35 were isolated (Fang *et al.* 1974).

32 $R_1=R_2=R_3=H$
33 $R_1=R_3=H$
    $R_2=$ glucopyranosyl

34 $R_2=R_3=H$
    $R_1=$ glucopyranosyl
35 $R_1=H$
    $R_2=R_3=$ glucopyranosyl

The alcoholic extract, puerarin and daidzein are now used not only in the treatment of stiffness of the neck in hypertensive patients, but also as a useful treatment for angina pectoris and such other vascular diseases as migraine and sudden deafness. No noticible side effect has been observed in patients taking this drug orally for several years.

From the pharmacological studies of the total isoflavones or its major component puerarin, the following actions were observed (Zeng *et al.* 1982): (1) decreasing the activity of the sympathetic nervous system by lowering the elevated catecholamine level of the hypertensive patients and the patients with severe angina pectoris, (2) increasing the cerebral and coronary blood flow and decreasing the coronary and cerebral vascular resistance, (3) inhibiting the platelet aggregation and the release of 5-HT from platelet, (4) improving myocardial ischemia through increasing oxygen content in the blood, decreasing myocardial oxygen consumption, and the lactate production in ischemic myocardium. These various physiological reactions may explain the therapeutic effects of these isoflavones obtained clinically. It seems that these isoflavones might act through a mechanism different from those of the other agents now used in the treatment of cardiac vascular disease, though more eleborate studies will be required to substantiate this assumption.

These 4 isoflavones all have the basic structure of daidzein. The total

Table I

Relative activity of the derivatives on endurance of mice under hypo-oxygen condition

Compound	Relative activity
$R = R_2 = H$ $R_1 = OH$	2.65
$R = R_2 = H$ $R_1 = OCH_3$	3.85
$R = CH_3, R_2 = H$ $R_1 = OCH_3$	4.67
$R = R_2 = H$ $R_1 = Cl$	1.71
$R = R_1 = R_2 = H$	1.57
$R = H, R_1 = OH$ $R_2 = CH_3$	1.33

isoflavones, puerarin and daidzein showed very similar therapeutic effects in clinical trial. Therefore, the derivatives of daidzein were prepared (Shao *et al.* 1980). Their effects on the endurance of mice under hypo-oxygen condition indicated methylation of 4'-ol or 7,4'-diol increased the activity significantly while introduction of methyl group on position 3 or replacing of the 4'-OH with H, NH_2, Cl, NO_1, etc., lowered the activity. Some of the results are listed in Table I. From the above studies, it is suggested that isoflavone may be a promising class of compounds for the cardiovascular diseases.

CONCLUSION

Each example given above reflected its own specific trend and strategy. Artemisinine is a rather straight forward case. Starting with a plant used as an antimalaria agent, led to an active principle with unique structure in the field concerned. Application of traditional theory achieved the discovery of the antileukaemic activity of indirubin and its related isomers. Study of Schizandrae not only verified its therapeutic value but made the accidental discovery of the antihepatitis agent DDB. *Radix Pueraria lobata* was used to treat the stiff neck symptom of hypertensive patients to start with, and further pharmacological study revealed it to be valuable for the cardiac and cerebro-vascular diseases. However, it should be emphasized that there is one fact shared by them all: The plants concerned had all been reported to be studied chemically before, but their biological activities had been ignored. Thus, the potential value of the leads for drug development, concealed in traditional medicine, is evident.

REFERENCES

Anonymous (1974) Clinical observation of taeniafuge effect of agrimophol. *Chinese Medical J. 54*, 344–345.
Anonymous (1977a) The structure of qinghaosu. *Kexue Tongbao 22*, 142.
Anonymous (1977b) Elucidation of the structure of agrimophol. *Acta Chim Sinica 35*, 87–96.
Anonymous (1979) Clinical and pharmacological studies of treatment of chronic myelocytic leukemia with indirubin. *Zhonghua Neike Zazhi 18*, 83–88.
Anonymous (1982a) The chemistry and synthesis of qinghaosu derivatives. *Trad. Chinese Med. 2*, 9–16.
Anonymous (1982b) Studies on the toxicity of qinghaosu and its derivatives. *Trad. Chinese Med. 2*, 31–38.
Anonymous (1982c) Antimalarial efficacy and mode of action of qinghaosu and its derivatives in experimental models. *Trad. Chinese Med. 2*, 17–24.

Anonymous (1982d) Metabolism and pharmacokinetics of qinghaosu and its derivatives. *Trad. Chinese Med. 2,* 25–30.

Anonymous (1982e) Clinical studies in the treatment of malaria with qinghaosu and its derivatives. *Trad. Chinese Med. 2,* 45–50.

Bao, T. T., Liu, G. T., Song, Z. Y., Xu, G. F. & Sun, R. H. (1980) A comparison of the pharmacologic action of 7 constutients isolated from *Fructus schizandrae. Chinese Med. J. 93,* 41–47.

Chen, Y. Y., Shu, Z. B. & Li, L. N. (1976a) Studies on *Fructus schizandrae* IV. *Scientia Sinica 19,* 276–290.

Chen, Y. Y. & Li, L. N. (1976b) Studies of *Fructus schizandrae. Acta Chimica Sinica 34,* 45–52.

Fang, Q. C., Ling, M., Sun, Q. M., Liu, X. M. & Lang, W. Y. (1974) The study of *pueraria flavones. Zhonghua Yixue Zazhi* 271–274.

Friedmann, E. & W. Jacobson (1946) Chemistry of leucaemia. *Nature 157,* 337.

Hsie, T. H., Chen, S. F. & Liang, X. T. (1975) The structure of chuanliansu. *Acta Chim. Sinica 33,* 35–47.

Huang, L., Wu, K. M., Zheng, M. Y. & Fang, Z. (1983) in press.

Ikeya, H., et al. (1979–1982) The constituents of *schizandra chinesis,* Raill I-XII. *Chem. Pharm. Bull. 27,* 1383–1394, 1395–1401, 1576–1582, 1583–1588, 2695–2709; ibid (1980) *28,* 2414–2421, 2422–2427, 3357–3361; ibid (1981) *29,* 2893–2898; ibid (1982) *30,* 132–139, 3202–3206, 3207–3211.

Ji, X. J., Zhong, F. R., Lei, J. L. & Xu, Y. T. (1981) Studies on the antineoplastic action and toxicity of synthetic indirubin. *Acta Pharm. Sinica 16,* 146–148.

Landsheere, B. C. (1951) Effect of indirubin on white blood cell count of the guinea pig. *Experientia 7,* 307–308.

Liang, X. T., Yu, D. Q., Wu, W. L. & Deng, H. C. (1979) The structure of yingzhaosu A. *Acta Chim. Sinica 37,* 216–230.

Liu, G. T., Wang, G. F., Wei, H. L., Bao, T. T. & Song, Z. Y. (1979) A comparison of the protective actions of biphenyl dimethyl-dicarboxylate, trans-stilbene, alcoholic extracts of *Fructus schzandrae* and ganodenma against experimental liver in mice. *Acta Pharm. Sinica 14,* 598–604.

Liu, K. T., T. Cresteil, Columelli, S. & Lesca, P. (1982) Pharmacological properties of dibenzo [a,c] cyclooctene derivatives isolated from *Fructus schzandrae sinensis* II. *Chem. Biol. Interactions 39,* 315–330.

Schmid, G. & Hofheinz, W. (1983) Total synthesis of qinghaosu. *J. Am. Chem. Soc. 105,* 624–625.

Shao, G. X., Mo, R. Y., Wang, C. Y., Zhang, D. Y., Yin, Z. Z., Ouyang, R. & Xu, L. N. (1980) Studies in the synthesis and structure-biological activity relationships of daidzein and its derivatives. *Acta Pharm. Sinica 15,* 538–547.

Tu, Y. Y., Ni, M. Y., Zhong, Y. R., Li, L. N., Cui, S. L., Zhang, M. Q., Wang, X. Z. & Liang, X. T. (1981) Studies on the constituents of *Artemisia annua* L. *Acta Pharm. Sinica 16,* 366–370.

Tu, Y. Y., Ni, M. Y., Zhong, Y. R., Li, L. N., Cui, S. L., Zhang, M. Q., Wang, X. Z., Ji, Z. & Liang, X. T. (1982) Studies on the constituents of *Artemisia annua* part II. *Planta Medica 44,* 143–145.

Wu, K. M., Zhang, M. Y., Fang, Z. & Huang, L. (to be published).

Xie, J. X., Zhou, J., Zhang, C. Z., Ying, J. H., Jin, H. G. & Chen, J. X. (1982) Synthesis of schzandrin C analogs. *Acta Pharm. Sinica 17,* 23–27.

Zeng, G. Y., Fan, L. L. & Zhou, Y. P. Pharmacologic study of *Radix Pueraria.* (to be published).

DISCUSSION

REUTRAKUL: Could you comment on the stability of the peroxide bond in artemisinine, or yingzhaosu A?

HUANG LIANG: The compound is stable under heat or light. This work has been carried out in the Shanghai district. The structure is supported by X-ray analysis.

ANAND: The peroxide bridge in qinghaosu is unusually stable; it can withstand even sodium borohydride reduction.

KROGSGAARD-LARSEN: You showed quisqualic acid in one of your slides. This is an analogue of glutamic acid. Would you elaborate on the pharmacology of this compound?

HUANG LIANG: This really is a very old compound. All the children having worm problems are just given the nuts to chew. In 1943 quisqualic acid was isolated from the nuts, but at that time more detailed pharmacological studies were not performed.

KROGSGAARD-LARSEN: You may know that this compound is a very powerful neurotoxic agent.

HUANG LIANG: Is that so?

KROGSGAARD-LARSEN: If quisqualic acid penetrates the blood-brain barrier it is a potentially dangerous compound to use.

HUANG LIANG: During the chewing of the nuts the patients probably get very low doses of quisqualic acid.

Recent Work on Some Thai Medicinal Plants

Vichai Reutrakul* & Pittaya Tuntiwachwuttikul

Zingiberaceous flora are widely distributed in Southeast Asia. More than 200 species are found in Thailand (Larsen 1980). Many of these plants are used in Thai traditional medicine, e. g., *Zingiber cassumunar* Roxb. is used for relieving asthmatic symptom, *Alpinia galanga* Sw. and *Curcuma longa* Linn. are used externally for the treatment of skin diseases, while *Curcuma xanthorrhiza* Roxb. is an emmenagogue. A number of plants of this family are commonly used as flavouring agents, e. g., *Amomum krervanh* Pierre, *Alpinia siamensis* Schum., *Alpinia galanga* Sw. and *Zingiber officinale.*

Recent investigations of many zingiberaceous plants yielded novel compounds which are of biological and chemical interest. Diarylheptanoids were isolated from *Alpinia officinarum* (compounds 1 to 9; Itokawa *et al.* 1981a, Kiuchi *et al.* 1982b). Compounds 1, 5, 7 and 8 were shown to be inhibitors of prostaglandin biosynthesis. Compound 8, also isolated from *Alpinia oxyphilla,* was reported to be 125 times more pungent than zingerone (Itokawa *et al.* 1981b). Methanolic extract from the rhizome of *Alpinia speciosa* significantly posseses inhibitory activities against histamine and barium chloride by the Magnus method, using excised guinea-pig ileum. Chemical investigations of the extract led to the isolation of compounds 10 to 18 (Itokawa *et al.* 1980, 1981c).

* Department of Chemistry, Faculty of Science, Mahidol University, Bangkok 10400, and Department of Medical Science, Ministry of Public Health, Bangkok 10100, Thailand.

NATURAL PRODUCTS AND DRUG DEVELOPMENT, Alfred Benzon Symposium 20.
Editors: P. Krogsgaard-Larsen, S. Brøgger Christensen, H. Kofod, Munksgaard, Copenhagen 1984.

1

2: R_1 = R_2 = H

3: R_1 = OH; R_2 = OMe

4: R_3=H; R_4=H; R_5=H
5: R_3=Me; R_4=OH; R_5=OMe
6: R_3=H; R_4=OH; R_5=OMe
7: R_3=H; R_4=OH; R_5=H

8

9   10   11

12   13   14: R = OCH_3
                                                         15: R = H

16   17   18

Hydroxyphenylalkanones 19 to 23 were isolated from *Amomum melegueta* (Tackie *et al.* 1975).

19: n=6, 6-Paradol
20: n=7, 7-Paradol

21: n=8, 8-Paradol
22: n=0, Zingerone

23: 6-Shogaol

The genus *Costus* has also been attracting a great deal of interest due to the presence of diosgenin, an important intermediate for the synthesis of steroidal drugs. More than 2% of diosgenin by dry weight has been isolated from the rhizomes of *Costus speciosus* (Gupta *et al.* 1981).

Zingiber officinale, commonly known as ginger, has long been valued for its flavour and pungency, and its use in food and in medicine has been recorded in ancient Sanskrit, Hebrew and Chinese scriptures. The existence of (3)-, (4)-, (5)-, (6)-, (8), 10- and (12)-gingerols 24 in this plant has been demonstrated (Denniff *et al.* 1981). The synthesis of some of these compounds and the biosynthesis of (6)-gingerol have been studied (Denniff *et al.* 1980). Kiuchi *et al.* (1982a), in their recent investigations, isolated potent inhibitors of prostaglandin biosynthesis from zingiberaceous plants. These compounds were identified as (6)- and (10)-dehydrogingerdione 25 and 26, and (6)- and (10)-gingerdione 27 and 28. The isolation of compounds 25 and 27 from *Z. officinale* along with compounds 26 and 28 gives strong support to the biosynthetic pathway for (6)-gingerol as proposed by Denniff *et al.* (1980).

n = 1, (3)-gingerol
n = 2, (4)-gingerol
n = 3, (5)-gingerol
n = 4, (6)-gingerol
n = 6, (8)-gingerol
n = 8, (10)-gingerol
n = 10, (12)-gingerol

25: n=4, (6)-dehydrogingerdione
26: n=8, (10)-dehydrogingerdione

27: n=4, (6)-gingerdione
28: n=8, (10)-gingerdione

Cytotoxic compounds 29 to 34 were isolated from *Zingiber zerumbet* (Matthes *et al.* 1980).

29

30

	R^1	R^2	R^3	R^4
31	OMe	OH	OMe	OH
32	OMe	OH	H	OH
33	H	OH	H	OH

34

As part of our systematic investigation of Thai medicinal plants in the Zingiberaceae family, *Boesenbergia pandurata* (yellow and red forms) and *Zingiber cassumunar* have been chosen for detailed investigations due to their interesting biological activities.

B. pandurata (yellow form)

This plant is widely distributed in Thailand and the fresh rhizome is used in cooking, also in folk medicine for the treatment of colic and as an aphrodisiac. Previous investigations of this plant were concerned mainly with the constituents of the essential oil obtained from its rhizomes (Lawrence *et al.* 1971). Mongkolsuk and Dean (1964) have isolated (±)-pinostrobin 35 and (±)-alpinetin 18 from an ether extract of the dried rhizome. Our re-investigation (Jaipetch *et al.* 1982) of the rhizomes of this plant led to the isolation of pinocembrin 36, pinostrobin 35 together with 2′,6′-dihydroxy-4′-methoxychalcone 37, cardamonin 15 and two new chalcones, (±)-boesenbergin A 38 and B 39.

	R^1	R^2
35:	Me	H
18:	H	Me
36:	H	H

	R^1	R^2	R^3
37:	Me	H	H
15:	H	H	Me

38

39

The structure of boesenbergin A was established on the basis of spectral data and x-ray diffraction analysis. A simple one-step synthesis of boesenbergin A has also been achieved. The reaction of citral with 2′,6′-dihydroxy-4′-methoxychalcone 37 in the presence of pyridine gave a product which proved to be identical with the natural product.

In view of the recent interest in the intramolecular 'citran' cyclization (Crombie *et al.* 1979), the acid catalyzed cyclization of compound 38 was studied. The acid-catalyzed reaction of compound 38 gave a mixture of compounds 40 and 41. Compound 41 was presumably derived from the acid-catalyzed cyclization of compound 40 and in fact further reaction of compound 40 with dilute acid gave compound 41. Methylation of compound 40 gave compound 43 which was identical with the product obtained from the acid-catalysed cyclization of compound 42.

The nmr spectrum of boesenbergin B is very similar to that of boesenbergin A. The comparative nmr data are shown in Table I.

Table I

NMR spectra of Boesenbergins A and B

Boesenbergin A		Boesenbergin B	
δ	Protons	δ	Protons
1.46, s	2×CH₃	1.42, s	3H
1.60, s	CH₃	1.58, s	3H
		1.66, s	3H
1.69–2.32, m	2×CH₂	1.71–2.30, m	4H
3.83, s	OCH₃	3.90, s	3H
5.09, t(J 6.0 Hz)	(CH₃)₂C=CHCH₂	5.10, t(J 6.0 Hz)	1H
5.40, d(J 10.0 Hz)	ArCH=CH	5.39, d(J 10.0 Hz)	1H
6.04, s	ArH	5.91, s	1H
6.62, d(J 10.0 Hz)	ArCH=CH	6.74, d(J 10.0 Hz)	1H
7.37, m	3×ArH	7.42, m	3H
7.60, m	2×ArH	7.60, m	2H
7.75, d(J 15.5 Hz)	ArCH=CHCO	7.92, d(J 15.5 Hz)	1H
8.13, d(J 15.5 Hz)	ArCH=CHCO	7.72, d(J 15.5 Hz)	1H
14.23, s	OH	14.50, s	OH

The mass spectra of boesenbergins A and B are identical. They show the molecular ion at m/e 404, the base peak at 217 and a prominent peak at 321.

Based on these evidences, the structures 39, 44 and 45 could be proposed for boesenbergin B.

44

45

As a very small quantity of boesenbergin B was isolated, it was then decided to synthesize this compound using the same procedure described for the synthesis of boesenbergin A. When a mixture of equivalent amounts of 2′,4′-dihydroxy-6′-methoxychalcone (cardamonin), distilled citral, pyridine and a few drops of dry dimethyl sulfoxide was heated at 90° for 24 h, boesenbergin B was obtained, upon purification, in 25% yield. The yield of the product could be improved up to 47% by carrying out the reaction in a sealed tube at 120° for 26 h. The NMR, IR spectra and TLC behavior of the synthetic sample are identical with those of the natural product.

Methylation of boesenbergin B with methyl iodide/potassium carbonate in boiling acetone gave a methyl ether derivative. The spectral data of this derivative differed from those of the methyl ether analogue obtained from the methylation of boesenbergin A.

On the basis of this evidence, structure 44 can be excluded. The structures 39 and 45 were differentiated by the following experiments. In the NOE experiment of boesenbergin B, there was a 32% increase in the integration of the aromatic signal at $\delta 5.9$ upon irradiation of the methoxy signal. This result, together with the fact that the natural product gave a positive Gibbs test, clearly indicated that 39 (not 45) is the structure of boesenbergin B.

B. pandurata (red form)
The rhizome of this plant is used in Thailand for the treatment of colic disorders.

Extraction of the rhizome with hexane followed by extensive chromatography of the extract led to the isolation of the new compound 46 (panduratin A), pinostrobin 35, pinocembrin 36 and 2 known chalcones, boesenbergin A 38 and rubranine 47.

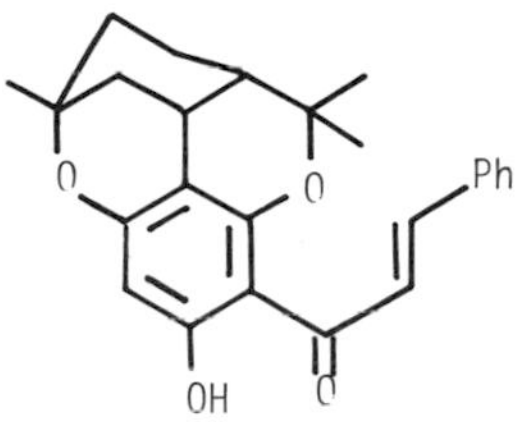

47 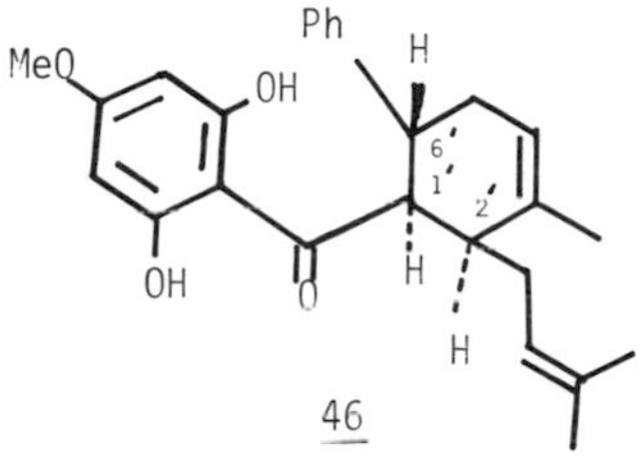   46

The structure of compound 46 was established on the basis of spectral data. The stereochemistries at C-1′, C-2′ and C-6′ were established on the basis of NMR decoupling experiments. The coupling constants for $J_{1,6}$, and $J_{1,2}$, are 11 and 4.4 Hz respectively. These values are comparable to those reported for saggenon D and saggenon C (partial structures shown) (Nomura et al. 1982).

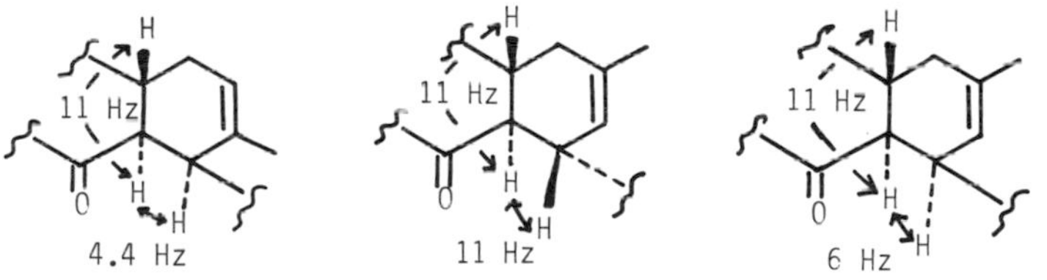

Panduratin A   Saggenon D   Saggenon C

The structure of rubranine 47 was established by comparing its melting point and spectral data with those published. The synthesis of compound 47 was first reported by Bandaranayake et al. (1969) by the reaction of citral with 5,7-dihydroxyflavanone (pinocembrin) 36 in refluxing pyridine. The product (the yield of which was not reported) of this reaction was tentatively assigned structure 47. Subsequent work (Combes et al. 1970) established the identity of compound 47 which was proved to be identical to a substance, named as rubranine, isolated from Aniba rosaeodora Ducke.

8*

116   REUTRAKUL & TUNTIWACHWUTTIKUL

We have repeated the synthesis of rubranine using the reported reaction conditions and were able to isolated rubranine 47 in 2.6% yield. However, when the reaction was carried out at 140°C in a sealed tube for 12 h, 25% yield of rubranine could be isolated. The product thus obtained, was identical to the natural product.

Z. cassumunar

This plant has been used as anti-inflammatory and relieving brochial congestion in Thai traditional medicine. The chemical investigations (Amatayakul *et al.* 1979, Kuroyanagi *et al.* 1980, Dinter *et al.* 1980a, b) led to the isolation of 13 compounds (compounds 48 to 60), 11 of which were new compounds (48 to 58).

	R^1	R^2
48:	OMe	OMe
49:	H	H
50:	H	OMe

51: R = H
52: R = Ac

54: R = H
55: R = OMe

53

56: R = H
57: R = OMe

58: R = $C_{15}H_{31}$

59: R = H
60: R = OMe

The structures of all the compounds isolated were established on the basis of spectral data. The structures of compounds 48 and 53 were also confirmed by x-ray diffraction analysis. The syntheses of compounds 48 to 50 have been achieved. The dimerization of a mixture of compounds 54 and 55 gave compounds 48, 49 and 50. The Wittig reaction between veratraldehyde and the ylide derived from 3-hydroxypropyl (triphenyl) phosphonium chloride gave compound 51. Acetylation of compound 51 gave the expected acetyl derivative 52.

The synthesis of compound 53 was achieved by a one-step regiospecific Diels-Alder reaction of the diene 54 with 2-methoxybenzo-1,4-quinone.

ACKNOWLEDGEMENTS

We thank Professor J. R. Cannon, Dr. L. T. Byrne and Dr. W. C. Taylor for NMR spectra, Dr. A. H. White for x-ray diffraction analysis and Professor N. R. Farnsworth for print-outs from the NAPRALERT data base. Financial support from the International Foundation for Science is gratefully acknowledged.

REFERENCES

Amatayakul, T., Cannon, J. R., Dampawan, P., Dechatiwongse, T., Giles, R. G. F., Huntrakul, C., Kusamran, K., Mokkhasamit, M., Raston, C. L., Reutrakul, V. & White, A. H. (1979) Chemistry and crystal structures of some constituents of *Zingiber cassumunar. Aust. J. Chem. 32,* 71–88.

Bandaranayake, W. M., Crombie, L. & Whiting, D. A. (1969) Selective introduction of mono-, sesqui- and di-terpenoid chromene residues: synthesis of Flemingin A, B and C methyl ethers. *Chem. Commun.* 58–59.

Combes, C., Vassort, Ph. & Winternitz, F. (1970) Structure de la Rubranine, Chalcone isolee de l'*Aniba Rosaeobora* Ducke. *Tetrahedron 26,* 5981–5992.

Crombie, L., Redshaw, S. D. & Whiting, D. A. (1979) The mechanism of intramolecular "Citran" bicyclization of Chromenes: stereochemistry of a forward (H$^+$ catalysed) and a related reverse (thermal) process. *J. Chem. Soc. Chem. Commun.,* 630–631.

Denniff, P., Macleod, I. & Whiting, D. A. (1980) Studies in the biosynthesis of [6]-Gingerol, pungent principle of Ginger *(Zingiber officinale). J. Chem. Soc. Perkin I,* 2637–2644.

Denniff, P., Maccleod, I. & Whiting, D. A. (1981) Syntheses of the (±)-[n]-Gingerols (pungent principles of Ginger) and related compounds through regioselective Aldol condensation: relative pungency assay. *J. Chem. Soc. Perkin I,* 82–87.

Dinter, H., Hansel, R. & Pelter, A. (1980a) The structure of Cassumunaquinones 1 and 2 from *Zingiber cassumunar. Z. Naturforsch. 35c,* 154–155.

Dinter, H., Hansel, R. & Pelter, H. (1980b) Isolation of two phenylbutadiene dimers and one monomeric 4-phenylbut-3-ene from *Zingiber cassumunar* Roxb. *Z. Naturforsch. 35c,* 156–158.

Gupta, M. M., Lal, R. N. & Shukla, Y. N. (1981) Aliphatic hydroxyketones and diosgenin from *Costus speciosus* roots. *Phytochemistry 20,* 2553–2555.

Itokawa, H., Morita, M. & Mihashi, S. (1980) Labdane and bisnorlabdane type diterpenes from *Alpinia speciosa* K. Schum. *Chem. Pharm. Bull. 28,* 3452–3454.

Itokawa, H., Morita, M. & Mihashi, S. (1981a) Two new diarylheptanoids from *Alpinia officinarum* Hance. *Chem. Pharm. Bull. 29,* 2383–2385.

Itokawa, H., Aiyama, R. & Ikuta, A. (1981b) A pungent diarylheptanoid from *Alpinia oxyphylla. Phytochemistry 20,* 769–771.

Itokawa, H., Morita, M. & Mihashi, S. (1981c) Phenolic compounds from the rhizomes of *Alpinia speciosa. Phytochemistry 20,* 2503–2506.

Jaipetch, T., Kanghae, S., Panchareon, O., Patrick, V. A., Reutrakul, V., Tuntiwachwuttikul, P. & White, A. H. (1982) Constituents of *Boesenbergia pandurata* (syn. Kaempferia pandurata): isolation, crystal structure and synthesis of (±) Boesenbergin A. *Aust. J. Chem. 35,* 351–361.

Kiuchi, F., Shibuya, M. & Sankawa, S. (1982a) Inhibitors of prostaglandin biosynthesis from Ginger. *Chem. Pharm. Bull. 30,* 754–757.

Kiuchi, F., Shibuya, M. & Sankawa, U. (1982b) Inhibitors of Prostaglandin biosynthesis from *Alpinia officinarum. Chem. Pharm. Bull. 30,* 2279–2282.

Kuroyanagi, M., Fukushima, S., Yoshihira, K., Natori, S., Dechatiwongse, T., Mihashi, K., Nishi, M. & Hara, S. (1980) Further characterization of the constituents of a Thai medicinal plant, *Zingiber cassumunar* Roxb. *Chem. Pharm. Bull. 28,* 2948–2959.

Larsen, K. (1980) Annotated key to the genera of Zingiberaceae of Thailand. *Nat. Hist Bull. Siam. Soc. 28,* 159–169.

Lawrence, B. M., Hogg, J. W., Terhune, S. J. & Pichitkul, N. (1971) The essential oil of *Kampferia pandurata* Roxb. *Appl. Sci. Res. Corp. (Thailand) Report no. 2,* 1–6.

Mattes, H. W. D., Luu, B. & Ourisson, G. (1980) Cytotoxic Components of *Zingiber zerumbet, Curcuma zedoaria* and *C. Domestica. Phytochemistry 19,* 2643–2650.

Mongkolsuk, S. & Dean, F. M. (1964) Pinostrobin and Alpinetin from *Kaemferia pandurata. J. Chem. Soc.,* 4654–4655.

Nomura, T., Fukai, T., Hano, Y. & Uzawa, J. (1982) Structure of Sanggenon D, a natural hypotensive Diels-Alder adduct from chinese drug 'Sang-Bai-Pi'" (Morus root barks). *Heterocycles 17,* 381–389.

Tackie, A. N., Dwuna-Badu, D., Ayim, J. S. K., Dabra, T. T., Knapp, J. E., Slatkin, D. J. & Schiff Jr., P. L. (1975) Hydroxyphenylalkanones from *Amomum melegueta. Phytochemistry 14,* 853–854.

DISCUSSION

RAZDAN: The structures of some of the chalcones are very similar to those of the cannabinoids we have been working with. In 1969, we and others published simultaneously a one-step synthesis of the cannabinoids concerned, starting with citral, and you have done the same type of reaction in your field. In the Cannabis plant similar compounds have not shown very exciting pharmacological profiles. I wonder what kind of activity was found in your series of compounds?

REUTRAKUL: We would like to subject the compounds to an *in vivo* test which we have set up recently.

BRØGGER CHRISTENSEN: You mentioned some compounds with flavanone structure. It has been shown that some compounds of this type affect cyclic AMP levels. Does your compound possess this activity?

REUTRAKUL: We don't know. We have not tested it.

ANAND: We have also isolated some coumarins exhibiting spasmolytic activity (1, 2).

NAKANISHI: You carried out an NOE experiment in order to determine the structure of boesenbergin B, and you said it had a 32% effect on the aromatic signal at δ 5.9. I was wondering whether that differentiates the 2 structures concerned, because on the other structure you also have a methoxy group in a similar position?

REUTRAKUL: In structure 39 the proton concerned is opposite to the hydroxyl. In compound 45, that you are referring to, this is not the case. We could also partially confirm structure 39 by X-ray. I did not mention that because our R-factor is very high, about 19%. But we did not question the structure. The problem with the R-factor was that the crystal used for X-ray analysis was not big enough to get a good set of data for computer analysis.

RAPOPORT: Were you surprised to find that your Diels-Alder reaction gave you only one regio-isomer?

REUTRAKUL: No, that was what we predicted. Subsequent theoretical calculations have indicated that this assumption was correct.

(1) Shoab, A., Manandhar, M. D., Kapil, R. S. & Popli, S. P. (1978) Clausmarins A. & B, *Chem. Comm. 281.*
(2) Lakshmi, V., Prakash, V., Raj, K., Kapil, R. S. & Popli, S. P. (1984) Chemical Constituents of C. *anisata, Phytochemistry, 24* (in press).

Some Recent Isolation and Synthetic Studies on the Constituents of Indigenous Medicinal Plants

Atta-ur-Rahman[1], G. A. Miana, Y. Ahmad, M. A. Khan, V. U. Ahmad, F. Zehra, A. A. Ansari, M. Bashir, M. Sultana, I. Hasan, Mehrun Nisa, S. Farhi, T. Zamir, M. Shamma[2], G. Blasko, N. Munugesan, J. Clardy[3], A. J. Freyer, S. A. Drexler, Wolfgang Voelter[4] & P. W. Le Quesne[5].

The bulk of the populations of the Afro Asian countries, particularly those living in villages, rely on the indigenous medical systems to provide relief from disease. Systematic scientific investigations, particularly during the current century, have resulted in the identification of a growing number of active constituents many of which are now routinely used in modern medicine. These include reserpine for the treatment of cardiac arrhythmias, vincamine as a vasodilator, and vinblastine and vincristine as anti-tumour agents, etc. Isolation, structural and synthetic studies have, accordingly, been directed in many laboratories around the world, including ours, to isolating new natural products which could prove to be valuable chemotherapeutic agents. Some of the recent studies carried out by my group at Karachi are briefly presented here.

ISOLATION AND STRUCTURAL STUDIES ON *BERBERIS ARISTATA*

Berberis aristata DC (Berberidaceae) is a shrub found in the northern mountainous regions of Pakistan and India as well as in the Nilgiri Hills of

[1]H. E. J. Research Institute of Chemistry, University of Karachi, Pakistan; [2]College of Science, Department of Chemistry, The Pennsylvania State University, and [3]Department of Chemistry, Baker Laboratory, Cornell University, U.S.A.; [4]Institute fuer Physiolog. Chem., Universitaet Tuebingen, Abteilung fuer Biophysikalische Chemie, West Germany; [5]Department of Chemistry, Northeastern University, Boston, U.S.A.

NATURAL PRODUCTS AND DRUG DEVELOPMENT, Alfred Benzon Symposium 20.
Editors: P. Krogsgaard-Larsen, S. Brøgger Christensen, H. Kofod, Munksgaard, Copenhagen 1984.

southern India. The extracts, made from the root bark are known as "rasaut" and are used in the traditional system of medicine for the treatment of jaundice and skin diseases. As a result of careful isolation studies, 2 new alkaloids, "Karachine" (1) and "Taxilamine" (2) have recently been isolated (G. Blasko *et al.* 1982a, G. Blasko *et al.* 1982b). Karachine is the first naturally occurring berbinoid of this skeletal system and is the most complex of more than 50 protoberberine alkaloids presently known. Its structure (1) has been elucidated largely on the basis of its high resolution mass and 360 MHz (FT) nmr spectra, and the positioning of groups confirmed by Nuclear Overhauser Effect studies.

The uv spectrum of karachine, λ_{max}EtOH 226 and 285 nm (log ε 3.90 and 3.62), was suggestive of a tetrahydroprotoberberine. The mass spectrum shows the molecular ion at m/e 433, and the base peak at m/e 336. The latter peak fits exactly for the molecular ion of berberine or epiberberine and is formed by loss

(2)   (5)   (19)

Papilamine (6) R=H
Papilicine (7) R=CH₃

Moenjodaramine (8) R=CH₃
I.R:ν_{max}1360, 2940 & 1595 cm⁻¹
U.V: λ_{max}207, 237, 254 nm
Mass: m/e 426.3609 (M⁺), 58.0650 (100%)
NMR: δ0.71 (s,3H), 0.75 (s,3H), 1.03 (s,3H),
      0.88 (d,3H).

Harappamine (9) R=H
I.R:ν_{max}3400, 2540, 1650 cm⁻¹
U.V:λ_{max}238, 246
Mass: m/e 412.3454 (M⁺), 58.0660 (100%)
NMR: δ1.03 (s,3H), 1.06 (s,3H), 1.12 (s,3H),
      0.72 (d,3H), 5.98 (s,1H), 5.56 (m,1H).

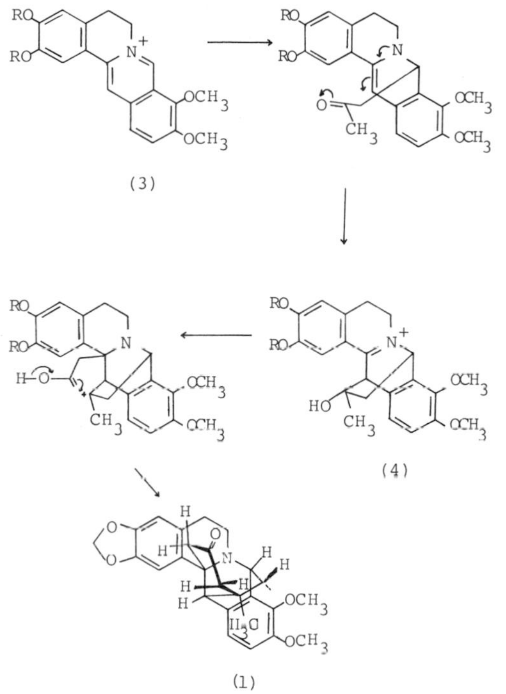

Scheme 1

of 97 mass units from the molecular ion via cleavage alpha to the nitrogen atom (C-14 to C-ε bond), followed by a retro-Diels-Alder process. The m/e 97 fragment corresponds to C_6H_9O, or, more specifically, to 2 moles of acetone minus the elements of water[3]. A sharp absorption band at 1710 cm^{-1} in the ir spectrum (CHCl$_3$) denoted the presence of a non-conjugated carbonyl.

The 360 MHz (FT) nmr spectrum in CDCl$_3$ presented a complex pattern, but allowed for the tentative assignment of expression 1 to karachine.

In order to settle conclusively the nature of the substitution pattern in aromatic-rings A and D, an n.o.e. study was carried out. Irradiation of the C-10 methoxyl singlet at δ 3.77 resulted in an overall 11.6% increase in the area of the δ 6.52 and δ 6.55 ring D aromatic doublet of doublets. Alternatively, irradiation of the H-1 singlet at δ 6.73 gave a 2.8% increase of the δ 2.70 and 2.72 doublet of doublets assigned to the C-ε protons, as well as to a 5.6% increase of the signal at δ 3.07 due to H-13. Significantly, irradiation of either the H-1 or H-4 singlets at δ 6.73 and δ 6.17 respectively led to no observable n.o.e. for the methoxyl absorptions. Further support for the structure of karachine has come from its borohydride reduction, and analysis of the mass and nmr spectra of the corresponding alcohol.

Karachine must arise by the condensation of berberine (3) with 2 moles of acetone and accompanying loss of water, as suggested in the Scheme (1). It is the first naturally occurring berbinoid incorporating acetone units (Govindachari *et al.* 1981). It is a true alkaloid and not an artefact of isolation since (a) optically active, as well as inactive, naturally occurring adducts of the related benzo-phenanthridine alkaloids with acetone are known (M. Shamma *et al.* 1972), (b) no acetone was used during the isolation process, and (c) various attempts on our part to obtain karachine by condensation of berberine with acetone at varying pH's were to no avail.

Taxilamine (2) was isolated by chromatography of the alkaloidal fraction (8 g) using neutral alumina. Besides a consistent u.v. spectrum, the 360 MHz (FT, CDCl$_3$) nmr spectrum of taxilamine shows H-5 and H-8 as singlets at δ 7.15 and δ 7.40, respectively; H-3 and H-4 as a doublet of doublets at δ 8.46 and δ 7.66 (J$_{vic}$ = 5.5 Hz); and H-5' and H-6' as another doublet of doublets at δ 6.44 and δ 7.28 (J$_{vic}$ = 9.1 Hz). The 4 methoxyl signals appear as singlets at δ 3.92, 3.96, 3.97 and 4.06. This spectrum bears a distinct resemblance to that reported for rugosinone (Wu *et al.* 1980). The mass spectrum of taxilamine confirmed the molecular formulation C$_{20}$H$_{19}$O$_6$N and the structure (2) assigned.

Taxilamine (2) is the fourth member of its class of pseudobenzyl isoquinoline alkaloids and must probably have been formed in nature through oxidative rearrangement of palmatine to supply initially polycarpine. Hydrolytic N-deformylation followed by further oxidation would then afford taxilamine (Murugesan *et al.* 1979).

ISOLATION AND STRUCTURAL STUDIES ON THE CHEMICAL CONSTITUENTS OF *FAGONIA INDICA*

Fagonia indica Linn. is a small spiny undershrub which is widely distributed in Pakistan. An aqueous decoction of the leaves and young twigs is a popular remedy for cancer in its early stages. A new sapogenin "Nahagenin" (5) (Atta-ur-Rahman *et al.* 1982a) has been isolated from the hydrolysed extracts of the aerial parts of the plant, and its structure has been elucidated on the basis of a 400 MHz NMR spectrum, a 100 MHz CMR spectrum and high resolution mass spectrum.

The substance analyzed for $C_{30}H_{48}O_4$ (confirmed by high resolution mass spectrometry, m/z$=$472.3740 mass, 472.3552 for $C_{30}H_{48}O_4$). Major peaks in the MS occurred at m/z 454, 436, 424, 409, 395 and 261. The IR spectrum ($CHCl_3$) showed peaks at 1740 cm^{-1} and 3460 cm^{-1} suggesting a δ-lactone and hydroxy groups. The substance readily afforded a diacetate (m/e$=$556), but was found to be remarkably inert to attempted hydrolysis of the lactone. The ^1H NMR showed no olefinic protons. The ^{13}C NMR recorded on a 400 MHz instrument confirmed the presence of 30 carbons. The carbon atoms in the A and B rings were readily recognised by comparison with corresponding signals of known pentacyclic triterpenoids (Knight *et al.* 1974). Eight quaternary centres and 6 methyl groups were also identified. The ^{13}C NMR displayed a resonance at δ 177.29 for the carbonyl carbon, and 3 resonances at δ 84.72 (s), 76.54 (dd) and 71.92 (d) for the oxygen-bearing carbons C(20), C(3) and C(23) respectively. On the basis of these spectral data, structure (5) was assigned to nahagenin which has been confirmed by an unambiguous structure determination by a single crystal X-ray diffraction analysis carried out by Prof. Clardy and co-workers at Cornell University.

ISOLATION AND STRUCTURAL STUDIES ON *BUXUS PAPILOSA*

Buxus papilosa (Buxaceae) is a shrub which occurs abundantly in the northern regions of Pakistan. Extracts of *Buxus* species have been used since ancient times for the treatment of a wide variety of diseases including malaria and venereal disease. *Buxus papilosa* has found use in the indigenous system of medicine as a febrifuge for relief of rheumatism and for the treatment of a number of other ailments. Four new alkaloids, papilamine (6) (Atta-ur-Rahman *et al.* 1983a), papilicine (7) (Atta-ur-Rahman *et al.* 1983b), moenjodaramine (8) (Atta-ur-Rahman *et al.* 1983c), and harappamine (9) (Atta-ur-Rahman *et al.* 1983d), have recently been isolated by us from the leaves of this plant and their structures elucidated on the basis of the spectral data of the alkaloids as well as their derivatives. The spectral data obtained for each alkaloid are given against each structure.

The uv spectrum of moenjodaramine showed absorption maxima at 207, 237, 245 and 254 nm, characteristic of the presence of a 9(10→19) *abeo*-diene system (Khuong *et al.* 1966). An identical u.v. spectrum is encountered in buxamine E, buxaminol E and papilamine (Atta-ur-Rahman *et al.* 1983a). The proton NMR spectrum ($CDCl_3$) showed 3 singlets, corresponding to the 3 tertiary methyl

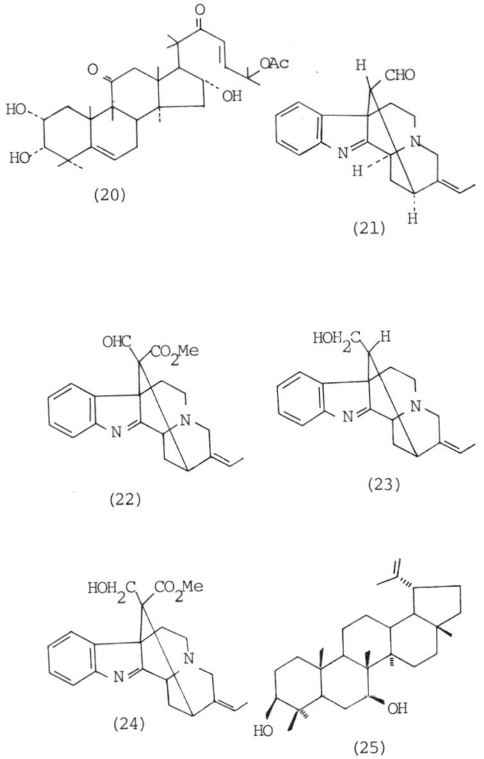

Fig. 1.

groups at δ 0.71, δ 0.75 and δ 1.03. The secondary (C-21) methyl group resonated as a doublet at δ 0.88 (J=6 Hz). A 3-proton singlet resonating at δ 2.1, was assigned to the $-NCH_3$ group, while another peak resonating at δ 2.2 and integrating for 6 protons was assinged to the $-N(CH_3)_2$ group attached to C-20. A set of AB doublets resonating at δ 3.24 and δ 3.82 was assigned to C-29 methylene protons α- to the C-3 nitrogen. A singlet at δ 5.98 was ascribed to the isolated olefinic proton at C-19 while a multiplet centred at δ 5.55 was assigned to the C-11 olefinic proton.

The mass spectrum of the compound afforded the molecular ion at m/z=426.3609 which corresponded to the formula $C_{28}H_{46}N_2O$ (calcd. 426.3609). The substance showed a base peak at m/z 58.0650 corresponding to the composition $C_3H_8N^+$ which suggested the loss of $CH_2N^+(CH_3)_2$ character- istically encountered in alkaloids bearing a $-N(CH_3)_2$ grouping on ring A, and which may be formed in moenjodaramine by intramolecular proton transfer and cleavage. Another peak at m/z 57.0625 corresponded to the fragment $CH_2=$

$^+$N(CH$_2$)CH$_3$. A peak at m/z 85.0883 was in accordance with the composition C$_5$H$_{11}$N (calc. 85.089) which was attributed to (CH$_2$)$_2$CH=N$^+$(CH$_3$)$_2$ formed by the cleavage of ring A along with the side chain. A peak at m/z 72.0810 having the composition C$_4$H$_{10}$N$^+$ corresponded to the loss of CH$_3$·CH=N$^+$(CH$_3$)$_2$ commonly encountered in alkaloids bearing a −CH(CH$_3$)−N(CH$_3$)$_2$ grouping on ring D (Waller *et al.* 1980). Another peak at m/z=71.0734 having formula C$_4$H$_9$N$^+$ was assigned to the fragment CH$_2$−CH=N$^+$(CH$_3$)$_2$ formed by cleavage of ring A along with the side chain.

In the light of the above studies, structure (8) has been assigned to moenjodaramine. This substance has previously been reported as a synthetic product prepared from desoxy-16-buxidienine C (Khuong *et al.* 1971), but it has not been isolated. A second alkaloid, harappamine was similarly established to have structure (9).

Moenjodaramine (8) and harappamine (9) are the first representative numbers of a new class of pentacyclic natural products bearing both a tetrahydrooxazine ring and a 9(10→19) *abeo*-diene system.

(a) ISOLATION AND STRUCTURAL STUDIES ON THE CHEMICAL CONSTI-
TUENTS OF *CATHARANTHUS ROSEUS*

Studies on the alkaloids of *Catharanthus roseus* have resulted in the isolation of a new alkaloid, to which structure (10) has been assigned. The substance afforded a u.v. spectrum which was typical of a dihydroindole system, showing absorption maxima at 212, 246 and 303 nm and minima at 276, 226 nm. The i.r. spectrum showed the presence of an ester carbonyl absorption at 1730 cm^{-1}. The mass spectrum was very similar to that reported for vindolinine (Djerassi *et al.* 1962) and 19-epi-vindolinine (Mehri *et al.* 1972). A high resolution mass measurement on the molecular ion afforded the exact mass to be m/z 336.1837 in agreement with the formula C$_{21}$H$_{24}$N$_2$O$_2$. The C-13 NMR spectrum of the alkaloid (10) (broad-band and off-resonance) showed interesting similarities to the C-13 NMR spectra reported for 19-R-vindoline (Ahond *et al.* 1974), 19-S-vindoline (Ahond *et al.* 1974), and 16-epi-19-R-vindolinine (Ahond *et al.* 1974). The ester carbonyl carbon resonated at δ 173.47, whereas the methyl of the ester group resonated at δ 52.6 (quartet). The substance afforded 4 doublets for the tertiary aromatic carbons, and 2 singlets for the 2 quaternary aromatic carbon atoms. A characteristic singlet appeared at δ 81.36 corresponding to the quaternary carbon atom α to the indoline nitrogen (Atta-ur-Rahman *et al.* 1983e).

The H-NMR spectrum of (10) recorded on a 200 MHz instrument showed the presence of a doublet at δ 0.62 (J = 7.4 Hz) which is assigned to the C-18 methyl protons. The proton adjacent to the carbomethoxyl function resonated as a double doublet at δ 3.18 (J_1 = 12.2 Hz, J_2 = 5.8 Hz). A double-doublet at δ 6.41 was assigned to the olefinic proton at C-15, showing coupling with the vicinal olefinic proton and an allylic coupling with the C-3 proton (J_1 = 10 Hz, J_2 = 2,8 Hz). The other olefinic proton at C-14 resonated as a doublet of double doublets at δ 5.84 (J_1 = 10 Hz, J_2 = 5.2 Hz, J_3 = 1.8 Hz). The chemical shift of δ 0.62 for the methyl group is consistent with a 19-S-configuration as the methyl group of 19-S-vindolinine resonates at δ 0.57 while the methyl group in 19-R-vindolinine resonates at δ 0.95.

Direct t.l.c. comparison with authentic samples of vindolinine and epi-vindolinene showed that the substance could be just separated from these 2 materials in 25% ethanol in ethylacetate on a silica gel plate. In order to confirm the structure, the alkaloid (10) was subjected to an oxidative cleavage reaction (Janot et al. 1962, Rasoanaivo et al. 1974) with iodine/THF/H_2O/Na_2CO_3 when it was found to be smoothly converted to the iodo compound (11). On hydrogenolysis with Raney Ni at 30°C for 2 h, the iodo compound was found to be transformed to (−)-vincadifformine (12). When the same hydrogenolysis experiment was repeated at 0°C for 5 min, quantitative conversion to tabersonine (13) was observed (Scheme 2). The identity of the synthetic hydrogenolysis products was established by direct chromatographic and spectroscopic comparison with authentic samples of tabersonine and vincadifformine.

16-Epi-19-S-vindolinine, when refluxed in benzene for 3 h in the presence of an equimolar amount of lead tetraacetate, was found to be smoothly transformed to 2 faster running products. The major product formed in 70% yield afforded a normal indolic u.v. spectrum. The i.r. spectrum (KBr) showed bands at 1655 cm^{-1} and 1730 cm^{-1}, which were assigned to N_b-CHO and -CO_2CH_3 groups respectively. The mass spectrum showed M$^+$ at 352.1783 (calc. for $C_{21}H_{24}N_2O_3$, 352.1786), and other major peaks at 320, 293, 214, 169 and 154. The PMR spectrum (CDCl$_3$) showed resonances at δ 1.23, (3H, d, J = 5.6 Hz, C=CH-CH$_3$), δ 3.67 (3H, s, OCH$_3$), δ 5.46 (1H, q, J = 5.6 Hz, C=CH-CH$_3$), δ 5.7–6.1 (2H, m, HC=CH), δ 7.6–6.9 (4H, m, aromatic), δ 8.00 (1H, s, N_b-CHO) and δ 8.35 (1H, s, NH). Irradiation at δ 5.46 resulted in the collapse of the methyl group at δ 1.23 to a singlet.

The above spectroscopic data were identical with those for (14), a product

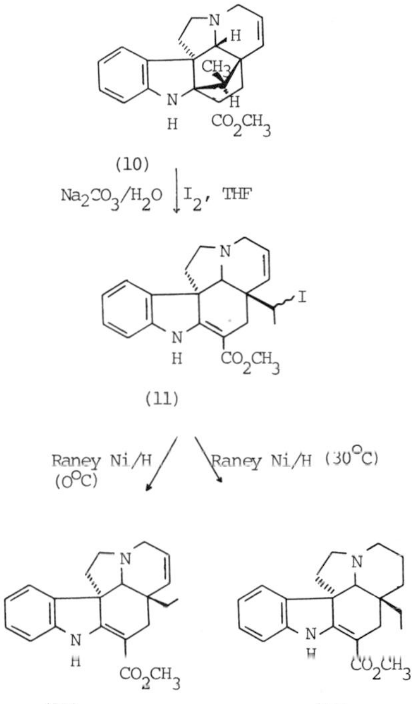

Scheme 2

(10), (11), (13), (12)

previously reported to be formed from 19-iodo-tabersonine on heating with sodium acetate in DMF (Diatta *et al.* 1976). In order to confirm the structure of the oxidation product, 16-epi-19-S-vindolinine (10) was oxidized with iodine under conditions previously described for the oxidation of its diastereo isomer (Rasoanaivo *et al.* 1974b). This afforded the corresponding 19-iodo-tabersonine in quantitative yields. Treatment of the latter with sodium acetate in hot DMF afforded (14). A direct spectroscopic and chromatographic comparison of the product formed by lead tetraacetate oxidation with that prepared from 19-iodotabersonine (Diatta *et al.* 1976) unambiguously established its structure. A plausible mechanism for the formation of (14) is presented in (Scheme 3).

The second minor product formed in the lead tetraacetate oxidation possessed a u.v. characteristic for the dihydroindole system. Further work on the structure of this material is under progress.

The facile formation of (14) from (10) is biogenetically intersting particularly in view of the occurrence of the binary indole alkaloids such as catharine (16) (Rasoanaivo *et al.* 1974c) in which one of the moieties bears a distinct

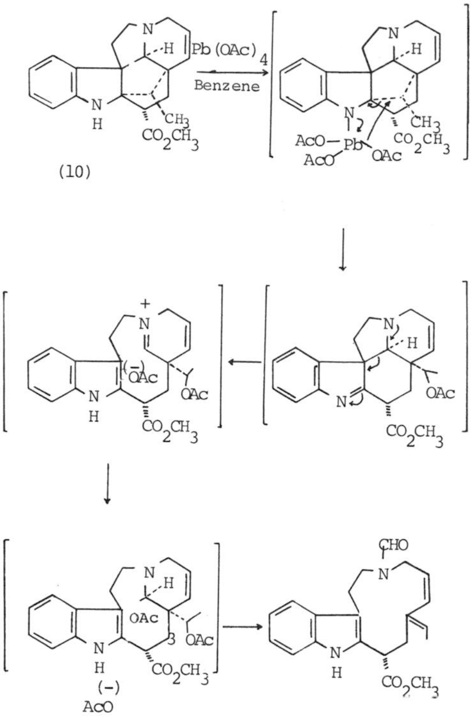

Scheme 3

resemblance to (14) & raises the interesting possibility that the indole moiety of catharine may arise by a parallel process occurring in a binary precursor alkaloid such as (15) (Scheme 4).

(b) A RAPID PROCEDURE FOR THE ISOLATION OF CATHARANTHINE, VINDOLINE AND VINBLASTINE

The binary indole alkaloids vinblastine (17) and vincristine (18) are among the most potent chemotherapeutic agents known to man, and are being used for the treatment of several different type of cancer including Hodgkins disease, acute leukaemia in children and choriocarcinoma. As both alkaloids occur only in minute traces in the leaves of *Catharanthus roseus,* they cost several thousand dollars per gram. This has attracted the attention of a number of groups towards their synthesis.

Our earlier efforts in this field (Atta-ur-Rahman *et al.* 1980) have led to 2

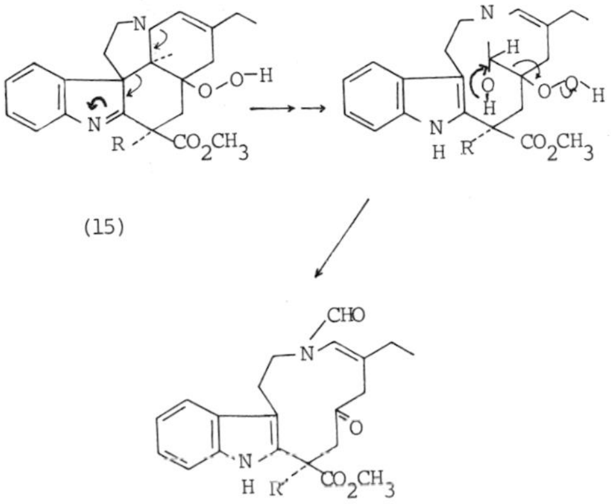

(15)

Scheme 4

(16): R-10-vindolinyl

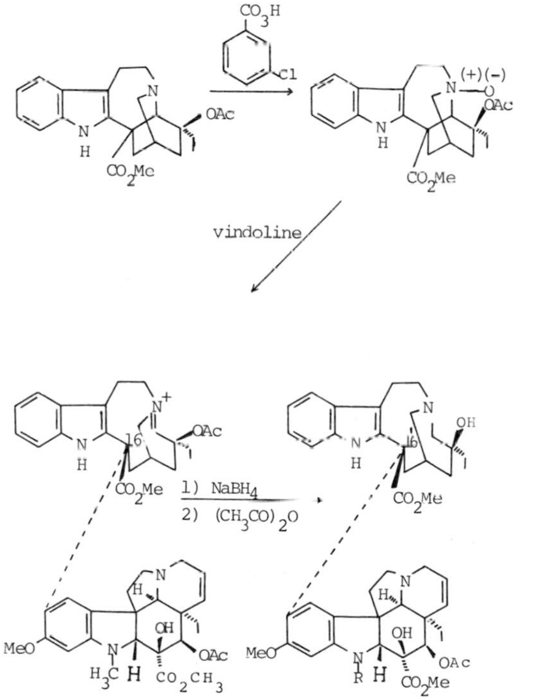

vindoline

1) NaBH$_4$
2) (CH$_3$CO)$_2$O

Scheme 5

vinblastine (17) R = CH$_3$
vincristine (18) R = CHO

different syntheses of vinblastine based on functionalisation of the olefinic bond of catharanthine before (Atta-ur-Rahman *et al.* 1976) (Scheme 5), or after (Atta-ur-Rahman *et al.* 1978) (Scheme 6) (Atta-ur-Rahman 1980b, 1981) coupling with vindoline. These syntheses employed a novel modification of the polonovski reaction developed by Potier and co-workers (Potier *et al.* 1975). A similar approach to vinblastine has also been reported by the French group (Manganey *et al.* 1979).

It is notable that we were the first to propose a novel biogenetic hypothesis that the tetracyclic indole moiety of vinblastine arises in the plant from the coupling of a pentacyclic iboga alkaloid such as catharanthine with the aspidosperma alkaloid vindoline, rather that from a tetracyclic cleavamine-like precursor. This approach led us to report the first analogue of vinblastine, 16-epi-anhydrovinblastine, ever prepared starting from catharanthine and vindoline (Atta-ur-Rahman 1971). The majority of the subsequent synthetic ap-

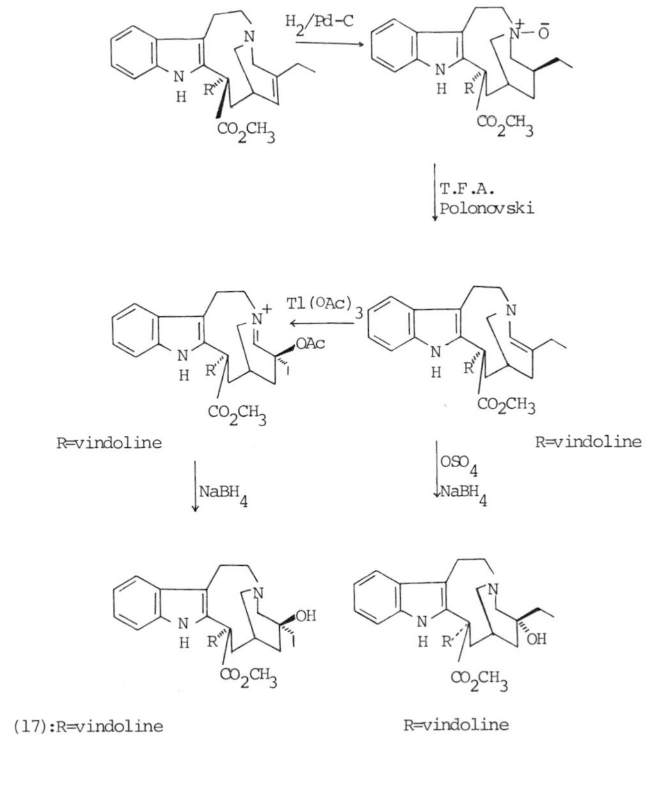

Scheme 6

proaches to vinblastine and its analogues published to date are all based on the biosynthetic route proposed by us.

As the above synthetic routes were all based on catharanthine and vindoline as starting materials, it was important to develop an isolation procedure which could afford these alkaloids in bulk without having to resort to extensive chromatography. We have now developed a rapid isolation procedure for the isolation of catharanthine, vindoline and vinblastine. This procedure has been tested and found to be extremely satisfactory both at laboratory and pilot-plant levels. This should produce catharanthine, vindoline and vinblastine much more readily, as well as stimulating further research on the development of new anti-tumoural derivatives of these oncolytic alkaloids. The procedure that we have developed (Atta-ur-Rahman et al. 1982b, Atta-ur-Rahman et al. 1983f), involves extraction of the alkaloids with pH 3 phosphate buffer, selective precipitations by use of appropriate solvents and selective extractions. For vinblastine, a direct and simple isolation procedure has been developed which does not involve any chromatography, but affords pure vinblastine sulphate in yields of 0.02% to 0.025% by weight of the dried leaves (8–10 gm of vinblastine from 40 Kg of leaves). Pilot plant investigations have proved very successful and commerciali-sation of the procedure is under active exploration.

ISOLATION AND STRUCTURAL STUDIES ON THE CHEMICAL CONSTITUENTS OF *BETULA UTILIS*

Betula utilis is a tree commonly found at high altitudes in the temperate Himalayas extending from Chitral eastwards to Azad Kashmir, and in Sikkim and Bhutan. The infusion of its bark has found wide use in indigenous medicine as an antiseptic, carminative, and for hysteria. Our interest in the systematic investigation of the chemical constituents of Pakistani medicinal plants has led us to a chemical investigation of the bark of *Betula utilis*. This has resulted in the isolation of a new triterpenoid, "Karachic acid" (19), the structure of which has been solved on the basis of chemical and spectroscopic studies (Atta-ur-Rahman & Khan 1975).

ISOLATION AND STRUCTURAL STUDIES ON THE CHEMICAL CONSTITUENTS OF *CUCUMIS PROPHETARUM*

The isolation of a number of cucurbitacins with cytotoxic properties prompted us to investigate the active principles present in the fruits of *Cucumis prophetarum* (Cucurbitaceae), a plant locally known as "Choti indrayan" or "Khar indrayan". It is a perennial trailing herb with ellipsoidal echinate fruits. The plant grows wild in various regions of Pakistan, Rajputana (India), Saudi Arabia and tropical Africa. The fruits are used in indigenous medicine as an emetic and purgative. It is known to contain cucurbitacins B and D and traces of cucurbitacins G and H.

As a result of isolation studies carried out on the fruits of this plant, we have isolated a new cucurbitacin, cucurbitacin Q-1 (20) which closely resembles cucurbitacins O and P in its structure (Atta-ur-Rahman *et al.* 1972). The cytotoxicity of these cucurbitacins against Eagles KB strain of human carcinoma of the nasopharynx has been demonstrated and it has been shown that

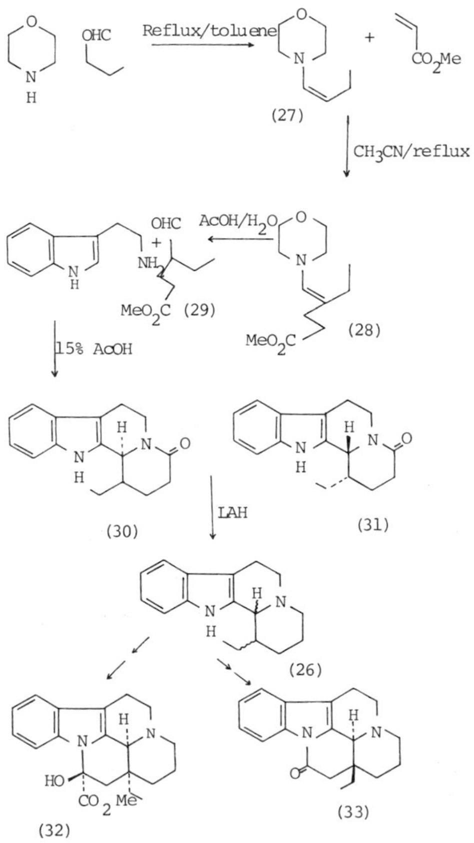

Scheme 7

the side-chain double bond and tertiary acetate are essential for cytotoxic activity. The activity of cucurbitacin Q-1 would, therefore, be of interest, and it is being studied by the National Institutes of Health, Bethesda, U.S.A.

ISOLATION AND STRUCTURAL STUDIES ON *RHAZYA STRICTA*

Rhazya stricta Decaisne (Apocynaceae) is a small glabrous erect shrub which grows profusely in the north-western region of the Indo-Pakistan subcontinent. It is used by the traditional practitioners as a bitter tonic for sore throat, in fever, in general debility and as a curative for chronic rheumatism. As a result of isolation and structural studies carried out by us, a number of new alkaloids have been isolated and their structures elucidated. These are strictalamine (21) (Knight 1974), rhazimal (22) (Atta-ur-Rahman *et al.* 1977), rhazinol (23) (Atta-ur-Rahman *et al.* 1979), and rhazimol (24) (Ahmad *et al.* 1983). Space does not permit a detailed discussion. The structures are shown in the Fig. 1).

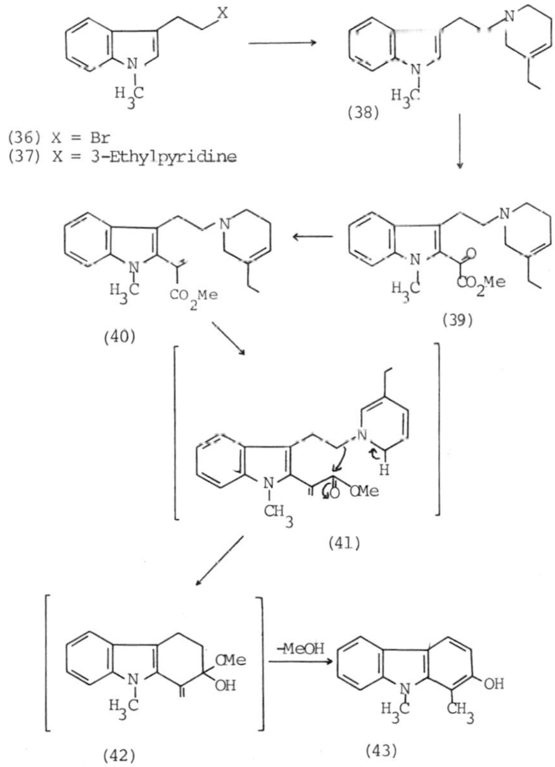

(36) X = Br
(37) X = 3-Ethylpyridine

(38)

(40)

(39)

(41)

(42)

(43)

Scheme 8

STUDIES ON THE CHEMICAL CONSTITUENTS OF *LORANTHUS GREWINKII*

Siddiqui and co-workers had previously reported a new triterpenoid, "loranthol" from the berries of *Loranthus grewinkii,* a parasite found widely distributed on pear, apricot and almond trees. The gum from these berries is widely used in the indigenous system of medicine as a general tonic, relaxant and laxative. This triterpenoid has been re-isolated and its structure (25) has been elucidated on the basis of chemical and spectroscopic studies (Atta-ur-Rahman *et al.* 1973b).

A FORMAL TOTAL SYNTHESIS OF (±)-VINCAMINE AND (±)-EBURNAMONINE

In view of the reported pharmacological properties of vincamine (32) and eburnamonine (Taylor *et al.* 1973), we have developed a new route to these alkaloids involving a novel synthesis of the key intermediate (26) a compound which contains 4 of the requisite 5 rings and 2 of the 3 chiral centers.

Butyraldehyde and morpholine were condensed by the method of Stork (Stork *et al.* 1963) to afford the morpholinoenamine (27). Alkylation of (27) with methyl acrylate gave the dialkylated product (28) which was hydrolysed with aq. acetic acid to give (29) in 45% yield.

Condensation of (29) with tryptamine afforded a gum which on purification through a silica column gave a mixture of 2 diastereoisomeric compounds, which could readily be separated by preparative layer chromatography as (30) and (31) (Scheme 7) each of which crystallised as white needles m.p. 185–186°C and 230°C respectively.

Lithium aluminium hydride reduction of the diastereoisomeric mixture of (30) and (31) afforded the amine (26) in 20% overall yield; (26) is convertible to vincamine and eburnamonine by one of several routes (Kuehne 1964, Wenkert & Wickberg 1965, Hermann *et al.* 1979). This, thus formally, constitutes a total synthesis of these alkaloids (Atta-ur-Rahman & M. Sultana 1982c).

A TOTAL SYNTHESIS OF N_a-METHYL SECODINE

The currently accepted biosynthetic route to the indole alkaloids envisages the mediation of 14, 21-dehydrosecodine (34) which can undergo intramolecular Diels-Alder reactions in 2 different ways to afford the Iboga alkaloids catharanthine (35), or the Aspidosperma alkaloid tabersonine (Wenkert 1962). Inspite of intensive efforts by several groups, the synthesis of dehydrosecodine has still not been accomplished because of its high susceptibility to oxidation, dimerization and polymerisation; the synthesis of N-benzyldehydrosecodine has recently been reported (Kutney *et al.* 1982). Secodine has, however, been synthesised (Kuehne *et al.* 1978, Kutney 1979, Raucher *et al.* 1981, Marazano *et al.* 1977), and a number of approaches to the indole alkaloids involving the intermediacy of the secodine system have been studied (Kuehne *et al.* 1979, Scott *et al.* 1974). We have recently developed a short and high yield synthesis of N-methyl secodine based on a facile Friedel-Crafts acylation reaction at the indole 2-position (Atta-ur-Rahman *et al.* 1983h) which is shown in Scheme 8.

N-methyl secodine (40) when refluxed in acetonitrile for 8 h afforded the 2-hydroxy carbazole (42) as a major product (yield 80%). The facile conversion of the secodine derivative to the carbazole system (43) (Scheme 8) suggests the intermediacy of N-methyl dehydrosecodine (41) in the reaction which may have been formed through aerial oxidation. The generation of carbazole derivatives has previously been reported (Kutney *et al.* 1982b, Scott & Cherry 1969), and it has been proposed that 2-hydroxy carbazole is formed via dehydro-secodine by an intramolecular rearrangement and hydrogen transfer mechanism. A parallel project aimed at synthesising N$_a$-benzylsecodine has also been carried out. This synthesis represents the shortest route (reported to date) to the secodine system. Attempts are presently underway to generate the corresponding dehydro-secodines for biomimetic transformations to the Aspidosperma and Iboga alkaloids.

REFERENCES

Ahmad, Y., Fatima, K., Le Quesne, P. W. & Atta-ur-Rahman (1983) Further alkaloidal constituents of the leaves of *Rhazya stricta. Phytochemistry, 22,* 1017.

Ahmad, Y., Fatima, K., Le Quesne, P. W. & Atta-ur-Rahman (1979) The isolation and structure of rhazimal, rhazimol and rhazinol from the leaves of *Rhazya stricta. J. Chem. Soc. Pak. 1,* 69–71.

Ahond, A., Janot, M. M., Langlois, N., Lukacs, G., Potier, P., Rasoanaino, P., Sangare, M., Neuss, N., Plat, M., Men, J. Le., Hagaman, E. W. & Wenkert, E. (1974) On the structure of vindolinine. *J. Am. Chem. Soc. 96,* 633–634.

Atta-ur-Rahman, Farhi, S., Miana, G. A., Nisa, M. & Voleter, W. (1983a) Isolation and structure of papilamine, a new alkaloid from *Buxus papilosa. Z. Naturforsch.* (in press).

Atta-ur-Rahman, Nisa, M. & Zamir, T. (1983b) The isolation and structure of papilicine, a new alkaloid from *Buxus papilosa. Z. Naturforsch.* (in press).

Atta-ur-Rahman & Nisa, M. (1983c) The isolation and structure of Moenjodaramine and harappamine – two new alkaloids from *Buxus papilosa. Z. Naturforsch.* (in press).

Atta-ur-Rahman & Nisa, M. (1983d) The isolation and structure of harappamine. *Heterocycles, 20,* 69–70.

Atta-ur-Rahman, Bashir, M., Kaleem, S. & Fatima, T. (1983e) Isolation and structure of 16-epi-19-S-vindolinine, A new dihydroindole alkaloid from *Catharanthus roseus. Phytochemistry 22,* 1021–1023.

Atta-ur-Rahman, Bashir, M., Hafeez, M., Perveen, N., Fatima, J. & Mistry, A. N. (1983f) Studies on the antitumour alkaloids of *Catharanthus roseus* – a rapid procedure for the isolation of catharanthine, vindoline and vinblastine. *Planta Medica 47,* 246.

Atta-ur-Rahman & Basha, A. (1983g) *Biosynthesis of Indole Alkaloids,* Oxford University Press, England.

Atta-ur-Rahman, Sultana, M. & Hasan, I. (1983h) A total synthesis of N-methyl secodine. *Tetrahedron Letters 24,* 1845–1848.

Atta-ur-Rahman, Ansari, A. A., Clardy, J. (1982a) The isolation and structure of nahagenin. *Heterocycles 19,* 217–220.

Atta-ur-Rahman, Bashir, M., Fatima, J. & Mistry, A. H. (1982b) A rapid procedure for the isolation of vinblastine from the leaves of *Catharanthus roseus. Pakistan Patent,* application No. 141/87.

Atta-ur-Rahman & Sultana, M. (1982c) A total synthesis of (±)-vincamine and (±)-eburnamonine. *Z. Naturforsch. 37b,* 793.

Atta-ur-Rahman (1981) Synthetic studies in the field of anticancer alkaloids, the synthesis of vinblastine and vincristine. *Proc. Asian Symp. Med. Plants and Spices 1,* 222–234; *Chem. Abstr. 95,* 98083 p.

Atta-ur-Rahman & Mason, J. H. (1980a) The total synthesis of (±)-16-hydroxydihydrocleavamine and the partial synthesis of demethoxycarbonyldeoxyvinblastine. *Tetrahedron 36,* 1063–1070.

Atta-ur-Rahman (1980b) The synthesis of vinblastine, vincristine, vinrosidine, coronaridine, and dihydrocatharanthine. *12th Int. Symp. on Chem. Nat. Prod. (IUPAC), C44,* 245.

Atta-ur-Rahman (1978) The total synthesis of vinblastine, vincristine, and vinrosidine. *Pakistan Patent* No. 126852, dated 14-2-1978.

Atta-ur-Rahman, Ahmad, Y., Fatima, K., Occolowitz, J. L., Solheim, B. A., Clardy, J., Garnick, R. L. & Le Quesne, P. W. (1977) Structure and absolute configuration of strictamine and strictalamine from *Rhazya stricta,* stereochemistry of Picralima alkaloids. *J. Am. Chem. Soc. 99,* 1943–1946.

Atta-ur-Rahman, Basha, A. & Ghazala, M. (1976) Synthetic studies towards anti-leukaemic alkaloids Part VIII. The synthesis of vinblastine and vincristine. *Tetrahedron Letters* 2351–2354.

Atta-ur-Rahman & Khan, M. A. (1975) Karachic acid, a new triterpenoid from *Betula utilis. Phytochemistry 14,* 789–791.

Atta-ur-Rahman, Ahmad, V. U., Khan, M. A. & Zehra, F. (1973a) Isolation and structure of cucurbitacin Q-1. *Phytochemistry 12,* 2741–2743.

Atta-ur-Rahman, Khan, M. A. & Khan, N. H. (1973b) Loranthol – a new hentacyclic triterpenoid from *Loranthus grewinkii, Phytochemistry 12,* 3004.

Atta-ur-Rahman (1971) Partial synthesis of Δ15,20-anhydrovinblastine, *Pakistan J. Sci. Ind. Res., 14,* 487; *Chem. Abs., 77,* 62204t.

Blasko, G., Mungesan, N., Freyer, A. J., Shamma, M., Ansari, A. A. & Atta-ur-Rahman (1982a) Karachine – An unusual protoberberine alkaloid. *J. Am. Chem. Soc. 104,* 2039–2041.

Blasko, G., Shamma, M., Ansari, A. A. & Atta-ur-Rahman (1982b) Taxilamine, A pseudobenzyl-isoquinoline alkaloid. *Heterocycles 19,* 257–259.

Diatta, L., Andriamialisoa, R. Z., Langlois, N. & Potier, P. (1976) Etude de la vindoline-v' reactivite des Iodo-19-tabersonines. *Tetrahedron 32,* 2839–2842.

Djerassi, C., Flores, S. E., Budzikiewicz, H., Wilson, J. M., Durham, L. J., Men, J. Le., Janot,

M. M. Plat, M., Gorman, M. & Neuss, N. (1962) Mass spectrometry in structural and stereo-chemical problems (IV)-vindolinine. *Proc. Nat. Acad. Sci. 84,* 113.

Govindachari, T. R., Pai, B. R., Rajeswari, S., Natarajan, S., Chandrasekaran, S., Premila, M. S., Charubala, R., Venkatesan, K., Bhadbhade, M. M., Nagarajan, K. & Richten, W. J. (1980) Studies in protoberberine alkaloids XVII – Neooxyberberine acetone. *Heterocycles 15,* 1463–1488.

Hermann, J. L., Gregge, R. J., Richman, J. E., Kieczykrwski, G. R., Normandin, S. N., Quesada, M. L., Semmelhack, C. L., Poss, A. J. & Schlessinger, R. H. (1979) Total synthesis of indole alkaloids d,1-eburnamonine and d,1-vincamine. *J. Am. Chem. Soc. 101,* 1540–1544.

Janot, M. M. & Goutarel, R. (1962) Steroid alkaloids (XIV) derivs. of 21-nor-E-homoconanine. *Bull. Soc. Chim. Fr.* 2234.

Khuong, H. F., Paris, R., Razafindrambao, R., Gave, A. & Goutarel, R. (1971) Steroidal alkaloids cxxxv. Alkaloids of *Buxus madagascarica* subspecies xeaophila f. Salicicola. cycloproto-buxines F and C, buxamine A, 16-deoxybuxidienine C, buxitrienine C. *C. R. Acad. Sci. Paris 273,* 558.

Khuong, H., Genlier, D. H., Huu, M. M. Q. K., Stanislas, E. & Goutarel, R. (1966) Alcaloids/steroidiques – LII alcaloids due *Buxus balearica* willd. cycloprotobuxine D, buxamine e , buxaminol-e, N-isobutyl-baleabuxidine-F, N-benzoyl-baleabuxidine-F, baleabuxoxazine-C, N-isobutyryl-baleahuxidicnine-F, N-benzoyl-baleabuxidienine-F, N-isobutyryl-baleabuxaline-F. *Tetrahedron 22,* 3321–3327.

Knight, S. A. (1974) *Organic Magnetic Resonance 6,* 603.

Kuehne, M. E., Matsko, T. H., Bohnert, J. C. & Kirkemo, C. H. (1979) Studies in biomimetic alkaloid synthesis 3. syntheses of ervincine and vincadifformine analogues from tetrahydro-β-carbolines through secodine intermediate. *J. Org. Chem. 44,* 1063–1068.

Kuehne, M. E., Roland, D. M. & Hafter, R. J. (1978) Studies in biomimetic alkaloid syntheses 2. Synthesis of vincadifformine from tetrahydro-β-carboline through a secodine intermediate. *J. Org. Chem. 43,* 3705–3710.

Kuehne, M. E. (1964) Synthesis of *Vinca minor* alkaloids. *Lloydia 27,* 435.

Kutney, J. P., Kartoon, Y., Kawammra, N. & Worth, B. R. (1982) Dihydropyridines in synthesis and biosynthesis. IV Dehydrosecodine, in-vitro precursor of indole alkaloids. *Can. J. Chem. 60,* 1269–1278.

Kutney, J. P., Badger, R., Beck, J. F., Basshardt, H., Mantough, F. S., Ridaura-Sanz, V. E., So, Y. H., Sood, R. S. & Worth, B. R. (1979) Dihydropyridines in Synthesis and Biosynthesis I. Secodine and precursors of dehydrosecodine. *Can. J. Chem. 57,* 289–299.

Manganey, P., Andriamialisoa, R. Z., Langlois, N., Langlois, Y. & Potier, P. (1979) Preparation of vinblastine, vincristine and leurosidine, antitumour alkaloids from catharanthus spp. (Apocynaceae). *J. Am. Chem. Soc. 101,* 2243–2245.

Marazano, C., Fourrey, J. L. & Das. B. C. (1977) Novel access to 2-substituted indoles and a convenient synthesis of secodine-type alkaloids. *J. C. S. Chem. Comm. 21,* 742–743.

Mehri, H., Koch, M., Plat, M. & Potier, P. (1972) Plants of New Caledonia. XIII. Structures of melobaline and baloxine, alkaloids of *Melodinus balansae. Ann. Pharm. Fr. 30,* 643–650.

Murugesan, N. & Shamma, M. (1979) A biogenetically patterned conversion of palmatine into polycarpine. *Tetrahedron Lett.* 4521.

Rasoanaivo, P., Langlois, N. & Potier, P. (1974a) Malgaches plants. VIII. Alkaloids of *Catharanthus longifolius. Tetrahedron Letters* 3369–3372.

Rasoanaivo, P., Ahond, A., Cosson, J. P., Langlois, N., Potier, P., Guilhem, J., Duerind, A., Riche, C. & Pascard, C. (1974b) Structure of catharine. *C. R. Acad. Sci. 79,* 279C.

Rasoanaivo, P., Langlois, N. & Potier, P. (1974c) Etude de la vindolinine II correlation avec la (–)-vincadifformine. *Tetrahedron Letters 42,* 3669–3672.

Raucher, S., MacDonald, S. E. & Lawrence, R. F. (1981) Indole alkaloid synthesis via Claisen rearrangement, total synthesis of secodine. *J. Am. Chem. Soc. 103,* 2419–2421.

Scott, A. I., Cherry, P. C. & Wei, C. C. (1974) Regio- and stereospecific models for the bio-synthesis of the indole alkaloids III. The Aspidosperma-Iboga-Secodine relationship. *Tetrahedron 30,* 3013–3019.

Scott, A. I. & Cherry, P. C. (1969) Further observations on the biogenetictype chemistry of the indole alkaloids. *J. Am. Chem. Soc. 91,* 5872–5874.

Shamma, M. & Moniot, J. L. (1978) *Isoquinoline Alkaloids Research.* pp. 287–288, Plenum Press, New York.

Stork, G., Brizzolara, A., Landesmann, H., Szmuskovics, J. & Terrel, R. (1963) The enamine alkylation and acylation of carbonyl compounds. *J. Am. Chem. Soc. 85,* 207–222.

Taylor, W. I. & Farnsworth, N. R. (1973) *The Vinca alkaloids,* Dekker, New York.

Waller, G. R. & Dermer, O. C. (1980) *Biochemical Applications of Mass Spectrometery* pp. 83 John Willy & Sons, New York.

Wenkert, E. & Wickberg, B. (1965) General methods of synthesis of indole alkaloids. IV. A synthesis of dl-eburnamonine. *J. Am. Chem. Soc. 87,* 1580–1589.

Wenkert, E. (1962) Biosynthesis of indole alkaloids. The Aspidosperma and Iboga bases. *J. Am. Chem. Soc. 84,* 98–102.

Wu, W. N., Beal, J. H. & Doskotch, R. W. (1980) Alkaloids of Thalictrum XXXI, eleven minor alkaloids from Thalictrum rugosum. *J. Nat. Prod. 43,* 143–150.

DISCUSSION

CASSADY: One comment relative to your work on anti-tumour compounds and your comment about the potential activity of the cucurbitacins. I think it would be fair to say that this may be either the most notorious group or the second most notorious group of compounds that have been picked-up in screening higher plants for anti-tumour activity. In general, I think, one can say that these are probably the most cytotoxic compounds that we have seen to date, however, there has never been any significant *in vivo* anti-tumour activity associated with any of these compounds. I don't think that the cucurbitacins have any potential as anti-tumour agents based on some 15 or 20 years experience with these compounds by a number of investigators.

KUTNEY: I guess, although your lead tetra-acetate mechanism on paper is an interesting one, it could not cope with the information available on the biosynthesis of catharantine.

ATTA-UR-RAHMAN: It is obvious that you don't have lead tetraacetate in the plant, but there may be a similar mechanism involving an enzyme, which couples with the nitrogen and promotes a fragmentation of the type that I have shown. In fact, if you look at one of Potier's earlier speculations on the biosynthesis of catharine this is what he proposes.

KUTNEY: Actually, we have shown that the speculation of Potier's is incorrect. We have demonstrated the existence of an enzyme, which has horseradish peroxidase-like activity. We actually have done the comparison with our system and commercial horseradish peroxidase and have shown that both our enzyme system and commercial horseradish peroxidase convert, in very high yields, anhydrovinblastine system to leurosine. The latter compound, in turn, on further incubation with the same enzyme system goes to catharine. Therefore, the horseradish peroxidase-type activity is clearly present in the enzymes from *Catharanthus roseus*.

II. Marine Sources for Active Constituents and Lead Structures

Modern Drug Research: The Potential and the Problems of Marine Natural Products

Joseph T. Baker

INTRODUCTION

I am honoured to be amongst those invited to participate in this Alfred Benzon Symposium No. 20, and have accepted the invitation in the belief that this contribution may be of value, because it illustrates my commitment to involvement in the search for biologically active substances from the sea, which will be of value to man, his animals and his crops, and reflects on my professional and practical experiences of the problems inherent in the multi-faceted path from interesting discovery to commercialisation as a drug or other beneficial product.

The topic is relevant to the objectives of the Alfred Benzon Symposia. Its presentation in the Royal Danish Academy of Sciences and Letters, which owes much of its security to the Carlsberg Foundation, whose strength, in turn, derives to a large extent from one man's scientific vision and subsequent success in a fermentation industry, may be most appropriate, in that "fermentation" involving marine micro-organisms is one of the fields of opportunity for development in the search for biologically active substances from the sea.

My presentation will cover the following aspects: – the involvement of Hoffmann-La Roche (Roche) – the novel potential of the oceans – Australia as a country of choice – operating practices and philosophy – examples of biologically active substances – specific problems for marine investigators – speculation on the future.

THE INVOLVEMENT OF HOFFMANN-LA ROCHE (ROCHE)

The Swiss-based pharmaceutical and fine chemicals company F. Hoffmann-La

Sir George Fisher Centre for Tropical Marine Studies, James Cook University of North Queensland, Townsville, Queensland 4811, Australia.

NATURAL PRODUCTS AND DRUG DEVELOPMENT, Alfred Benzon Symposium 20.
Editors: P. Krogsgaard-Larsen, S. Brøgger Christensen, H. Kofod, Munksgaard, Copenhagen 1984.

Roche (Roche) established the Roche Research Institute of Marine Pharmacology (RRIMP) which began operations in April 1974, at Dee Why, a suburb of
Sydney, Australia.

Their original concept of a unit with one or two scientists involved in a
collection and extraction operation with major studies being conducted in the
Basle laboratories, was subsequently modified, and, under the Basle co-
ordinator Dr Klaus von Berlepsch with the keen support of the Research
Director, Professor Alfred Pletscher, a research structure was developed. My
belief as Director-designate was that the RRIMP required a core of high quality
research staff in biology, microbiology, chemistry, biochemistry and pharmacology, with at least 10 years security of tenure, efficient laboratories and
modern equipment, to ensure the essential collaboration with Australian
universities and museums, as well as with the Roche research colleagues in
Switzerland, USA, Japan and England.

Hoffmann-La Roche provided excellent support for RRIMP in the period
1974 to December 1980 when the management decision was made to close the
Institute. The company generously allowed the period January 1981 to June
1981 to conclude research projects.

THE NOVEL POTENTIAL OF THE OCEANS

Roche looked to the sea for novel biologically active substances for several basic
reasons:

– all life has derived from the oceans – it is estimated that 90 % of all the species
of living organisms are to be found in the oceans – totally different biosynthetic
conditions exist in the marine environment, from those encountered on land –
many marine organisms have retained or attained a different evolutionary stage
than have land-based plants and animals.

Therefore, a high probability existed that the oceans would yield as yet
unknown chemical substances with novel structures and with a wide range of
biological activities. This projection, made in the mid-1960's, has certainly been
justified on the basis of research findings.

AUSTRALIA AS A COUNTRY OF CHOICE

Australia has a relatively small population per unit area. The country is
politically homogeneous; has a distribution from tropical to cold-temperate

areas; a coastline of length at least 20,000 km (much more if you trace each coastal bay and inlet); distinctive marine features such as the Great Barrier Reef, the Great Australian Bight, the North-West Shelf and many less well known; and a claim on Antarctic land and seas. Additionally, there is little marine pollution in Australia.

OPERATING PHILOSOPHY AND PRACTICES OF RRIMP

Our decision on staffing related to the belief that novel problems were to be faced by this new Institute. The problems varied from reliability of collection and re-collection, to development of biological screens, and to establishment of professional interaction within Australia and within Roche. Australia had a history of unhappy research associations with overseas companies.

We therefore took great care in staff selection. It took 2 years to locate a Head of the Pharmacology Section and a little longer to locate the best person to lead the Microbiology Section. During this time the Chemistry Section, under Dr Bob Wells, worked actively with the collaboration of the Biology Section, under Ian Skinner, and many substances were provided to Basle screening programs, perhaps, with too little information on activity to attract the necessary attention of our overseas Roche colleagues.

By early 1976 our RRIMP basic staffing level and screening program were effected and the basis for the Institute's operation firmly established. It was to become a closely integrated interdisciplinary program of 3 biologists, 5 chemists, 3 microbiologists, 6 pharmacologists, one biochemist at Ph.D. level, and good technical support, with maximum provision for feed-back of information and for double-checking on all aspects of biology chemistry, microbiology and pharmacology. The program was very much under "biological" control, but provision was made to check for the existence of novel chemical substances. Table I illustrates the system practiced. It is important to note that our supply of marine samples was both of macro-organisms and of micro-organisms. The latter gave a particularly high percentage of interesting leads. Table II lists the broad areas of screening in microbiology and pharmacology in RRIMP.

When activities were detected in the primary screens, the substances were initially forwarded to a Roche Basle group for further consideration. In about 1979, the Roche-international system was modified to allow direct scientist-to-scientist interaction on promising leads and this arrangement led to a much

Table I

Screening philosophy for marine natural product research

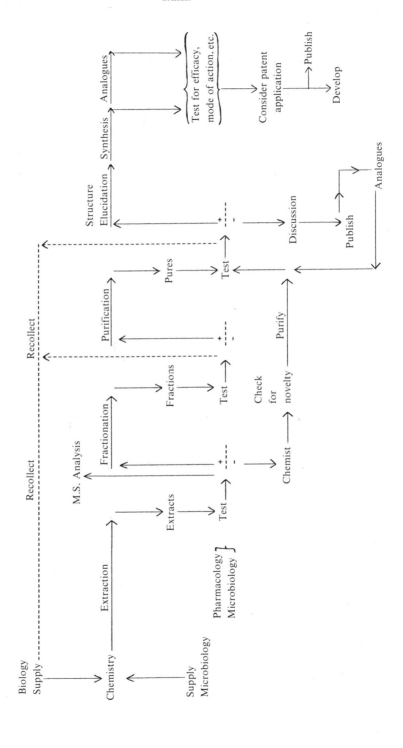

Table II

Pharmacology screening	Microbiology screening	
Gross observation: toxicity	Gram-positive bacteria	(3 spp)
Central nervous system	Gram-negative bacteria	(3 spp)
Cardiovascular	Yeasts	(2 spp)
Autonomic – *in vitro*	Fungi	(1 sp)
Neurophysiology	Protozoan	(1 sp)
Biochemical		
Marine Preparations		

(Agrochemical, anthelmintic, anti-viral and anti-tumour screens were conducted in other Roche centres.)

better acceptance of RRIMP substances in the other Roche research centres. More direct links were established with scientists in Roche at Nutley, Welwyn and Kamakura, as well as at Basle.

However, it was already obvious that the Roche clinical laboratories were under heavy demand and it was decided to extend testing in Australia to allow for evaluation of promising substances in 28-day studies in 2 species, one of which must be a non-rodent. Such studies would generally be in rats and in dogs. If such studies showed results with no adverse side effects, Australian regulations allowed limited dosage of the test compounds in man, provided the substances under test had been isolated and/or synthesized in Australia.

There is no doubt that extension of such testing facilities, to the level which allows human trials, is an essential development for a viable involvement in the search for therapeutic substances.

Table III shows the level of development finally available at RRIMP and compares it with the more extensive evaluation program necessary in a major drug company. It is this latter more involved program which results in the estimate of cost of development of a drug from discovery-to-market at being between (US)$50 million and $70 million.

Much has been said about the probability of a marine-derived substance becoming a drug. One must analyze this question in the context of drug development from traditional synthetic programs, based on known drugs or on proposed mechanisms of action and receptor sites. A most recent estimate on synthetic programs is that the probability of obtaining a successful drug is about 1 in 10,000. We do not have enough experience in marine natural products to

Table III

Typical process to drug development

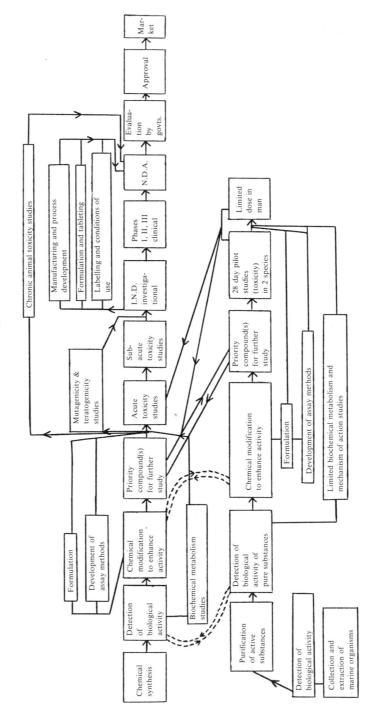

Natural product drug research possible stages for input

allow valid comparison on this scale. At a later point I will analyze whether "all things are equal" in drug evaluation.

EXAMPLES OF RRIMP BIOLOGICALLY ACTIVE SUBSTANCES

RRIMP analyzed many marine organisms prior to the establishment of the program eventually developed, as shown in Table I. We analysed only 1059 species in a definitive manner. A broad breakdown among different types of organisms is shown in Table IV. The column "% giving activity" is that percentage giving activity at a level justifying evaluation to the pure substance or at least to significant purified constituents, with high molecular weight peptides and/or proteins. This process was not followed as extensively in the case of the micro-organisms where many active fractions remained un-analysed at termination.

As a consequence of the RRIMP program more than 400 novel marine natural products were reported in the scientific literature. The following substances represent examples of marine natural products which showed promising biological activity, but for one reason or another were not developed.

(a) *Potential anti-convulsant*

$$R_1 = R_2 = H \qquad 1$$
$$R_1 = H; R_2 = Ac \qquad 2$$

This diterpene was isolated from the dichloromethane extract of a soft coral of the genus *Lobophyton*. It gave excellent protection against the tonic-extensor phase of metrazole-induced convulsions with and ED_{50} of ~ 85 mg/kg i.p. in mice. The LD_{50} (24 h) was ~ 600 mg/kg in the same test situation. Oral activity was weak.

A program of structural modification and analogue synthesis did not significantly enhance the oral activity or the therapeutic ratio. The most active candidate prepared was the monoacetate **2** ($R_1 = H; R_2 = Ac$), which is orally active and is not toxic at active dosage. However, the activity level did not attract development support, nor the approval of a more extensive synthetic program.

Table IV
RRIMP collections

Common name	Number collected	~%	~% Giving activity
Sponges	391	37.0	9
Soft corals and gorgonians	142	13.0	7
Hard Corals	2	0.2	50*
Other coelenterates	48	5.0	0
Holothurians	6	0.6	33
Other echinoderms	21	2.0	5
Molluscs	39	4.0	8
Ascidians	39	4.0	0
Fish	22	2.0	0
Sea grasses	10	1.0	0
Microalgae & bacteria	23	2.0	83
Blue-green algae	9	0.8	22
Green algae	40	4.0	13
Brown algae	102	10.0	8
Red algae	135	13.0	7
Other	30	3.0	0
	1059		

(*Not statistically significant)

(b) *Potential anti-inflammatory, anti-arthritic, anti-fungal agent*
The tetracyclic compound dendalone-3-hydroxybutyrate (3) was isolated from a sponge, *Phyllospongia dendyi.*

3   Dendalone-3-hydroxybutyrate

This compound was active in the carrageenan-induced rat-paw oedema test, showed excellent results in the cotton-pellet granuloma test, and in the adjuvant arthritis test. As an anti-inflammatory its potency was similar to that of phenylbutazone, and **3** was orally active; **3** was an inhibitor of prostaglandin synthetase, a potent inhibitor of platelet aggregation, *in vitro,* and of ^{3}H-serotonin release *ex vivo.* However, it had a poor therapeutic ratio and extensive modification of functional groups did not provide a therapeutically more acceptable candidate.

In agrochemical screening **3** showed excellent anti-fungal activity in 2 commercial crop species. The substance was not further developed for anti-fungal application because of the estimation that cost of synthesis would preclude commercial market entry.

(c) *Potential anti-depressant*

Our first major activity came as early as our first year of operation – 1974. This substance, methylaplysinopsin **4** was isolated from a sponge *Aplysinopsis reticulata,* and was a potent reversible monoamine oxidase (MAO) inhibitor. Therefore, it was of potential interest as an anti-depressant in humans. Within 3 weeks of discovery, Bob Wells and Peter Murphy had prepared some 36 analogues (all novel), and the analogue program continued on-and-off, in Australia and elsewhere in Roche, for 7 years.

4   (*E*-isomer)

This substance attracted interest because of its novel structure, but in 1974 Roche marketing did not support development of MAO-inhibitors. However, by 1978 this attitude had changed and **4** underwent intensive evaluation. Finally Roche decided to not proceed to the clinic with **4** when marked liver damage was observed in dogs and in rats following dosage of 25 mg.kg.$^{-1}$ day^{-1} p.o. over the 13 weeks trial. Doses of 1.0 mg.kg.$^{-1}$ day^{-1} i.v. for 2 weeks did not cause any significant liver damage in rats or dogs, but a dose of 3.32 mg.kg.$^{-1}$ day^{-1} i.v. produced some evidence of slight liver toxicity. In the Ames test for mutagenicity **4** was inactive at all concentrations tested (63 to 2000 µg per plate).

Many internal reports were written on **4**. Liver toxicity has sounded the death-knell of many MAO-inhibitors and this result was a great disappointment after so many years of effort. Roche had invested a great deal of time, effort and money in the analysis of **4** but eventually went to the clinic with a synthetic MAO-inhibitor not modelled on the marine natural product.

(d) *A Broadly active isoguanosine*

Another sponge isolate, 1-methylisoguanosine **5** from *Tedania digitata* showed a very broad pharmacological activity profile, with anti-inflammatory, skeletal muscle relaxant, hypothermic and cardiovascular effects (lowering of blood pressure and of heart rate).

5   1-methylisoguanosine

The problem with this substance was to try to separate the different activities in preparation of analogues and derivatives.

Several years work followed in RRIMP and in other Roche centres, where specific aspects of the program are still in progress. As with the methyl-aplysinopsin **4**, the substance **5** has been protected under patent.

The analogue program has been really extensive and several reports have appeared in the literature. The screening of analogues has been extended beyond the range originally indicated, but to date, no commercial product has emerged.

(e) *Active bi-indoles*

A series of novel active bi-indoles was isolated from a marine blue-green algae. One of the major constitutents was (+)-7′-methoxy-2,3,5,5′-tetrabromo-3,4′-bi-1H-indole **6**.

The compound **6** was active in the carrageenan-induced rat-paw oedema test, reducing oedema at doses of 1 mg.kg.$^{-1}$: **6** was also active in the kaolin rat-paw oedema test, markedly relieving pain induced by kaolin paw inflammation in the dose range 2.4–10 mg.kg.$^{-1}$, both prophylactically and therapeutically.

Other tests for analgesic activity include phenylquinone- and acetic acid-

6

[Chemically the substance is interesting because the optical activity derives from the lack of planarity of the molecule, due to the bulky bromine atoms in the 2,5′ positions.]

induced writhing in rats, and the hot plate test for mice. In these 3 tests, compound 6 had no significant activity. Compound 6 also showed no beneficial effects on adjuvant arthritis in rats (using preinjected Freund's complete adjuvant containing 10 mg.ml.$^{-1}$ of *Mycobacterium tuberculosis* and dosing each rat with 3 mg.kg.$^{-1}$ of 6 twice daily for 20 days).

Compound 6 is a potent inhibitor of passive paw and passive cutaneous anaphylaxis at doses in the range of 2–5 mg.kg.$^{-1}$: 50% inhibition of anaphylaxis was observed at 2 mg.kg.$^{-1}$ dosage of 6 in Oxford Hooded rats. This result suggests that 6 merits attention as a potential anti-allergic substance.

Compound 6 was also active in CNS tests, being active at 5 mg.kg.$^{-1}$ against amphetamine-induced activity. However, the substance 6 produced tremors in both rats and mice. Tremors commenced within 15 min of injection and persisted for at least 4 h in mice dosed at 10 mg.kg.$^{-1}$. The tremors were inhibited by propanalol, indicating a tremorigenic mechanism similar to that of harmaline.

Studies in rats showed that oral doses of 6 up to 10 mg.kg.$^{-1}$ were well tolerated. Some deaths were noted when rats were dosed at 15–20 mg.kg.$^{-1}$ and marked toxicity was noted at doses of 25–50 mg.kg.$^{-1}$. The therapeutic ratio for 6 is, therefore, rather low.

For this substance, 6 there are obvious valuable pharmacological indications.

However, the tremorigenic effect and the relatively high toxicity are unfavourable characteristics.

Looking at positive aspects, the substance **6** is most promising in combining anti-inflammatory and analgesic properties, and as a potential antiallergic substance. The potent anti-amphetamine activity is of interest, provided it can be dissociated from the tremorigenic activity.

Table V summarises the activity and potential. To further evaluate the potential of the substance as a pharmacological agent, synthesis of the parent **6**, of derivatives, and of analogues is necessary. In such a program, one would take note of known characteristics of drugs with an indole nucleus, e.g., among harmaline alkaloids, a methoxy group on the indole nucleus enhances tremors, whereas a hydroxyl group diminishes the effect. Therefore, conversion of the methoxy group in **6**, to a hydroxy group may be valuable in seeking to reduce the tremorigenic effects. Also on the basis of other known drugs, introduction of a 6-hydroxyl group may be beneficial. Additionally, "amino NH" groups can be readily acetylated.

All of these proposals require time, effort and involve significant expense. The priority areas of a particular drug company would determine whether a compound such as **6** merited further development. Roche did not indicate a development interest in this substance.

In the case of *Rivularia firma,* other bi-indoles were isolated. These included **7**, **8**, **9** and **10**. Additionally, a monoacetate and diacetate of **6** were prepared; the diacetate is shown as **11**. Whereas **6** gave significant tremorigenic effects, a

Table V

Activity:	
Carragenan rat-paw oedema	1 mg.kg.$^{-1}$
Kaolin rat-paw oedema	2.5 mg.kg.$^{-1}$
Passive paw and passive cutaneous anaphylaxis	2 mg.kg.$^{-1}$
C.N.S. (anti-amphetamine)	5 mg.kg.$^{-1}$
Toxic p.o.	$25–30$ mg.kg.$^{-1}$
Tremorigenic	10 mg.kg.$^{-1}$

Potential:
Anti-inflammatory
Analgesic
Anti-allergy
Anti-amphetamine

BLUE-GREEN ALGA *RIVULARIA FIRMA*

monoacetate gave only slight tremorigenic effect, and for both the monoacetate and diacetate the anti-amphetamine activity was approximately the same. Also, unlike the parent compound **6**, **11** was active in the acetic acid writhing test. In any detailed evaluation it would be necessary to isolate and test the individual mono- and di-acetates.

An encouraging aspect of this series of natural products is that structural variations can be shown to result in different activities. Considering the natural bi-indoles **6–10** one can exemplify activity differences in table form (Table VI). No doubt some group will follow the leads provided by **6–11**.

(f) *Adenosine analogues*

The final 2 substances I would illustrate have come from different organisms but may be grouped together because of structural similarities, in being halogenated pyrrolopyrimidine analogues of adenosine: The simpler substance, 4-amino-5-bromopyrrolo[2,3-d]pyrimidine **12** was isolated from a sponge of the genus *Echinodictyum*.

12

The second substance 5′-deoxy-5-iodotubercidin **13** was isolated from a red alga *Hypnea valentiae*.

13 $R_1 = I$
        $R_2 =$

Tubercidin   **14** $R_1 = H$
                $R_2 =$

Table VI

Bi-indole	Activity		
	Carrageenan-induced inflammation	Anti-amphetamine	Tremorigenic
(6)	+	+	+
(7)	+	−	−
(8)	+	−	−
(9)	−	−	−
(10)	−	−	−

The biochemical pharmacology of **12**, **13** and **14** was conducted by Dr Les Davies in RRIMP. Substance **12** has about twice the bronchodilator activity (p.o. guinea-pigs) of theophylline on a molar basis but has a different biochemical profile: **12** shows no antagonist activity at CNS adenosine receptors and is, like **13**, a potent inhibitor of adenosine uptake and adenosine kinase in brain tissue.

5′-Deoxy-5-iodotubercidin **13** – which appears to be the first naturally occurring 5′-deoxyribosyl nucleoside, and the first naturally occurring specifically iodinated nucleoside – causes potent muscle relaxation and hypothermia when injected i.p. into mice *in vivo*.

Neither **12** nor **13** was a substrate for, or an inhibitor of, adenosine deaminase. Both **12** and **13** are the subject of continuing studies.

The examples given are not "all-inclusive"; they show some reasons why biologically active substances may not progress to drugs. There are several other examples which could be illustrated from RRIMP investigations. However, it may be best to look instead at some general aspects of marine natural products as potential drugs.

SOME PROBLEMS FOR MARINE INVESTIGATORS

Previously, I mentioned some of the local practices that had to be developed to maximise the chance of success of RRIMP. Experience has revealed that there are additional factors that the marine natural product medicinal chemist must face. The very features which attracted Roche to the sea (as summarised above) create difficulties: the resultant natural products were often novel, very frequently involving halogen substitution, and with potentially different mechanisms of action to existing drugs. A question of importance is "are the traditional screens of the pharmaceutical industries adequate to ensure the detection of novel substances with novel mechanisms of action?" The answer in many cases will almost surely be "no".

If one takes as an example anti-inflammatory screens, which are basic to every major drug company, there is currently great concern for the validity of the assumption that the classical screens are indeed satisfactory. The screens have been accepted because they detect KNOWN drugs and do not reveal too many spurious activities. However, it is very doubtful if they will detect anti-inflammatory substances with novel mechanisms of action.

The obvious result is that there is a strong move from innovative drug evaluators to (for anti-inflammatories) test the molecular mechanism of tissue injury so that a "new" drug may be found which will prevent damage to the tissue.

This one example can be expanded to other areas of pharmacology. In many cases, screening for activity may be regarded as an art more than a science at this time.

In such existing circumstances, the prospects of introducing novel substances, with structures often far removed from those of existing drugs, as competitors for the existing drugs, may be expected to be of very low probability.

Therefore, the marine natural product input into human health therapy may be unfairly constrained. Direct testing involving, e.g., receptor binding and displacement studies, and effects on tissue culture preparations, may provide more reliable evaluations of potential therapeutic application.

One recognizes that such tests may not take into consideration the possible metabolism of an introduced substance before it reaches the site of action, in the practical application to a patient. Given the recognition of that factor, for which other methods are available to help solve the problem, the more modern methods of testing activity at the cellular or reactive site level may give a more accurate assessment of the potential of drugs from the sea.

Marine biomedical research is a comparatively new concept. It has been designated as the study of "marine derived physiologically active substances effective on mammalian tissues or organisms, and on pathogenic microbes affecting the mammalian system". The definition itself points the way towards initial testing on selected tissues or organisms, and those who work with marine-derived substances must recognize the potential inadequacy of traditional screens to detect biological activity in substances of novel composition. It is also obvious that physiological activity studies should be extended beyond human

Table VII
The "top 10" therapeutic groupings

Therapeutic group	Market share ~%	Market growth (77–81) ~%
Antibiotics	11.4	6.7
Antirheumatics	6.8	13.0
"Cough and cold"	6.0	6.9
Antihypertensives	5.2	5.5
Analgesics	4.7	7.5
Psycholeptics	4.4	1.9
Vitamins	3.8	5.6
Cardiac therapy	3.8	8.5
Peripheral vasodilators	3.7	7.2
Sex hormones	2.9	5.7
Others" with spectacular growth rates:		
β-Blockers		32.1
Anti-ulcerants		46.9
Cytostatics		22.0
Anti-coagulants		25.6

health to animal health, and to plant tissues and pathogenic microbes affecting plant systems, to maximize the potential of commercial utilization of marine-derived substances.

SPECULATION ON THE FUTURE

In the drug industry most major companies have their specialisations which result in a "products profile". Obviously it is important to work within a company which has products in the range of activities on which the market indicates growth.

Table VII shows the major therapeutic groupings by sales value with their market share in 1981 and their market growth in the 5 years 1977–81. The Table also shows other therapeutic groupings, not in the "top 10", but with spectacular growth rates in the 5 year period of review.

The company marketing division wants to have products in the "top 10" and, preferably, to see candidates in the areas of spectacular growth rate. That division must make money for the company, from the research output.

Therefore, a close interaction must develop between the marketing division and the research division, so that marketing of new products can be planned, and, particularly, so that "marketing" understands the time lag from discovery through development to market. If this interaction does not evolve the marketing division may turn increasingly to licensing activities in buying-in research from other companies. Obviously, such a situation has a potentially demoralising effect on the in-house research and of serious misunderstanding by management of the competence of the in-house research.

For the marine natural product resource developer, it is almost impossible to fit into the systematic regulated program of drug development in prescribed indication objectives. There is, at this time, inadequate background information to predict what activity one will find in the next organism extracted. But there are natural indications in species interactions and behaviour to maximize our chances of finding biologically active molecules.

There is no doubt that the Roche decision to close RRIMP has impeded the search for biologically active substances from the sea. However, there is also no doubt that the basis on which RRIMP was built, was justified, and, provided one utilises the marine resource, both macro- and micro-, as a potential to provide fine chemicals, agrochemicals, and animal health products, as well as drugs for human well-being, other ventures based on marine natural products will be initiated and will prosper.

It is a great pleasure to record the names of those scientists, who, aided by some excellent technicians, and periodically by a few postdoctoral workers, conducted with me, the work of RRIMP.

Biologists: Dr. M. Borowitzka, Mr. P. Alderslade, Mr. K. Harada, (Mr. I. Skinner)*. *Chemists:* Dr. R. Wells, Dr. R. Quinn, Dr. P. Murphy, Dr. R. Kazlauskas, Dr. R. Gregson. *Biochemist:* Dr. R. Norton. *Mass Spectroscopist:* Mr. R. Lidgard. *Pharmacologists:* Dr. B. Baldo, Dr. J. Marwood, Dr. I. Spence, Dr. J. Baird-Lambert, Dr. L. Davies, Mrs. D. Jamieson, (Dr. K. Taylor)*. *Microbiologists:* Dr. J. Reichelt, Dr. L. Borowitzka, Dr. L. Sanders, (Mrs. B. Kinsela)*. *Laboratory Manager:* Mr. F. O'Neil. *Electronics:* Mr. D. Edwards, (Mr. D. Melley)*.

(*Persons who left RRIMP prior to 1981 but who spent a considerable number of years in the Institute.)

DISCUSSION

DJERASSI: What efforts were tried, and why didn't anyone continue this work?

BAKER: Australia has no pharmaceutical research industry, and no other was interested in continuing the group.

DJERASSI: That is actually why I think you could have done something about it.

BAKER: There is very little high-risk capital in Australia, and this is still high-risk work. We approached the Government, we approached one industry which was big enough, but they were not interested. Roche closed the institute because of a management decision to maintain research costs at a constant figure, yet still expand their research effort in the interferon field.

RAPOPORT: Did you find any structural patterns for the constituents of the investigated organisms?

BAKER: I don't think we have gone far enough to find structural patterns in the majority of organisms. Compounds, in which intensive research appeared to be of no profit to the company, were not investigated further. Photographs of all species worked on, and summary records, are kept in the Australian Museum in Sydney, Australia. Research reports have appeared in refereed journals. Dr. Boh Wells did some excellent work on chemotaxonomy of sponges. This has been reported.

Marine Sterols

Carl Djerassi

INTRODUCTION

The isolation and structure elucidation of novel plant sterols from terrestrial sources peaked in the 1950's and within another decade had declined in terms of academic interest, since the majority of unusual structures had been encountered by then. Economically, sterols have played a major role. Cholesterol, from animal sources, was the first economically viable starting material for the synthesis of the medicinally important steroid hormones, to be displaced by the plant steroidal sapogenins (Djerassi 1959). In the 1970's partly for political reasons (Djerassi 1976), their importance declined at the expense of the conventional plant sterols, sitosterol and stigmasterol, which have proved to be excellent starting materials for microbiological conversions to intermediates in corticosteroid synthesis as well as for the preparation of other, medicinally useful, steroids.

Given the decline of activity in the plant sterol field and the greatly reduced number of new plant sterols reported in the literature, it was particularly surprising to encounter a veritable explosion of new sterol structures from marine sources in the 1970's and early 1980's; probably prompted by the structure elucidation (Ling *et al.* 1970) of the marine sterol gorgosterol (14) with its totally unexpected features: the presence of a cyclopropane ring and the fact that every carbon atom of the cholesterol side chain bore a carbon substituent. If we recall that plant and animal sterols possess either unsubstituted side chains (1 R=H) or a carbon substituent at C-24 (1, R=Me or Et) and that the biosynthesis of such side chains had been studied in exquisite detail (Lederer 1969), it was indeed surprising to encounter a sterol side chain substitution pattern based on 2, especially since the pioneer of marine sterol chemistry,

Department of Chemistry, Stanford University, Stanford, California 94305, U.S.A.

NATURAL PRODUCTS AND DRUG DEVELOPMENT, Alfred Benzon Symposium 20.
Editors: P. Krogsgaard-Larsen, S. Brøgger Christensen, H. Kofod, Munksgaard, Copenhagen 1984.

Werner Bergmann (for leading references see Scheuer 1973) in his extensive studies of marine sterols had only encountered variants of 1. As the field of marine sterols has grown so rapidly since 1970, I shall focus in the present paper on unusual variations in the sterol side chain and in ring A, with primary emphasis on results from our own laboratory.

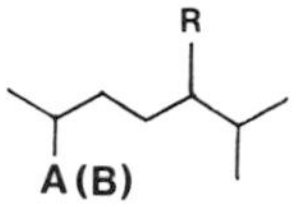

R

A(B)

1 R = H, Me, Et

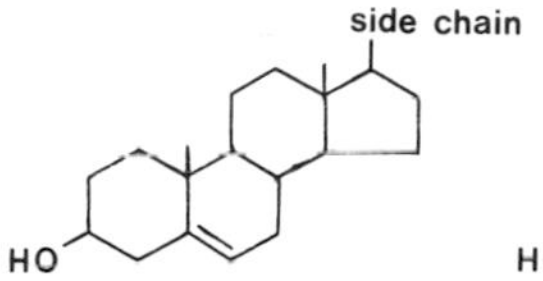

side chain

side chain

HO

A

HO
H

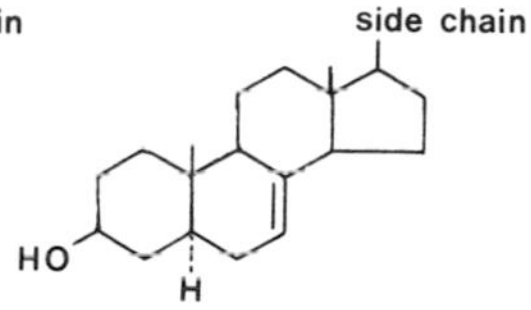

B

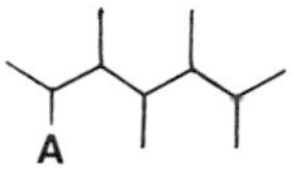

2

UNUSUAL STRUCTURAL FEATURES OF MARINE STEROLS

Marine sterols are distinguished from their terrestrial counterparts by 3 unique features: (a) unprecedented bioalkylation patterns in the side chain; (b) existence of three-membered rings in the side chain; (c) nuclear variations in ring A, which had previously not been found in nature. Each of these have interesting biosynthetic implications, not encountered previously in terrestrial counterparts, and some may also be of potential economic utility.

Examples of unusual bioalkylation

Work performed since 1970, notably in Italy, Japan and the U.S., has produced such a plethora of unusual side chain substitution patterns that even recent reviews (Schmitz 1978, Goad 1978, Djerassi 1981) are already outdated. As well over 100 new sterols have been isolated from marine sources, notably sponges (a recent report by Itoh *et al.* 1983, describes the characterization of 74 sterols from a *single* animal), it will suffice to illustrate the range of bioalkylation possibilities by giving the structures (Fig. 1) of a few marine sterols isolated in our laboratory which arise by triple (e.g., 5–7) and quadruple (e.g., 9–11) biomethylation sequences. With one exception (Kikuchi *et al.* 1982) such multiple biomethylations have not been encountered in terrestrial sterols. Except for pulchrasterol (5 in Fig. 1), which possesses a different nucleus (Crist *et al.* 1983), it

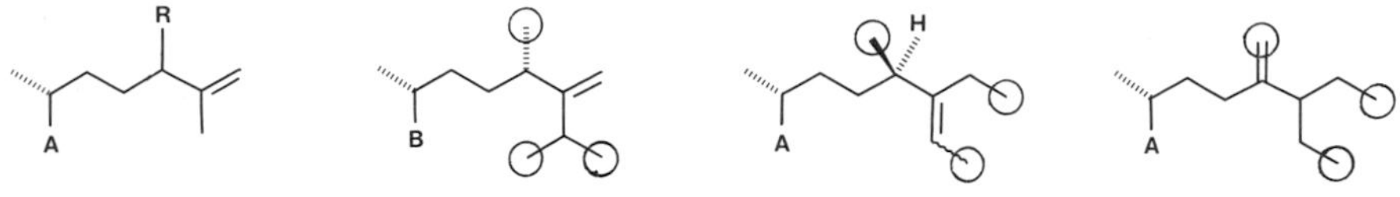

Epicodisterol (3 R=Me)   Pulchrasterol (5)   Verongulasterol (6)   Xestosterol (7)
Epiclerosterol (4 R=Et)

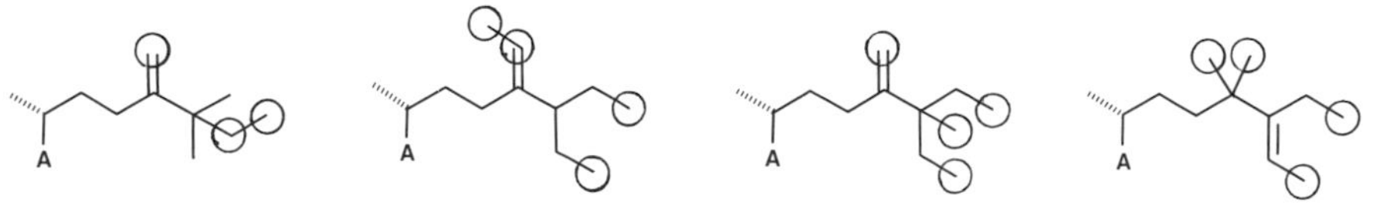

Mutasterol (8)   28-Methylxestosterol (9)   25-Methylxestosterol (10)   Xestospongesterol (11)

Fig. 1.

is likely that all of the other sterols described in Fig. 1 arise, directly or indirectly, from an epicodisterol (3) or epiclerosterol (4) precursor as discussed in more detail below.

Sterol side chains with cyclopropane and cyclopropene rings
This sub-group of marine sterols contains not only entirely unprecedented examples of sterol side-chain substitution, but they also raise biosynthetic questions (Djerassi *et al.* 1979) for which there is little precedent except for studies in the fatty acid field (Buist & MacLean 1982). With the exception of 23-demethylgorgosterol (13, Schmitz & Pattabhiraman 1970), petrosterol (15, Mattia *et al.* 1978, Ravi *et al.* 1978) and calysterol (16, Fattorusso *et al.* 1975, Li *et al.* 1982), all other sterols summarized in Fig. 2 were isolated and structurally characterized in our laboratory. Even cursory inspection of Fig. 2 makes evident the wide range of cyclopropyl substitution, which can be found among marine sterols, but 2 special points merit emphasis. The first refers to the cyclopropanes: with the exception of 24, 26-cyclocholesterol (20, Catalan *et al.* 1982) and papakusterol (21, Bonini *et al.* 1983a), the three-membered ring invariably includes an "extra" carbon atom introduced into the cholesterol side chain by S-adenosylmethionine (SAM)biomethylation. The 2 cyclopropanes 20 and 21 are biosynthetically distinct in that no additional carbon atom is involved in the generation of the three-membered ring. The second comment refers to the three-cyclopropenes calysterol (16), (23R)-23H-isocalysterol (17, Li *et al.* 1982), and (24S)-24H-isocalysterol (18, Itoh *et al.* 1983b). The cyclopropene functionality is one of the rarest among natural products, the best known example being

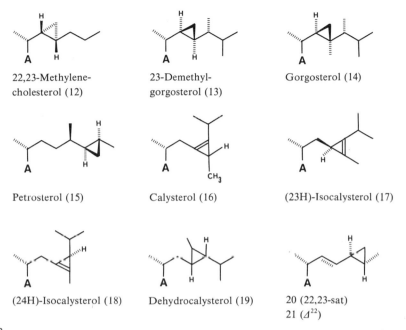

22,23-Methylene-
cholesterol (12)

23-Demethyl-
gorgosterol (13)

Gorgosterol (14)

Petrosterol (15)

Calysterol (16)

(23H)-Isocalysterol (17)

(24H)-Isocalysterol (18)

Dehydrocalysterol (19)

20 (22,23-sat)
21 (Δ^{22})

Fig. 2.

sterculic acid and its congeners (Carter & Frampton 1964). Biosynthetically, the origin of the steroidal and the fatty-acid cyclopropene is similar. Thus, Yano *et al.* (1972) have shown that the double bond in sterculic acid is introduced as the last step by biochemical dehydrogenation of the corresponding cyclopropane. Similarly, we have recently been able to show (Catalan *et al.* to be published) by radioactive tracer studies that the recently isolated (Li *et al.* 1982) 23,24-dihydrocalysterol (19) is the biosynthetic precursor of the steroidal cyclopropenes 16–18. The possible biosynthetic role of steroidal cyclopropanes has already been speculated upon (Djerassi 1981) and will be discussed below.

Nuclear variations in ring A
Three types of nuclear alterations have been observed, which are unique to the marine sterol field. The first are 9,11-seco sterols of Type C, which were first encountered (Enwall *et al.* 1972) in the gorgosterol series (cf. 14 in Fig. 2). Recent work in our laboratory (Bonini *et al.* 1983b) has shown that such 9,11-seco sterols can also have a variety of other and more conventional side chains, but that both the 8α- and 8β-isomers are naturally occurring, an observation that

DJERASSI

may be of significance when the hitherto unknown biosynthetic origin of these seco sterols is eventually unravelled.

The other 2 types of nuclear variants are both of potential practical use and have first been discovered by Minale's group in Italy (cf. Minale & Sodano 1977 for leading references), namely the A-nor sterols of Type D and 19-nor stanols of type E. In each case, the associated side chains were of the conventional type, but subsequent work in our laboratory has shown that almost every conceivable side chain, including the most unusual ones including cyclopropane rings, can be associated with the A-nor skeleton D (for leading references see Eggersdorfer *et al.* 1982, Bohlin *et al.* 1982). Both direct (DeStefano & Sodano 1980), and indirect (Bohlin *et al.* 1982), evidence has been presented to show that sterols with a variety of side chains but the conventional cholesterol nucleus (A) are acquired by the sponge through dietary intake and then transformed efficiently into the A-nor skeleton D.

Similar generalizations can be made about the 19-nor stanols of type E, where both direct, i. e., radioactive incorporation studies (Minale & Sodano 1977), and indirect, i. e., observation of wide variety of different side chains (Minale & Sodano 1977, Crist & Djerassi, to be published), evidence has been provided to show that sponges can efficiently transform dietary sterols into 19-nor steranes (E).

BIOSYNTHETIC ASPECTS

In contrast to the enormous amount of work that has been performed during the past quarter century on the biosynthesis of terrestrial animal and plant steroids, relatively little has been accomplished among marine species (for leading references see Goad 1981), and especially lower marine animals like sponges. The work of Minale and Sodano (1977) has shown that sponges can efficiently carry out ring A nuclear modifications (A→D; A→E) and Minale *et al.* (1977) have also noted the incorporation (albeit in poor yield) of fucosterol into calysterol (16 in Fig. 2). The reasons for the paucity of relevant experiments are of a technical nature, how to keep a sponge alive while feeding precursors, as well as lack of availability of many potentially relevant precursors. A considerable effort has been expended in our laboratory along these lines and as an example of an unambiguous experiment, we can cite the high yield incorporation of radioactive epicodisterol (3) into 25-dehydroaplysterol (22) and, thence, into aplysterol (23), whereas codisterol (3a) was not utilized by the sponge (Catalan *et al.* 1983). Low, though definite, incorporation into verongulasterol (24) in the same sponge (*Aplysina fistularis*) was also demonstrated. The results are, thus, consistent with the expected sequence summarized in Fig. 3 and, as earlier work by Minale and Sodano (1977) had shown that *de novo* sterol synthesis does not occur in this sponge genus, the efficient side chain modification of dietary sterols by the sponge is established. Feeding experiments with a variety of other precursors and other sponges are now under way in our laboratory and the preliminary results indicate that the course of the multiple bioalkylation of the sterol side chain will soon be completely clarified. Recently, we have also succeeded (Kokke *et al.* to be published) in incorporating deuterated methionine into cultured unicellular organisms which produce gorgosterol (14 in Fig. 2) thus opening the way to the elucidation of the biosynthetic pathway to such cyclopropyl-containing sterols.

This brings us to the question of the role of such cyclopropyl-containing sterols. Are these metabolic end-products or are they themselves active intermediates to some other sterol structures? We have speculated earlier

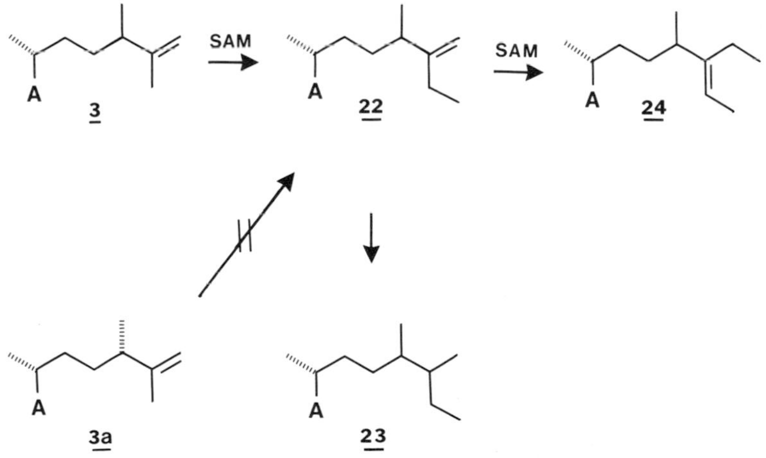

Fig. 3.

(Djerassi *et al.* 1979) that such cyclopropanes may be enzymatically isomerized to allylic methyl functionalities and, thus, provide an alternative to conventional SAM methylation of olefins. While no direct evidence has so far been provided to settle this question, 2 biomimetic experiments (Fig. 4) from our laboratory are relevant. Lang and Djerassi (1982) were able to show that mild acid treatment of petrosterol (15) led to 26-dehydro-25-epiaplysterol (25), which had been isolated earlier by us from the same sponge (Khalil *et al.* 1980). Even more intriguing is the observation by Catalan and Djerassi (1983) that acid treatment of 24,26-cyclocholesterol (20) yields as the major product 24-methyl-27-nor-5,25-cholestadien-3β-ol (26). The latter has the 27-norergostene side chain, which has been encountered (Kobayashi & Mitsuhashi 1974) in various marine organisms and whose biosynthetic origin is as yet unknown.

BIOLOGICAL FUNCTION OF MARINE STEROLS WITH UNUSUAL STRUCTURES
While nothing can be said at the present time about the possible biological role of unusual trace sterols in marine animals, speculation is much more justified (Carlson *et al.* 1980) in those instances where practically no "conventional" sterols such as cholesterol are present and where the latter is replaced by one or more marine sterol(s) of unusual structure. We have suggested (Carlson *et al.* 1980) that such sterols replace cholesterol in cell membranes and that they, thus, play a functional role. As most of the unusual structural features reside in the

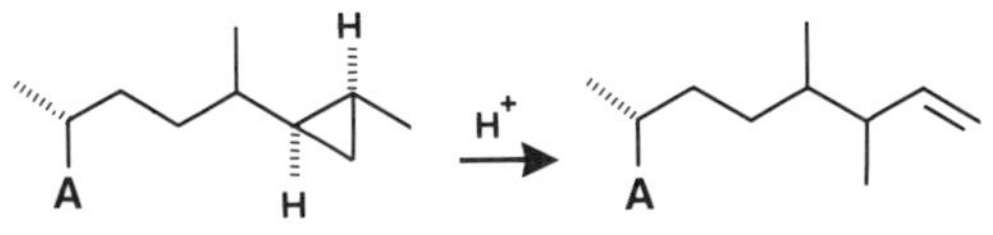

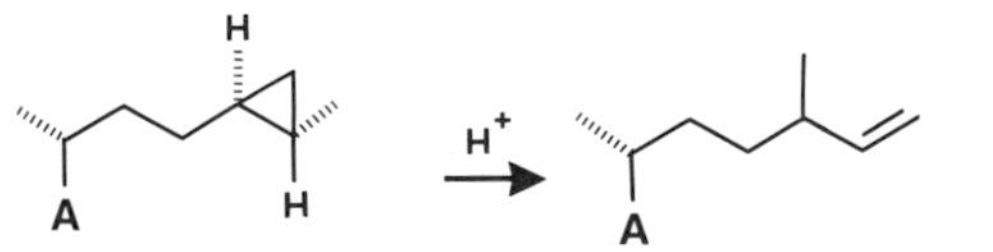

Fig. 4.

side chain (see above) which would be situated deep within the lipophilic portion of the phospholipid bilayer of cell membranes, we have examined several such sponges for unusual phospholipid fatty acids. In point of fact, every one of the sponges examined by us contained unusual fatty acids, never encountered before in terrestrial organisms (Walkup *et al.* 1981, Ayanoglu *et al.* 1982, Ayanoglu *et al.* 1983). Current work in our laboratory deals with the synthesis of phospholipids containing these usual fatty acids, preparation of model membranes and examination of membrane properties by comparing the appropriate marine sterols with cholesterol. These experiments should shed light on the question of the biological role of these unusual sterols.

POTENTIAL PRACTICAL SIGNIFICANCE OF MARINE STEROLS

The sterols with unusual side chains or ring A substitution cited in this paper are unlikely to possess intrinsic medicinal properties that would make them of economic significance. Antagonism to cholesterol deposition may be a theoretical possibility, but none of them have been examined in this regard. However at least theoretically, some of them may be of economic significance as starting materials for the synthesis of medicinally important drugs, similar to the present utilization of terrestrial plant sterols (see Djerassi 1976). Two possible applications are cited below.

Corticosteroid synthesis

A number of marine sterols (cf. Schmitz 1978) as well as marine steroids, such as the pregnene 27 (*inter alia* Sheikh *et al.* 1972), possess a 9,11-double bond, which offers a convenient entry into 11-oxygenated steroids. In fact, the conversion of the pregnene 27 derived from the star fish *Acanthaster planci* into 4,9(11)-pregnadiene-3,20-dione (28) has been accomplished in our laboratory (Gurst *et*

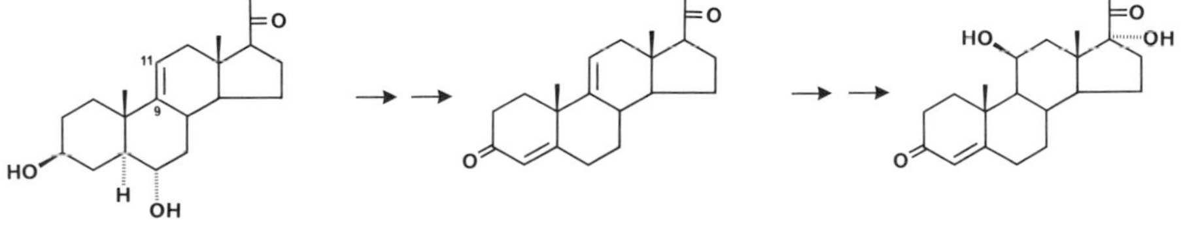

<table>
<tr><td>27</td><td>28</td><td>Cortisol</td></tr>
</table>

Fig. 5.

al. 1973) and, as 28 has already been transformed earlier into cortisone, cortisol and corticosterone, this represents a feasible synthesis of corticosteroids from a marine steroid precursor, provided a readily available and preferably cultivatable marine source became available. This seems unlikely at the present time.

19-Norsteranes for oral contraceptive synthesis

Virtually all currently used oral contraceptives are of the 19-norandrostene type, with approximately half of them bearing an angular methyl (norethindrone type 32) and the other half an angular ethyl group (norgestrel type) at C-18. The latter must be synthesized by total synthesis, since no naturally occurring steroids with an angular C-18 ethyl group are known. Members of the norethindrone type, on the other hand, are accessible by total or partial synthesis (Djerassi 1976). A very

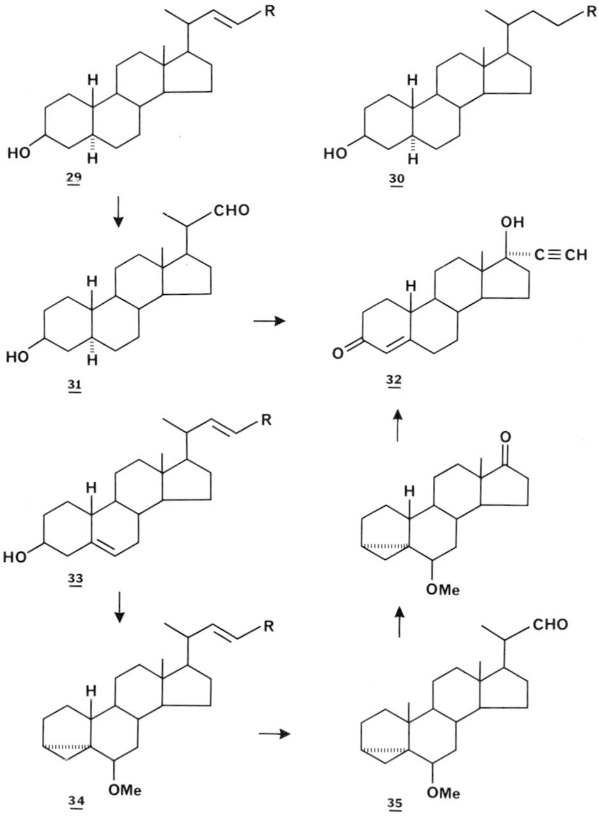

Fig. 6.

conveniently available, naturally occurring 19-nor steroidal starting material might well tip the balance in favor of partial synthesis. In this respect, the 19-nor marine sterols (nucleus E) are a viable possibility. A detailed re-examination in our laboratory (Crist & Djerassi, to be published) of the sterol content of the sponge *Axinella polypoides,* first studied by Minale and Sodano (1977), showed that 15 different side chains were attached to the 19-norandrostane nucleus E. However, from a practical standpoint these 15 side chains can be divided into 2 subgroups, 29 and 30 (Fig. 5), depending upon the presence or absence of a Δ^{22} double bond. Approximately 40% of the sterol mixture falls into category 29 and 60% into category 30, with the cholestane, ergostane and sitostane side chains being the most prevalent.

For purposes of a feasible partial synthesis of norethindrone (32) and its congeners, all that would be necessary is to subject the total 19-norsterane mixture (29 and 30) to ozonolysis and then to isolate the aldehyde 31, which would lend itself readily to further transformation to the oral contraceptive 32.

Another potential alternative is to consider the corresponding 19-nor-Δ^5-3β-hydroxy sterols (Type 33) as starting materials. Such 19-nor sterols are also naturally occurring (Popov *et al.* 1976) among marine organisms, although in much lower yield than the saturated steranes (29, 30); protection of the Δ^5-3β-hydroxy system via the i-methyl ether 34 followed by ozonolysis to the aldehyde 35 and conventional degradation to the ketone 36 would provide a second attractive intermediate for the synthesis of norethindrone (32).

It should immediately be recognized that these are only hypothetical routes to oral contraceptives and that major hurdles would have to be overcome to convert them into reality. First and foremost – even if a sponge, or other marine invertebrate, could be found that is rich in 19-nor sterols with unsaturated side chains (Types 29 or 33) – it would be ecologically unacceptable to harvest them considering their slow growth and capacity for regeneration. What would be needed is to isolate the enzyme system(s) responsible for the sponge's efficient conversion of Δ^5-3β-hydroxy sterols into their 19-nor equivalents. If this can be done and if an immobilized enzyme system could be constructed that works efficiently on a substrate such as stigmasterol, then a potentially very interesting route to 29 or 33 could be developed which could have real economic potential.

ACKNOWLEDGEMENTS
Deep appreciation is expressed to my numerous collaborators, both at Stanford

University and elsewhere, for their outstanding contributions. Their names are listed in the bibliography. Generous and long-term financial support was provided by the National Institutes of Health (Grants No. GM 06840 and GM 28352).

REFERENCES

Ayanoglu, E., Walkup, R., Sica, D. & Djerassi, C. (1982) Phospholipid studies of marine organisms 3. New phospholipid fatty acids from *Petrosia ficiformis. Lipids 17,* 617–625.

Ayanoglu, E., Kornprobst, J. M., Aboud-Bichara, A. & Djerassi, C. (1983) Phospholipid studies of marine organisms 4. (2R,21Z)-2-Methoxy-21-octacosenoic acid from a phospholipid. *Tetrahedron Letters,* 1111–1114.

Bergmann, W., MacLean, M. J. & Lester, D. J. (1943) Contributions to the study of marine products. XIII. Sterols from various marine invertebrates. *J. Org. Chem. 8,* 271–282.

Bohlin, L., Sjostrand, U., Sodano, G. & Djerassi, C. (1982) Sterols in marine invertebrates. 33. structures of five new 3β-(hydroxymethyl)-A-nor steranes: Indirect evidence for transformation of dietary precursors in sponges. *J. Organ. Chem. 47,* 5309–5314.

Bonini, C., Kinnel, R. B., Li, M., Scheuer, P. J. & Djerassi, C. (1983a) Minor and trace sterols in marine invertebrates. 38. Isolation, structure elucidation and partial synthesis of papakusterol, a new biosynthetically unusual marine sterol with a cyclopropyl-containing side chain. *Tetrahedron Letters,* 277–280.

Bonini, C., Cooper, C. B., Kazlawkas, R., Wells, R. J. & Djerassi, C. (1983b) Minor and trace sterols in marine invertebrates. 41. Structure and stereochemistry of naturally occurring 9,11-seco sterols. *J. Org. Chem. 48,* 2108–2111.

Buist, P. H. & MacLean, D. B. (1982) The biosynthesis of cyclopropane fatty acids. II. Mechanistic studies using methionine labelled with one, two and three deuterium atoms in the methyl group. *Can. J. Chem. 60,* 371–378.

Carlson, R. M. K., Tarchini, C. & Djerassi, C. (1980) "Biological implications of recent discoveries in the marine sterol field." In: *Frontiers of Bioorganic Chemistry and Molecular Biology,* ed. Ananchenko, S. N., pp. 211–224. Pergamon Press, N.Y.

Carter, F. L. & Frampton, V. L. (1964) Review of the chemistry of cyclopropene compounds. *Chem. Rev. 64,* 497–525.

Catalan, C. A. N., Lakshmi, V., Schmitz, F. J. & Djerassi, C. (1982) Minor and trace sterols in marine invertebrates. 39. 24ζ. 25ζ-24, 26-cyclocholest-5-en-3β-ol, a novel cyclopropyl sterol. *Steroids 40,* 455–463.

Catalan, C. A. N. & Djerassi, C. (1983) Chemical proof of absolute configuration by biometric conversion to 27-nor ergostenes. *Tetrahedron Letters,* (in press).

Catalan, C. A. N., Kokke, W. C. M. C., Sodano, G., Sica, D. & Djerassi, C. Biosynthesis of calysterol. (To be published).

Catalan, C. A. N., Thompson, J. E., Kokke, W. C. M. C. & Djerassi, C. (1983) Experimental demonstration of the course of side chain extension in marine sterols. *Tetrahedron Letters* (in press).

Crist, B. V., Djerassi, C., Li, X. & Bergquist, P. (1983) Sterols of marine invertebrates. 44. Isolation, structure elucidation, partial synthesis and determination of absolute configuration of pulchrasterol – the first example of double bioalkylation of the sterol side chain at position 26. *J. Org. Chem.* (in press).

Crist, B. V. & Djerassi, C. Minor and trace sterols in marine invertebrates. 47. 19-Nor-stanols from the sponge *Axinella polypoides*. A re-investigation. (To be published).

DeStefano, A. & Sodano, G. (1980) Metabolism in Porifera. XII. Further informations on the biosynthesis of 3β-hydroxymethyl-A-nor-steranes in the sponge *Axinella verrucosa*. *Experientia 36*, 630–632.

Djerassi, C. (1959) Plant steroids and related substances. *Fourth International Congress of Biochemistry IV*, 1–19, Pergamon Press, London.

Djerassi, C. (1976) The manufacture of steroidal contraceptives: technical versus political aspects. *Proc. Royal Soc. of London B195*, 175–186.

Djerassi, C., Theobald, N., Kokke, W. C. M. C., Pak, C. S. & Carlson, R. M. K. (1979) Recent progress in the marine sterol field. *Pure Appl. Chem. 51*, 1815–1828.

Djerassi, C. (1981) Recent studies in the marine sterol field. *Pure Appl. Chem. 53*, 873–890.

Eggersdorfer, M., Kokke, W. C. M. C., Crandell, C. W., Hochlowski, J. E. & Djerassi, C. (1982) Sterols in marine invertebrates. 32. Isolation of 3β-(hydroxymethyl)-A-nor-5α-cholest-15-ene, the first naturally occurring sterol with the 15–16 double bond. *J. Org. Chem. 47*, 5304.

Enwall, E. L., vanderHelm, D., Hsu, I. N., Pattabhiraman, T., Schmitz, F. J., Spraggins, R. L. & Weinheimer, A. J. (1972) Crystal structure and absolute configuration of two cyclopropane containing marine steroids. *Chem. Soc. J. Chem. Comm.*, 215–216.

Fatturosso, E., Magno, S., Mayol, L., Santacroce, C. & Sica, D. (1975) Calysterol: a C_{29} cyclopropene-containing marine sterol from the sponge *Calyx nicaensis*. *Tetrahedron 31*, 1715–1716.

Goad, L. J. (1978) "The sterols of marine invertebrates." In: *Marine Natural Products II*, P. J. Scheuer, ed., chapter 2, Academic Press, NY.

Goad, L. J. (1981) Sterol biosynthesis and metabolism in marine invertebrates. *Pure Appl. Chem. 51*, 837–852.

Gurst, J. E., Sheikh, Y. M. & Djerassi, C. (1972) Synthesis of corticosteroids from marine sources. *J. Amer. Chem. Soc. 95*, 628–629.

Itoh, T., Sica, D. & Djerassi, C. (1983a) Minor and trace sterols in marine invertebrates. Part 35. Isolation and structure elucidation of seventy four sterols from the sponge *Axinella cannabina*. *J. Chem. Soc. Perkin. Trans. I*, 147–153.

Itoh, T., Sica, D. & Djerassi, C. (1983b) (24S)-24H-Isocalysterol: a new steroidal cyclopropene from the marine sponge *Calyx niceaensis*. *J. Org. Chem. 48*, 890–892.

Khalil, M. W., Djerassi, C. & Sica, D. (1980) Minor and trace sterols in marine invertebrates. XVII. (24R)-24,26-Dimethylcholesta-5,26-dien-3β ol, a new sterol from the sponge Petrosia ficiformis. *Steroids 35*, 707–720.

Kikuchi, T., Kadota, S., Suehara, H. & Namba, T. (1982) Occurrence of non-conventional side chain sterols in an orchidaceous plant, *Nervilia purpurea Schlechter* and structure of nervisterol. *Chem. Pharm. Bull. 30*, 370–373.

Kobayashi, M. & Mitsuhashi, H. (1974) Marine sterols IV. Structure and synthesis of amuresterol, a new marine sterol with unprecedented side chain, from *Asterias amurensis Lütken*. *Tetrahedron 30*, 2147–2150.

Kokke, W. C. M. C., Bothner-by, A., Shoolery, J. & Djerassi, C. Biosynthesis of gorgosterol. (To be published).

Kobayashi, M. & Mitsuhashi, H. (1974) Marine sterols IV. Structure and synthesis of amuresterol, a new marine sterol with unprecedented side chain, form *Asterias amurensis Lütken. Tetrahedron 30*, 2147–2150.

Kokke, W. C. M. C., Bothner-by, A., Shoolery, J. & Djerassi, C. Biosynthesis of gorgosterol. (To be published).

Lang, R. W. & Djerassi, C. (1982) Stereospecific cyclopropane ring-opening of petrosterol. A possible biomimetic process. *Tetrahedron Letters*, 2063–2066.

Lederer, E. (1969) Some problems concerning biological C-alkylation reactions and phytosterol biosynthesis. *Chem. Soc. Quart. Rev. 22*, 453–481.

Li, L. N., Li, H., Lang, R. W., Itoh, T., Sica, D. & Djerassi, C. (1982) Minor and trace sterols in marine invertebrates. 31. Isolation and structure elucidation of 23H-isocalysterol, a naturally occurring cyclopropene. Some comparative observations on the course of hydrogenolytic ring opening of steroidal cyclopropenes and cyclopropanes. *J. Amer. Chem. Soc. 104*, 6726–6732.

Ling, N. C., Hale, R. L. & Djerassi, C. (1970) The structure and absolute configuration of the marine sterol gorgosterol. *J. Amer. Chem. Soc. 92*, 5281–5282.

Mattia, C. A., Mazzarella, L., Puliti, R., Sica, D. & Zollo, F. (1978) X-Ray crystal structure determination of petrosterol *p*-bromobenzoate. A revision. *Tetrahedron Letters*, 3953–3954.

Minale, L., Riccio, R., Scalona, O., Sodano, G., Fattorusso, E., Magno, S., Mayol, L. & Santacroce, C. (1977) Metabolism in Porifera VII. Conversion of [7,7-^{3}H$_2$]-fucosterol into calysterol by the sponge *Calyx niceaensis. Experientia 33*, 1550–1552.

Minale, L. & Sodano, G. (1977) "Non-conventional sterols of marine organisms." In: *Marine Natural Products*, eds. Faulkner, D. J. & Fenical, W. H., pp. 87–109. Plenum Press, NY.

Popov, S., Carlson, R. M. K., Wegmann, A. & Djerassi, C. (1976) Occurrence of 19-nor cholesterol and homologs in marine animals. *Tetrahedron Letters*, 3491–3494.

Ravi, B. N., Kokke, W. C. M. C., Delseth, C. & Djerassi, C. (1978) Isolation and structure of 26,27-cycloaplysterol (petrosterol), a cyclopropane containing marine sterol. *Tetrahedron Letters*, 4379–4380.

Scheuer, P. J. (1973) "Sterols." In: *Chemistry of Marine Natural Products.* pp. 58–87, Academic Press, NY.

Schmitz, F. J. (1978) "Uncommon marine steroids." In: *Marine Natural Products I*, Scheuer, P. J. ed., pp. 241–297, Academic Press, NY.

Schmitz, F. J. & Pattabhirman, T. (1970) New marine sterol possessing a side chain cyclopropyl group: 23-Demethylgorgosterol. *J. Am. Chem. Soc. 92*, 6073–6074.

Sheikh, Y. M., Tursch, B. M. & Djerassi, C. (1972) 5α-pregn-9(11)-ene-3β,6α-diol-20-one and 5α-cholesta-9(11), 20(22)-dine-3β, 6α-diol-23-one. Two novel steroids from the starfish *Acanthaster planci. J. Amer. Chem. Soc. 94*, 3278–3280.

Walkup, R. D., Jamieson, G. C., Ratcliff, M. R. & Djerassi, C. (1981) Phospholipid studies of marine organisms 2. Phospholipids, phospholipid bound fatty acids and free sterols of the sponge *Aplysina fistularis*. Isolation and structure elucidation of unprecedented branched fatty acids. *Lipids 16*, 631–646.

Yano, I., Morris, L. J., Nichols, B. W. & James, A. T. (1972) The biosynthesis of cyclopropane and cyclopropene fatty acids in higher plants (Malvaceae). *Lipids 7*, 35–45.

DISCUSSION

NAKANISHI: First question, does an empirical method exist, enabling you to identify the absolute stereochemistry of C(24) and C(25), and second question: is there a difference in the biosynthetic incorporation of C(24) or C(25) epimeric precursors into the sponges?

DJERASSI: The answer is yes to both of your questions. By very high field NMR (360 or better 500 MHz), you can distinguish the C(24) and C(25) epimers and establish the configuration by empirical rules. The most informative signal is that of H(21), which by a long-range effect is influenced by the stereochemistry of C(24) and C(25). You have different effects, depending on where, and if, you have double bonds in the side chain. We now have enough pairs of epimers to determine the stereochemistry of any isolated compound. When it comes to the incorporation question, in the case of codisterol and epicodisterol we get exclusively incorporation of epicodisterol into 25-dehydroaplysterol. However, biosynthetic studies are complicated by poor knowledge of how to get the precursors into the organism. Frequently, we don't even know if the bio-synthesis is performed by the marine organism from which it was isolated, if it is made by a symbiont that is present, or if it is a dietary constituent.

KUTNEY: Has anybody started to do any tissue culture work on these marine sources?

DJERASSI: We are starting this now.

KUTNEY: That is excellent, that really is the way to overcome the mentioned problems.

KROGSGAARD-LARSEN: Are the biosynthetic pathways for the production of these long-chain branched fatty acids in the marine organisms different from those producing the normal fatty acids?

DJERASSI: We have done nothing along these lines yet, but intend to synthesize radioactive branched fatty acids found in bacteria, feed them to the sponge, and see if they are homologated.

KROGSGAARD-LARSEN: Have you isolated these long-chain fatty acids containing cyclopropane or cyclopropene rings?

DJERASSI: We have not isolated any of the cyclopropenes, we have isolated one of the cyclopropane-containing acids having a much longer chain than the acids found in lactobacillus. Here, again, the cyclopropane ring is in that vulnerable position roughly 7 carbon atoms from the terminus.

Biologically-Active Compounds from British Marine Algae

Gerald Blunden, David J. Rogers & Clive J. Barwell

Of the large number of species of marine algae only a very small proportion have been utilised by man. In the British Isles, the only species collected in substantial quantity is *Ascophyllum nodosum,* which is used primarily for the extraction of alginate, although some is used in animal feedstuffs and for the manufacture of seaweed extracts for use in agriculture. Stormcast *Laminaria hyperborea* is harvested in Ireland, the stipes being used for the extraction of alginate and the laminae for various purposes, including animal feedstuffs. Small quantities of *Fucus serratus* and *F. vesiculosus* are collected for use in the health food industry and for the manufacture of seaweed extracts, and total drift weed, made up mainly of *Fucus* species, *A. nodosum* and *Laminaria* species, is harvested for use, primarily as animal feeds. Small quantities of the red algae *Chondrus crispus, Gigartina stellata, Palmaria palmata* and *Porphyra umbilicalis* are collected for human consumption (Guiry & Blunden 1981), and calcareous red algae, known collectively as maërl, are harvested for use as a soil conditioning agent (Blunden *et al.* 1981a).

Little attention seems to have been paid to British marine algae as sources of medicinal agents or of other biologically-active compounds. An early study by Chesters & Stott (1956) showed the presence of antimicrobial activity in several species, but no compound was characterised. A more detailed study was undertaken by Hornsey & Hide (1974), who observed also that the level of antimicrobial activity varied with the season (Hornsey & Hide 1976).

As a result of the lack of published data, a study of the occurrence of biologically-active compounds in British marine algae has been undertaken in

School of Pharmacy, Portsmouth Polytechnic, Hampshire, PO1 2DZ, England.

NATURAL PRODUCTS AND DRUG DEVELOPMENT, Alfred Benzon Symposium 20.
Editors: P. Krogsgaard-Larsen, S. Brøgger Christensen, H. Kofod, Munksgaard, Copenhagen 1984.

the School of Pharmacy at Portsmouth Polytechnic. Extracts have been tested for anti-viral activity (Blunden *et al.* 1981b), as potential sources of hypoglycaemic agents, as inhibitors of selected enzyme systems and for pharmacological activity towards the rat fundus strip and isolated guinea pig ileum (Barwell *et al.* 1981). The inhibition of mammalian digestive enzymes by algal extracts has been investigated in more detail by us recently, in particular the reported inhibition of α-amylase by extracts of *Ascophyllum nodosum* (Barwell *et al.* 1981). Extracts of this alga were demonstrated to inhibit α-amylase, trypsin and lipase. The inhibitors were found to have molecular weights in the range 30,000 to 100,000 daltons. The active compounds were isolated and characterised, primarily by ^{1}H nuclear magnetic resonance spectroscopy, and shown to be polyphenols. These are non-selective inhibitors which interact irreversibly with the enzymes. Thus, they are of no potential value, but are probably important in determining the usefulness of algae as feedstuffs, health foods and fermentable material.

Two areas of study which have shown particular promise are marine algae as sources of betaines and of lectins. The former appear to have interesting plant-growth regulatory activity. Some results from these 2 areas of study are presented in this communication.

BETAINES AND THEIR POTENTIAL AS PLANT-GROWTH REGULATORS
Extracts from commercially-available marine brown algae are marketed for use in agriculture and horticulture. A wide range of beneficial effects have been reported from the use of seaweed extracts including increased crop yields, increased resistance of plants to frost, increased uptake of inorganic constituents from the soil, increased resistance to stress conditions, and reductions in storage losses of fruit (Blunden 1977). Only small quantities of material are applied to a hectare and hence the active substances present in the seaweed extracts must be capable of having an effect in low concentrations. As a result, plant hormones were considered, and it was demonstrated that commercially-available seaweed extracts have high levels of cytokinin-like activity (Brain *et al.* 1973, Williams *et al.* 1981). More detailed investigation has revealed that, although in some bioassay systems high levels of cytokinin activity are recorded, in others, for example, the *Amaranthus* seedling assay (Biddington & Thomas 1973), low levels are found. These discrepancies indicate that the extracts contain, in addition to

true cytokinins (Jones 1979), other compounds which behave like them in certain respects.

Wheeler (1973) assayed extracts of sugar-beet for cytokinins by the oat-leaf senescence test. He found that one of the constituents of the extracts, glycine betaine, caused chlorophyll retention in the oat leaves. Glycine betaine was found also to have activity reminiscent of cytokinins in several other growth tests and so some of the cytokinin-like activity of the sugarbeet extracts was thought to be due to glycine betaine.

Glycine betaine has been shown to be a major cytoplasmic osmoticum in certain higher plant families adapted to salt or water stress and it has been suggested that other betaines and tertiary sulphonium compounds have a similar function in other species (Wyn Jones 1980, Wyn Jones & Storey 1981). It has been claimed also that glycine betaine has a role in frost resistance (Bokarev & Ivanova 1971, Sakai & Yoshida 1968).

Glycine betaine, other betaines and tertiary sulphonium compounds, all of which react with Dragendorff's reagent, have been recorded for a number of marine algae (see references in Blunden et al. 1981c). Extracts of all British marine algae tested by us to date have showed the presence of Dragendorff-positive compounds, many in high yield. Because of the reported effects produced after the application of commercial seaweed extracts and the known properties of compounds such as glycine betaine, the circumstantial evidence for at least part of the activity of the seaweed extracts being due to compounds of this type is strong. Moreover, the presence of these compounds in the extracts might account for the discrepancies in the results obtained for the cytokinin contents when the extracts are bioassayed using different procedures.

Most commercially available seaweed extracts are prepared from *Ascophyllum nodosum,* although some utilise other species as well, such as *Fucus serratus* and *Laminaria* species. The *Laminaria* species have been studied by us earlier. All 4 British species examined, *L. digitata, L. hyperborea, L. ochroleuca* and *L. saccharina,* yielded glycine betaine, γ-aminobutyric acid betaine (γ-butyrobetaine), laminine and lysine betaine, with laminine being the predominant component (Blunden et al. 1982). More recently, *Ascophyllum nodosum, Fucus serratus,* and commercial seaweed extracts used in agriculture have been studied for their content of betaines.

For this study, all the collections of *Ascophyllum nodosum* were made from Farlington Marshes, Hampshire, U.K. and *Fucus serratus* from Southsea, Hampshire, U.K. Each fresh alga was extracted with methanol and the extract purified, as described by Blunden *et al.* (1981c). The semi-purified extracts were examined by thin-layer chromatography (TLC) before the detected compounds were isolated by preparative TLC (Blunden *et al.* 1981c). Each isolated material, after recrystallisation, was characterised by cochromatography with reference compounds, and from both infra-red (Gordon *et al.* 1981), and ^{1}H nuclear magnetic resonance (^{1}H NMR) spectroscopy (D$_2$O, 270 MHz) (Table I).

Regardless of the time of year when collected, *Ascophyllum nodosum* yielded γ-aminobutyric acid betaine, δ-aminovaleric acid betaine (δ-valerobetaine) and laminine. In addition to these 3 compounds, collections made at certain times of the year contained other, as yet unidentified, Dragendorff-positive components. *Fucus serratus* yielded γ-aminobutyric acid betaine in all collections; δ-aminovaleric acid betaine was never detected. In some collections, other compounds were found including glycine betaine. The compounds found in the 2 algal species studied, change markedly with the season. This is the first time that δ-aminovaleric acid betaine has been isolated from a plant source, although it has

Table I

Proton chemical shift assignments for betaines found in Ascophyllum nodosum *and* Fucus serratus

Compound (as hydrochloride)	Group		Assignments Shift[a]
Glycine betaine	Me$_3$N	(9H)	3.23 (s)
	α CH$_2$	(2H)	4.11 (s)
γ-Aminobutyric acid betaine	Me$_3$N	(9H)	3.05 (s)
	α CH$_2$	(2H)	3.25 (m,W$_{1/2}$≈19 Hz)
	β CH$_2$	(2H)	2.00 (m,W$_{1/2}$≈22 Hz)
	γ CH$_2$	(2H)	2.22 ("t",J≈7.5 Hz)
δ-Aminovaleric acid betaine	Me$_3$N	(9H)	3.02 (s)
	α CH$_2$	(2H)	3.27 (m,W$_{1/2}$≈20 Hz)
	β CH$_2$	(2H)	1.75 (m,W$_{1/2}$≈25 Hz)
	γ CH$_2$	(2H)	1.58 (m,W$_{1/2}$≈15 Hz)
	δ CH$_2$	(2H)	2.28 ("t",J≈10 Hz)
Laminine	Me$_3$N	(9H)	3.04 (s)
	α CH$_2$	(2H)	3.84 ("t",J≈6 Hz)
	β CH$_2$	(2H)	1.95 (m,W$_{1/2}$≈23 Hz)
	γ CH$_2$	(2H)	1.47 (m,W$_{1/2}$≈30 Hz)
	δ CH$_2$	(2H)	1.84 (m,W$_{1/2}$≈27 Hz)
	ε CH$_2$	(2H)	3.27 (m,W$_{1/2}$≈20 Hz)

[a] Chemical shifts are measured in ppm from DSS (internal reference), using D$_2$O as solvent. All spectra were recorded using a Brüker WH-270 MHz spectrometer.

been recorded previously for the ovary of the shell fish, *Callista brevishiphonata,* by Yasumoto & Shimizu (1977).

A commercial seaweed extract prepared from *A. nodosum,* and *Fucus* and *Laminaria* species (SM3, manufactured by Chase Organics Ltd., Shepperton, Middlesex, U.K.) was examined for its content of Dragendorff-positive compounds. γ-Aminobutyric acid betaine, δ-aminovaleric acid betaine and glycine betaine were isolated and fully characterised (TLC, ir, ^{1}H NMR). Chromatographic data was obtained for the presence of laminine and lysine betaine.

The regular occurrence of betaines and tertiary sulphonium compounds in marine algae would seem to be related strongly to the marine habitat of the plants. The circumstantial evidence appears strong for the role of the betaines found in commercial seaweed extracts in producing some, if not many, of the cytokinin-like activities of these extracts. If this is the case, a detailed study of the

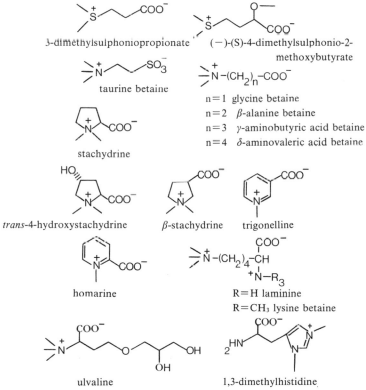

Fig. 1. Betaines and tertiary sulphonium compounds found in marine algae.

activity of a wide range of betaines and related compounds in suitable test systems would seem desirable. Many different betaines and tertiary sulphonium compounds have been isolated already from various marine algae (Fig. 1). These compounds may form a basis for a programme of chemical modification to produce substances which have economic potential for use in alleviating the effects of certain stress conditions of plants.

LECTINS FROM MARINE ALGAE

Since the early 1970s, work has been in progress at Portsmouth Polytechnic on the detection and characterisation of lectins in marine algae, using human erythrocytes as indicator cells. Low titre agglutinins were found in the extracts of a number of the species tested (Blunden *et al.* 1975, 1978), but all were non-specific for human erythrocytes with the exception of the red alga *Ptilota plumosa,* which showed specificity for erythrocytes carrying the blood-group B antigen (Rogers *et al.* 1977). Extracts of *P. plumosa* agglutinate foetal group B red blood cells (Rogers *et al.* 1977), but do not react with clinical examples of acquired B antigens (Rogers *et al.* 1979).

In addition to their use in blood grouping, lectins are of value in studies of the cell-surface chemistry of leucocytes, platelets, spermatozoa, mitochondria, tissue cells, tumour cells, viruses, fungi and bacteria. Some cells, tissues and organisms can be typed or differentiated on the basis of their surface carbohydrate chemistry. Lectins have the capacity to bind to specific sugar moieties and can, thus, be used to help in this typing or differentiation. For example, blood group B-erythrocytes differ from blood group A-erythrocytes by the presence of a terminal α-(1→3)-linked-D-galactose unit on the surface of the former, whereas group A erythrocytes have a terminal N-acetylgalac-tosamine unit. The lectin in extracts of *P. plumosa* reacts specifically with the α-(1→3)-linked-D-galactose unit and, hence, agglutinates blood group B-erythro-cytes preferentially. The lectin does not bind to terminal α-(1→4)-linked-D-galactose units and, therefore, fails to react with P system antigens, unlike the anti-group B preparations from Salmonidae ova (Voak *et al.* 1974).

In one of the surveys of British algae for haemagglutinins, extracts of the red alga *Solieria chordalis* did not agglutinate erythrocytes in 0.9% sodium chloride solution, but produced high titres after the addition of bovine albumin (Blunden *et al.* 1978). However, when erythrocytes pre-treated with papain were used no haemagglutination was observed. Further work on this alga was not possible at the time because of its rarity in the U.K., but subsequent collections have enabled a detailed study to be made by Rogers & Topliss (1983).

The extract of *S. chordalis,* when titrated against native (untreated) erythrocytes of blood groups A, B and O, gave a titre of 1:2048, but only after bovine albumin had been added to the medium. The results were identical with each blood group, which indicates that the receptor for the haemagglutinin is common to all normal human erythrocyte surfaces. Significant reductions in titration values were achieved when enzyme-treated erythrocytes were used, the effect being most pronounced with neuraminidase-treated cells (1:64). The ability of the extract to agglutinate neuraminidase-treated erythrocytes was studied during a 30 min period of enzyme treatment and the sialic acid released at various times during this period was assayed. The extract showed a gradual decrease in titration value in direct correlation to sialic acid release, and, hence, the common receptor for the haemagglutinin is probably sialic acid.

The haemagglutination produced by *S. chordalis* extract was inhibited most strongly by the sialoglycoproteins fetuin, bovine submaxillary gland mucin and porcine mucin; α-D(+)-melibiose was also highly inhibitory. The inhibitory sialoglycoproteins carry terminal sialic acid residues $(2\rightarrow6)$-linked to N-acetylgalactosamine. N-acetylneuramin-lactose, which is composed of 85% N-acetylneuraminic acid-$(2\rightarrow3)$-D-galactose-β-$(1\rightarrow4)$-D-glucose and 15% N-acetylneuraminic acid-$(2\rightarrow6)$-D-galactose-β-$(1\rightarrow4)$-D-glucose, was noninhibitory. This indicated that a subterminal N-acetylgalactosamine residue may be a prerequisite of haemagglutination inhibition. Neuraminidase-treatment of the sialoglycoproteins reduced their inhibitory powers significantly, which suggests that inhibition can be assigned to the sialic acid content of the substances rather than to any dysfunction of the lectin as a result of protein-protein interactions.

Porcine mucin, which contains predominantly N-glycoylneuraminic acid, inhibits the *S. chordalis* lectin to a similar degree to the N-acetylneuraminic acid-containing sialoglycoproteins. This suggests that the N-substituted group at carbon 5 of sialic acid does not influence the receptor site of the lectin. All the inhibitory sialoglycoproteins used carry terminal sialic acid, but solutions of N-acetylneuraminic acid were non-inhibitory.

The evidence available suggests that the receptor site for *S. chordalis* haemagglutinin involves a $(2\rightarrow6)$-linkage to the penultimate sugar. The preference of the lectin for a subterminal N-acetylgalactosamine and not a galactose residue infers that the N-acetyl group may confer a more rigid conformation on the penultimate sugar, which in turn, has a more stabilising

influence on the linkage to the terminal residue. The receptor site for the
haemagglutinin may, therefore, incorporate a structure involving sialic acid, the
glycosidic bond and carbons 6 and 2 of N-acetylgalactosamine. A similar
situation is apparent in the binding of wheatgerm agglutinin to sialoglycoproteins (Maget-Dana *et al.* 1981), where the exact arrangement of N-acetylneuraminic acid and N-acetylglucosamine in glycoconjugates and cell surfaces is
important for the formation of a stable association between the lectin and its
receptor. A complex receptor site has been proposed also for the antisialic acid
lectin from *Limulus polyphemus* involving an N-acetylneuraminic acid and N-
acetylglucosamine complex (Cohen & Rozenberg 1974).

The anti-sialic acid specificity of *S. chordalis* is very unusual. The most
obvious area of application for this lectin is in studies of cell surfaces, for which
L. polyphemus lectin has been used in the past (Cohen *et al.* 1976).

Molecular weight determination of the purified *S. chordalis* lectin showed it to
exist in a variety of oligomeric forms. On polyacrylamide gel electrophoresis 5
protein bands were found with calculated molecular weights of 70,000, 140,000,
200,000, 290,000 and 360,000 daltons. Sodium dodecylsulphate polyacrylamide
gel electrophoresis produced a single band with a calculated molecular weight of
35,000 daltons. A comparison of the molecular weights and chemical specificities of the *S. chordalis* lectin and other marine algal lectins is given in Table II.

Table II
Molecular weights and chemical specificities of marine algal lectins

Species	Molecular weight (daltons)	Chemical specificity	Reference
Solieria chordalis	35,000	sialic acid	Rogers & Topliss 1983
Ptilota plumosa	65,000 and 170,000	α-D-galactose	Rogers *et al.* 1977 and Rogers *et al.* 1980
Agardhiella tenera	12,000	unknown	Shiomi *et al.* 1979
Cystoclonium purpureum	6,000	unknown	Kamiya *et al.* 1980
Serraticardia maxima	25,000	unknown	Shiomi *et al.* 1980
Gracilaria verrucosa	tetramer consisting of 2×12,000 and 2×10,500	unknown	Shiomi *et al.* 1981
Palmaria palmata	20,000	D-glucuronic acid and N-acetylneuraminic acid	Kamiya *et al.* 1982

REFERENCES

Barwell, C. J., Blunden, G. & Jewers, K. (1981) An investigation of British marine algae as sources of biologically-active substances. *Proc. 3rd EMPRA Symp.* pp. 73–84. EMPRA, University Botanic Garden, Cambridge.

Biddington, N. L. & Thomas, T. H. (1973) A modified *Amaranthus* betacyanin bioassay for the rapid determination of cytokinins in plant extracts. *Planta 111,* 183–186.

Blunden, G. (1977) Cytokinin activity of seaweed extracts. In: *Marine Natural Products Chemistry* eds. Faulkner, D. J. & Fenical, W. H., pp. 337–344. Plenum Press, New York.

Blunden, G., Farnham, W. F., Jephson, N., Barwell, C. J., Fenn, R. H. & Plunkett, B. A. (1981a) The composition of maërl beds of economic interest in Northern Brittany, Cornwall and Ireland. *Proc. 10th Intern. Seaweed Symp.* pp. 651–656. Walter de Gruyter & Co., Berlin.

Blunden, G., Barwell, C. J., Fidgen, K. J. & Jewers, K. (1981b) A survey of some British marine algae for anti-influenza virus activity. *Bot. Mar. 24,* 267–272.

Blunden, G., El Barouni, M. M., Gordon, S. M., McLean, W. F. H. & Rogers, D. J. (1981c) Extraction, purification and characterisation of Dragendorff-positive compounds from some British marine algae. *Bot. Mar. 24,* 451–456.

Blunden, G., Gordon, S. M. & Keysell, G. R. (1982) Lysine betaine and other quaternary ammonium compounds from British species of the Laminariales. *J. Nat. Prod. 45,* 449–452.

Blunden, G., Rogers, D. J. & Farnham, W. F. (1975) Survey of British seaweeds for hemagglutinins. *Lloydia 38,* 162–168.

Blunden, G., Rogers, D. J. & Farnham, W. F. (1978) Haemagglutinins in British marine algae and their possible taxonomic value. In: *Modern Approaches to the Taxonomy of Red and Brown Algae* eds. Irvine, D. E. G. & Price, J. H., pp. 21–45. Academic Press, London & New York.

Bokarev, K. S. & Ivanova, R. P. (1971) The effect of certain derivatives and analogs of choline and betaine on content of free amino acids in leaves of two species of potato differing with respect to frost resistance. *Sov. Plant Physiol. 18,* 302–305.

Brain, K. R., Chalopin, M. C., Turner, T. D., Blunden, G. & Wildgoose, P. B. (1973) Cytokinin activity of commercial aqueous seaweed extract. *Plant Sci. Lett. 1,* 241–245.

Chesters, C. G. C. & Stott, J. A. (1956) Production of antibiotic substances from seaweeds. *Proc. 2nd Intern. Seaweed Symp.* pp. 49–53.

Cohen, E. & Rozenberg, M. (1974) Agglutinins of *Limulus polyphemus* (horseshoe crab) and *Birgus latra* (coconut crab). *Ann. N.Y. Acad. Sci. 234,* 28–33.

Cohen, E., Monowada, J., Pliss, M., Pliss, L. & Blumenson, L. E. (1976) Differentiation of human leukaemic from normal lymphocytes by Limulus serum agglutination. *Vox. Sang. 31,* 117–123.

Gordon, S. M., Blunden, G., McLean, W. F. H. & Barwell, C. J. (1981) Isolation and characterisation of Dragendorff-positive compounds from marine algae. *First International Conference on Chemistry and Biotechnology of Biologically Active Natural Products,* Vol. 3.1, pp 248–252, Bulgarian Academy of Sciences.

Guiry, M. D. & Blunden, G. (1981) The commercial collection and utilisation of seaweeds in Ireland. (1981) *Proc. 10th Intern. Seaweed Symp.* pp. 675–680. Walter de Gruyter & Co., Berlin.

Hornscy, I. S. & Hide, D. (1974) The production of antimicrobial compounds by British marine algae. I Antibiotic-producing marine algae. *Br. phycol. J. 9,* 353–361.

Hornsey, I. S. & Hide, D. (1976) The production of antimicrobial compounds by British marine algae. II Seasonal variation in production of antibiotics. *Br. phycol. J. 11,* 63–67.

Jones, E. M. (1979) Studies on the cytokinin activities of seaweed extracts. M. Phil. thesis, C.N.A.A. (Portsmouth Polytechnic), 144 pages.

Kamiya, H., Shiomi, K. & Shimizu, Y. (1980) Marine biopolymers with cell specificity III. Agglutinins in the red alga *Cystoclonium purpureum:* isolation and characterisation. *J. Nat. Prod.* 43, 136–139.

Kamiya, H., Ogata, K. & Hori, K. (1982) Isolation and characterization of a new agglutinin in the red alga *Palmaria palmata* (L.) O. Kuntze. *Bot. Mar.* 25, 537–540.

Maget-Dana, R., Yeh, R. W., Sander, M., Roche, A., Schauer, R. & Monsigny, W. (1981) Specificities of limulin and wheat-germ agglutinin towards derivatives of GM3 gangliosides. *Eur. J. Biochem.* 114, 11–16.

Rogers, D. J., Blunden, G. & Evans, P. R. (1977) *Ptilota plumosa,* a new source of a blood group B-specific lectin. *Med. Lab. Sci.* 34, 193–200.

Rogers, D. J., Topliss, J. A. & Blunden, G. (1979) Reactions of anti-B lectins with erythrocytes sensitised with lipopolysaccharide from *Escherichia coli* O_{86}. *Med. Lab. Sci.* 36, 79–84.

Rogers, D. J. & Blunden, G. (1980) Structural properties of the anti-B lectin from the red alga *Ptilota plumosa* (Huds.) C.Ag. Bot. Mar. 23, 459–462.

Rogers, D. J. & Topliss, J. A. (1983) Purification and characterisation of an anti-sialic acid agglutinin from the red alga *Solieria chordalis* (C.Ag.) J.Ag. *Bot. Mar.* 26, 301–305.

Sakai, A. & Yoshida, S. (1968) Protective action of various compounds against freezing injury in plant cells. *Teion Kagaku, Seibutsu-Hen 26,* 13–21; from *Chem. Abstr. 71:* 934y.

Shiomi, K., Kamiya, H. & Shimizu, Y. (1979) Purification and characterisation of an agglutinin in the red alga *Agardhiella tenera. Biochim. Biophys. Acta 576,* 118–127.

Shiomi, K., Yamanaka, H. & Kikuchi, T. (1980) Biochemical properties of hemagglutinins in the red alga *Serraticardia maxima. Bull. Japan. Soc. Sci. Fish. 46,* 1369–1373.

Shiomi, K., Yamanaka, H. & Kikuchi, T. (1981) Purification and physicochemical properties of a haemagglutinin (GVA-1) in the red alga *Gracilaria verrucosa. Bull. Japan. Soc. Sci. Fish. 47,* 1079–1084.

Voak, D., Todd, G. M. & Pardoe, G. I. (1974) A study of the serological behaviour and nature of the anti-B/P/P^k activity of Salmonidae roe protectins. *Vox Sang. 26,* 176–188.

Wheeler, A. W. (1973) Endogenous growth substances. *Rep. Rothamsted Exp. Stn.* Part 1, pp. 101–102.

Williams, D. C., Brain, K. R., Blunden, G., Wildgoose, P. B. & Jewers, K. (1981) Plant growth regulatory substances in commercial seaweed extracts. *Proc. 8th Intern. Seaweed Symp.* pp. 760–763, Marine Science Laboratories, Menai Bridge.

Wyn Jones, R. G. (1980) An assessment of quaternary ammonium and related compounds as osmotic effectors in crop plants. In: *Genetic Engineering of Osmoregulation. Impact on Plant Productivity for Food, Chemicals, and Energy,* eds. Rains, D. W. & Valentine, R. C., pp. 155–170. Plenum Press, New York.

Wyn Jones, R. G. & Storey, R. (1981) Betaines. In: *The Physiology and Biochemistry of Drought Resistance in Plants,* eds. Paleg, L. G. & Aspinall, D., pp. 171–204. Academic Press, Sydney.

Yasumoto, T. & Shimizu, N. (1977) Identification of δ-valerobetaine and other betaines in the ovary of shellfish *Callista brevishiphonata. Bull. Japan. Soc. Sci. Fish. 43,* 201–206.

DISCUSSION

DAVIES: Is anything known about the mechanism by which the betaine is protecting the plant against frost.

BLUNDEN: As far as I can see from the literature, there is not. However, it may have something to do with the protection of enzymes produced by betaines (1).

PORTOGHESE: Has anyone looked at the methylases that actually are involved in the methylation of the amino acids that you were talking about?

BLUNDEN: To my knowledge this has not been done with marine algae. However, Kjær and co-workers have studied this in higher plants (2).

RAPOPORT: Your betaines are reminiscent of a substance known as antho-pleurine, which is pheromone for the sea anemone having the structure 2,3-dihydroxy-4-aminobutyric acid betaine. I wonder if you have found any similar compounds?

BLUNDEN: We have found γ-aminobutyric acid betaine in several algae, and hydroxy derivatives of these have been found in a number of marine animals, but I am not aware of the detection of 2,-3-dihydroxy-4-aminobutyric acid betaine in an alga.

RAPOPORT: So this means that if the sea anemone is using 4-aminobutyric acid betaine as a precursor it is getting hydroxylated?

NAKANISHI: Do you run the betaines on TLC?

BLUNDEN: Yes. They are easily separated and detected by TLC (3). The betaines are frequently isolated by preparative TLC.

BAKER: Have your actually sprayed the plants with the betaines alone, or have you sprayed them with the extract?

BLUNDEN: Most of our work has been done with the extract, although limited trials have been conducted with the betaine alone.

BAKER: Do you note any additional uptake with the crude extract, compared with the extracts heated with base, perhaps due to the polysaccharide or mucopolysaccharide, which may give additional protection by forming a film which lowers the temperature at which ice would form?

BLUNDEN: We have studied only an extract that was prepared by simple aqueous extraction of the seaweeds.

———————

(1) Pollard, A. & Wyn Jones, R. G. (1979) *Planta 144,* 291–298.
(2) Grue-Sørensen, G., Kelstrup, E. & Kjær, A. (1980) *J. Chem. Soc. Chem. Commun.* 19–21.
(3) Blunden, G., El Barouni, M. M., Gordon, S. M., McLean, W. F. H. & Rogers, D. J. (1981) (see p. 187).

III. Antimicrobial and Antitumour Compounds

The Search for New Antimicrobial Agents:
Unusual Sources

Lester A. Mitscher & G. S. Raghav Rao

Despite what one might imagine to be the case after forty years of highly organized and intensive industrial research on antibiotics from soil micro-organisms, new chemical entities are being discovered at a higher annual rate than ever before. In early years, the bacteria, *Fungi Imperfecti* and soil streptomycetes accounted for the vast majority of reports; whereas in recent years, newer and less usual sources are being explored increasingly (Berdy 1980). These conclusions can be supported by an examination of Fig. 1 and Tables I and II.

One notes that thirty years ago, 57 antibiotics were described belonging to 11 different structural types. Most (35, 61%) of these were isolated from streptomycetes. By 1982, 230 new antibiotics were being described but only 46% (106) of these were from streptomycetes. Tables I and II contrast the relationship between type of antibiotic and producing organism for these same two years. The differences are dramatic. In 1952, antibiotics were isolated only from bacteria, streptomycetes, nocardiae, fungi and micromonosporae. By 1982, antibiotics were also being isolated from streptosporangiae, actinomadurae, kitasatoae, actinoplanetes, dactylosporangia, saccharopolysporae, streptoalloteichi and streptoverticilliae as well. On the other hand, the structural classes were essentially the same (15 structural families). From Fig. 1, one sees that the move toward exploitation of rare micro-organisms became quite discernable by 1977 and is now quite pronounced. It is also apparent that the rarer organisms are mostly producing new antibiotics classifiable into the same well established structural types.

At the present it is estimated that there are about 4000–9000 known natural

Medicinal Chemistry Department, Kansas University, Lawrence, Kansas, U.S.A.

NATURAL PRODUCTS AND DRUG DEVELOPMENT, Alfred Benzon Symposium 20.
Editors: P. Krogsgaard-Larsen, S. Brøgger Christensen, H. Kofod, Munksgaard, Copenhagen 1984.

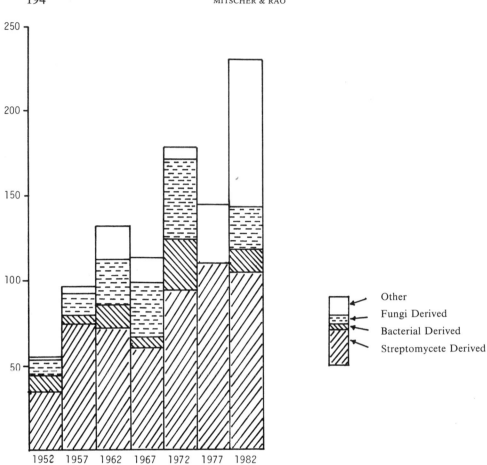

Fig. 1 Pattern of Antibiotic New Entry Discovery 1952–1982.

Table I

New antibiotic entities reported in 1952 arranged by producing organism and by structural type.

	1	2	3	4	5	6	7	8	9	10	11	12	13	14	15	Sum	%
Bacterium						5						3				8	14
Fungus				1		1					1	4			5	12	21
Micromonospora														2		2	4
Nocardia														1		1	2
Streptomyces	2			4	6	1		5			1	4	9		3	35	61
	2	0	0	5	6	2	5	5	0	1	5	4	12	0	11	57	

Key: 1=Aminocyclitol, 2=Ansamycin, 3=Beta-lactam, 4=Heterocycle, 5=Macrolide, 6=Nucleoside, 7=Peptide, 8=Polyene Macrolide, 9=Polyether, 10=Quinone, 11=Sugar, 12=Terpene, 13=Unknown, 14=Glycopeptide, 15=Miscellaneous.

Table II

New antibiotic entities reported in 1982 arranged by producing organism and by structural type.

	1	2	3	4	5	6	7	8	9	10	11	12	13	14	15	Sum	%
Actinomadura							1		1	1					1	4	2
Actinoplanes							2			1	2					5	2
Bacterium		1	6				1				3				2	13	6
Dactylosporangium	1															1	1
Fungus		1		7	1		3			2		7			5	25	11
Kitasatoa													1			1	1
Micromonospora	15			1			2						1		1	20	9
Nocardia		17		1	1								1			20	9
Saccharopolyspora	1															1	1
Streptoalloteichus							21									21	9
Streptomyces	6	5	6	5	4	6	22	2	2	25	2		18	1	2	106	46
Streptosporangium		2														2	1
Streptoverticillium										1						1	1
	23	26	12	14	6	6	52	2	3	30	7	7	21	1	11	230	

Key: 1=Aminocyclitol, 2=Ansamycin, 3=Beta-lactam, 4=Heterocycle, 5=Macrolide, 6=Nucleoside, 7=Peptide, 8=Polyene Macrolide, 9=Polyether, 10=Quinone, 11=Sugar, 12=Terpene, 13=Unknown, 14=Glycopeptide, 15=Miscellaneous

antibiotics. When one adds to this number the vast quantity of semisynthetic analogues now being prepared, the grand total is a very impressive one. In the USA, fully 15% of the top 200 most frequently prescribed drugs are antibiotics.

As gratifying as this picture appears at first glance, unfortunately, we cannot say that mankind's needs for anti-infective agents are largely satisfied. The combination of the genetic versatility of microbes and widespread overuse of antibiotics has led to increasing clinical resistance of previously sensitive microorganisms and the emergence of previously uncommon infections. One can mention in this regard, anaerobes, amoebae, fungi, legionellae, toxogenic staphylococci, the unknown agent responsible for the aquired immune deficiency syndrome (AIDS), and so on. Infectious diseases still are estimated to rank fourth on the list of causes of death in the US. Despite the level of effort described, infectious diseases still account for 7% of all deaths and a very substantial morbidity.

There are various ways of trying to deal with this problem. One of these involves the search for antibiotics of a chemical and biological type not previously explored. This, in the hope that novel activity spectra, novel modes of action and less cross-resistance will be seen than with presently utilized

13*

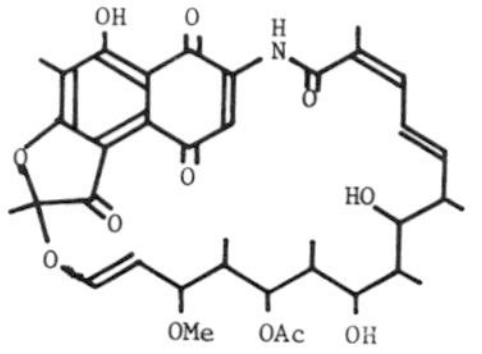

(1)

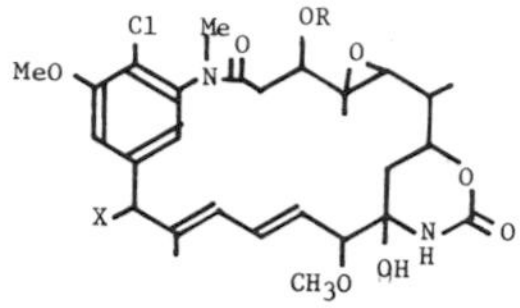

(2), X=H, R=COCHMeNMeCOMe
(3), X=OH, R=H
(4), X=OH, R=CO-aliphatic

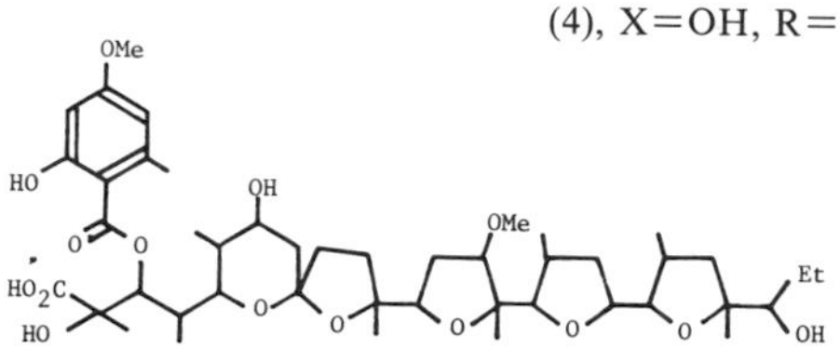

(5)

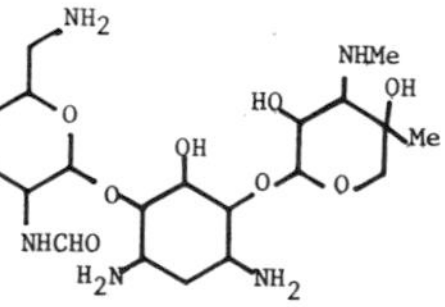

(6)

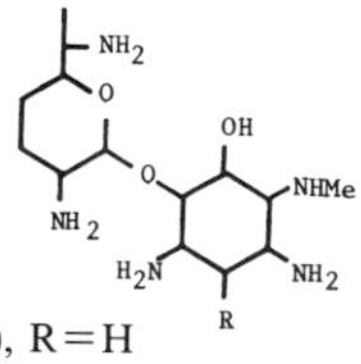

(7), R=H
(8), R=OH

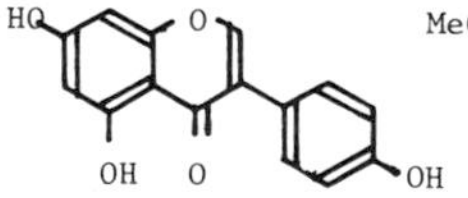

(9)

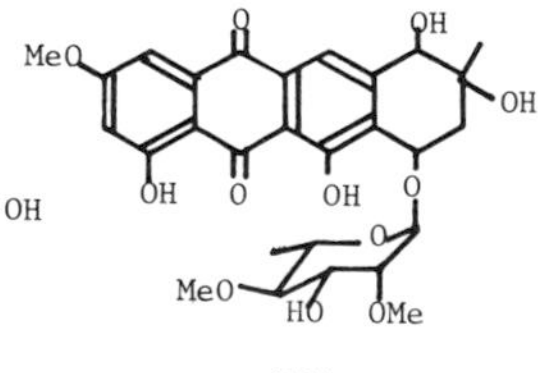

(10)

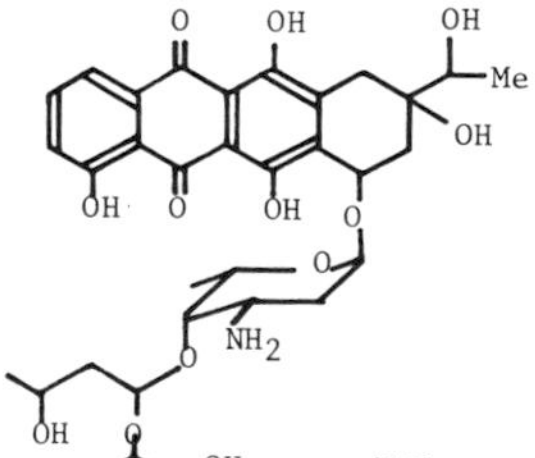

(11)

antibiotics. Ideally such novel agents would go to the clinic directly. Less ideally, but still usefully, they would serve as leads for medicinal chemists to modify to enhance potency, alter spectrum, sharpen selectivity, reduce toxicity or enhance pharmacodynamic character.

In industrial laboratories a conservative approach which makes maximal use of existing equipment and human resources emphasizes fermentation of less commonly explored genera and use of unusual habitats (soils from sea bed, mine shafts, deserts, etc.). This approach became popular in the last decade and has

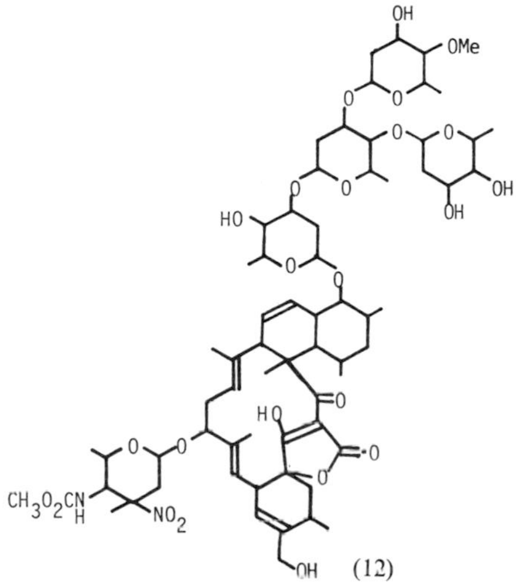

(12)

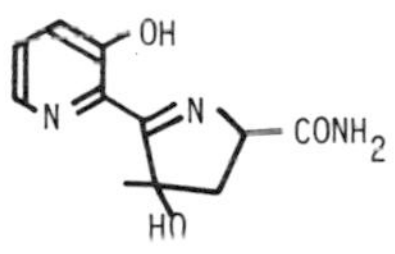

(13)

been fruitful. Most of the antibiotics so discovered represent structural variations on themes familiar to antibiotic chemists. The following specific examples from the literature of 1981 are sufficient to document this point.

The discovery of the antibacterial and antitumor agent maytansine (2) from the Ethiopian shrub *Maytenus ovatus* has awakened considerable interest in the properties of this subfamily of ansamacrolides, distantly related to rifamycin (1). The ansamitocins (4) (Izawa *et al.* 1981), including 3-deacetylmaytanbutacine (3) (Tanida *et al.* 1981; Nakahama *et al.* 1981) are, amazingly, not only isolated from several streptomycetes (*S. sclerotialus, S. castaneus, S. flavochromogenes, S. olivaceiscleroticus, S. flavoscleroticus,* and *S. luridus*) but also from *Chainia nigra,* an unspeciated *Nocardia,* and *Streptosporangium roseum* as well. Considering that they are also related to a compound from a higher plant, these are remarkable examples of the point being made.

Cationomycin (5) (Nakamura *et al.* 1981), isolated from *Actinomadura azurea,* is a rather typical example of the ionophorous polyether antibiotics more commonly associated with the streptomycetes. Aminocyclitol antibiotics such as streptomycin, neomycin and kanamycin are quite common among the streptomycetes and the gentamicins are common among the micromonosporae, however, the aminocyclitols are not limited by any means to these genera. For example, 2'-N-formylsisomycin (6) (Fuji *et al.* 1980, 1981) is produced by *Dactylosporangium thailandense,* and sporaricin E (7) (Iwasaki *et al.* 1982) is produced by *Saccharopolyspora hirsuta.* The latter is the C-2 deoxy analogue of the micromonospora antibiotic fortimicin B (8) (Egan *et al.* 1977).

Differinol A (9) (Asahi *et al.* 1981) represents another example of an apparently widespread antibiotic type. Isoflavones are widely distributed amongst higher plants extracts. Differinol A is isolable from *Micromonospora halophytica* as well as from the fungus *Aspergillus niger.* It has been suggested that differinol A may occur as a glucoside (genistin) in soya beans (Chimura *et al.* 1975). Soya bean meal is a medium constituent in these fermentations so the possibility exists that differenol A is an artifact produced by those microbes which have the appropriate glycosidase.

Antitumor and antibacterial anthracycline antibiotics such as doxorubicin are produced by streptomycetes. Close relatives are produced by rarer soil micro-organisms. One may cite the dihydrosteffimycins (10) (Marshall *et al.* 1980) from *Actinoplanes utahensis* and 4-hydroxybaumycinols (11) (Matsuzawa *et al.* 1981) from an *Actinomadura* species.

The reader should not be led to the impression that all antibiotics from rare organisms fall into well precedented classes. For example, kijanimycin (12), from *Actinomadura kijaniata* (Mallams et al. 1981), and siderochelin A (13), from a *Nocardia* species (Liu *et al.* 1981), have no obvious streptomycete-derived counterparts as yet. Still, the basic point remains that in most instances published recently, the structures produced by rare organisms are related to previously explored substances.

From this brief analysis, one concludes that if one is to discover truly unusual structural types, one must look more closely at fermentation residues, make use of novel screening methodologies, or make some more fundamental alteration in approach. Amongst the alternate approaches being examined at present is the search for antimicrobial agents from marine organisms where such agents appear to be common (Faulkner 1977; Kaul 1982).

In our case, we have been examining the relatively neglected and surprisingly plentiful antimicrobial agents from terrestrial higher plants. Plants are subject to infections by bacteria, fungi and viruses. The specific organisms involved are rarely the same as those infecting animals, but the overall phenomenon has many similarities. While plants lack an immune system and an efficient circulatory system, they possess several means of defense. Amongst these is the pre-infection elaboration of antimicrobial agents and the ability to produce phytoalexins (Gross 1977; Ingham 1983). (A number of apparently innocuous substances are present in plants. Enzymes brought in by plant pathogens can effect structural changes on these compounds. Occasionally, these changes result in amplification of the quantity of a previously minor antimicrobial constituent or in formation of a new antimicrobial agent. Post-infectional antibiotics are known as phytoalexins and many are known). For practical reasons, phytoalexins are hard to deal with in broad screening programs and, despite the many fascinating co-evolutionary relationships they represent, there is less opportunity for man to exploit these for his own protection than there is for use of preformed agents. Fortunately the latter are plentiful.

The literature dealing with antimicrobial agents from higher plants is somewhat hard to evaluate because it is widely scattered, is often found in relatively obscure journals, and has emerged with no uniformity in the choice of test organism or in the means used to report potency. In our work, we have developed a useful screening system which uses indicator organisms predictive of possible utility against human bacterial diseases (Mitscher et al. 1972). By this approach, as many as 1 in 5 extracts of higher plants shows reproducable antimicrobial activity. On the other hand, following up literature reports and folkloric accounts results in detection of activity in 1 in 4 extracts. A wide variety of plant genera are involved.

Using a standardized fractionation scheme devised for the purpose, bioassay-directed methods usually produced the active agent(s) (Mitscher 1977). The structures of pre-infectional higher-plant antimicrobial agents are usually quite different than those from fermentation of soil micro-organisms. They are not very different from the structures of the phytoalexins suggesting that the distinction is not a particularly useful one for our purposes. For example, the active agent from the Bolivian coral tree, *Erythrina crista-galli,* is the pterocarpene erycristagallin (14) (Mitscher et al. 1983a). A very similar antimicrobial agent was discovered from the leaves of *E. abyssinica* and named erythrabyssin II (15) (Kamat et al. 1981). Pterocarpans are quite often identified as phytoalexins and many of the structures are very similar to that of erycristagallin (Ingham 1983). This underlines another important point. The structures of antibiotics from higher plants are types usually familiar to natural products chemists. Such well-studied classes as flavanoids, quinones, coumarins, aliphatics, terpenes, phenolics, and the like, are involved. Among specific examples from our recent work are the indole alkaloid harmine (16) from *Peganum harmala* seeds (AlShamma et al. 1981b), the phenanthroquinolizidine alkaloid cryptopleurine (17) from *Boehmeria cylindrica* var. *drummondiana* (AlShamma et al. 1981b), the piperidine alkaloid 3,4-dimethoxy-ω-(2'-piperidyl) acetophe-

(14)   (15)

(16)   (17)

(18)   (19)

(20)   (21)   (22)

(23), R=H
(24), R=CH₂CH=CMe₂

none (18) from the same plant, the flavan derivatives dracorhodin (19) and dracorubin (20) from *Daemonorops draco* resin (Rao *et al.* 1982), the diterpene acids trachyloban-19-oic (21) and (-)-kaur-16-enoic (22) acids from the stems of the prairie sunflower, *Helianthus annuus* (Mitscher *et al.* 1983b), and the novel bibenzyls amorfrutin A (23) and B (24) from the fruits of the false indigo plant, *Amorpha fruticosa* (Mitscher *et al.* 1981a).

While disappointing from the standpoint of structural excitement, this indicates that many compounds whose structures are known to the literature have unsuspected antimicrobial activity and that testing of congeners be a worthwhile effort. It is also clear that these molecules should be readily accessible to synthesis. The structures are relatively simple and one rarely has significant optical isomerism to worry about. Also, as the compounds have been co-evolutionarily optimized against different pathogens than those infecting humans, it seems quite likely that synthetic analogues would possess usefully altered antimicrobial spectra and, perhaps, enhanced activity. These thoughts are supported by studies on the antifungal antibiotic tryptanthrin (25). *Strobilanthes cusia* has a folkloric reputation as a topical antidermatophytic agent in Taiwan. The active constituent is tryptanthrin (Mitscher *et al.* 1981b). This compound, remarkably, has also been isolated from the unrelated species *Polygonum tinctorium, Isatis tinctoria* (Honda *et al.* 1980), and *Candida lipolytica* (Fiedler *et al.* 1976). Synthetic studies and directed biosyntheses have allowed the preparation of a number of analogues (Fiedler *et al.* 1976). The flexibility of these processes and the alterations in spectra and potency of the unnatural analogues produced, support the optimistic view that persistance might produce a clinically useful agent.

For illustrative purposes, our synthesis of the tryptanthrin ring system, conceptually very similar to that developed independently by Bergman (Bergman *et al.* 1977), follows: Of the many unnatural analogues prepared in this way,

(25), X=Y=H

Table III

Bioactivity in vitro of some synthetic tryptanthrin analogues.

X	Y	Bioactivity (Microorganism*) minimum inhibitory conc. in mcg/ml
H	H	(1)50(4)100(5)6.25(6)100
4-Cl	H	(1)0.5(5)0.4(6)0.8
3-Cl	H	Inactive
5-Cl	H	(5)6.25

*(1)=*Staphylococcus aureus*, (4)=*Klebsiella pneumoniae*, (5)=*Mycobacterium smegmatis*, (6)=*Candida albicans.*

the following are particularly instructive: The first substance (X=Y=H) is tryptanthrin. In this *in vitro* test, tryptanthrin is broad spectrum at a modest potency level. When a halogen atom is added to the C-3, 4 or 5 positions, the effect on potency and spectrum is quite variable. The C-4 chloro analogue has a somewhat narrower anti-microbial spectrum but is at least 100-fold more

Route A

Route B

potent. The C-5 chloro analogue has retained significant potency against mycobacteria but has a dramatically narrowed spectrum. Another positional isomer, the C-3 chloro analogue, is not active at all. Thus, at least in this series, co-evolution has not produced the optimal structure for human purposes and encourages the belief that the availability of simple syntheses can occasionally provide dramatically more interesting substances for further evaluation than the naturally occuring lead substance.

To illustrate how far afield such studies can take one, pteleatinium chloride (26), a quaternary quinolinium alkaloid, is the constituent responsible for the ancient use of the leaves of the false hop tree, *Ptelea trifoliata,* in brewing beer (Mitscher *et al.* 1975a). We developed a new synthesis as a laboratory exercise, but the products were usually devoid of significant antibacterial activity (Mitscher *et al.* 1975b). This work did, however, draw our attention to the chemically related synthetic urinary tract antimicrobial agents typified by oxolinic acid (27, R=H). Our synthesis (route b) was more powerful in scope than that classically used (route a) so we were able to undertake a systematic study of some previously unexplored structure-activity relationships. We quickly showed that the previously unknown C-2-substituted analogues were all less active than the lead substance (Mitscher *et al.* 1978) and that the methylenedioxy moiety was optimally placed at C-6,7 (Mitscher *et al.* 1979). At about this time it was discovered that the molecular target of the action of this antimicrobial agent class was the newly discovered enzyme DNA-gyrase (Cozzarelli 1980). This fascinating enzyme presents an important new target for chemotherapy. As it seems to have no counterpart in human biochemistry, an outstanding opportunity for selective toxicity is presented. Thus, we were encouraged to continue this effort. In order to investigate the putative mode of action of oxolinic acid, we undertook a synthetic evaluation of the importance of the N-1 atom and its pendent groups. For this it was necessary to develop different synthetic routes. The following schemes lead to the bio-inactive 1-carba (Högberg et al. 1983a), and 1-oxa (Högberg et al. 1983b) analogues. From the properties of these compounds both in bacteria and against the purified enzyme, it is apparent that the N-1 linkage plays a vital role in upsetting the workings of DNA-gyrase.

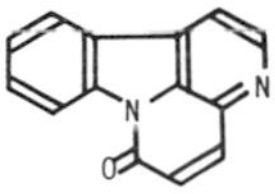

(28) 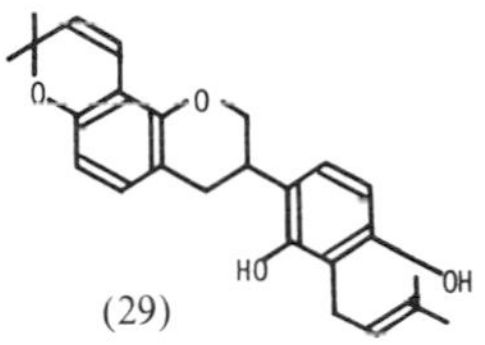   (29)

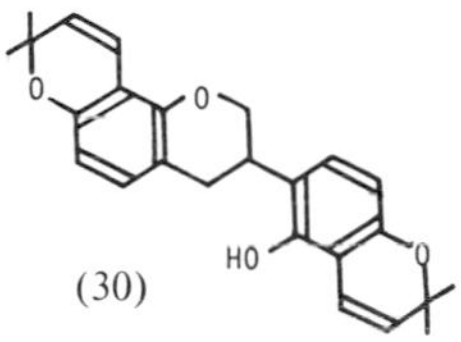

(30) 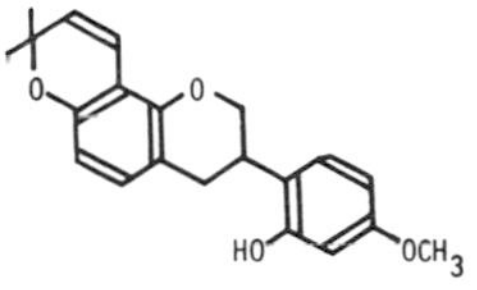   (31)

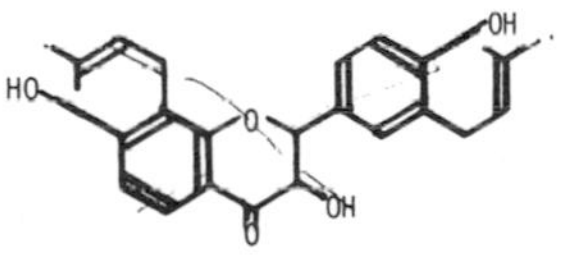

(32)

As one of the advantages of bioassay-directed fractionation, even quite thoroughly studied plants can produce interesting new findings. While the active principle of the Jamaican plant *Zanthoxylum elephantiasis* turned out to be the previously known alkaloid canthin-6-one (28), it had not been known to have antibiotic activity (Mitscher *et al.* 1972b). Ptelea trifoliata had been the subject of at least 5 previous investigations, but the major alkaloid, pteleatinium chloride, had been missed (Mitscher *et al.* 1975a). Few plants have been as thoroughly studied as licorice, *Glycyrrhiza glabra* var. Spanish. Licorice has been used as a sweetening and flavoring agent since prehistoric times. A study of the roots resulted in the isolation of numerous active antimicrobial agents,

Putative molecular mode of action

1-Carba Analogues

1-Oxa Analogues

(34)

(35)

(37)

(38)

several of which were new to the literature. These were hispaglabridin A (29), B (30), 4'-0-methyl-glabridin (31) and 3-hydroxyglabrol (32). The most significant agent, glabrol (33), was previously known to be present in *Glycyrrhiza* species, but was not known to be an antibiotic (Mitscher *et al.* 1980).

Interestingly, the only American *Glycyrrhiza* species, *G. lepidota*, grows wild in Kansas. It is not usefully sweet. Extracts were found by us to be antibiotically active and fractionation showed that these agents, except for glabranin (35, R = prenyl), were different from those of *G. glabra*. While 3,5-dihydroxy-4-(3-methyl-2-butenyl)-bibenzyl (34) and pinocembrin (36) were known from other plants, glepidotin A (37) and glepidotin B (38) were new (Mitscher *et al.* 1983c).

As yet, few antimicrobial agents from higher plants have received biochemical study with a view to understanding their mode of action. Berberine has been subject of a number of studies, but its molecular mode of action remains obscure. A number of alkaloids are known to be inhibitors of ribosomal protein biosynthesis. The main target of the aminocyclitol and tetracycline antibiotics is the 30S ribosomal subparticle. It is interesting to note that emetine, tubulosine, cryptopleurine, tylophorine and tylocebrine are also inhibitors of the ribosomal 30S subparticle in susceptible bacteria. Less likely to show a satisfactory safety margin are a group of natural products which inhibit protein biosynthesis by interfering with the proper functioning of the 60S subpartical of eucaryotes. These agents include narciclasine, harringtonine, pederine and bruceantin (Gale *et al.* 1981). Considering the well-known utility of antibiotics as probes of cell function and the very large and structurally diverse number of antimicrobial agents from higher plants which have received no study at all, it seems highly likely that this would prove to be a fruitful field for exploration.

One of the disappointing aspects of antimicrobial agents from higher plants is their often weak potency and narrow spectrum. The threshhold of meaningful antibiosis lies at about 50 mcg/ml. One does not normally get very excited about an agent that is not active at less that 10 mcg/ml. Many commercially significant antibiotics are potent at less than 1 mcg/ml. Few antimicrobial agents from higher plants are active at less than 1 mcg/ml. In our test system, sulfonamides and a number of other synthetic agents show activities at more than 1 mcg/ml, so many of the higher plant agents are not hopelessly out of the race, but greater potency would be a helpful characteristic. One needs, however, also to point out that many agents produced by soil micro-organisms (e.g., siderochelin A, differenol A) are also of such low potency. The narrowness of spectrum is a more open question. Classically, broadness of antimicrobial spectrum has usually been regarded as a useful characteristic. This of course eases the pressure on accurate diagnosis. The more recent recognition of antibiotic-facilitated resistence emergence and the ever increasing emergence of new opportunistic pathogens are causing some reconsideration of the uncritical acceptance of broad spectrum as a deciding factor in commercialization of new antibiotics. One can defend the thesis that the ideal antibiotic would be rapidly and uniformly effective against only certain pathogenic micro-organisms and not disturb bacteria which were not at that moment part of the disease process. One must balance the intellectual appeal of this strategem against the difficulties of diagnosis in real life. If this newer idea gains strength, then the relative narrowness of antimicrobial agents from higher plants would transfer from a weakness to a strength.

One other important philosophical question raised by the relative common-ness of these agents is why man has not made greater use of them during the course of history. Infectious diseases are of ancient origin. Thus, the need for antimicrobial agents has been with us for a very long time. Along with discovering opium, etc., why did man not discover penicillin or one of the agents from higher plants? One part of the answer is that man did find some such agents. Almost every primitive society has records of the use of crude extracts for this purpose and some of the materials have found their way into modern medicine. Quinine for the treatment of malaria and emetine for amoebiasis are examples. Berberine has been used, though less successfully, as an anti-infective agent.

Nevertheless, nothing as significant as penicilin or tetracycline was found. Partly the soil-produced substances which have transformed modern medicine are present in extremely small quantities, if at all, in untreated soil. It seems very unlikely that accidental discovery could have occurred under these conditions. It is also important to point out that soil micro-organisms are unevenly distributed so that the discovery would have been extremely difficult to reproduce once it had been made.

Antimicrobial agents from higher plants are also relatively minor constituents in many cases and are present only in certain plant parts and at certain seasons. This would have made their discovery more difficult, but did not, after all, prevent the discovery of the opiates, quinine, etc. Another complicating factor, which may have been more important, is the episodic nature of infectious disease. Whereas the pharmacological effects of the opiates find perceptable expression in healthy individuals at any time, and malaria and, to a lesser extent, amoebiasis are chronic infections whose symptoms are present in infected individuals for long periods of time, most bacterial infections are acute and resolve in a favorable or unfavorable sense in a week or two. It would be much more difficult to discover an anti-infective agent during that time and associate it with cause and effect, than it would be to make a useful discovery for a chronic infection.

Finally, what are the prospects for the future discovery of a clinically useful antimicrobial agent from a higher plant source? The answer is that they are uncertain. Active agents are clearly plentiful. They are amenable to convenient synthesis and the synthetic analogues are sometimes more exciting than the natural lead substances. Nevertheless no agent presently in hand looks like a clear threat to the position of penicillin in medicine. I personally believe that there are grounds for cautions optimism that such agents can be found, given that the harvest is plentiful and the laborers few, but I certainly would continue soil-screening programs and the search for alternate sources of antimicrobial agents. Perhaps the prospects of agricultural applications or use in the form of extracts in capital-starved third world areas will be the first area of economic penetration for these fascinating substances. Less problematic is that the presence of these agents raises important evolutionary and ecologic questions for further study.

ACKNOWLEDGEMENT
We thank the National Institute of Health, U.S.A., for financial support for the majority of this work under grant No. AI-13155.

REFERENCES
AlShamma, A., Drake, S., Flynn, D. L., Mitscher, L. A., Park, Y. H., Rao, G. S. R., Simpson, A., Swayze, J. K. Veysoglu, T. & Wu, T.-S. (1981a) Antimicrobial agents from higher plants. Antimicrobial agents from *Peganum harmala* seeds. *J. Nat. Prods. 44*, 745–747.

AlShamma, A., Drake, S. D., Guagliardi, L. E., Mitscher, L. A. & Swayze, J. K. (1981b) Antimicrobial alkaloids from *Boehmeria cylindrica*. *Phytochem. 21*, 485–487.

Asahi, K.-I., Ono, I., Kusakabe, H., Nakamura, G. & Isono, K. (1981) Studies on differentiation inducing substances of animal cells. I. Differenol A, a differentiation inducing substance against mouse leukemia cells. *J. Antibiotics 34*, 919–920.

Berdy, J. (1980) Recent advances and prospects of antibiotic research. *Process Biochem.* 28–35.

Bergman, J., Egestad, B. & Lindstroem, J. O. (1977) The structure of some indolic constituents in *Couroupita guaianensis* Abul. *Tetrahedron Letters*, 2625–2626.

Chimura, H., Sawa, T., Kumada, Y., Naganawa, H., Matsuzaki, M., Takita, T., Hamada, M., Takeuchi, T. & Umezawa H. (1975) New isoflavones, inhibiting catechol-0-methyltransferase, produced by Streptomyces. *J. Antibiotics 28,* 619–626.

Cozzarelli, N. R. (1980) DNA gyrase and the supercoiling of DNA. *Science 207* 953–960.

Egan, R. S., Stanaszek, R. S., Cirovic, M., Mueller, S. L., Tadanier, J., Martin, J. R,. Collum, P., Goldstein, A. W., deVault, R. L., Sinclair, A. C., Fager, E. E. & Mitscher, L. A. (1977) Fortimicins A and B, new aminoglycoside antibiotics. III. Structural identification. *J. Antibiotics 30,* 552–563.

Faulkner, D. J. (1977) Interesting aspects of marine natural products. *Tetrahedron 33,* 1421–1443.

Fiedler, E., Fiedler, H.-P., Gerhard, A., Keller-Schierlein, W., Konig, W. A., & Zahner, H. (1976) Stoffwechselprodukte von Mikroorgansimen. 156 Mitteilung. Synthese und biosynthese substituierter tryptanthrine. *Arch. Microbiol. 107,* 249–256.

Fuji, T., *et al.* (1980) *Japan Kokai 80,* 133, 394.

Fuji, T., *et al.* (1981) *United States Patent 4,* 297, 486.

Gale, E. F., Cundliffe, E., Reynolds, P. E., Richmond, M. H. & Waring, M. J. (1981) *The Molecular Basis of Antibiotic Action, Second Edition.* Wiley, New York.

Gross, D. (1977) Phytoalexine und verwandte Pflanzenstoffe. *Fortsch. der Chem. Org. Naturstoffe 34,* 188–247.

Hogberg, T., Khanna, I., Drake, S. D., Mitscher, L. A. & Shen, L. L. (1983a) Structure-activity relationships among DNA-gyrase inhibitors. Synthesis and biological evaluation of 4,4-dimethyl-1-naphthalenone-2-carboxylic acids as 1-carba bioisosteres of oxolinic acid. Submitted.

Hogberg, T., Vora, M., Drake, S. D., Mitscher, L. A. & Chu, D. T. W. (1983b) Structure-activity relationships among DNA-gyrase inhibitors. Synthesis and antimicrobial evaluation of chromones and coumarins related to oxolinic acid. Submitted.

Honda, G. & Tabata, M. (1979) Isolation of antifungal principle tryptanthrin, from *Strobilanthes cusia* O. Kuntze. *Planta Medica 36,* 85–86.

Ingham, J. L. (1982) Phytoalexins from the Leguminosae. In: *Phytoalexins.* pp. 21–80, ed. J. A. Bailey & J. W. Mansfield. Wiley, New York.

Iwasaki, A., Deushi, T., Watanabe, I., Okuchi, M., Itoh, H. & Mori, T. (1982) A new broad-spectrum aminoglycoside antibiotic complex. Sporaricin. V. Sporaricin E. *J. Antibiotics 35,* 517–519.

Izawa, M., Wada, Y., Kasahara, F., Asai, M. & Kishi, T. (1981) Hydroxylation of ansamitocin P-3. *J. Antibiotics 34,* 1591–1595.

Kamat, V. S., Chuo, F. Y., Kubo, I. & Nakanishi, K. (1981) Antimicrobial agents from an East African medicinal plant *Erythrina abyssinica. Heterocycles 15,* 1163–1170.

Kaul, P. N. (1982) Biomedical potential of the sea. *Pure and Applied Chem., 54,* 1963–1972.

Liu, W.-C., Fischer, S. M., Wells, J. S., Jr., Ricca, C. S., Principe, P. E. Trejo, W. H., Bonner, D. P., Gougoutos, J. Z., Toeplitz, B. K. & Sykes, R. B. (1981) Siderochelin, a new ferrous-ion chelating agent produced by *Nocardia. J. Antibiotics 34,* 791–799.

Mallams, A. K., Puar, M. S. & Rossman, R. R. (1981) Kijanimicin. 1. Structures of the individual sugar components. *J. Am. Chem. Soc. 103,* 3938–3940.

Marshall, V. P., *et al.* (1980) *United States Patent 4,* 209, 611.

Matsuzawa, Y., Yoshimoto, A., Kouno, K. & Oki, T. (1981) Baumycin analogs isolated from *Actinomadura sp. J. Antibiotics 34,* 774–776.

Mitscher, L. A., Leu, R.-P., Bathala, M. S., Wu, W.-N., Beal, J. L. & White R. (1972a) Antibiotics from higher plants. I. Introduction, rationale and methodology. *J. Nat. Prods. 35,* 157–166.

Mitscher, L. A., Showalter, H. D. H., Shipchandler, M. T., Leu, R. P. & Beal, J. L. (1972b) Antimicrobial agents from higher plants. IV. *Zanthoxylum elephantiasis* Macf. Isolation and identification of canthin-6-one. *J. Nat. Prods. 35,* 177–180.

Mitscher, L. A., Bathala, M. S., Clark, G. W. & Beal, J. W. (1975a) Antimicrobial agents from higher plants. The quaternary bases of *Ptelea trifoliata. J. Nat. Prods. 38,* 109–116.

Mitscher, L. A., Clark, G. W., Suzuki, T. & Bathala, M. S. (1975b) A new synthesis of quinol-2,4-diones. *Heterocycles 3,* 913–919.

Mitscher, L. A. (1977) Plant-derived antibiotics. In: *Isolation, Separation and Purification of Antibiotics.* pp. 463–477, ed. G. Wagman and C. Weinstein. Elsevier, Amsterdam.

Mitscher, L. A., Graccy, H. E., Clark, G. W. & Suzuki, T. (1978) Quinolone antimicrobial agents. 1. Versatile new synthesis of 1-alkyl-1,4-dihydro-4-oxo-3-quinoline carboxylic acids. *J. Med. Chem., 21,* 485–489.

Mitscher, L. A., Flynn, D. L., Gracey, H. E. & Drake, S. D. (1979) Quinolone antimicrobial agents. 2. Methylenedioxy positional isomers of oxolinic acid. *J. Med. Chem. 22,* 1354–1357.

Mitscher, L. A., Park, Y. H., Clark, D. & Beal, J. L. (1980) Antimicrobial agents from higher plants. Antimicrobial isoflavanoids and related substances from *Glycyrrhiza glabra* L. (*var.* Spanish). *J. Nat Prods. 43,* 259–269.

Mitscher, L. A., Park, Y. H., AlShamma, A., Hudson, P. G., & Haas, T. (1981a) Amorfrutin A and B, bibenzyl antimicrobial agents from *Amorpha fruticosa. Phytochem. 20,* 781–783.

Mitscher, L. A., Wong, W.-C., DeMeulenaere, T., Sulko, J. & Drake, S. (1981b) Antimicrobial agents from higher plants. New synthesis and bioactivity of tryptanthrin (indolo-[2,1-b]-quinazolin-6,12-dione) and its analogues. *Heterocycles 15,* 1017–1021.

Mitscher, L. A., Ward, J. A. & Rao, G. S. R. (1983a) Antimicrobial agents from higher plants. Erycrystagallin, a new pterocarpene from the roots of the Bolivian coral tree, *Erythrina cristagalli.* In preparation.

Mitscher, L. A., Rao, G. S. R., Veysoglu, T., Drake, S. & Haas, T. (1983b) Isolation and identification of trachyloban-19-oic and (-)-kaur-16-en-oic acids as antimicrobial agents from the prairie sunflower, *Helianthus annuus. J. Nat. Prods.* (in press).

Mitscher, L. A., Rao, G. S. R., Khanna, I., Veysoglu, T. & Drake, S. D. (1983c) Antimicrobial agents from higher plants. Prenylated phenols from *Glycyrrhiza lepidota. Phytochemistry 22,* 573–576.

Nakahama, M., Izawa, M., Asai, M., Kida, M. & Kishi, T. (1981) Microbial conversion of ansamitocin. *J. Antibiotics 34,* 1581–1586.

Nakamura, G., Kobayashi, K., Sakurai, T. & Isono, K. (1981) Cationomycin, a new polyether ionophore antibiotic produced by *Actinomadura nov. sp. J. Antibiotics 34,* 1513–1516.

Rao, G. S. R., Gerhart, M. A., Lee, R. T., II, Mitscher, L. A. & Drake, S. (1982) Antimicrobial agents from higher plants. Dragon's blood resin. *J. Nat. Prods. 45,* 646–648.

Tanida, S, Izawa, M. & Hasegawa, T. (1981) Ansamitocin analogs from a mutant strain of *Nocardia.* I. Isolation of the mutant, fermentation and antimicrobial properties. *J. Antibiotics 3,* 489–495.

DISCUSSION

ANAND: Of over 2500 plants that we have screened, those showing promising antimicrobial activity have been the lowest in number; we have many more with CNS activity, cardiovascular activity and anti-inflammatory activity. Therefore, I believe that in areas such as antimicrobials, where highly active synthetic compounds or antibiotics are already available, we have to depend upon them for clinical practice.

MITSCHER: The specific screening methodology used is extremely important in work of this type. We should exchange our specific protocols in order to identify the sources of the differences in our findings.

ANAND: I believe that synthetic antimicrobial agents which are of definite composition and are stable, are the most suitable for use in developing nations and that is the source which we depend upon.

MITSCHER: Are you talking about chloramphenicol? Chlormaphenicol is often available in developing nations even without a prescription.

ANAND: Not chloramphenicol, because it can have serious side-effects, but many other synthetic antibacterials and antibiotics that are now available.

FARNSWORTH: Did I understand you to say that you isolated aspirin in your studies?

MITSCHER: Yes. We found it in relatively small amounts in our work on *Glycyrrhiza glabra*. It was not active as an antimicrobial agent. We have not found any indication in the literature that aspirin has been isolated previously as a natural product.

FARNSWORTH: Do you believe that any of the compounds whose structures you showed could be used systemically, perhaps after chemical modifications, without having prominent side effects.

MITSCHER: I think that it is possible, based on the wide diversity of activities and structures encountered, but none of the ones mentioned today is an obvious candidate for such use at present.

ARCAMONE: As a chemist involved in the screening of antibiotics for almost 30 years now, I would like to make a comment. I feel that the new, non-classical beta-lactams will cover practically all modern needs of bacterial infections in clinical interest in the next 20 years. Screening should be directed either to β-lactams, in order to add new structural models to this group, or to those infections that may not be treated with β-lactams like viral infection. There is no clinical evidence that plant-derived antibiotics should be effective. They can only be leads for work in universities.

MITSCHER: The new, third generation, β-lactam antibiotics are remarkably active substances with very wide antibiotic spectra, but they are ruinously expensive even for industrialized nations.

ARCAMONE: I don't think that the cost of the drug by itself, if it can reduce the number of days of recovery or prevent hospitalization of the patient, is a great a problem in the case of the new cefalosporins or classical β-lactams.

MITSCHER: I share your enthusiasm for these agents in principle, but in practice the very high cost of these drugs is an important factor to the patients and will discourage them from using their prescriptions. In addition, there are still gaps in their coverage, such as tuberculosis, some anaerobes, fungi, and the viruses you mentioned, for example. Experience also tells us that the antibiotics lose some of their effectiveness after a time, when used in the clinic. There is and will be a continuous need for new classes of antibiotics into the foreseeable future.

ALBUQUERQUE: I think one should be very careful about dumping drugs and chemicals into the third world that would find no use either in The United States or in European countries.

MITSCHER: I agree with you. I would not endorse this either. If they were introduced by third world nations themselves to meet their own needs, then that would be quite another proposition.

BAKER: With regard to your comment on marine sources of antibiotics, we had found the literature virtually useless in determining which organisms would be valuable. Too many reports of antibiotic activity in the literature are not definitive and many are due to frequently occurring substances such as phenols.

14*

Using the systematic technique developed at RRIMP we tested 584 extracts, and, of those, 211 gave positive *in vitro* activity, but only 9 gave positive, valuable *in vivo* activity. However, I would suspect that more study of red algae is merited.

DAVIES: If you look at the most popular antibiotics of long standing, tetracyclines, streptomycin, neomycin, erythromycin, chloramphenicol, etc., you realize that a lot of the structural studies that were done in an attempt to improve their activity were done before one really knew how these antibiotics worked. Would it be worth while going back to do rational modifications, now one has a much better idea of how those particular compounds act in terms of biochemical activity?

MITSCHER: Certainly that is a valuable approach and much work of this type is presently going on. In the chloramphenicol case mentioned previously, there is great difficulty in properly testing new analogues to ensure the lack of devastating idiosyncratic side effects of relatively low incidence.

DJERASSI: Can one develop a clinical or non-clinical assay that will identify the particular side-effects of chloramphenicol?

MITSCHER: I don't know of any such test at present. Curiously, this test may not be necessary any longer. An analogue of chloramphenicol, named thiamphenicol, is available in Europe. It has been used in many patients and has not been reported, as yet, to cause aplastic anemia.

Chemistry of Danomycin, an Iron Containing Antibiotic

Walter Keller-Schierlein, Peter Huber & Hiroshi Kawaguchi[1]

SIDEROPHORES

Many hydrophilic antibiotics have molecules too large to penetrate the cell-membrane barrier by simple diffusion. Active transport mechanisms are necessary for the uptake of antibiotics by bacteria. However, the development of particular mechanisms for the uptake of cell-killing compounds would be contraselective in an evolutionary process.

On the other hand, the organisms had to develop uptake mechanisms for nutrients and other factors necessary for bacterial growth. It has been found in the last twenty years that the uptake of many antibiotics is coupled to the uptake of nutrients: the antibiotics misuse mechanisms developed for the incorporation of sugars, amino acids and lower peptides, and other compounds useful for the bacteria. A particularly illustrative example is the pathway by which some iron-containing antibiotics, the *sideromycins,* enter the bacterial cells. It is the pathway originally developed for the uptake of iron. The uptake of iron, an essential constituent of many enzymes catalyzing redox reactions, is a very difficult task for micro-organisms, because iron is present in the inorganic world predominantly as insoluble hydroxide complexes. Most micro-organisms (possibly all) synthesize compounds which form highly stable and soluble complexes with iron, the *siderophores,* which show a high preference for iron in comparison with other metals (Neilands 1973, Neilands 1981, Keller-Schierlein *et al.* 1964). Bacterial as well as fungal cells have on their cell surfaces membrane-bound proteins acting as specific receptors for the siderophore-iron complexes (*sideramines*).

Organisch-chemisches Laboratorium der Eidg. Technischen Hochschule, Zurich, Switzerland.
[1]Bristol-Banyu Research Institute, Ltd., Tokyo, Japan.

NATURAL PRODUCTS AND DRUG DEVELOPMENT, Alfred Benzon Symposium 20.
Editors: P. Krogsgaard-Larsen, S. Brøgger Christensen, H. Kofod, Munksgaard, Copenhagen 1984.

1    $H_2N-(CH_2)_5-N\overset{|}{\underset{OH}{}}-\overset{O}{\underset{||}{C}}-(CH_2)_2-CO-NH-(CH_2)_5-N\underset{OH}{|}-\overset{O}{\underset{||}{C}}-(CH_2)_2-CO-NH-(CH_2)_5-N\underset{OH}{|}-\overset{O}{\underset{||}{C}}-CH_3$

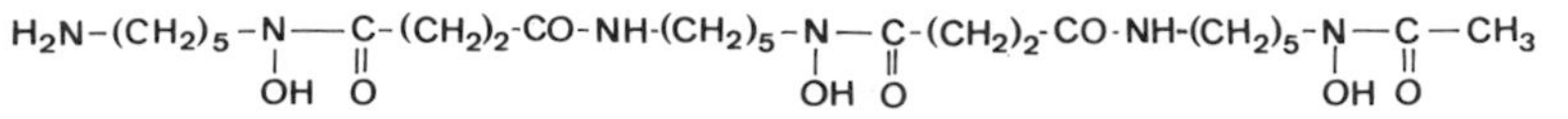

2    $H_2N-(CH_2)_5-N\underset{OH}{|}-\overset{O}{\underset{||}{C}}-(CH_2)_2-CO-NH-(CH_2)_5-N\underset{OH}{|}-\overset{O}{\underset{||}{C}}-(CH_2)_2-CO-NH-(CH_2)_5-N\underset{OH}{|}-\overset{O}{\underset{||}{C}}-(CH_2)_2-COOH$

3

```
      NH-CH₂-CO-NH-CH₂-CO-NH-CH₂-CO
       |            |            |
       |    L       |    L       |    L
      CO-CH-NH-CO-CH-NH-CO-CH-NH
       |            |            |
       CH₂          CH₂          CH₂
       |            |            |
       CH₂          CH₂          CH₂
       |            |            |
       CH₂          CH₂          CH₂
       |            |            |
       N-OH         N-OH         N-OH
       |            |            |
       C=O          C=O          C=O
       |            |            |
       CH₃          CH₃          CH₃
```

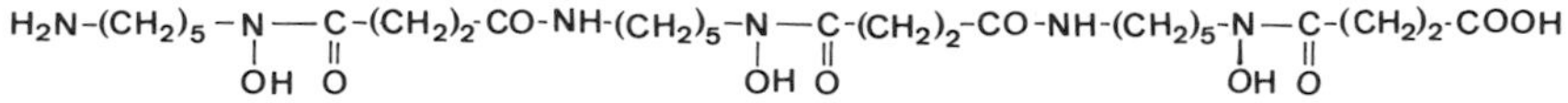

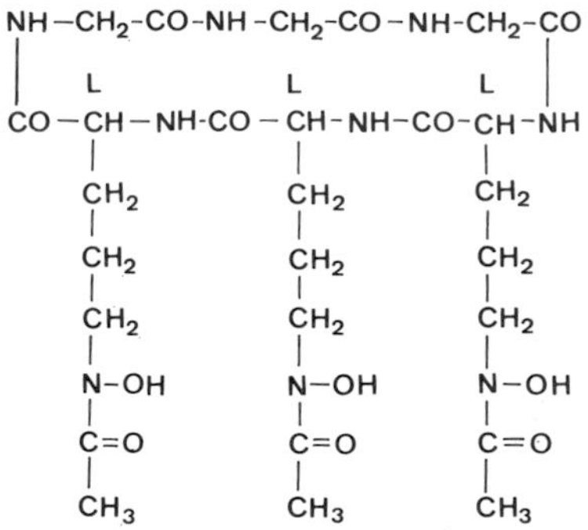

Fig. 1. Structural formulae of deferri-ferrioxamine B (1), deferri-ferrioxamine G (2), and deferri-ferrichrome (3).

Some other membrane proteins of unknown structures, but well-defined genetically, are responsible for the transport of the iron through the membranes (Winkelmann 1982, Winkelmann & Braun 1981, Hantke & Braun 1975). More than 50 different siderophores are known from various species of micro-organisms, many of them being trihydroxamic acids. Three examples are given in Fig. 1. Deferri-ferrioxamine B (1) is the major component of the siderophore mixture of actinomycetes and some groups of bacteria (Müller & Zähner 1968). Deferri-ferrioxamine G (2), a minor component of the same mixture, will play a role in connection with the structure elucidation of danomycin (see below). Deferri-ferrichrome (3) is a typical siderophore of fungal origin. The iron complexes (sideramines) can be depicted in a planar projection as in Fig. 2. It is noteworthy that some entero-bacteria, although their own siderophores are of considerably different structures, have specific receptors for ferrichrome and some closely related cyclohexapeptides and can incorporate iron which is present in the form of ferrichrome (Hantke & Braun 1975).

SIDEROMYCINS

A few antibiotics have been found which are iron complexes of trihydroxamic acids. The first one, *albomycin,* was isolated as early as 1954 (Brazhnikova *et al.*

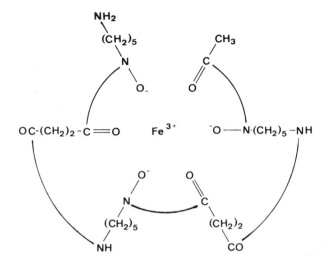

4

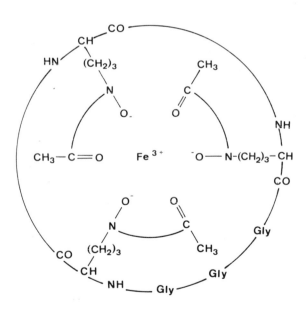

5

Fig. 2. Structural formulae of ferrioxamine B (4) and ferrichrome (5).

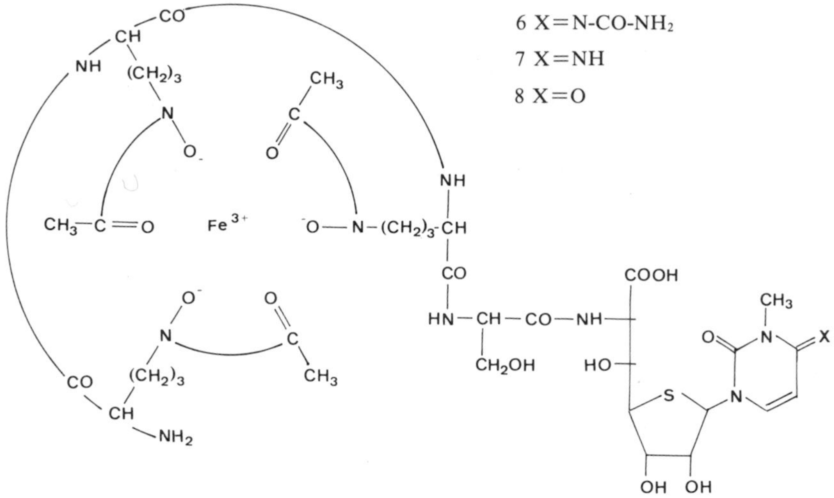

KELLER-SCHIERLEIN ET AL.

6 X=N-CO-NH₂

7 X=NH

8 X=O

Fig. 3. Structural formulae of albomycines δ_2 (6), ε (7), and δ_1 (8).

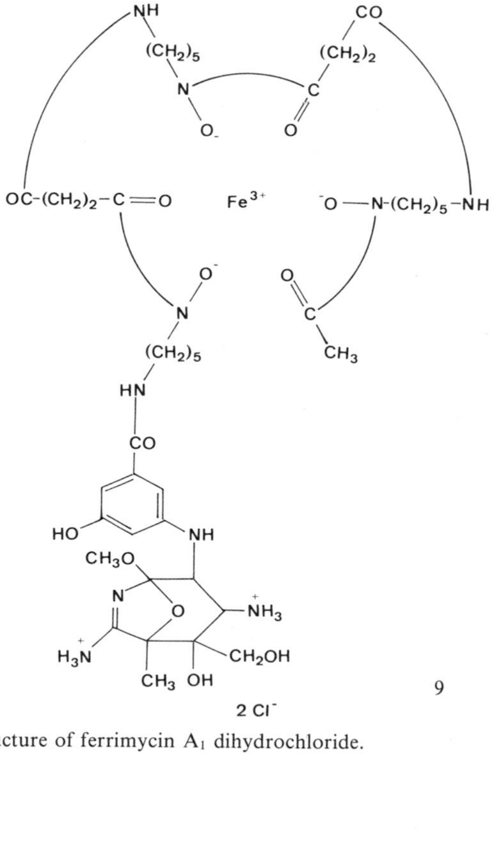

Fig. 4. Tentative structure of ferrimycin A₁ dihydrochloride.

1954) and was later found to be the same as grisein (Stapley & Ormond 1957). Despite considerable efforts to elucidate its structure in the 1960's (Turkovà *et al.* 1964), a complete structure was established only recently (Benz *et al.* 1982). The iron-containing part is similar in its structure to ferrichrome. However, the peptide moiety contains only 4 amino acid residues and is not closed to a large ring (Fig. 3). Albomycin is obviously recognized by the bacterial ferrichrome receptors as a ferrichrome-like sideramine, and is transported into the cells through the ferrichrome pathway. Once in the cell, the unusual nucleoside moiety evolves its inhibitory activity (Hartmann *et al.* 1979).

A second sideromycin, also known for more than 20 years (Bickel *et al.* 1960), is ferrimycin A. The structure given in Fig. 4 differs somewhat in the region of the heterocyclic ring system from that originally proposed by Prelog and his co-workers (Bickel *et al.* 1965). This revision is based on recent spectroscopic investigations carried out in our laboratory. On the other hand, the new spectra fully confirm the structure of the iron-complexing moiety. This part is a perfect copy of the molecule of the major sideramine from actinomycetes, ferrioxamine B.

DANOMYCIN

A third sideromycin, first isolated in 1964 in the Bristol-Banyu Laboratories (Tsukiura *et al.* 1964), is *danomycin*. A compound isolated at about the same

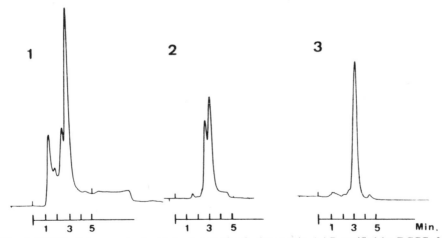

Fig. 5. HPLC of danomycin: 1. crude danomycin; 2. danomycin A+B purified by DCCC; 3. danomycin A purified by prep. HPLC. Column: Merck Lichrosorb RP 8, 10μ; 5 mm×250 mm; uv detector 254 nm, CH$_3$CN - MeOH - 0.2 M NH$_4$OAc - H$_2$O 15:5:15:90; 2 ml/min.

time in Umezawa's group (Ogawara *et al.* 1966) proved to be identical with danomycin, as well as an antibiotic called A 22765, isolated in the Ciba-Geigy Laboratories (Knüsel & Zimmermann 1975). Preliminary chemical investigations on danomycin were reported by Ogawara *et al.* (1966). However, the preparation used for these investigations proved later to be of doubtful purity. A series of amino acids detected in the hydrolysates must originate from peptidic impurities, as we now know that amino acids are not constituents of the antibiotic. On the other hand, the detection of succinic acid, cadaverine, and $FeCl_3$ among the hydrolysis products showed that danomycin is more related to ferrimycin A_1 than to albomycin.

When we began our investigations on danomycin in Zurich, the purification of the antibiotic proved to be a troublesome task. The crude preparation, present as the sulphate (Bristol-Banyu Inst.), contained not only 2 deeply coloured brown-red iron complexes, the danomycins A and B, but also several UV-absorbing iron-free impurities with low retention time (RP-HPLC; acetonitrile - MeOH - 0.2 M NH_4OAc - H_2O 15:5:15:90; UV detector, 254 nm), as shown in Fig. 5, plot 1. By droplet countercurrent chromatography (DCCC; $CHCl_3$-MeOH-PropOH-H_2O 45:60:14:40) we could remove the impurities, but the danomycins A and B were not separated by this procedure (Fig. 5, plot 2). A small sample of pure danomycin A (Fig. 5, plot 3) sufficient for a spectroscopic characterization could, however, be obtained as the free base by preparative HPLC in the system mentioned above.

After the DCCC purification, we observed that the peak of danomycin A had diminished in favour of the first peak (danomycin B). It was obvious that danomycin A had been partly transformed into danomycin B during this procedure. Indeed, when crude danomycin mixture was heated during several hours in aqueous solution, the product contained danomycin B as the predominant coloured iron compound, whereas danomycin A had disappeared. From this mixture it was easy to prepare pure danomycin B in substantial amount by DCCC (BuOH-AcOH - H_2O 4:1:5). The spectroscopic properties of the danomycins A and B were very similar to one another. The ir spectra with major maxima at 3400, 1735, 1645 and 1575 cm^{-1} are nearly superimposable. The UV/vis. spectra (H_2O) show a broad maximum at 430 nm ($E_{1\ cm}^{1\%}$ ca. 20) in accordance with those of the ferrioxamines and ferrichrome. Nmr spectra cannot be measured with the paramagnetic iron complexes. However, the iron can be removed by precipitation with 8-hydroxyquinoline (Keller-Schierlein *et al.* 1964). The deferridanomycins A and B form colourless or pale-brown powders, which gave nearly identical ^{13}C-nmr spectra. The only remarkable difference is a signal at 153.5 ppm in the spectrum of deferridanomycin A which is lacking in deferridanomycin B. This suggested the presence of a carbamate group (-O-CO-NH$_2$) in danomycin A which is replaced by an OH group in danomycin B. Both antibiotics exhibit a high antibacterial activity against *Bacillus subtilis;* danomycin A is slightly more active than danomycin B.

DANOXAMINE

During the transformation of danomycin A into danomycin B the occurrence of a small peak of an additional iron complex was observed, showing a much shorter retention time in our HPLC system (1.5 min versus 2.7 min and 3.1 min for the danomycins B and A, resp.). This compound became the major product when danomycins A or B were subjected to mild hydrolysis with 0.05 N sodium hydroxide at room temperature (7 h).

After purification (DCCC), it was obtained as a brown powder with the composition $C_{27}H_{46}N_5O_{11}Fe. 2 H_2O$. This compound was no longer an antibiotic, but exhibited growth-promoting activity similar to that of the ferrioxamines, albeit at about 10–20 times higher concentration than ferrioxamine B. The compound was named *danoxamine.*

Deferridanoxamine, a colourless powder with mp 139°, gave ^{1}H- and ^{13}C-nmr spectra very similar to those of the known deferriferrioxamines, particularly

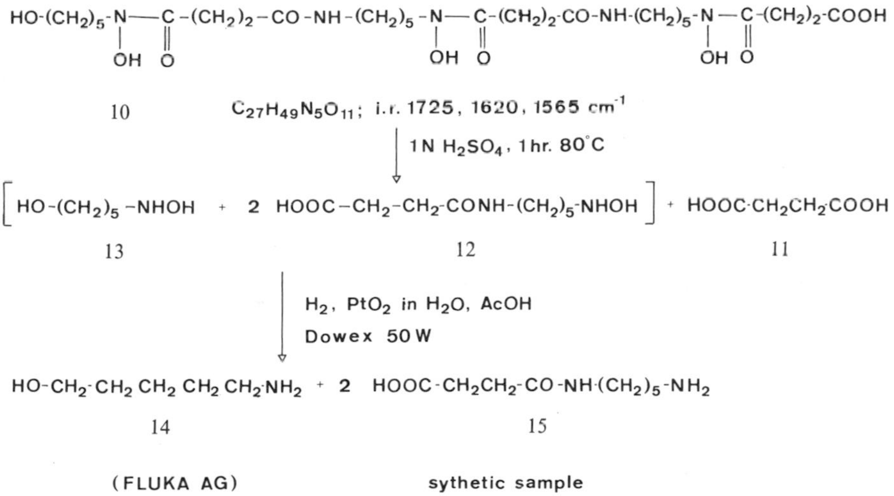

HO-(CH$_2$)$_5$-N—C-(CH$_2$)$_2$-CO-NH-(CH$_2$)$_5$-N—C-(CH$_2$)$_2$-CO-NH-(CH$_2$)$_5$-N—C-(CH$_2$)$_2$-COOH ,
          | || | || | ||
          OH O   OH O   OH O

    10           $C_{27}H_{49}N_5O_{11}$; i.r. 1725, 1620, 1565 cm^{-1}

                       | 1N H$_2$SO$_4$, 1hr. 80°C
                       ↓

[HO-(CH$_2$)$_5$-NHOH + 2 HOOC-CH$_2$-CH$_2$-CONH-(CH$_2$)$_5$-NHOH] + HOOC-CH$_2$CH$_2$-COOH

    13   12   11

                       | H$_2$, PtO$_2$ in H$_2$O, AcOH
                       | Dowex 50 W
                       ↓

HO-CH$_2$-CH$_2$ CH$_2$ CH$_2$ CH$_2$-NH$_2$ + 2 HOOC-CH$_2$CH$_2$-CO-NH-(CH$_2$)$_5$-NH$_2$

      14   15

     (FLUKA AG)   sythetic sample

Fig. 6. Chemical degradation of deferri-danoxamine (10).

^{13}C - NMR. SPECTRA IN DMSO-D$_6$ (75 MHz.)

Deferri-danoxamine	Deferri-ferrioxamine G	Assign.
22.6 ppm	22.9 ppm	C(3)
23.4	23.5	
	25.7	C(4)
26.0	26.0	
26.1	26.5	
27.0	27.0	
27.5	27.6	C(7)
28.3	28.1	C(8)
29.9	29.0	
28.7	28.7	C(2)
32.1	?	
38.4	38.5	C(1)
	38.7	
47.1	47.1	C(5)
60.5	---	CH$_2$OH
171.3	171.5	CON
171.6		
171.9	172.0	
173.9	172.9	COOH

$$-NH-CH_2-CH_2\cdot CH_2-CH_2-CH_2-\underset{\overset{|}{OH}}{N}- \qquad -CO-CH_2-CH_2-CO-$$

$$1 \qquad 2 \qquad 3 \qquad 4 \qquad 5 \qquad\qquad 6 \quad 7 \quad 8 \quad 9$$

deferriferrioxamine G (2 in Fig. 1). The only remarkable difference in the ^{13}C-nmr spectrum was a signal at 60.5 ppm (off-resonance: t; Table I) suggesting the presence of a primary alcohol group. The hypothesis that deferridanoxamine is represented by formula 10 (Fig. 6) could easily be confirmed by chemical

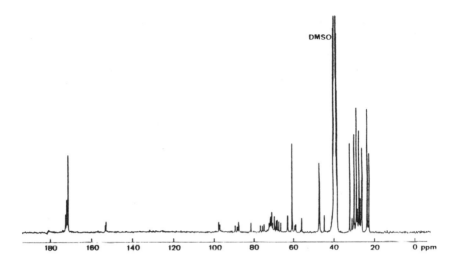

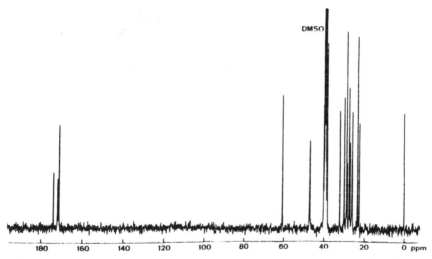

Fig. 7. ^{13}C-nmr spectra in DMSO-d$_6$, noise decoupled, 75 MHz. Top: deferridanomycin A; bottom: deferridanoxamine.

methods. The microanalyses were in accordance with an elementary composition $C_{27}H_{49}N_5O_{11}$. The presence of a carboxylic acid group could be shown by an ir absorption band at 1725 cm^{-1} and the formation of a sodium salt (mp 150°) and a methyl ester. Finally, several degradation products were in best agreement with formula **10** (Fig. 6).

Under mild acidic conditions (1 N H_2SO_4, 1 h., 80°C) which have been shown to cleave completely the hydroxamic acid bonds of ferrioxamine B, whereas amide bonds are not attacked, deferridanoxamine yielded 3 hydrolysis products. From an ether extract nearly 1 mole of pure succinic acid was obtained by crystallization. In the aqueous phase 2 hydroxylamines (12) and (13), giving red spots with triphenyl-tetrazolium reagent, were found by tlc. After reduction of the hydroxylamines to the more stable amines the mixture could be separated by ion exchange chromatography, and the amines (14) and (15) identified by comparison with authentic samples (Fig. 6).

SUGAR COMPONENTS

The nature of the non-sideramine moiety of danomycin is partly clarified by a ^{13}C-nmr comparison of danomycin and danoxamine (Fig. 7). In additon to the signals of danoxamine we find a series of signals in the range 60–80 ppm, characteristic for alcoholic carbon atoms, and several signals in the 90–100 ppm region, characteristic for acetal or hemiacetal carbon atoms. This suggested that the remainder of the danomycin molecule is built up of sugars.

Indeed, when deferridanomycin (520 mg, mixture of A and B) was hydrolysed with 0.12 M barium hydroxide (30 min, room temperature) and the barium removed by neutralization with 0.1 N H_2SO_4 and centrifugation, in addition to deferridanoxamine several fractions were obtained by chromatography on Sephadex G 10 which showed in their ^{13}C-nmr spectra predominantly the signals of sugar- and deoxysugar-like compounds. One particular fraction (7 mg) seemed to be a mixture of 2 or 3 disaccharides with signals at 30.9, 31.4, 56.4, 56.6, 59.6, 60.1, 67.0, 70.3, 70.5, 71.7, 74.4, 76.2, 92.7, and 96.9 ppm. However, other fractions showed much more complex spectra. In order to identify the sugar components we applied a method proposed by Albersheim et al. (1967). Particular carbohydrate fractions (usually ca. 2 mg) from danomycin hydrolysis or deferridanomycin itself were hydrolysed by means of 2 N aq. trifluoroacetic acid (1 h, 120°C), the residues after evaporation were dissolved in 1 N aq. ammonia (0.5 ml) and reduced with 10 mg $NaBH_4$ (1 h, room temp.), and the alditols formed were acetylated (Ac_2O, 3 h, 120°C). The alditol acetates were extracted with ether and analysed by gas-liquid chromatography (Carlo Erba Fractovap G1/450, capillary column Ucon HB-5100, 20 m×0.3 mm; temperature 150°C; He: 3 ml/min.). Samples for comparison were prepared by reduction and acetylation of commercial aldohexoses. From a particular carbohydrate fraction from danomycin equal amounts of the hexaacetates of mannitol ($t_R = 54.4$ min) and glucitol ($t_R = 64.4$ min) were obtained. Another fraction gave mannitol hexaacetate, glucitol hexaacetate, and an unidentified sugar derivative ($t_R = 73.6$ min) in about the same quantity. The disaccharide fraction mentioned above gave glucitol hexaacetate and the unknown derivative ($t_R = 73.6$ min), but no mannitol hexaacetate. However, other fractions of the carbohydrate mixture, and particularly deferridanomycin itself, gave much more complex mixtures by hydrolysis, reduction, and acetylation. In addition to glucitol hexaacetate (major product, 35% of the mixture), mannitol hexaacetate (7%), and the unidentified product ($t_R = 73.6$ min, 24%), peaks with $t_R = 59.0$ min (2%), 60.8 min (30%) and 62.4 min (2%), all different from the derivatives from allose (44.8 min), talose (53.6 min), and galactose (63.2 min), were observed.

Some of these unidentified peaks probably represent derivatives of sugar methyl ethers, because ^{13}C signals (quartets in the off-resonance spectrum) at 58.7 and 59.2 ppm in the spectrum of deferridanomycin (Fig. 7) indicate the presence of O-methyl groups in some of the sugars. This large variety of sugar derivatives is in contrast to the elemental composition of deferridanomycin. The FAB-m.s. shows a quasimolecular ion peak $(M+H)^+$ at 1000 mass units and an ion $(M+Na)^+$ at 1022, in agreement with the composition $C_{41}H_{73}N_7O_{21}$[1]. When we substract from this a deferridanoxamine residue, $C_{27}H_{48}N_5O_{11}$ (618), there remains for the sugar part a residue $C_{14}H_{25}N_2O_{10}$. If one of the sugars is an aldohexose, only 8 carbon atoms are left for the remainder, just sufficient for one additional sugar component containing a carbamate group, an O-methyl group and a free amino group.

In addition to mannose and glucose, deoxyhexoses seem to be present in danomycin, since the quasimolecular peak at 1000 is accompanied by a second peak 16 mass units lower, at m/z 984 (MH^+; $MNa^+ = 1006$). Minor contaminants of the composition $C_{41}H_{73}N_7O_{20}$ must therefore be present. These deoxysugars give rise to some minor signals in the 30 ppm region of the ^{13}C-nmr spectrum of deferridanomycin (Fig. 7).

This preliminary investigation of the sugar components of danomycin shows that glucose, mannose, and the deoxysugars cannot be constituents of one single danomycin molecule. This means that chromatographically pure danomycin is

---

[1] Elemental analysis of a danomycin A sample purified by prep. HPLC, an amorphous brown powder: found C 43.80 H 6.26 N 8.60 Fe 4.52%; calcd. for $C_{41}H_{70}N_7O_{21}Fe.3\,H_2O$: C 44.48 H 6.92 N 8.86 Fe 5.04%.

still a mixture of compounds containing the same iron-complexing moiety - danoxamine -, but various sugar components in a disaccharide moiety. This makes this investigation so difficult: no single disaccharide could be obtained upon mild alkaline hydrolysis of danomycin, and no pure monosaccharide could be isolated in sufficient amount for a complete spectroscopic characterization.

CONCLUSIONS

At the provisional end of this investigation we can say that danomycin (Fig. 8) is a mixture of sideromycins containing as the sideramine moiety, responsible for the uptake into bacterial cells, a danoxamine residue which is related to the bacterial siderophore ferrioxamine G. The moiety responsible for the antibacterial activity is a non-uniform disaccharide consisting of an aldohexose (glucose, mannose, deoxysugar) and a non-identified amino sugar, carrying a carbamate group, a methoxy residue, and a free amino group.

ACKNOWLEDGEMENT

We are grateful to Ciba-Geigy AG, Basel, for financial support, to Bristol-Banyu Institute, Tokyo, for crude danomycin, and to Prof. H. Zähner, Tübingen, for biological tests.

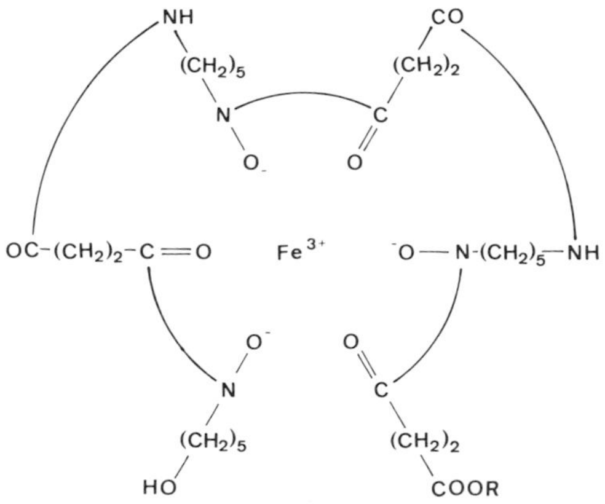

16 Danoxamine, $R = H$

17 Danomycin B, $R = C_{13}H_{24}NO_9$ ($C_{13}H_{24}NO_8$)

18 Danomycin A, $R = C_{13}H_{23}NO_8$-OCONH$_2$ ($C_{13}H_{23}NO_7$-OCONH$_2$)

Fig. 8. Structure of danoxamine (16); partial structures of danomycin B (17) and danomycin A (18).

REFERENCES

Albersheim, P., Nevins, D. J., English, P. D., & Karr, A. (1967) A method for the analysis of sugars in plant cell-wall polysaccharides by gas-liquid chromatography. *Carbohydrate Research* 5, 340–345.

Benz, G., Schröder, T., Kurz, J., Wünsche, Ch., Karl, W., Steffens, G., Pfitzner, J., & Schmidt, D, (1982) Konstitution der Desferriform der Albomycine δ_1, δ_2 und ε. *Angew. Chem. 94*, 552–553.

Bickel, H., Gäumann, E., Nussberger, G., Reusser, P., Vischer, E., Voser, W., Wettstein, A. and Zähner, H. (1960) Ueber die Isolierung und Charakterisierung der Ferrimycine A_1 und A_2, neuer Antibiotica der Sideromycin-Gruppe. *Helv. Chim. Acta 43*, 2105–2118.

Bickel, H., Mertens, P., Prelog, V., Seibl, J., & Walser, A. (1966) Ueber die Konstitution von Ferrimycin A_1. *Tetrahedron Suppl. 8, Part I*, 171–179.

Brazhnikova, M. G., Lomakina, N. N. & Muravieva, L. I. (1954) Albomycin, its properties and chemical nature. *Doklady Akad. Nauk (USSR) 99*, 827–830.

Hantke, K. & Braun, V. (1975) Membrane receptor dependent iron transport in *Escherichia coli. FEBS Letters 49*, 301–305.

Hartmann, A., Fiedler, H.-P., & Braun, V. (1979) Uptake and conversion of the antibiotic albomycin by *Escherichia coli* K-12. *Eur. J. Biochem. 99*, 517–524.

Keller-Schierlein, W., Prelog, V., & Zähner, H. (1964) Siderochrome (natürliche Eisen (III)-trihydroxamat-Komplexe). In: *Progress in the Chemistry of Organic Natural Products*, ed. L. Zechmeister, Vol. 22, pp. 279–322. Springer, Wien.

Knüsel, F. & Zimmermann, W. (1975) Sideromycins. In: *Antibiotics. Mechanisms and Action of Antimicrobial and Antitumor Agents*, ed. J. W. Corcoran & F. E. Hahn, Vol. III, pp.653–667. Springer-Verlag, Berlin, Heidelberg, New York.

Neilands, J. B. (1981) Microbial iron compounds. *Ann. Rev. Biochem. 50*, 715–731.

Neilands, J. B. (1973) Microbial iron transport compounds (siderochromes). In: *Inorganic Biochemistry*, ed. G. L. Eichhorn, Vol. 1, pp. 167–202. Elsevier, Amsterdam.

Ogawara, H., Maeda, K., & Umezawa, H. (1966) Degradation studies on danomycin *J. Antibiotics (Tokyo), Ser. A, 19*, 190–192.

Stapley, E. O. & Ormond, R. E. (1957) Similarity of albomycin and grisein. *Science 125*, 587–589.

Tsukiura, H., Okanishi, M., Ohmori, T., Koshiyama, H., Miyaki, T., Kitazima, H., & Kawaguchi, H. (1964) Danomycin, a new antibiotic. *J. Antibiotics (Tokyo), Ser. A, 17*, 39–47.

Turková, J., Mikeš, O., & Sorm, F. (1964) Chemical composition of the antibiotic albomycin. VI. Determination of the structure of the peptide moiety of the antibiotic albomycin. *Collect Czech. Chem. Comm. 29*, 280–288.

Winkelmann, G. (1982) Specificity of siderophore iron uptake by fungi. In: *The Biological Chemistry of Iron*, eds. H. B. Dunford, D. Dolphin, K. N. Raymond & L. Sieker, pp. 107–116.

Winkelmann, G. & Braun, V. (1981) Stereoselective recognition of ferrichrome by fungi and bacteria. *FEMS Microbiology Letters 11*, 237–241.

DISCUSSION

ANAND: What is the action of danomycin or the iron-containing antibiotics on blood cells?

KELLER-SCHIERLEIN: I think this has not been investigated very much. These antibiotics are very untoxic. On the other hand, deferri-ferrioxamine-B is used in medicine in order to remove pathological deposits or iron from patients who have some iron overload either by blood transfusions or, also, by some metabolic diseases. No negative effect on blood has been observed. Intense pharmacological and biochemical investigations with deferri-ferrioxamine-B have shown that it does not remove iron from hemin, hemoglobin, or from the iron-containing blood proteins like transferrin.

DAVIES: Do bacteria resistant to these antibiotics have defective iron-uptake pathways?

KELLER-SCHIERLEIN: Yes. This loss is not at all lethal, because most bacteria have different iron-uptake mechanisms at high iron supply. Even citrate is often sufficient for supplying the cells with iron. The bacteria which have lost the ferrichrome iron-uptake mechanisms are resistant also to sideromycins.

DAVIES: Since you say that the modes of action of the 3 compounds are different, can you give us any ideas as to the mechanism of action?

KELLER-SCHIERLEIN: For danomycin it has been recently demonstrated that it acts on the ribosome. For the other 2, albomycin and ferrimycin A, we only know that it has nothing to do with the ribosome or protein synthesis.

RAZDAN: How specific is danomycin iron-(III) complexing?

KELLER-SCHIERLEIN: The ability of danomycin to complex with other metals than iron has not been investigated, but ferrioxamine and also ferrichrome form complexes with many metals, aluminum, lantanides, and many others, but the preference for iron (III) is very high. Iron has a stability constant of about 10^{30}, the next one then is aluminium with about 10^{22}[1,2].

NAKANISHI: In the danomycin B, do you get 2 molecular iron peaks in the mass spectra, and was the DCCC done on the ferro compound?

KELLER-SCHIERLEIN: The DCCC was done with the iron complexes. The mass spectrum was made of the de-ferri compound of pure danomycin A, and we observed predominantly one peak, but also a smaller side peak 16 units lower, which indicates that de-oxy sugars could also be present as building stones.

(1) Anderegg, G., F. l'Eplattenier & G. Schwarzenbach (1936a) *Helv. Chim. Acta 46,* 1400–1408.
(2) Anderegg, G., F. l'Eplattenier & G. Schwarzenbach (1936b) *Helv. Chim. Acta 46,* 1409–1422.

Antineoplastic Agents from Higher Plants: Novel Xanthones from *Psorospermum Febrifugum*

John M. Cassady, C.-J. Chang, A. M. Habib, David Ho, Ashok Amonkar & S. Masuda

Psorospermum febrifugum Sprach. is a woody plant of tropical Africa which occurs in the family Guttiferae. The Guttiferae is composed of forty genera and members occur mainly in tropical areas. Members of the family have been reported to have a variety of medicinal properties (Streelman 1977, Sultanbawa 1980). Previous chemical studies on *Psorospermum* led to the isolation (Kupchan *et al.* 1980) of a novel xanthone named psorospermin **1**. Psorospermin was isolated in very low yield (0.004%) using an activity directed isolation procedure. Based on chemical and spectroscopic evidence, structure **1** was proposed for psorospermin, however, lack of sufficient material precluded establishment of the stereochemistry at the 2',3' positions in the unique epoxydihydrofuran moiety. Insufficient material also limited testing, however, **1** was shown to have significant effects in several systems and is one of a very limited group of natural xanthones which show significant antitumor activity (Douros & Suffness 1981, Cassady *et al.* 1981). Psorospermin was cytotoxic in cell culture (9KB cells, $ED_{50} = 10^{-1}$ μg/ml) and inhibited mitosis in sea urchin eggs at 10^{-6} M. In addition, and more significantly, psorospermin showed activity in the P-388 mouse leukemia model with T/C ranging from 140–165% at doses from 0.1 to 8 mg/kg. The highest dose tested was 8 mg/kg due to limited material and its toxic dose was not reached at this level. In addition, psorospermin was active in 2 solid tumors, a mammary (CD) and colon (C_6) model (Suffness 1979).

Department of Medicinal Chemistry and Pharmacognosy, School of Pharmacy, Purdue University, West Lafayette, IN 47907 U.S.A.

NATURAL PRODUCTS AND DRUG DEVELOPMENT, Alfred Benzon Symposium 20.
Editors: P. Krogsgaard-Larsen, S. Brøgger Christensen, H. Kofod, Munksgaard, Copenhagen 1984.

Based on this observation, our research group initiated an investigation of *Psorospermum febrifugum* in order to re-isolate **1** to complete the assignment of the stereochemistry of the compound and its biological evaluation. A recollection of the plant from Nigeria was fractionated and led to the isolation of the novel antileukemic anthrone **2** (Amonkar *et al.* 1981), however, no trace of **1** was contained in this plant source. A recollection of the plant from the original source in Tanzania has now been examined and has yielded trace amounts of **1** (0.0002%) and a series of related, novel xanthones including 3',4'-deoxypsorospermin **3**, 3',4'-deoxypsorospermin-3',4'-diol **4**, and 3',4'-deoxypsorospermin-3',4'-chlorohydrin **5** (Fig. 1).

The dried, ground woody portions of *P. febrifugum* from Tanzania were defatted with hexane and extracted with ethanol. The resulting extract (1.38 kg from 15 kg of plant) was partitioned between chloroform and water with the activity being concentrated in the chloroform layer. The chloroform extract was then partitioned between hexane and 10% aqueous methanol to give an active methanol extract and an active interface. Chromatography of the methanol extract on silica gel with chloroform and chloroform containing increasing amounts of methanol gave a fraction eluted with 3% methanol in chloroform which on rechromatography on silica gel with 20–50% ethyl acetate in benzene followed by repeated preparative-tlc gave **1** in 0.0002% yield.

Analysis of the fraction eluted from the first silica gel column with 2% methanol in chloroform, and the interface, by tlc indicated that these fractions

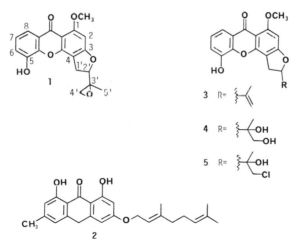

Fig. 1. Structures of xanthones and anthrones isolated from *Psorospermum febrifugum*.

contained compounds related to **1**. Partition fractions from these mixtures which contained 2 major fluorescent spots were combined and chromatographed on an alumina column. Fractions from this column yielded 3',4'-deoxypsorospermin **3**. High resolution mass spectrometry showed a molecular ion at m/e 324.0996 and established a molecular formula of $C_{19}H_{16}O_5$ (324.0997) for **3**. Evidence of a close relationship the **1** included the optical rotation $[\alpha]_D^{20}$ $-46°C$ (c=0.1, MeOH), and a strong band at $1647 \, cm^{-1}$ in the infrared typical for a xanthone carbonyl. The ultraviolet spectrum was also typical of a substituted xanthone, and very similar to **1**, with λ_{max}^{MeOH} (log ε) 247 (4.59) and 310 nm (4.13) (Kupchan *et al.* 1980). Comparison of the ^{1}Hnmr spectrum of **1** and **3** led to the structural assignment (Table I). The major differences in the spectra occurred in the position and pattern of the protons at 2', 4', and 5'. The pair of doublets at 2.68 and 2.93 ppm in **1**, typical for the geminal protons of an *a,a*-disubstituted epoxide were replaced by a pair of doublets at 4.97 and 5.12 ppm typical of terminal vinyl methylene protons. The appearance of the 5' protons at 1.8 ppm and the downfield shift of the 2'-H from 4.87 in **1** to 5.4 ppm in **3** were consistent with those expected for 3',4'-deoxypsorospermin **3**.

A chloroform partition fraction was derived from adsorption of the ethanol extract on cellulose, followed by successive extractions with toluene-hexane and acetone, then methanol and aqueous methanol. The methanol extracts were back-partitioned into chloroform and triturated with toluene-hexane. The residue was then chromatographed on a silica column to give a fraction which on

Table I
^{1}H-NMR spectral data, psorospermin and related xanthones

Proton	Cmpd. **1**†	Cmpd. **3**†	Cmpd. **4**‡	Cmpd. **5**‡
1-OCH₃	3.96 s	3.96 s	3.84 s	3.84 s
2-H	6.37 s	6.37 s	6.51 s	6.57 s
6-H	7.22 dd (7.8, 1.7)	7.23 dd (7.8, 1.8)	7.21 dd (7.3, 2.1)	7.22 dd (7.3, 2.2)
7-H	7.19 t(7.8)	7.19 t (7.8)	7.15 t (7.3)	7.15 t (7.3)
8-H	7.80 dd (7.8, 1.7)	7.80 dd (7.8, 1.8)	7.48 dd (7.3, 2.1)	7.48 dd (7.3, 2.2)
1'-Ha	3.49 dd (15,9.9)	3.53 dd (15.5, 7.5)	3.31 d (8.7)	3.3 d (8.7)
1'-Hb	3.30 dd (15,7.2)	3.18 dd (15.5. 9.0)		
2'-H	4.85 dd (9.9, 7.2)	5.40 dd (9.0, 7.5)	5.0 t (8.7)	5.08 t (8.7)
4'-Ha	2.98 d (4.5)	4.97 d (1)	3.57 dd (10.6, 5.0)	3.80 d (10.7)
4'-Hb	2.73 d (4.5)	5.12 d (1)	3.34 dd (10.6, 5.0)	3.63 (10.7)
5'-H	1.43 s	1.80 s	1.11 s	1.24 s

†470 MHz, CDCl₃
‡200 MHz, DMSO-D₆

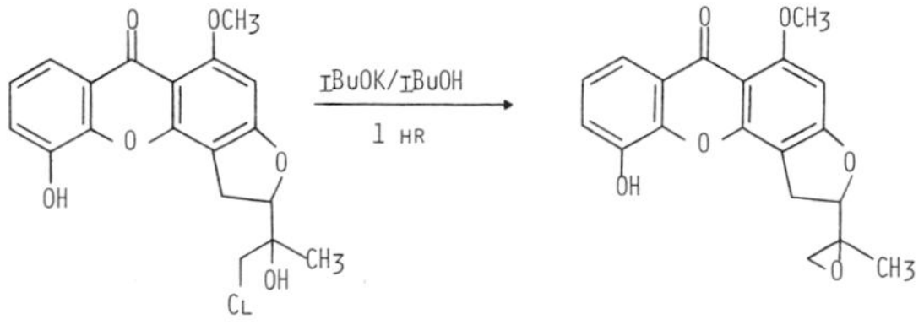

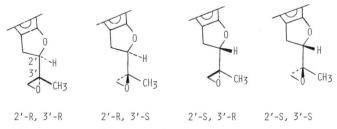

Fig. 2. Chemical conversion of chlorohydrin to psorospermin.

repeated crystallization yielded the chlorohydrin **5**. The diol, **4**, was obtained by absorbing a subsequent fraction on celite, followed by extraction into chloroform, partition into aqueous methanol, and finally partition into chloroform-isopropanol from water. Chromatography of the chloroform-isopropanol fraction on silica gel gave a fraction enriched in diol **4**.

Compound **4** melted at 278–279°C and showed a negative optical rotation, $[a]_D^{20}$ −114°C (c=0.1, MeOH). The molecular formula of **4** was $C_{19}H_{18}O_7$ (359.1131 for M+H$^+$) based on a molecular ion at m/e 359.1123 (M+H'). The xanthone carbonyl group was revealed by the infrared absorption at 1640 cm^{-1}. Absorption in the ultraviolet at λ_{max}^{MeOH}(log ε) 247 (4.57) and 310 nm (4.13) was again typical of the xanthone chromophore. Assignment of the structure to the 3',4'-diol corresponding to **1** was confirmed by the ^{1}Hnmr spectrum of **4** (Table I). Again the major differences occurred in the positions of the aliphatic protons at 1', 2', 4', and 5' of the substituted furan moiety. The 4'-methylene signals in **1** at 2.68 and 2.93 ppm were absent and replaced by signals at 3.57 (dd, J=10.6, 5.0) and 3.34 ppm (dd, J=10.6, 5.0) in DMSO-d$_6$. A hydroxyl proton appeared at 4.82 ppm (t, 5.0) and supported presence of a terminal -CH$_2$-OH group. The singlet for the 5' protons at 1.11 ppm suggested a methyl on carbon attached to the other (tertiary) alcohol group. These data are consistent with the assignment of **4** to the structure 3',4'-deoxypsorospermin-3',4'-diol.

2'-R, 3'-R   2'-R, 3'-S   2'-S, 3'-R   2'-S, 3'-S

Fig. 3. Possible stereoisomers of psorospermin.

Compound **5** crystallized from methanol-ether and showed a mp at 269–270°C and an optical rotation $[a]_D^{20} = -114°C$ (c=0.1, MeOH). High resolution mass spectrometry established a molecular formula of $C_{19}H_{17}O_6Cl$ (found 377.0786, calculated for $M+H^+$, 377.0792). Absorption in the ultraviolet at λ_{max}^{MeOH} (log ε) 247 (4.67) and 311 nm (4.26) coupled with the typical carbonyl absorption in the infrared at 1642 cm^{-1} again supported the presence of the xanthone chromophore and suggested a compound closely related to **1, 3,** and **4**. The aromatic region of the nmr spectrum of **5** was very similar to **1, 3,** and **4**. Again the epoxide methylene signals were missing and were replaced with a two proton AB pattern at 3.63 and 3.80 ppm (J=10.7) consistent with a terminal - CH$_2$-Cl grouping. Final confirmation of structure **5** was obtained by converting **5** to **1** by treatment with *t*-butoxide (Fig. 2).

As indicated previously, the absolute stereochemistry of psorospermin **1** at the 2' and 3' centers of the epoxydihydrofuran moiety remains to be established. The compound can exist as one of 4 possible isomers as illustrated in Fig. 3. Psorospermin and related compounds exhibit plain negative Cotton curves and, thus, appear to belong to the 2'-R series of compounds which are related to (-)-rotenone and derived compounds such as tubaic acid and the epoxytubaic acids (Unai *et al.* 1973a, 1973b, Begley *et al.* 1975). Tubaic acid is obtained by degradation of (-)-rotenone (Buchi *et al.* 1961), and can be converted to separable diastereoisomeric epoxides as outlined in Fig. 4, and 5. Compounds **1,**

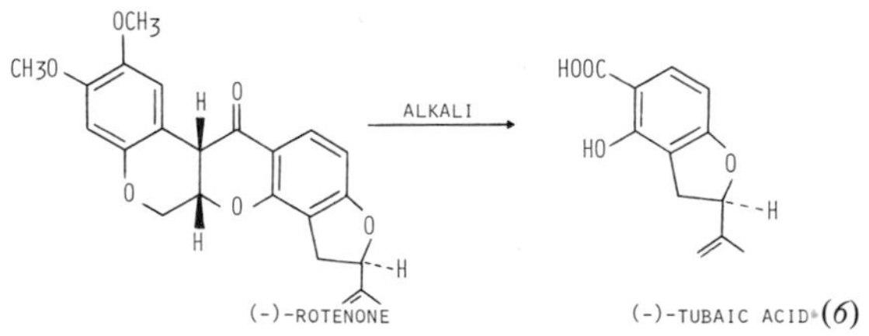

Fig. 4. Conversion of rotenone to tubaic acid.

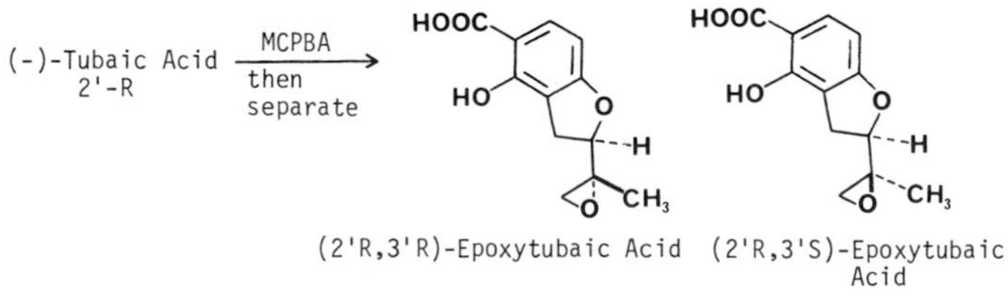

Fig. 5. Conversion of tubaic acid to epoxytubaic acids (**7a, 7b**).

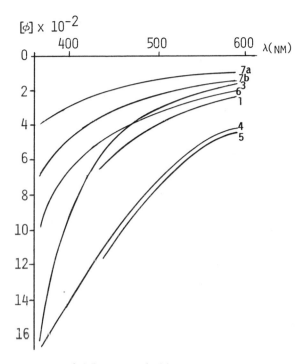

Plain negative cotton curves of a) Psorospermin (**1**),
b) 3',4'-Deoxypsorospermin (**3**), c)3',4'-Deoxy-psorospermin-3',4'-diol (**4**),
d) 3',4'-Deoxypsorospermin-3',4'-chlorohydrin (**5**),
e) Tubaic acid (**6**), f) Epoxytubaic Acid-lower R_f isomer (**7a**),
and g) Epoxytubaic acid-higher R_f isomer (**7b**).

Fig. 6. Cotton curves of 2'-R series and psorospermin and related xanthones.

3, 4, 5 and the tubaic acid derivatives which are related to rotenone display similar Cotton curves as illustrated in Fig. 6, and in contrast to those shown by compounds in the 2'-S series such as fomannoxin (Fig. 7) which exhibits a plain positive curve (Donnelly & O'Reilly 1980).

The terminal 3',4'-epoxide is unique among natural products of this type although a mixture of diastereoisomeric epoxides have been prepared from rotenone by epoxidation with m-chloroperbenzoic acid and separated into individual isomers (Unai *et al.* 1973a). Epimers of this type can be differentiated by ^{1}Hnmr spectra based on the relative chemical shifts for the 4'-methylene protons. Psorospermin **1** shows an nmr pattern which is very similar to one of the diastereoisomeric epoxides derived by epoxidation of (-)-tubaic acid (Table

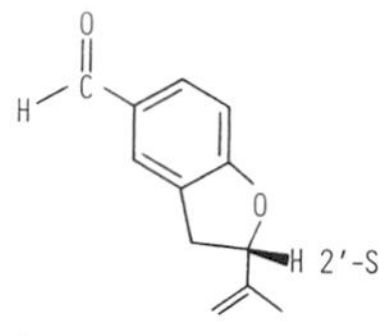

Fig. 7. (+)-Fomannoxin from *Fomes Annosus*.

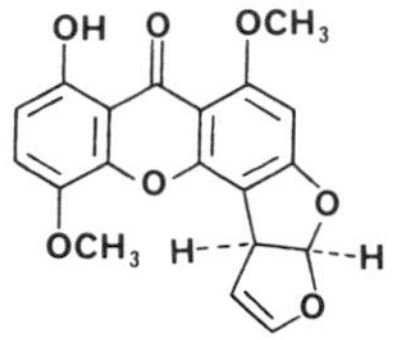

5-methoxysterigmatocystin 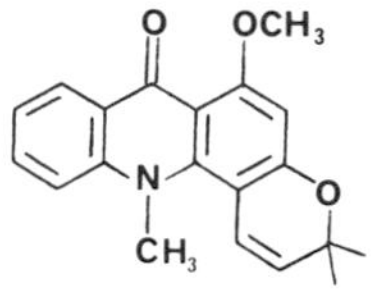   acronycine 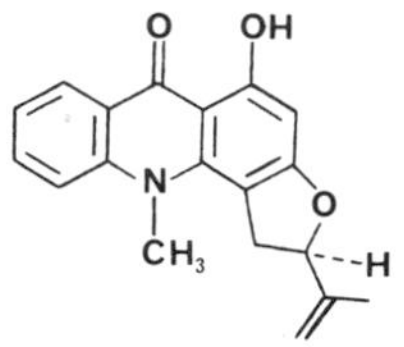   rutacridone

Fig. 8. Structures of xanthone and acridones with potential anticancer activity.

II). Establishment of the relative configuration of either epoxytubaic acid would in turn allow assignment of the complete stereochemistry of **1**.

The significant preliminary anticancer acitivity shown by **1** places it among a very small number of substituted xanthones which have been established to have anti-cancer effects. The carcinogenic fungal metabolite, 5-methoxysterigmato-cystin, which was isolated from *Aspergillus versicolor* (Bradner *et al.* 1975, Essery *et al.* 1976) has also shown significant activity (Fig. 8).

Sterigmatocystin shares one of its primary biological effects, inhibition of nucleoside transport, with another structurally related anti-cancer agent with an acridone structure, acronycine (Liska 1972, Svoboda *et al.* 1966, Kurimoto *et al.* 1974, Tan & Aversperg 1973) which was isolated from the plant *Acronychia*

Table II
Comparison of 470 MHz ^{1}H-NMR data (CDCl$_3$)

| Proton | Psorospermin | Epoxytubaic Acids | |
		Lower R$_f$ Isomer	Higher R$_f$ Isomer
1'	3.30 (dd, J=7.2, 15.0)	3.11 (dd, J=7.4, 15.7)	3.07 (dd, J=7.6, 15.7)
	3.49 (dd, J=15.0, 9.9)	3.30 (dd, J=9.9, 15.7)	3.23 (dd, J=9.9, 15.7)
2'	4.85 (dd, J=7.2, 9.9)	4.78 (dd, J=7.4, 9.9)	4.83 (dd, J=7.6, 9.9)
4'	2.73 (d, J=4.5)	2.70 (d, J=4.7)	2.71 (d, J=4.6)
	2.98 (d, J=4.5)	2.94 (d, J=4.7)	2.82 (d, J=4.6)
5'	1.43 (s)	1.38 (s)	1.41 (s)

bauerii by a research group at Eli Lilly and Co. Acronycine received clinical trial but was dropped due to lack of broad spectrum activity. Another natural product with the acridone structure which has never been evaluated for anti-cancer acitivity is the compound rutacridone (Fig. 8) which bears a striking resemblance to **1**. This compound can serve as a semi-synthetic intermediate to acridone analogs of **1** and arrangements have been made with Gröger (Halle) to obtain this compound which is produced in plant cell cultures of *Ruta graveolens* (Baumert *et al.* 1982).

Results of testing the natural analogs of **1** including **2**, **3**, **4** and **5** have established the importance of the configuration and functionality of the substituent attached to the xanthone system. Compound **1** is clearly the most active *in vivo*. Both **2** and **5** show borderline activity in P388 *in vivo*, and **3** and **4** are inactive. Further research is underway to establish the mechanism of the anti-tumor action of **1** and related compounds and also to establish structure-anti-tumor activity relationships in this series.

ACKNOWLEDGEMENT

The authors would like to thank the Economic Botany Laboratory, USDA, Beltsville, MD, for the collection and identification of *P. febrifugum*. High resolution (470 MHz) NMR spectra were recorded at the Purdue University Biological Magnetic Resonance Laboratory supported by NIH Grant RR01077 from the Division of Research Resources. This work was funded by Grant No. CA33326 from PHS, NCI, Bethesda, MD.

REFERENCES

Amonkar, A., Chang, C.-j., & Cassady, J. M. (1981) 6-Geranyloxy-3-methyl-1,8-dihydroxyan-throne, a novel antileukemic agent from *Psorospermum febrifugum* Sprach. *Experientia 37,* 1138.
Baumert, A., Kuzovkina, I. N., Krauss, G., Hieke, M. & Gröger, D. (1982) Biosynthesis of Rutacridone in Tissue Cultures of *Ruta Graveolens*. L. *Plant Cell Reports 1,* 168.
Begley, M. J., Crombie, L., and Whiting, D. A. (1975) Conformation and Absolute Configuration of Rotenone: Examination of 8'-Bromorotenone by X-Ray Methods. *J. Chem. Soc.* 850.
Bradner, W. T., Bush, J. A., Myelymaki, R. W., Nettleton, D. E. & O'Herron, F. A. (1975) Fermentation, Isolation and Antitumor Activity of Sterigmatocystins. *Antimicrobial Agents and Chemotherapy, 8,* 159.
Buchi, G., Crombie, L., Godin, P. J., Kaltenbronn, J. S., Siddalingaiah, K. S. & Whiting, D. A. (1961) The Absolute Configuration of Rotenone. *J. Chem. Soc.* 2843.
Cassady, J. M., Chang, C.-j., & McLaughlin, J. L. (1981) Recent Advances in the Isolation and

Structural Elucidation of Antineoplastic Agents of Higher Plants. In: *Natural Products as Medicinal Agents,* ed. J. L. Beal and E. Reinhard. Hippokrates Verlag, Stuttgart, pp. 93–124.

Donnelly, D. M. X. & O'Reilly, J. (1980) Synthesis of (±)-Fomannoxin: Absolute Configuration of (+)-Fomannoxin. *J. Chem. Res.* (M) 0124.

Douros, J. & Suffness, M. (1981) New Antitumor Substances of Natural Origin. *Cancer Treatment Reviews 8,* 63.

Essery, J. M., O'Herron, F. A., McGregor, D. N. & Bradner, W. T. (1976) Preparation and Antitumor Activities of Some Derivatives of 5-Methoxysterigmatocystin. *J. Med. Chem. 19,* 1339.

Kurimoto, T., Kurimoto, Y., Aibara, K. & Miyaki, K. (1974) Inhibition of Nucleoside Transport by Aflatoxins and Sterigmatocystin. *Cancer Res. 34,* 968.

Kupchan, S. M., Streelman, D. R. & Sneden, A. T. (1980) Psorospermin, A New Antileukemic Xanthone from *Psorospermum Febrifugum. J. Nat. Products 43,* 296.

Liska, K. J. (1972) Preparation and Antitumor Properties of Analogs of Acronycine. *J. Med. Chem. 15,* 1177.

Streelman, D. R. (1977) The Chemistry of Some Potent Antileukemic Principles from Plants, Ph. D. Thesis, University of Virginia, Charlottesville, August.

Suffness, M. (1979) Private communcation of NCI files documenting antitumor acitivity of xanthones.

Sultanbawa, M. U. S. (1980) Xanthanoids of Tropical Plants. *Tetrahedron 36,* 1465.

Svoboda, G., Poore, G. A., Simpson, P. J. & Boder, G. B. (1966) Alkaloids of *Acronychia Baueri* Schott. I. Isolation of the Alkaloids and A Study of the Antitumor and Other Biological Properties. *J. Pharm. Sci. 55,* 758.

Tan, P. & Aversperg, N. (1973) Effects of the Antineoplastic Alkaloid Acronycine on the Ultrastructure and Growth Patterns of Cultured Cells, *Cancer Res 33,* 2320.

Unai, T., Yamamoto, I., Cheng, H.-M. & Casida, J. E. (1973a) Synthesis and Stereochemical Characterization of Hydroxy- and Epoxy-derivatives of Rotenone. *Agr. Biol. Chem. 37,* 387.

Unai, T. & Yamamoto, I. (1973b) Synthesis of the Stereoisomers of Natural Rotenone. *Agr. Biol. Chem. 37,* 897.

DISCUSSION

WALL: The basic difference between the xanthone and the acronycine is the substitution of a nitrogen for the oxygen. That nitrogen will give you an extended conjugation, which you lack in the xanthone, and predictably, I don't think the xanthones could ever be very active because normally you need at least 3 conjugated rings.

CASSADY: It is also very clear that there are some very active xanthones, for example the sterigmatocysins have shown encouraging T/C values at higher doses. I agree with you that moving to the acridone series might actually improve things and these studies are underway in our research group.

RAZDAN: Could the activity be explained by the alkylating properties of the epoxide, or maybe a combination of the properties of the epoxide and the rings?

CASSADY: In general, what has been found with simple epoxides is that they produce a cytotoxic effect, but not an anti-tumour effect. A compound of this type must be bifunctional in order to have significant anti-tumour activity. The activity of psorospermin does require both the intact xanthone nucleus and the reactive epoxide. In compounds of this type, one alkylating group is sufficient.

WAGNER: Do your compounds have anti-malaria activity as the botanic name *febrifuga* might suggest.

CASSADY: We have not isolated enough compound to really do extensive testing of anti-malerial activity.

KUTNEY: As you indicated, the biological activity seems to be related to the chirality of the epoxide. Have you considered synthesizing analogous epoxides?

CASSADY: Yes, we are working in that direction. We don't want to move too quickly until we have established the stereo-chemistry.

FARNSWORTH: How would you select a class of anti-tumour agents for initiating synthesis and structure activity studies? Would a T/C value of 158 be encouraging?

CASSADY: This question is a very important one and it is not easy to propose an exact formula for the medicinal chemist to use. One factor certainly would be the novelty of the class compound. Other factors would include the level of activity in the P388 pre-screen as you suggest but also the spectrum of activity, especially in animal tumour models. A word of caution must be added here, based on recent developments in the clinical use of derivatives of podophyllotoxin, a plant lignan which was established to be cytotoxic by J. Hartwell, including the epimeric analogue VP-16 which was developed by Sandoz. VP-16 has shown significant clinical effects in treatment of solid tumours including resistant testicular cancer. Here is a dramatic example of modifying weakly active (cytotoxic in cell culture, no activity in animal tumour models) and highly toxic lead compounds and developing highly active, clinically significant drugs.

NAKANISHI: We are using a modified Ames test, about 5–600 plants have been screened, and 5 anti-mutagens have been identified, only one has been published. We are using *E. coli* and observing the ability of extracts to prevent mutagenesis.

CASSADY: I think that what you are talking about falls into the general area of chemo-prevention, and there is a developing and strong interest at the National Cancer Institute in this area, including an interest in natural products with chemopreventive potential.

Bleomycin and Its Derivatives

Tomohisa Takita & Hamao Umezawa

Bleomycin (BLM) is a name of a group of glycopeptide antibiotics and has been used in the treatment of Hodgkin's lymphoma, carcinomas of the skin, head, neck, and cervix and tumors of the testis mostly in combination with radiation or other chemotherapeutic agents. Various BLMs produced by a BLM-producing strain which belongs to *Streptomyces verticillus* are different from one another in the terminal amine moiety. As described in a previous review (Umezawa & Takita 1980), the following antibiotics which are structurally related to BLM have been isolated: phleomycin, YA56X, YA56Y, zorbamycin (identical with YA56X), zorbonomycin B and C, victomycin, platomycin A and B and tallysomycin A and B. Thereafter, cleomycin (Umezawa *et al.* 1980), SF-1961 (Shomura *et al.* 1980), SF-1771 (Ohba *et al.* 1980) have been added. The structural similarity of these antibiotics to BLM suggests that the mechanism of action of these antibiotics should be essentially the same as that of BLM. It is characteristic that BLM has not bone-marrow toxicity but has pulmonary toxicity. The mechanism of its action causing DNA strand scission, and the relationships between structures and renal or pulmonary toxicity, have been studied in detail. In this chapter, the mechanism of antitumor action of BLM, preparation of new BLMs, and selection of more improved BLMs are described.

MECHANISMS OF ANTITUMOR ACTION OF BLEOMYCIN
In 1978, the conslusive structures of BLM and its copper complex, the natural form produced by fermentation, were presented (Figs. 1, 2, Table I) (Takita *et al.* 1978a, Takita *et al.* 1978b). On the basis of these structures, it became possible to discuss the mechanisms of antitumor action of BLM on a molecular level. BLM is a bifunctional compound consisting of the binding site to DNA and the

Institute of Microbial Chemistry, Tokyo 141, Japan.

NATURAL PRODUCTS AND DRUG DEVELOPMENT, Alfred Benzon Symposium 20.
Editors: P. Krogsgaard-Larsen, S. Brøgger Christensen, H. Kofod, Munksgaard, Copenhagen 1984.

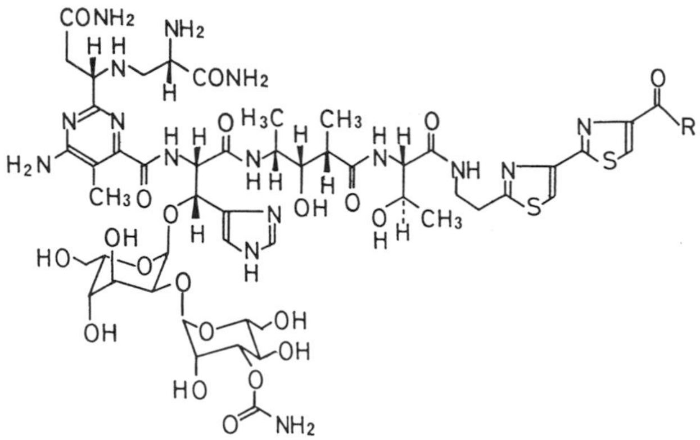

Fig. 1. Structure of bleomycin (R: terminal amine, see Table I)

reaction site with DNA (Fig. 3) (Takita *et al.* 1978b). The planar bithiazole moiety intercalates between bases of double-stranded DNA (Povirk *et al.* 1979), and the terminal amine is also involved in the binding by electrostatic attraction (Kasai *et al.* 1979). The activated oxygen on the iron complex of BLM appears to cleave DNA strand (Sausville *et al.* 1976). The structure of the active ternary complex has been suggested to be BLM-Fe(III)-O_2^{2-}, and the scheme of the regeneration cycle of the active complex was proposed (Fig. 4) (Kuramochi *et al.* 1981). The important points are: 1) the active complex is formed by one electron transfer to the adduct of molecular oxygen and BLM-Fe(II) complex, and 2) DNA is catalytically cleaved by iron-complex of BLM and molecular oxygen in the presence of reducing agents. The DNA fragments cleaved by the active BLM have been isolated, and the degradation process shown in Fig. 5 has been suggested from these fragments (Giloni *et al.* 1981).

Metal-free BLM injected in animals binds to cupric ion in blood to form the stable BLM-Cu(II) complex, and after penetration into the cells, the copper of the complex is removed reductively and the cuprous ion, thus liberated, is trapped by an intracellular protein (Takahashi *et al.* 1977). Thus, BLM is dynamically trapping and releasing copper ions in the body. All kinds of human and animal cells contain BLM hydrolase which hydrolyzes the amide bond of the α-aminocarboxamide of metal-free BLM resulting in inactivation of the BLM (Umezawa *et al.* 1974). BLM-Cu(II) complex is resistant to this enzyme, and it also does not cause DNA strand scission *in vitro.* Thus, the Cu(II) complex of BLM has 2 biological roles: one is resistance to the inactivation enzyme and the other is protection against manifestation of the biological activity (Sugiura *et*

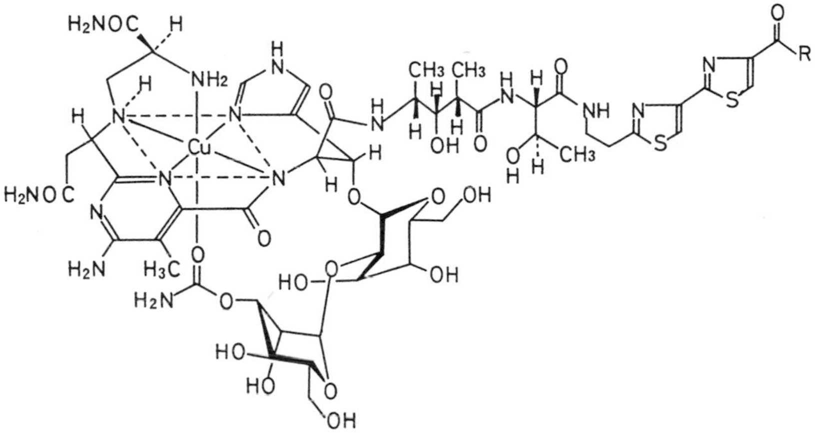

Fig. 2. Structure of copper-complex of bleomycin (R: terminal amine, see Table I)

al. 1979). The tumor cells in which the amount of BLM hydrolase is small compared with other cells should be susceptible to BLM treatment. Reasons why BLM is effective in the treatment of carcinomas of the skin, head, neck and cervix has been suggested to be due to a low content of BLM hydrolase and a high concentration of this antibiotic in the tumor cells of these types.

It has also been shown that the degree of renal and pulmonary toxicity is

Table I
Terminal Amines of Natural Bleomycins

Bleomycin	Terminal amine	Bleomycin	Terminal amine
A1*	NH_2-$(CH_2)_3$-$\overset{\overset{O}{\|\|}}{S}$-$CH_3$	A2'-c	NH_2-$(CH_2)_2$- (imidazole ring)
Demethyl-A2*	NH_2-$(CH_2)_3$-S-CH_3	A5	NH_2-$(CH_2)_3$-NH-$(CH_2)_4$-NH_2
A2	NH_2-$(CH_2)_3$-$\overset{X^-}{\underset{+}{S}}$-$(CH_3)_2$	A6	NH_2-$(CH_2)_3$-NH-$(CH_2)_4$-NH-$(CH_2)_3$-NH_2
A2'-a	NH_2-$(CH_2)_4$-NH_2	B2	NH_2-$(CH_2)_4$-NH-$\overset{\overset{}{C}}{\underset{\|\|}{}}$-$NH_2$ (C=NH)
A2'-b	NH_2-$(CH_2)3$-NH_2	B4	NH_2-$(CH_2)_4$-NH-C-NH-$(CH_2)_4$-NH-C-NH_2 (both C=NH)

* Derived from bleomycin A2 spontaneously.

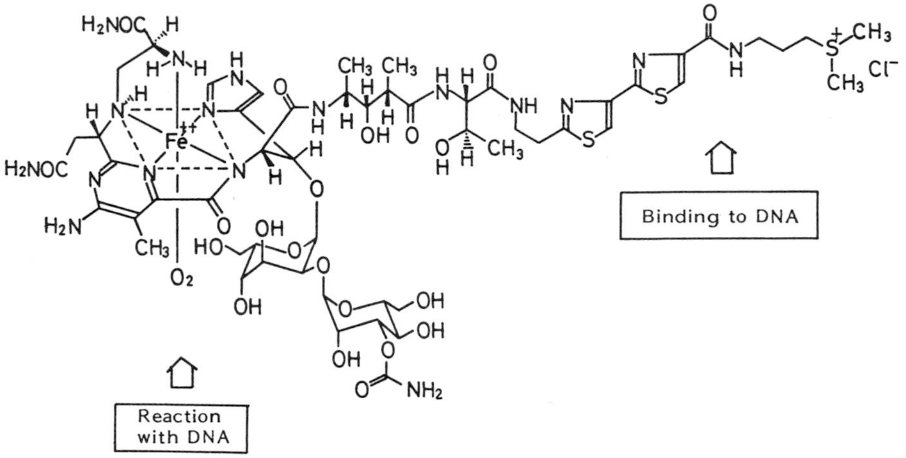

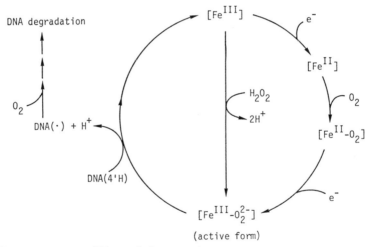

Fig. 3. Interaction of bleomycin with DNA

Fig. 4. Iron-oxygen states of bleomycin iron-complex

different among various BLMs containing different terminal amines. For instance, BLM B4 and B6 which contain 2 or more guanidine groups in the terminus have strong renal toxicity. As described later, artificial BLMs which contain various terminal amines have been prepared and among them those which have low pulmonary toxicity in animals have been found.

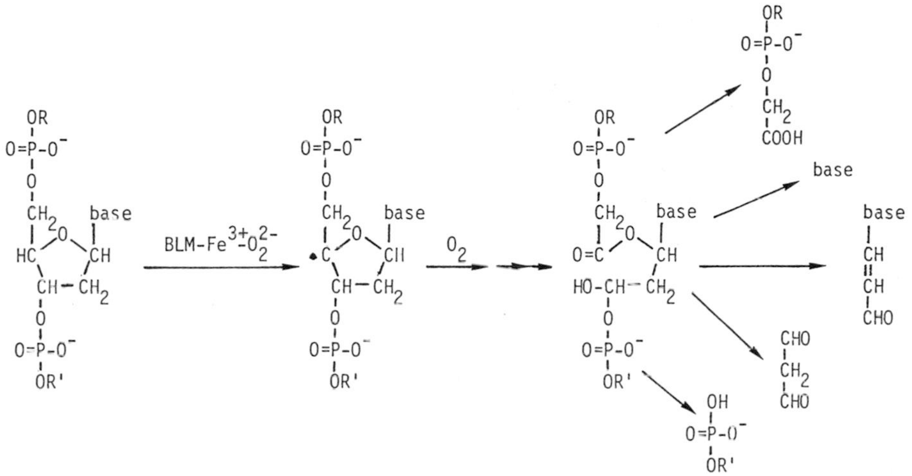

$$
\begin{array}{c}
OR \\
| \\
O=P-O^- \\
| \\
O \\
| \\
CH_2 \\
| \\
HC\diagdown \overset{O}{\diagup}CH \\
CH-CH_2 \\
| \\
O \\
| \\
O=P-O^- \\
| \\
OR'
\end{array}
\quad\xrightarrow{BLM-Fe^{3+}-O_2^{2-}}\quad
\begin{array}{c}
OR \\
| \\
O=P-O^- \\
| \\
O \\
| \\
CH_2 \\
| \\
\bullet C\diagdown \overset{O}{\diagup}CII \\
CH-CH_2 \\
| \\
O \\
| \\
O=P-O^- \\
| \\
OR'
\end{array}
\quad\xrightarrow{O_2}\quad
\begin{array}{c}
OR \\
| \\
O=P-O^- \\
| \\
O \\
| \\
CH_2 \\
| \\
O=C\diagdown \overset{O}{\diagup}CH \\
HO-CH-CH_2 \\
| \\
O \\
| \\
O=P-O^- \\
| \\
OR'
\end{array}
$$

base

$$
\begin{array}{c}
OR \\
| \\
O=P-O^- \\
| \\
O \\
| \\
CH_2 \\
| \\
COOH
\end{array}
$$

base

$$
\begin{array}{c}
base \\
| \\
CH \\
\| \\
CH \\
| \\
CHO
\end{array}
$$

$$
\begin{array}{c}
CHO \\
| \\
CH_2 \\
| \\
CHO
\end{array}
$$

$$
\begin{array}{c}
OH \\
| \\
O=P-O^- \\
| \\
OR'
\end{array}
$$

Fig. 5. Main degradation pathway of DNA by bleomycin-iron-O_2 complex

PRINCIPLES FOR PREPARATION OF NEW BLEOMYCINS

Preparation by fermentation

More than 10 natural BLMs have been isolated from the culture filtrate of ordinary fermentation of *Streptomyces verticillus* (Fujii *et al.* 1973). They are different from one another in the terminal amine moiety. Biogenetically, all of these amines originate from amino acids such as methionine, arginine and histidine (Table I).

When the BLM-producing micro-organism is cultured in a medium containing a special amine, which is not present in nature, the amine is incorporated into BLM, and a new BLM, which has the added amine in its terminal amine moiety, is produced. The structural requirement of the amine for the incorporation is to have a primary amino group at the end of a short alkyl chain, which forms the amide bond with the carboxylic acid of bleomycinic acid (*vide post*), and also to have at least one more basic functional group such as amino, guanidium, imidazole, sulfonium *etc.*, (Fujii *et al.* 1974) (Fig. 6, Table I).

Bleomycinic acid from bleomycin B2 by enzymatic hydrolysis

The BLM derivative which does not contain the terminal amine is called bleomycinic acid (BLM-acid). It was an imaginary derivative when we started searching for the enzyme to cleave BLM B2, the second major component of natural BLMs, into BLM-acid and agmatine, the terminal amine of BLM B2, from microbial origin. We found the presence of the enzyme in the mycelium of *Fusarium anguioides* (Umezawa *et al.* 1973). It was purified and found to be a new kind of enzyme, acylagmatine amidase (EC 3.5.1.40). BLM-acid is a staring material suitable for preparation of new semi-synthetic BLMs, because it has only one free carboxyl group which is connected with the terminal amine, and the free primary amino group present in BLM-acid can be readily protected by copper-coordination (Takita *et al.* 1978b). Actually, Cu(II)-complex of BLM-acid was reacted with an amine in the presence of a coupling reagent for peptide synthesis such as dicyclohexylcarbodiimide-1-hydroxybenzotriazole (DCC-HOBt) to afford a new semi-synthetic BLM in a good yield.

Bleomycinic acid from bleomycin A2 by chemical cleavage
During the structural study of BLM, we found that the amide bond connecting the terminal amine is most resistant to acid hydrolysis among the amide bonds present in BLM. In order to cleave this amide bond selectively, some modification by participation of a neighboring functional group is necessary prior to the hydrolysis. Thus, BLM A2, which is the major component of natural BLMs and has the reactive dimethylsulfonium group at the end, was treated with sodium thiocyanate to give BLM demethyl-A2 (Fig. 7). It was dissolved in 1% trifluoroacetic acid and was reacted with cyanogen bromide at room temperature overnight. The main product was not the expected cyclic iminoether, but the 3-aminopropyl ester of BLM-acid, the hydration product of the former. The newly formed primary amino group was selectively acylated with acyl chloride after the Cu(II)-complexation. Mild alkaline hydrolysis of the product afforded BLM-acid in good yield. Thus, selective chemical cleavage of the terminal amide bond of BLM A2 was achieved by participation of repeated elimination of the methyl group as methyl thiocyanate from the dimethyl-sulfonium group at the end (Takita *et al.* 1973). New semi-synthetic BLMs were also derived directly from the acylaminopropyl ester of BLM-acid, an intermediate of the chemical cleavage of BLM A2, by aminolysis.

Derivatives resistant to bleomycin hydrolase
All human and animal cells have BLM hydrolase which inactivates BLM by hydrolysis of the carboxamide bond adjacent to the primary amino group. This enzyme is a kind of aminopeptidase. The primary amino group is the recognition

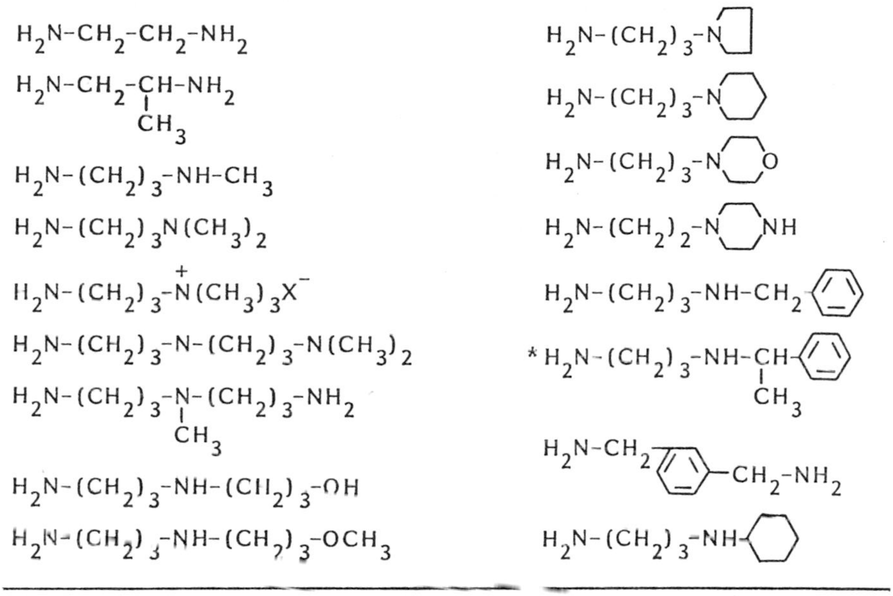

$H_2N-CH_2-CH_2-NH_2$

$H_2N-CH_2-CH-NH_2$
$\qquad\qquad \underset{CH_3}{|}$

$H_2N-(CH_2)_3-NH-CH_3$

$H_2N-(CH_2)_3N(CH_3)_2$

$H_2N-(CH_2)_3-\overset{+}{N}(CH_3)_3X^-$

$H_2N-(CH_2)_3-N-(CH_2)_3-N(CH_3)_2$

$H_2N-(CH_2)_3-\underset{\underset{CH_3}{|}}{N}-(CH_2)_3-NH_2$

$H_2N-(CH_2)_3-NH-(CH_2)_3-OH$

$H_2N-(CH_2)_3-NH-(CH_2)_3-OCH_3$

$H_2N-(CH_2)_3-N\square$

$H_2N-(CH_2)_3-N\bigcirc$

$H_2N-(CH_2)_3-N\bigcirc O$

$H_2N-(CH_2)_2-N\bigcirc NH$

$H_2N-(CH_2)_3-NH-CH_2-\langle \rangle$

$*H_2N-(CH_2)_3-NH-\underset{\underset{CH_3}{|}}{CH}-\langle \rangle$

$H_2N-CH_2-\langle \rangle-CH_2-NH_2$

$H_2N-(CH_2)_3-NH-\bigcirc$

*Peplomycin (S-configuration)

Fig. 6. Unnatural amines well-incorporated into the terminal amine moiety of bleomycin

site of this enzyme. While, the co-ordination of this amino group to Fe(II)-ion appears to be essential in the manifestation of the BLM activity (Sugiura et al. 1979).

The N-alkylation of the primary amino group diminished the BLM activity greatly, except the monomethyl derivative (Fukuoka et al. 1980) (Scheme I). This should be due to difficulty of the co-ordination of the amino group by bearing the bulky alkyl group. The monomethyl derivative was resistant to BLM hydrolase but had stronger toxicity and lower therapeutic index against Ehrlich carcinoma in comparison with original BLM.

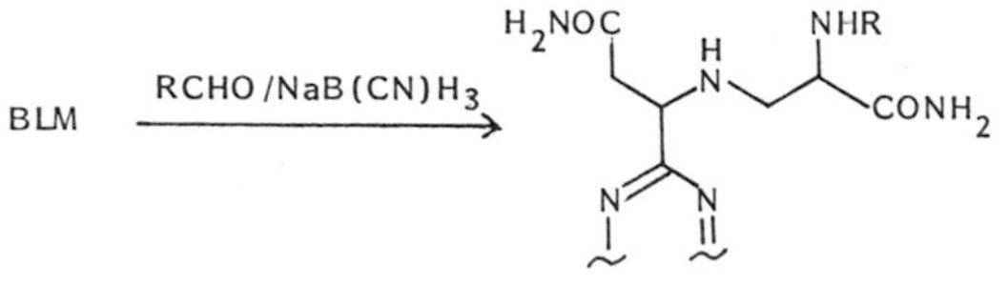

$$BLM \xrightarrow{\text{RCHO /NaB(CN)H}_3} $$

Scheme I

The acylation of the primary amino group (Scheme II) also eliminated the activity in causing DNA strand scission *in vitro,* but the N-L-α-aminoacyl derivatives showed the antitumor activity *in vivo*, because the aminoacyl groups in these derivatives were removed by aminopeptidases. The velocity of the hydrolysis is different depending on the amino-acyl groups and organs. For instance, the hydrolysis of the N-glycyl-BLM is lower in lung homogenates than in those of the other organs.

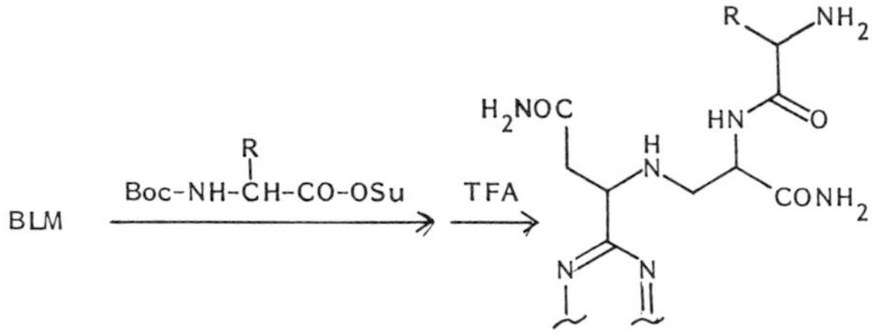

Scheme II

It is expected that if the scissile primary amide by BLM hydrolase is transformed to the secondary amide, this secondary amide bond will be more resistant to BLM hydrolase. These derivatives were prepared as follows. BLM was first treated with BLM hydrolase isolated from bovine liver to give deamide-BLM. After the Cu(II)-complexation, the free carboxyl group of deamide-BLM was coupled with an amine to afford the desired derivative (Scheme III). Many of these derivatives were resistant to BLM hydrolase, and showed strong activities against Ehrlich ascites carcinoma and P388 leukemia.

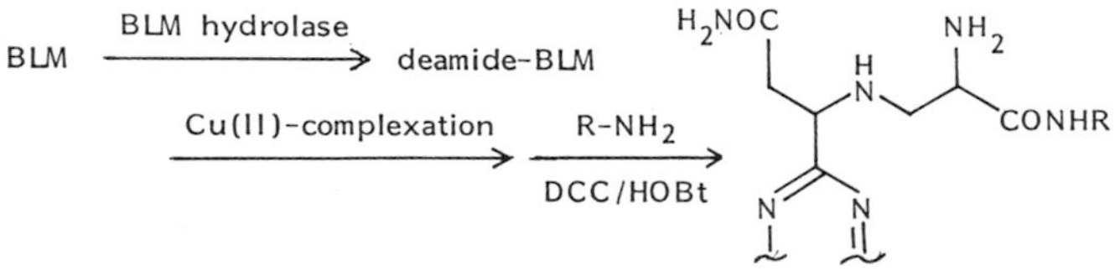

Scheme III

Preparation by chemical synthesis
In 1981, the total synthesis of BLM was achieved for the first time (Takita *et al.* 1981), and in 1982, the improved total synthesis has been established (Saito *et al.* 1982). On the basis of this synthesis, the reconstruction of BLM molecule has

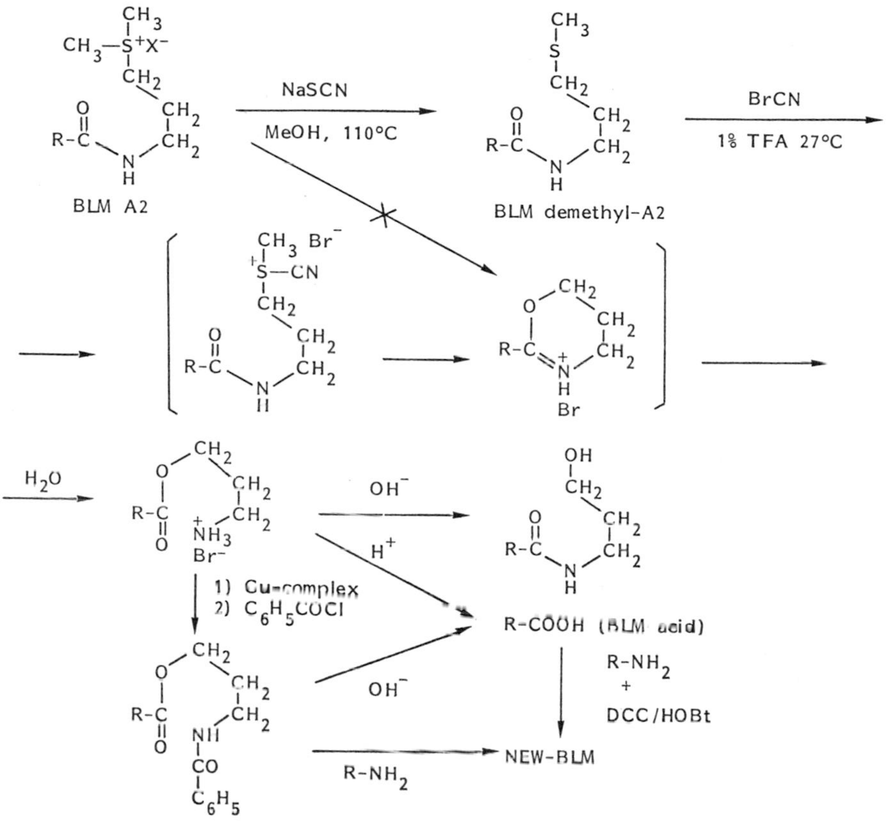

Fig. 7. Chemical transformation of bleomycin A2 into bleomycinic acid and other bleomycins

become feasible from the fragments derived from BLM (Fig. 8). Boc-pyrimido-blamic acid (2, in Fig. 9), which is a key compound to synthesize BLM, has been derived from pyrimidoblamic acid (1, in Fig. 8) by esterification, Cu-complexation followed by butoxycarbonylation and ammonolysis. The key reaction is a selective hydrolysis by Cu-complexation (Fig. 9). The stereo-selective synthesis of *erythro-β*-hydroxyhistidine, the central part of BLM molecule, was also achieved by Cu-mediated coupling of 4-formylimidazole and N-pyruvylideneglycinato-Cu(II) (Fig. 10) (Yoshioka 1977). The success of these synthetic studies enabled us to prepare the desirable derivatives which could not be prepared by the former methods. These analogues will contribute to the elucidation of the mechanism of action of BLM in more detail and to obtaining new synthetic BLMs more effective than natural BLMs. For example, the

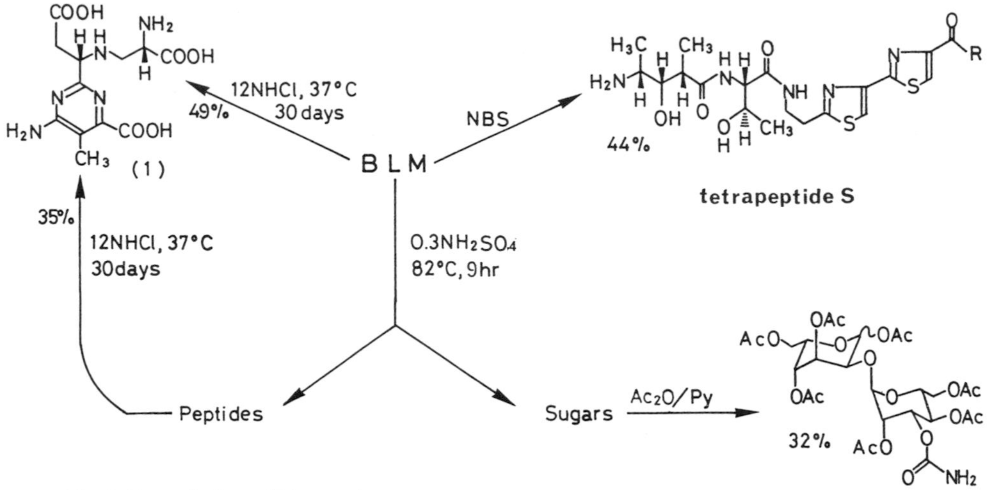

Fig. 8. Degradation of bleomycin

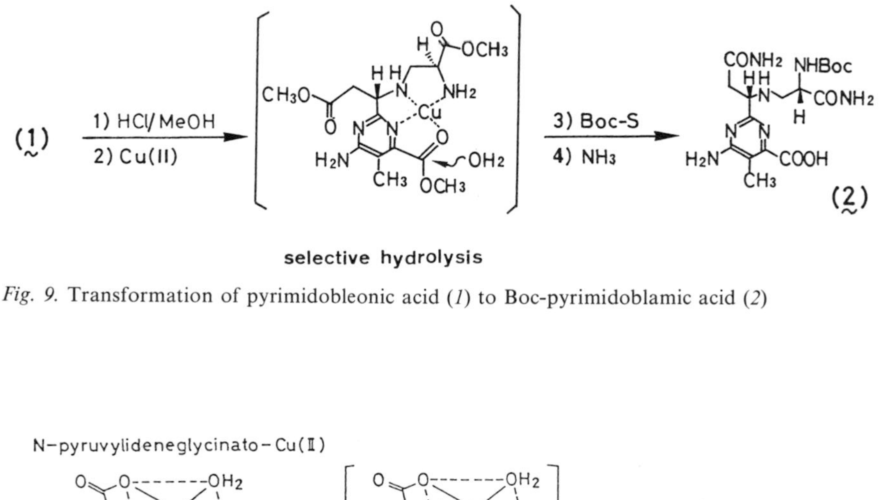

Fig. 9. Transformation of pyrimidobleonic acid (*1*) to Boc-pyrimidoblamic acid (*2*)

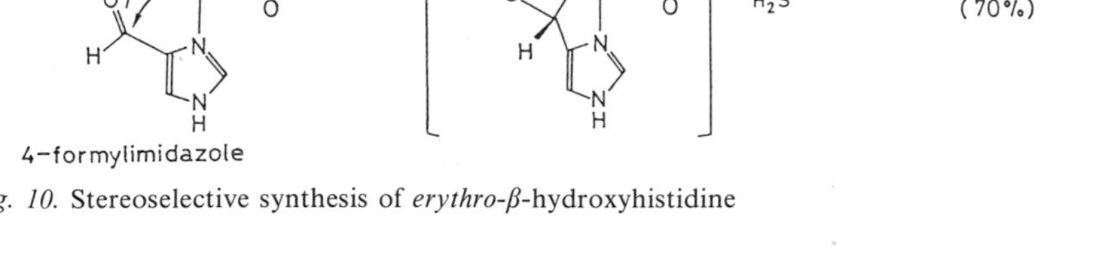

Fig. 10. Stereoselective synthesis of *erythro-β*-hydroxyhistidine

importance of the terminal methyl group of the 4-amino-3-hydroxy-2-methyl-pentanoic acid moiety of BLM in the manifestation of the antitumor activity was elucidated by these synthetic studies of the analogues (Saito *et al.* unpublished).

SELECTION OF BLEOMYCIN ANALOGUES USEFUL IN CANCER TREATMENT

Pulmonary toxicity limits the total dose of the present BLM in one course treatment of carcinomas of the skin, head, neck, cervix and lung. Therefore, the BLM analogues which have the same or higher degree of antitumor activity and lower pulmonary toxicity have been studied.

In order to predict the antitumor effect of BLM analogues in cancer patients, the effects on Hela S_3 cells, ascites and solid types of Ehrlich carcinoma in mice *etc.*, have been tested. The high therapeutic index has been taken as an important point for the selection. The distribution of BLM analogues in various organs of mice and rats has also been tested to predict the sensitivity of tumor in the target organs. Because, BLM distributes in skin at a high concentration without decomposition, and it shows therapeutic effect against skin tumors.

The testing method of the pulmonary toxicity in mice after the local or

Table II
Biological Properties of Peplomycin and Bleomycin*

	Peplomycin	Bleomycin*
Antitumor activity		
Hela S_3 cell (ID_{50})	0.82 mcg/ml	1.70 mcg/ml
Ehrlich solid carcinoma (ID_{50})	0.35 mg/kg×10	0.49 mg/kg×10
Percent inhibition of lymph node	90%	46%
metastasis of AH66 rat hepatoma at a dose		
of 1.25 mg/kg		
MNNG-induced gastric cancer in rats	Effective	Not effective
DMBA-induced mammary carcinoma in rats	Effective	Weakly effective
Distribution in rats		
(at a dose of 100 mg/kg SC)		
Lung	2.1 mcg/gm	1.1 mcg/gm
Skin	4.1 mcg/gm	2.7 mcg/gm
Mesenteric lymph node	1.9 mcg/gm	0.5 mcg/gm
Lumbar lymph node	1.5 mcg/gm	0.4 mcg/gm
Prostate	0.4 mcg/gm	0 mcg/gm

* BLM clinically used: A2~70%, B2~30% and trace of other BLMs

systemic application of BLM analogues has been established (Matsuda *et al.*
1978). This test using aged mice has been shown to be useful to predict the degree
of pulmonary toxicity in cancer patients.

Thus, peplomycin (PEP), of which the terminal amine is 3-(S-1-phenylethyl-
amino)-propylamine, has been selected (Fig. 6). It was also selected from its
effect on N-methyl-N'-nitro-N-nitrosoguanidine(MNNG)-induced gastric cancer in rats, which was resistant to the BLM clinically used (BLM^c, Table II). The
antitumor activity and distribution of PEP in comparison with those of BLM^c
are shown in Table II.

Antitumor activities of PEP in various tumor systems were 1.2–2.0 times
stronger than BLM^c. PEP had a highly inhibitory action on tumor metastasis to
lymph nodes. It suggests that PEP may be effective for metastasised patients.
PEP was distributed in 1.5–3.0 times higher than BLM^c in all organs except
spleen. The inhibitory action of PEP on tumor metastasis to lymph node may be
due to distribution in a high concentration in this organ. PEP has also been
confirmed to be effective in the treatment of prostatic carcinoma, which is
insensitive to BLM^c. In animal experiments, PEP was also effective to 9,10-
dimethyl-1,2-benzanthracene(DMBA)-induced mammary carcinoma in rats,
resistant to BLM^c. Here, it may be necessary to note that human gastric cancer
inoculated into the skin of nude mice is almost equally sensitive to both PEP and
BLM^c, although they are both ineffective in gastric cancer patients.

It seems to be most reasonable for the development of new BLMs to select the
one which has a low pulmonary toxicity, has no strong renal toxicity, has a wider
antitumor spectrum than the present BLM, and has a high therapeutic index
against Ehrlich carcinoma or other experimental tumors susceptible to BLM
treatment.

REFERENCES

Fujii, A., Takita, T., Maeda, K. & Umezawa, H. (1973) New components of bleomycin. *J. Antibiot.*
   26. 396–397.
Fujii, A., Takita, T., Shimada, N. & Umezawa, H. (1974) Biosyntheses of new bleomycins. *J.*
   Antibiot. 27, 73–77.
Fukuoka, T., Muraoka, Y., Fujii, A., Naganawa, H., Takita, T. & Umezawa, H. (1980) Reductive
   methylation of bleomycin. *J. Antibiot. 33,* 114–117.
Giloni, L., Takeshita, M., Johnson, F., Iden, C. & Grollman, P. (1981) Bleomycin-induced
   strand-scission of DNA. Mechanism of deoxyribose cleavage. *J. Biol. Chem. 256,* 8608–8615.
Kasai, H., Naganawa, H., Takita, T. & Umezawa, H. (1978) Interaction of bleomycin with
   nucleic acids, preferential binding to guanine base and electrostatic effect of the terminal amine.
   J. Antibiot. 31, 1316–1320.

Kuramochi, H., Takahashi, K., Takita, T. & Umezawa, H. (1981) An active intermediate formed in the reaction of bleomycin-Fe(II) complex with oxygen. *J. Antibiot. 34,* 576–582.

Matsuda, A., Yoshioka, O., Takahashi, K., Yamashita, T., Ebihara, K., Ekimoto, H., Abe, F., Hashimoto, Y. & Umezawa, H. (1978) Preclinical studies on bleomycin-PEP (NK-631). In: *Bleomycin: Current Status and New Development,* eds. Carter, S. K., Crooke, S. T. & Umezawa, H., pp. 311–332. Academic Press, New York.

Ohba, K., Shomura, T., Tsuruoka, T., Omoto, S., Kojima, M., Hisamatsu, T., Inoue, S. & Niida, T. (1980) SF-1771, a new antibiotic related to bleomycin. *J. Antibiot. 33,* 1236–1242.

Povirk, L. F., Hogan, M. & Dattagupta, N. (1979) Binding of bleomycin to DNA: Intercalation of the bithiazole ring. *Biochemistry 18,* 96–101.

Saito, S., Umezawa, Y., Yoshioka, T., Muraoka, Y., Takita, T. & Umezawa, H. (1982) An improved total synthesis of bleomycin. In: *Peptide Chemistry 1982,* ed. Sakakibara, S., pp. 133–138. Protein Research Foundation, Osaka.

Sausville, E. A., Peisach, J. & Horwitz, S. B. (1976) A role for ferrous ion and oxygen in the degradation of DNA by bleomycin. *Biochem. Biophys. Res. Comm. 73,* 814–822.

Shomura, T., Omoto, S., Ohba, K., Ogino, H., Kojima, M. & Inoue, S. (1980) SF-1961, a new antibiotic related to bleomycin. *J. Antibiot. 33,* 1243–1248.

Sugiura, Y., Muraoka, Y., Fujii, A., Takita, T. & Umezawa, H. (1979) Deamidebleomycin from viewpoint of metal coordination and oxygen activation. *J. Antibiot. 32,* 756–758.

Takahashi, K., Yoshioka, O., Matsuda, A. & Umezawa, H. (1977) Intracellular reduction of the cupric ion of bleomycin copper complex and transfer of the cuprous ion to a cellular protein. *J. Antibiot. 30,* 861–869.

Takita, T., Fujii, A., Fukuoka, T. & Umezawa, H. (1973) Chemical cleavage of bleomycin to bleomycinic acid and synthesis of new bleomycins. *J. Antibiot. 26,* 252–254.

Takita, T., Muraoka, Y., Nakatani, T., Fujii, A., Umezawa, Y., Naganawa, H. & Umezawa, H. (1978a) Revised structures of bleomycin and phleomycin. *J. Antibiot. 31,* 801–804.

Takita, T., Muraoka, Y., Nakatani, T., Fujii, A., Iitaka, Y. & Umezawa, H. (1978b) Metal-complex of bleomycin and its implication for the mechanism of bleomycin action. *J. Antibiot. 31,* 1073–1077.

Takita, T., Umezawa, Y., Saito, S., Morishima, H., Umezawa, H., Muraoka, Y., Suzuki, M., Otsuka, M., Kobayashi, S., Ohno, M., Tsuchiya, T., Miyake, T. & Umezawa, S. (1981) Total synthesis of bleomycin. In: *Peptides: Synthesis-Structure-Function,* eds. Rich, D. H. & Gross, E., pp. 29–39. Pierce Chemical Company, Illinois.

Umezawa, H., Takahashi, Y., Fujii, A., Saino, T., Shirai, T. & Takita, T. (1973) Preparation of bleomycinic acid: Hydrolysis of bleomycin B2 by a Fusarium acylagmatine aminohydrolase. *J. Antibiot. 26,* 117–119.

Umezawa, H., Hori, S., Sawa, T., Yoshioka, T. & Takeuchi, T. (1974) A bleomycin-inactivating enzyme in mouse liver. *J. Antibiot. 27,* 419–424.

Umezawa, H. & Takita, T. (1980) The bleomycins: Antitumor copper-binding antibiotics. *Structure and Bonding 40,* pp. 73–99. Springer-Verlag, Berlin.

Umezawa, H., Muraoka, Y., Fujii, A., Naganawa, H. & Takita, T. (1980) Cleomycin, a new family of bleomycin-phleomycin group. *J. Antibiot. 33,* 1079–1082.

Yoshioka, T. (1977) Dissertation. pp. 151. Faculty of Pharmaceutical Sciences, University of Tokyo.

DISCUSSION

HUANG LIANG: First question: Can you, by changing the terminal amine, influence the organ specificity? Second question: In China a mixture of bleomycins, containing primarily bleomycin A5, is preferred by physicians. Have you tested bleomycin A5?

TAKITA: Generally speaking, the terminal amine is more lipophilic, the affinity to the organ is stronger. But we can not explain why the organ distribution is different among the bleomycins. To your second question: in Japan we have also tested the bleomycin A5, but it is less effective than the bleomycin mixture clinically used at present.

HUANG LIANG: According to your results, the organ distribution in the lung is relatively higher for peplomycin than for bleomycin. What do you know about toxicity?

TAKITA: The activity of peplomycin is stronger but the toxicity to the lung is smaller. This has been proved experimentally and clinically.

HUANG LIANG: Do you have any clinical results of the peplomycin?

TAKITA: Peplomycin has already been marketed. So, there are a lot of clinical results available.

RAPOPORT: Do you plan on changing the peptide residue to something else?

TAKITA: We changed the hydroxyaminovaleric acid moiety to GABA, but it does not show any activity. We will study this series of the analogues more, and then we will change the bithiazole moiety.

NAKANISHI: Can you explain the dramatic effect of the exchange of hydroxy-aminovaleric acid on the basis of your model?

TAKITA: The chemical shifts of the protons of this part in the metal complex are unusual, so maybe some part of this amino acid is spatially very near the metal. This conformation may be important for the bioactivity.

Antineoplastic Structure-Activity Relationships of Camptothecin and Related Analogs

Monroe E. Wall & M. C. Wani

INTRODUCTION

This lecture will review recent and previous studies relating to structure activity relationships (SAR) of camptothecin (**1**) and analogs with respect to antineoplastic activity. Camptothecin and its analogs are aromatic, planar alkaloids which are found in a very narrow segment of the Plant Kingdom. Most of the work has been done on the alkaloids of *Camptotheca acuminata* (Nyssaceae), which is a native of China. Because of the high activity exhibited by camptothecin in the mouse leukemia L1210 assay, the compound was given clinical trial. Because of the extremely water insoluble nature of (**1**), it was tested clinically as the water soluble sodium salt (**2**), which is readily obtained by hydrolysis of the lactone moiety. The clinical trials were negative. As will be shown subsequently, the water soluble salt (**2**) is much less potent than the parent compound. As a consequence, we decided to make a detailed study of the factors required for antineoplastic activity in the camptothecin series. Our findings are reported in this paper.

CAMPTOTHECIN

This alkaloid was first isolated from the wood, bark and fruits of *Camtotheca acuminata,* DECAISNE (Nyssaceae) (Wall *et al.* 1966). The taxonomy, occurrence and the interesting manner in which the seeds of this Chinese tree were collected from Szechwan Province and sent to the United States many years ago

---

Chemistry and Life Sciences, Research Triangle Institute, North Carolina 27709, U.S.A.

NATURAL PRODUCTS AND DRUG DEVELOPMENT, Alfred Benzon Symposium 20.
Editors: P. Krogsgaard-Larsen, S. Brøgger Christensen, H. Kofod, Munksgaard, Copenhagen 1984.

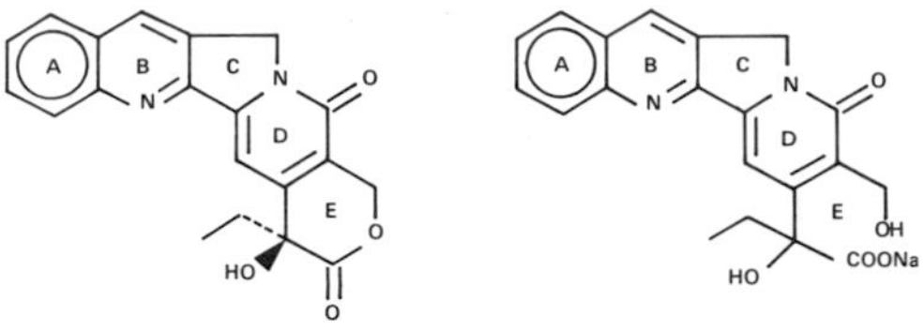

Camptothecin (1)   Camptothecin Sodium (2)

Fig. 1. Camptothecin and camptothecin sodium

has been reported (Perdue *et al.* 1970). The structure of camptothecin, an alkaloid which has been shown to be related to the commonly occurring indole alkaloid group (Heckendorf *et al.* 1976) is shown in Fig. 1. It will be noted that the compound has a pentacyclic ring structure with only one asymmetric center in ring E with the 20S configuration. Other notable features are the presence of the α-hydroxy lactone system in ring E, the pyridone ring D moiety and the conjugated system which links rings A, B, C and D. Because of its noteworthy activity in the rat leukemia L1210 system, camptothecin was of great interest from the time of its initial isolation. The compound demonstrated L1210 activity between 0.25 mg to 3.0 mg/kg with T/C values frequently in excess of 200. It is one of the few antineoplastic alkaloids that has shown consistent high activity in the resistent L1210 mouse leukemia assay, most of the others showing rather low L1210 but high P388 activity. In addition, camptothecin has great activity in inhibition of the growth of solid tumors in animals.

Camptothecin SAR studies

Initial activity studies quickly revealed some interesting SAR relationships (Wall 1969). These are outlined in Fig. 2. The important features noted were as follows: hydroxylation of ring A of camptothecin is compatible with activity, and indeed this compound, 10-hydroxycamptothecin 3, has the highest activity of all the various natural or synthetic analogs of camptothecin, showing L1210 activity at 0.5–2 mg/kg as high as T/C 230, and in the PS leukemia system values frequently exceed T/C of 300 at concentrations as low as 2–4 mg/kg. Camptothecin reacts readily with bases or amines to give water-soluble salts or amides, formed by reaction with the lactone moiety with conconcomitant opening of ring E. Reaction of the lactone moiety with nitrogenous bases analogous to amide formation may possibly be involved in the antitumor activity and potency of **1**. The water soluble sodium salt, which is the form used in the clinic, has a potency 8–10 times less than that of the natural product. The

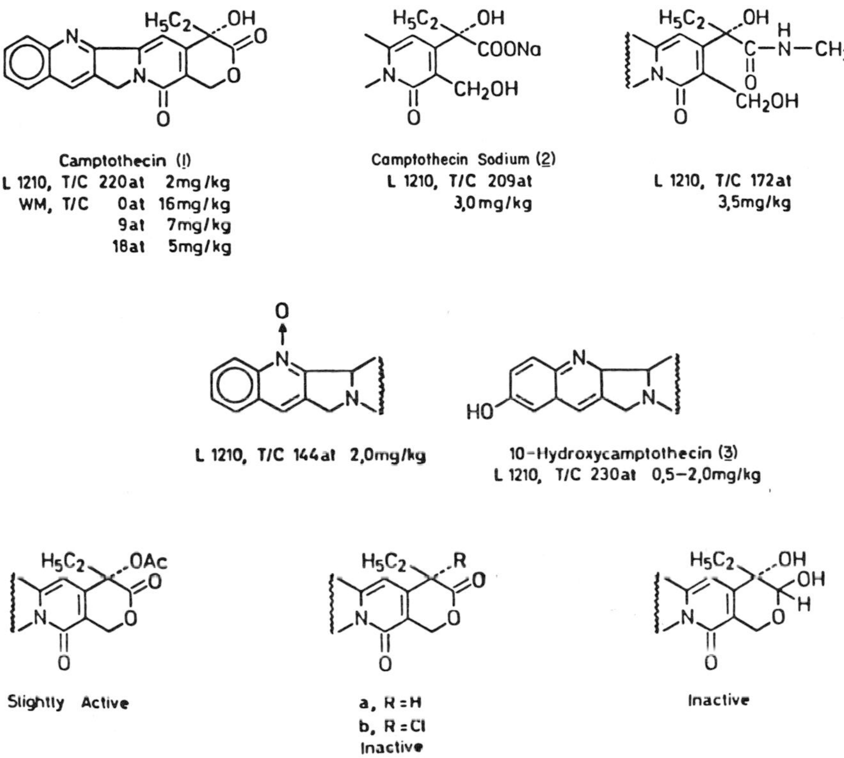

Camptothecin (1)
L 1210, T/C 220at   2mg/kg
WM, T/C   0at   16mg/kg
             9at   7mg/kg
            18at   5mg/kg

Camptothecin Sodium (2)
L 1210, T/C 209at
             3,0mg/kg

L 1210, T/C 172at
             3,5mg/kg

L 1210, T/C 144at 2,0mg/kg

10-Hydroxycamptothecin (3)
L 1210, T/C 230at 0,5-2,0mg/kg

Slightly Active

a, R=H
b, R=Cl
Inactive

Inactive

Fig. 2. Structure activity relationships in the camptothecin series

salt is inactive when administered intravenously at pH 7.2 and shows activity only after intraperitoneal administration, probably due to limited recyclization.

Major reduction of antineoplastic activity was noted as a result of reactions involving the hydroxyl or lactone moiety in ring E, (Fig. 2). After acetylation of camptothecin, the resultant acetate is virtually inactive. Other reactions also point to the absolute requirement for the α-hydroxyl group as shown by the fact that after replacement of this group by chlorine, both the resultant chloro analog and the corresponding hydrogenolysis product, desoxycamptothecin, are inactive in L210 and PS leukemia. Reduction of the lactone under mild conditions to give the lactol also results in complete loss of activity. Our early studies, hence, clearly indicated the absolute requirement for the α-hydroxy lactone moiety. It is, thus, quite clear that the activity of the sodium salt is due entirely to the ability of this compound to recyclize at least to a limited extent under physiological conditions.

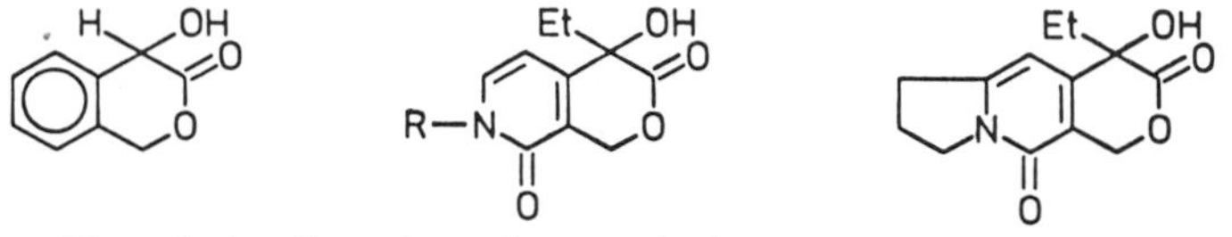

Fig. 3. Mono-, Bi- and tricyclic analogs of camptothecin

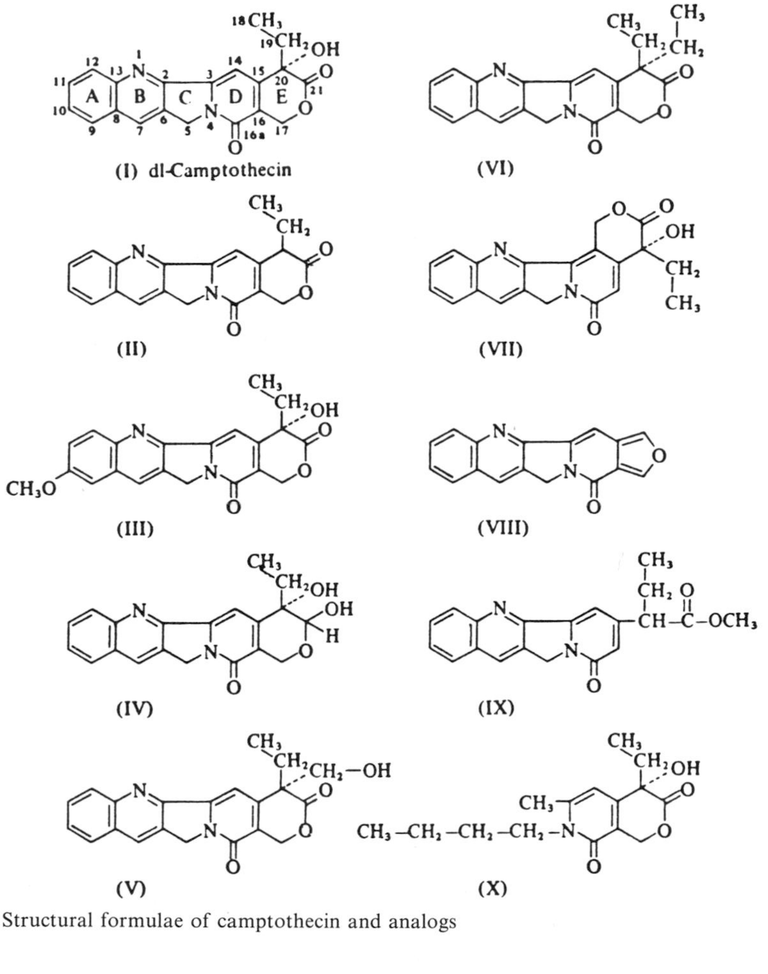

Fig. 4. Structural formulae of camptothecin and analogs

Synthetic analogs

Our initial synthetic studies were designed to determine whether the α-hydroxy lactone moiety was the sole factor involved in the antineoplastic activity of camptothecin. Some simple monocyclic ring E, bicyclic DE and tricyclic CDE analogs containing the α-hydroxy lactone moieties were prepared (Fig. 3). We

Table I

Effect of camptothecin and analogs on inhibition of RNA synthesis and DNA molecular weight

Inhibitor Added	50% Inhibition of RNA Synthesis (μM)	"High Molecular Weight" DNA (%)
None	–	93
Camptothecin (I)	1	14
Desoxycamptothecin (II)	2	20
10-Methoxycamptothecin (III)	5	5
Camptothecin Lactol (IV)	30	77
Homocamptothecin (V)	1	62
Diethylcamptothecin (VI)	6	88
Isocamptothecin (VII)	8	84
Furan Derivative (VIII)	4	81
Camptothecin Monoester (IX)	5	89
Camptothecin Analog-1 (X)	*	93

* 40% Inhibition at 70 μM.

Taken from S. B. Horwitz, in Antibiotics III. Mechanism of Action of Antimicribial and Antitumor Agents, John W. Corcoran & Fred E. Hahn, Eds., Springer-Verlag, New York, 1975.

found that the compounds were inactive *in vivo*. Similar compounds were studied *in vitro* by procedures involving the depolymerization of DNA or the inhibition of RNA synthesis (Horwitz 1975), and were again found inactive. It should be noted that camptothecin and its sodium salt have become an important tool for molecular biologists studying macromolecular processes because of its rapid onset of action, rapid reversibility, and selective action. Fig. 4 and Table I are taken from Horwitz (1975) and reproduced here with the consent of both the author and the publisher, Springer-Verlag. Fig. 4 shows the structures of a variety of compounds of camptothecin and its analogs, a number of which came from our laboratories. Table I presents the results found by Horwitz both in terms of the inhibition of high molecular weight RNA synthesis and the polymerization of DNA. It can be seen that many compounds which lack the α-hydroxy lactone moiety, show activity in the inhibition of RNA synthesis and depolymerization of high molecular weight DNA. Compare, for example, camptothecin and desoxycamptothecin in Table I. Note that the bicyclic analog, compound 10 in this table, is inactive both *in vivo* and *in vitro*. The earlier *in vivo* studies carried out by our group and the latter *in vitro* studies on DNA from the work of Horwitz permit the following generalizations: inhibition of RNA synthesis seems to be a general property of camptothecin and

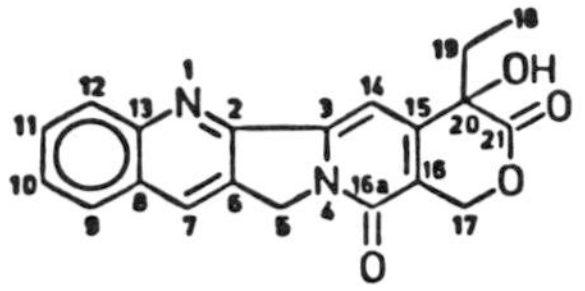

(±)–Camptothecin

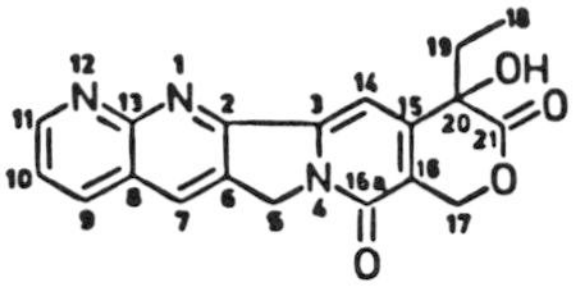

(±)–12–Azacamptothecin

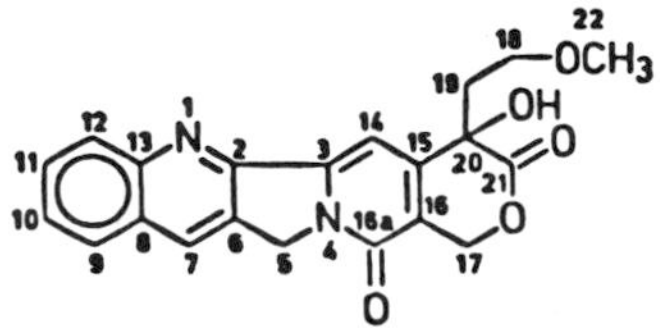

(±)–18–Methoxycamptothecin

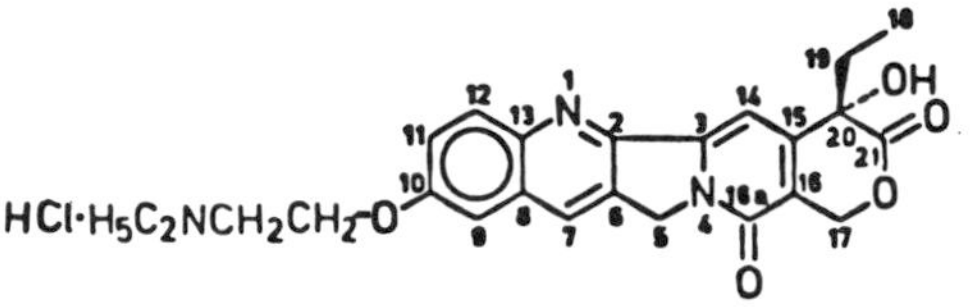

10–(2'–Diethylaminoethoxy)–20(S)–camptothecin, hydrochloride

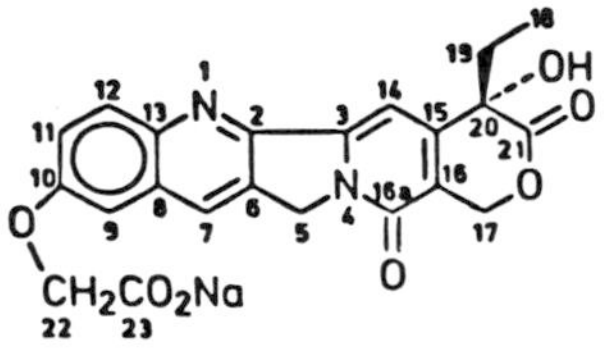

Sodium Salt of 10–Carboxymethyloxy–20(S)–camptothecin.

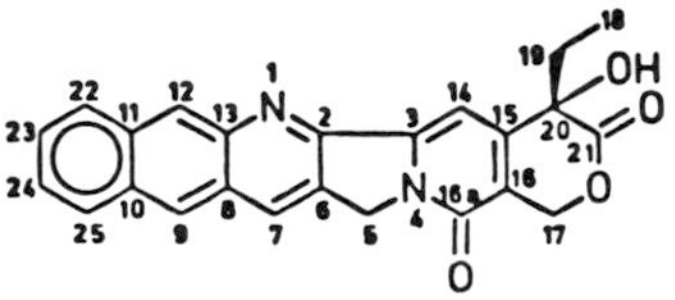

(±)–Benz(j)camptothecin

Fig. 5. Structures of synthetic camptothecin analogs

all analogs with the conjugated A, B, C, D ring system. Conversion of cellular DNA to lower molecular weight species seems to be more sensitive to alterations in ring E. Only compounds with structures close to camptothecin are active in this test. Note, however, that desoxycamptothecin, which is quite active in its effects on RNA and DNA, is completely inactive *in vivo*. From our *in vivo* studies and the *in vitro* data from Horwitz's laboratory, we conclude that several structural features are required in the *in vivo* antineoplastic activity observed in the camptothecin series: (1) the necessity for a flat, planar structure which would be required for binding with nucleic acids, possibly by a mechanism related to or identical to intercalation; (2) the presence of the α-hydroxy lactone moiety in ring E is an absolute requirement as this moiety in all likelihood is involved in a covalent reaction, conceivably with one of the nitrogen bases of the nucleic acids.

Total synthesis studies

The above considerations became an important factor in subsequent synthetic

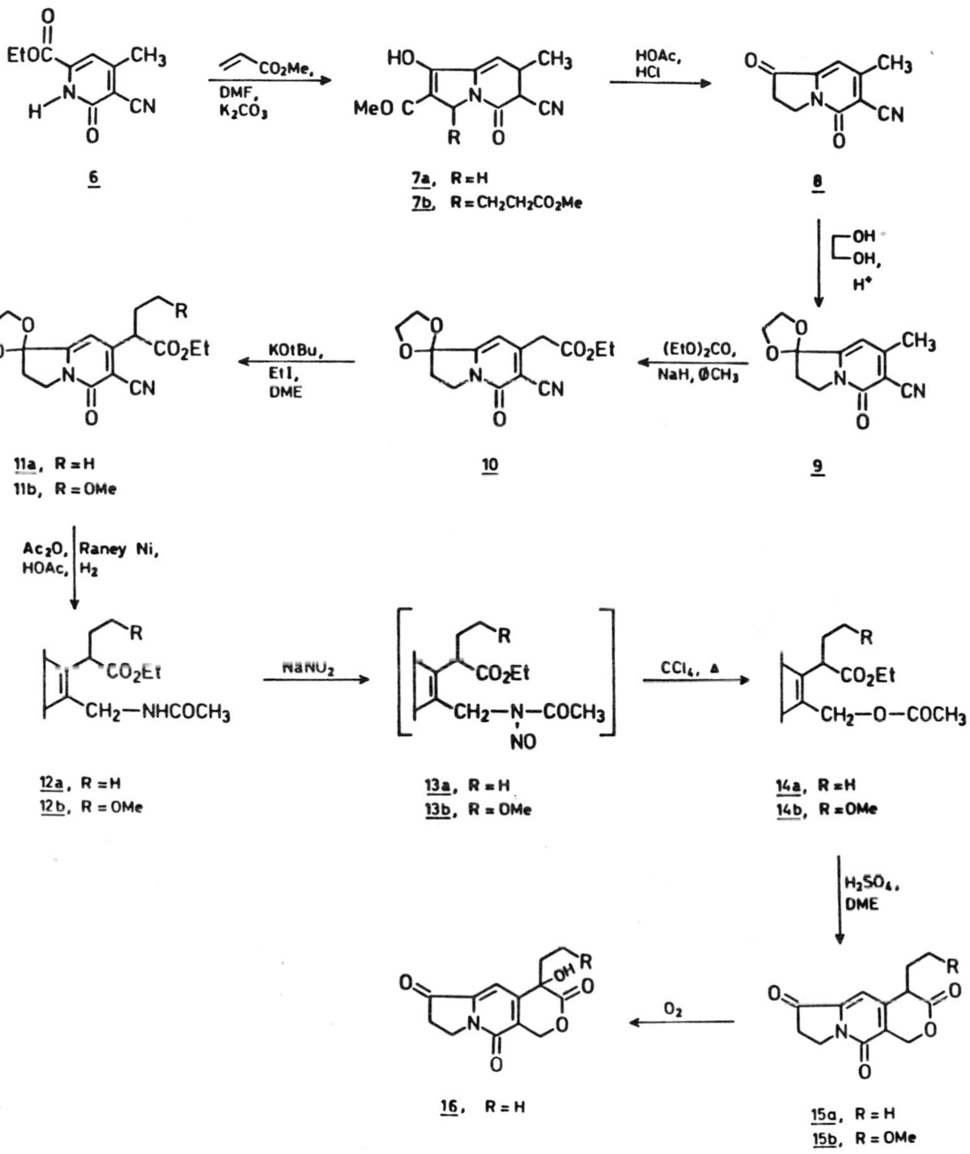

Fig. 6. Synthesis of tricyclic ring C, D, E intermediates

efforts to further delineate the mode of action of camptothecin and its analogs. Our synthetic studies were designed to obtain a general procedure from which a variety of camptothecin analogs could be prepared in high enough yield to permit *in vivo* testing and, thus, determine whether structural modifications

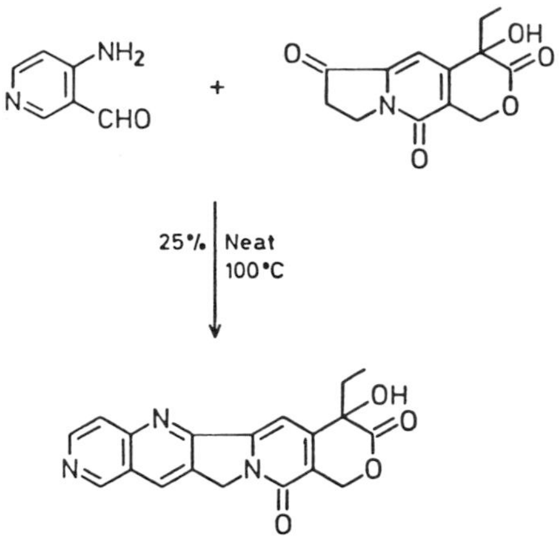

Fig. 7. Synthesis of 10-azacamptothecin

might result in even more active compounds. This latter consideration is all important; for example, in spite of the many total syntheses of camptothecin and analogs which have appeared in the literature, until our work, not even racemic camptothecin (the usual final product) had received any testing. Another target was to see if we could produce water-soluble compounds without opening the important α-hydroxy lactone ring. These types of compounds were produced by partial synthesis from 10-hydroxycamptothecin. The various procedures utilized to obtain our goals have been published in detail (Wani *et al.* 1980). The target compounds are shown in Fig. 5. The key to the successful synthesis of camptothecin and its analogs was based on the development of a method which made available on a large scale the tricyclic intermediate as outlined in Fig. 6. Subsequent reaction of this key intermediate with any one of a number of an appropriate ortho-aminobenzaldehyde analogs yields, via the Friedlander reaction, the desired camptothecin analog as exemplified for the synthesis of 10-azacamptothecin shown in Fig. 7.

Camptothecin analogs with a solubility function in ring A were prepared by partial synthesis from naturally occurring 10-hydroxycamptothecin. The synthesis of appropriate ether derivatives which could then be converted to water-soluble sodium salt or the diethylamino hydrochloride, is shown in Fig. 8. These compounds were completely water soluble, and their activity will be discussed subsequently.

Table II presents both the antileukemic *in vivo* activity in the P388 system and the 9KB cytotoxicity activity of camptothecin and a number of its analogs. All

Table II

Antileukemic activity against P388 system and cytotoxicity against 9KB cells of camptothecin and its analogs

Compound	Dose Range (mg/kg)	Optimal % T/C	Optimal Dose (mg/kg)	Lowest Toxic Dose (mg/kg)	Therapeutic Index	9KB ED$_{50}$ (μg/ml)
1	8.0–0.5	197	4.0	8.0	8	2×10^{-2}
2	80.0–2.5	212	40.0	80.0	4	2×10^{-1}
3	8.0–0.5	314	4.0	8.0	8	2×10^{-2}
4	4.0–0.5	145	0.5	1.0	1	2×10^{-2}
17	16.0–1.0	222	8.0	16.0	8	1×10^{-1}
24	32.0–4.0	Inactive	–	–	–	$>1 \times 10^{0}$
26	32.0–2.0	234	32.0	–	16	$>1 \times 10^{0}$
29	32.0–2.0	175	32.0	–	2	$>1 \times 10^{0}$
36	32.0–1.0	198	16.0	–	4	2×10^{-1}
38	8.0–0.5	160	4.0	8.0	2	2×10^{-1}

assays were conducted with camptothecin as a positive control. The naturally occurring camptothecin series shown in this table are compounds *1–4* and are respectively camptothecin **1**, camptothecin sodium salt **2**, 10-hydroxycampto-thecin **3**, and 10-methoxycamptothecin **4**. It will be noted that all of these compounds, with the exception of the sodium salt, show 9KB activity of the order of 10^{-2}. 10-Hydroxycamptothecin is obviously the most active compound in this series, having both significantly higher T/C and lower optimal dose than any other compounds. The sodium salt **2** is active, but it is evident that it is about ten-times less potent than the others. The 9KB activity of the sodium salt also is lower by an order of magnitude from activities of other naturally occurring compounds. Compounds **17, 29, 36** and **38** are synthetic camptothecin analogs, respectively racemic camptothecin **17**, 12-aza-camptothecin **29**, 18-methoxy-camptothecin **36** and the benz(j)camptothecin **38**. All of the synthetic campto-thecin analogs show some degree of activity. It will be noted that racemic camptothecin **17** is a highly active compound *in vivo* and has about half the potency of the naturally occurring compound. In adition, the cytotoxicity is about a power of 10 lower. Similar 9KB activities were noted for the racemic synthetics **36** and **38**. The 12-aza compound **29**, which is weakly active *in vivo*, is essentially inactive in 9KB.

We conclude that the stereochemistry of the hydroxyl group in natural camptothecin is specifically essential for activity. The racemic mixture, of

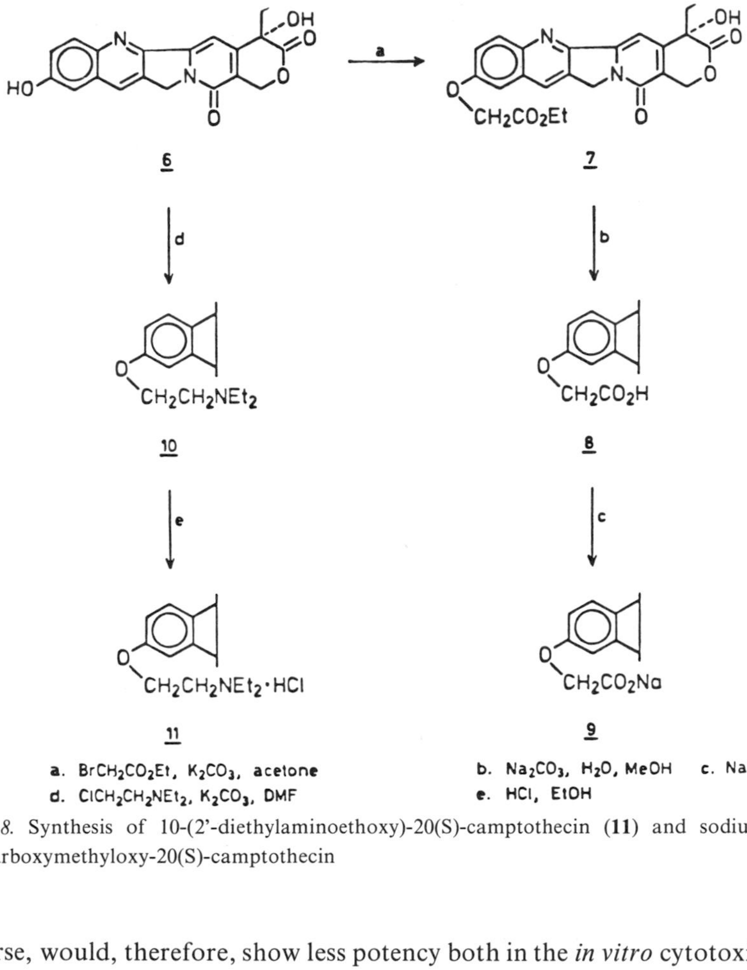

a. BrCH₂CO₂Et, K₂CO₃, acetone   b. Na₂CO₃, H₂O, MeOH   c. NaHCO₃
d. ClCH₂CH₂NEt₂, K₂CO₃, DMF   e. HCl, EtOH

Fig. 8. Synthesis of 10-(2'-diethylaminoethoxy)-20(S)-camptothecin (**11**) and sodium salt of 10-carboxymethyloxy-20(S)-camptothecin

course, would, therefore, show less potency both in the *in vitro* cytotoxicity and in the *in vivo* leukemia systems. If one allows for the fact that all of the compounds produced by a total synthesis are racemic, it can be concluded that the optically active form of analogs **36** and **38** would be of the same order of potency and activity as natural camptothecin both *in vivo* and *in vitro*. However, none of the synthetics show any greater activity than natural camptothecin. The relative inactivity of 12-aza-camptothecin may well be due to the fact that 1,8-naphthyridines forms complexes with metal ions (Hendricker *et al.* 1970). Hence, the 12-aza analog **29** may form a complex which prevents intercalation with the base pairs of DNA and hence would result in reduced activity. We have prepared the corresponding 10-aza analog, and it is quite active, of the same order as racemic **1** in the *in vivo* P388 assay.

The water-soluble hydroxycamptothecin analogs **24** and **26** showed no cytotoxicity. The sodium salt **24** was completely inactive *in vivo*. The diethyl-amino hydrochloride showed high T/C activity in P388 leukemia but with 8-fold less potency than the parent compound. We have evidence that the latter compound slowly hydrolyzes to give 10-hydroxycamptothecin **3**. Hence, this compound may have some use as a prodrug. Its lack of cytotoxicity is quite encouraging in this regard. As an interesting conclusion, it is evident from the relative inactivity of these water soluble derivatives that there are definite structural restrictions to ring A modifications. These may be both steric and electronic, i.e., the formation of ionic-charged species as in **24** and **26** may give rise to electronic interaction with the phosphoric acid moieties in nucleic acids and, thus, prevent intercalation or binding. Conceivably steric factors may also be involved. For example, whereas 10-methoxycamptothecin **4** is active, it is less active than the corresponding 10-hydroxy analog **3**, and recently we prepared 10,11-dimethoxycamptothecin and found that it was inactive.

There is an excellent correlation between 9KB *in vitro* activity and the *in vivo* PS leukemia activity, (Table II). It will be noted that all the inactive or weakly active compounds *in vivo* are also inactive in the 9KB cytotoxicity screen. The racemic synthetic camptothecin analogs which are active *in vivo* have a reduced activity and/or potency, more or less proportional to the fact that half of the administered compounds is, in all likelihood, inactive. This is also borne out by

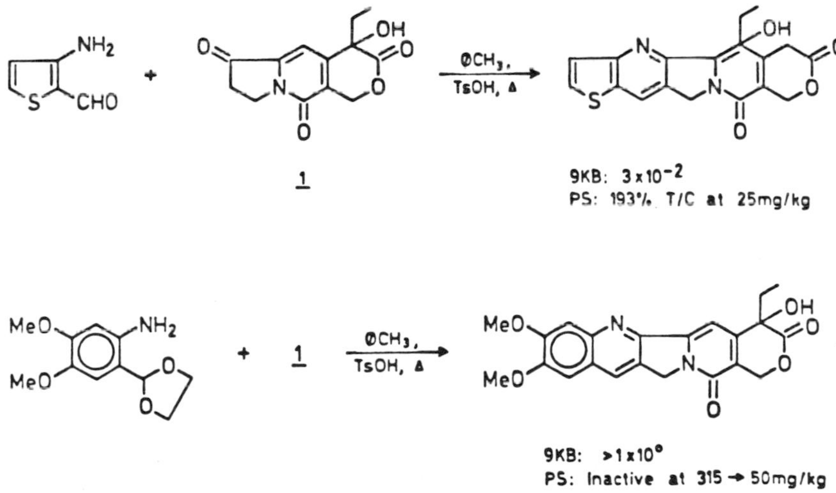

Fig. 9. Recent new synthetic analogs of camptothecin

the cytotoxicity which is *always* reduced by an order of magnitude for all of the racemic forms.

The correlation between cytotoxicity and *in vivo* activity in the camptothecin series was recently demonstrated in a rather amusing fashion by certain recent synthetic studies in our laboratory. The 10,11-dimethoxy analog of camptothecin and the thiopene analog were synthesized from appropriate orthoamino-aldehyde precursors as described previously. The structures and biological activity of these compounds are shown in Fig. 9. When the PS leukemia data arrived from the biological screener, we felt certain that the compounds in some manner had been interchanged. After receiving the original vials and confirming the structures, we obtained the 9KB data. This showed that indeed the dimethoxy analog was inactive; whereas, the thiopene analog was highly active, in accord with the *in vivo* data. In this case undoubtedly steric interaction interfering with binding must be responsible for the inactivity of the dimethoxy analog.

SUMMARY

In summary, we have shown that the α-hydroxy lactone moiety and the conjugated linkage in rings ABCD are requisite for antineoplastic activity. Although the addition of another aromatic ring, hexacyclic-camptothecin **38**, permits retention of activity, there are restrictions on the size or number of substituents in ring A. Whereas the 10-hydroxy analog is highly active, the 10-methoxy analog is less active, and the 10,11-dimethoxy analog is inactive. Camptothecin exerts its antineoplastic activity in 2 modes; one via binding of the aromatic rings to nucleic acids, possibly by intercalation; the other involving covalent bond reactions of the α-hydroxy lactone moiety, possibly with nitrogen bases of nucleic acids.

REFERENCES

Heckendorf, A. H., Mattes, K. C., Hutchinson, C. R., Hagaman, E. W. & Wenkert, E. (1976) Stereochemistry and conformation of biogenetic precursors of indole alkaloids. *J. Org. Chem.* *41*, 2045–2047.

Hendricker, D. G. & Bodner, R. L. (1970) Complexes of 1,8-Naphthyridines. III. Transition metal-perchlorate complexes of 2,7-dimethyl-1,8-naphthyridine. *Inorg. Chem., 9*, 273–277.

Horwitz, S. B. (1975) Camptothecin. In: *Antibiotics. III. Mechanism of Action of Antimicrobial and Antitumor Agents,* eds. J. W. Corcoran & F. E. Hahn, pp. 48–57. Springer-Verlag, New York.

Perdue, R. E., Jr., Smith, R. L., Wall, M. E., Hartwell, J. L. & Abbott, B. J. (1970) *Camptotheca acuminata* Decaisne (Nyssaceae). Source of camptothecin. U. S. Dept. Agr., Agr. Research Service, Technical Bulletin N. 1415, 1–26.

Wall, M. E., Wani, M. C., Cook, C. E., Palmer, K. H., McPhail, A. T. & Sim, G. A. (1966) Plant antitumor agents. I. The isolation and structure of camptothecin, a noval alkaloidal leukemia and tumor inhibitor from *Camptotheca acuminata. J. Amer. Chem. Soc., 88,* 3888–3890.

Wall, M. E. (1969) Plant antitumor agents. V. Alkaloids with antitumor activity. Symposiums-berichtes, 4. Internationales Symposium, Biochemie und Physiologie der Alkaloide, eds. K. Mothes, K. Schreiber & H. R. Schütte, pp. 77–87, Akademie-Verlag, Berlin.

Wani, M. C., Ronman, P. E., Lindley, J. T. & Wall, M. E. (1980) Plant antitumor agents. 18. Synthesis and biological activity of camptothecin analogs. *J. Med. Chem., 23,* 554–560.

DISCUSSION

BRØGGER CHRISTENSEN: If the lactone ring is open at physiological pH it is difficult to understand the different activities of the lactone and its sodium salt.

WALL: The lactone ring recyclizes quite readily at acidic pH values.

KROGSGAARD-LARSEN: The N-methyl-amide is as potent as the natural product, but the lactone ring appears to be a prerequisite for a biological activity. How do you explain the activity of the N-methyl-amide?

WALL: These compounds were administered intraperitoneally, which means they have to go to the liver first. It is my hypothesis that during this process you possibly enzymatically get a small amount of lactone.

KUTNEY: Have you tested other readily available alkaloids containing lactam rings, for example some of the products isolated from Catharanthus.

WALL: No, we haven't. We were trying to find out what we can do in the rings of camptothecin. We have recently succeeded in making the 10-amino compound, and that compound makes a water-soluble hydrochloride. If that compound has activity, then we may have something that can go into man.

Anthracyclines with Antitumor Activity

Federico Arcamone & Giuseppe Cassinelli

The anthracycline glycosides and their aglycones, the anthracyclinones, have been known for thirty years and the compounds of this class, originally of interest as antibiotic pigments produced by micro-organisms belonging to the genus Actinomycetes, are now receiving considerable attention since doxorubicin (Adriamycin) was introduced in cancer chemotherapy in 1972 (Arcamone 1981). Typical anthracyclinones, as described by Brockmann (Brockmann 1963) are presented in Fig. 1. They were obtained from 2 different micro-organisms namely *Streptomyces purpurescens* (the rhodomycinones) and *Streptomyces DOA 1205* (the pyrromycinones). The biologically active compounds are the glycosides derived from the said anthracliones. The sugar moieties appearing most frequently are 3-dimethylamino-2,3,6-trideoxy-L-*lyxo*-hexopyranose (rhodosamine), 2,6-dideoxy-L-*lyxo*-hexopyranose(2-deoxy-L-fucose), and 2,3,4-trideoxy-L-*glycero*-hexopyran-4-ulose (cinerulose A).

The novel compounds originally isolated in our laboratories from cultures of *Streptomyces peucetius var. caesius* and *carneus* are shown in Fig. 2. Doxorubicin as an antitumor agent was demonstrably more effective than the more easily available daunorubicin, itself a clinically useful drug (Arcamone 1981). Further evidence of doxorubicin superiority over daunorubicin in experimental solid tumors of the mouse has been published recently (Casazza 1982). The development of a convenient procedure for the chemical conversion of daunorubicin in doxorubicin made the latter compound promptly available for clinical use (Arcamone *et al.* 1974).

Doxorubicin is now a well-established chemotherapeutic agent, and more than one and half million patients were treated with the drug by 1982 (Praga 1982). However, human tumors of major importance such as colorectal cancer,

Farmitalia Carlo Erba Ricerca & Sviluppo Chimico, 20146 Milano, Italy

NATURAL PRODUCTS AND DRUG DEVELOPMENT, Alfred Benzon Symposium 20.
Editors: P. Krogsgaard-Larsen, S. Brøgger Christensen, H. Kofod, Munksgaard, Copenhagen 1984.

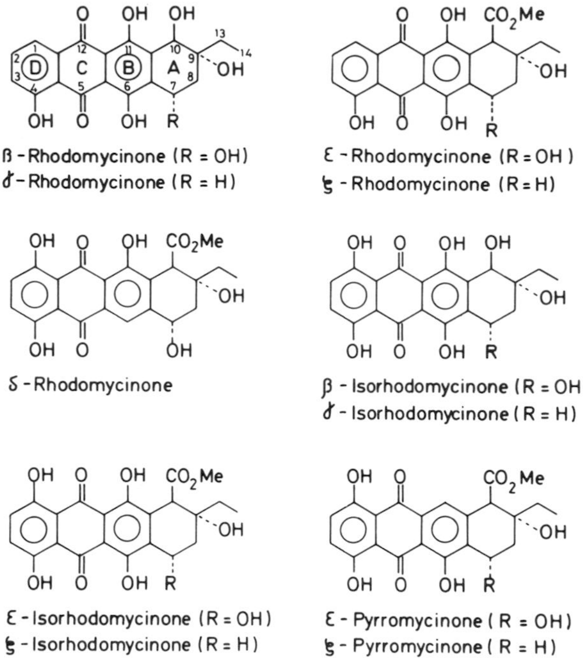

ARCAMONE & CASSINELLI

β -Rhodomycinone (R = OH)
δ -Rhodomycinone (R = H)

ε -Rhodomycinone (R = OH)
ζ -Rhodomycinone (R = H)

δ -Rhodomycinone

β - Isorhodomycinone (R = OH)
δ - Isorhodomycinone (R = H)

ε -Isorhodomycinone (R = OH)
ζ -Isorhodomycinone (R = H)

ε - Pyrromycinone (R = OH)
ζ - Pyrromycinone (R = H)

Fig. 1. Typical anthracyclinones.

pancreatic and renal cancers, lung tumors, are not generally responsive to doxorubicin. Moreover, toxic side effects impose limitations to dosage both in terms of single medication and of cumulative treatment (Carter 1975). Therefore, research activity aimed at the improvement of anthracycline antitumor agents either by synthetic methods, or through the search of biosynthetic analogues was started in 1972 in our laboratory. A particular attention was devoted to the synthesis of new aminoglycosides related to doxorubicin, possessing selected modifications in the sugar moiety.

Clearly, as daunosamine was promptly available upon acid hydrolysis of biosynthetic daunorubicin, it was a starting material for the semisynthesis of related aminosugars such as acosamine or 4-deoxydaunosamine. Other isomers of daunosamine such as ristosamine (L-ribo configuration) and the L-xylo analogues, as well as the 6-hydroxylated analogues of all four L-stereosiomeric aminohexoses were instead synthetized starting from L-arabinose or L-glucose (Arcamone 1981). Glycosidation of daunomycinone with the protected 4'-epi and 4'-deoxy daunosaminyl halide in the presence of silver triflate followed by deblocking afforded 4'-epi and 4'-deoxydaunorubicin. These compounds were

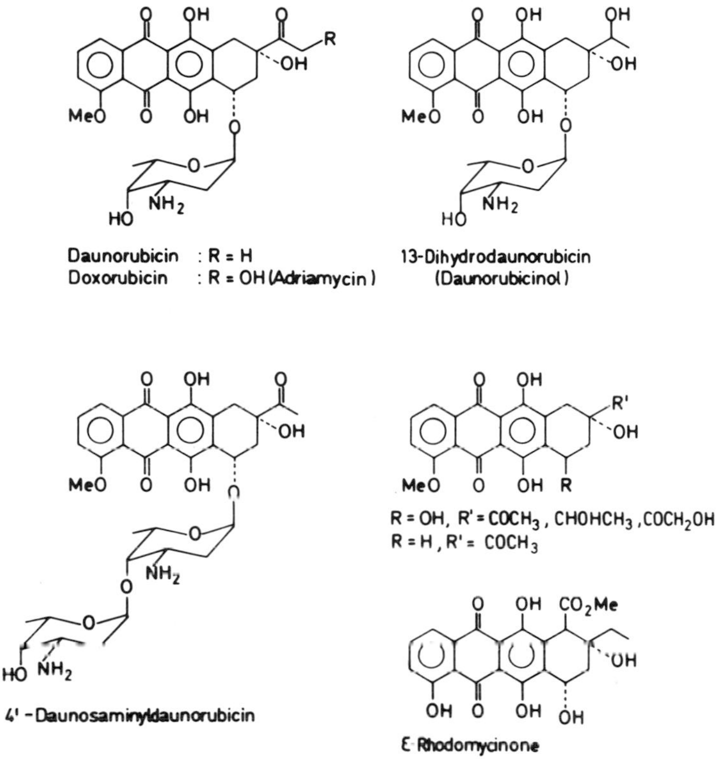

Daunorubicin : R = H
Doxorubicin : R = OH (Adriamycin)

13-Dihydrodaunorubicin
(Daunorubicinol)

$R = OH, R' = COCH_3, CHOHCH_3, COCH_2OH$
$R = H, R' = COCH_3$

4'-Daunosaminyldaunorubicin

ε Rhodomycinone

Fig. 2. Anthracycline derivatives from *S. peucetius var. caesius* and *var. carneus*.

converted to the corresponding doxorubicin analogues, showing promising pharmacological properties in experimental murine systems (Arcamone 1981). The silver triflate procedure or, alternatively, the glycal-acid-catalyzed condensation method, was also used for the synthesis of the other aminoglycosides. The stereoisomeric variants and the 6'-hydroxy derivatives resulted less biologically active than the parent biosynthetic compounds, or their 4'-epi and 4'-deoxy analogues (Arcamone 1981). Starting from daunosamine, new aminosugar derivatives modified at C-4 were obtained and coupled with daunomycinone. The 4'-O-methyl and 4'-C-methyl analogues of the antitumor anthracyclines exhibited interesting biological activity. The inhibition of L1210 murine leukemia by 4'-O-methyldoxorubicin (Figure 3) was noteworthy (Cassinelli *et al.* 1979).

Recent studies (Suarato *et al.* 1981) have provided a procedure for the direct conversion of biosynthetic daunorubicin into 4'-epidoxorubicin (epirubicin)

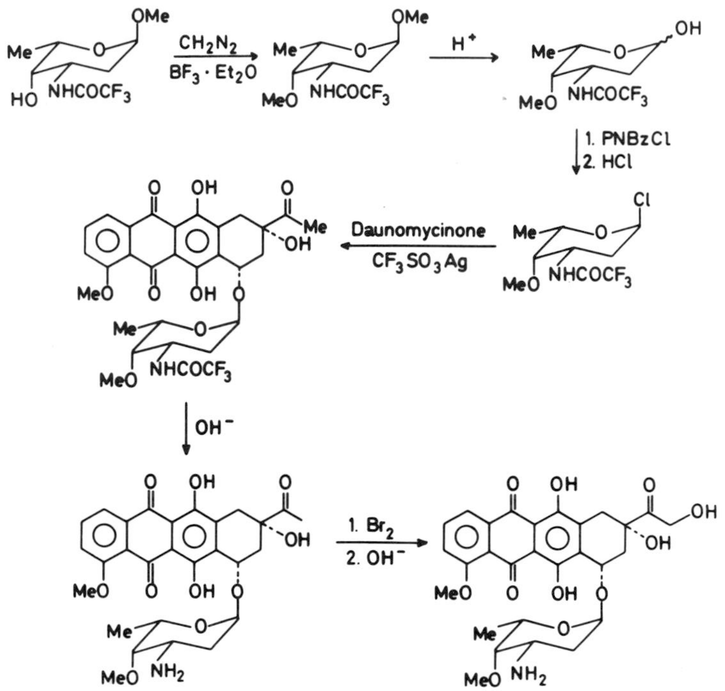

Fig. 3. Synthesis of 4'-O-methyldoxorubicin.

and 4'-deoxydoxorubicin (Fig. 4). The new procedures clearly represent a substantial improvement in respect to the previous ones reported above. The availability of the new compounds has allowed extended clinical trials for both new analogues. 4'-Epidoxorubicin displays an antitumor spectrum similar to that of doxorubicin, albeit with lower incidence and severity of toxic side effects. After doses up to 90 mg/m^2, the pattern of acute toxicity in Phase 1 studies was similar to that observed after comparable doses of doxorubicin, however, a lower incidence of vomiting, stomatitis and myelo suppression was recorded. When 4'-epidoxorubicin was administered every 3 weeks using single iv doses in the range 60 to 90 mg/m^2 results presented in Table I were obtained in different studies (Ganzina 1983). On the other hand, interest in 4'-deoxydoxorubicin is mainly based on its activity on human colon tumor xenografts in nude (immunodeficient) mice (Giuliani et al. 1981), and on the absence of cardio-toxicity at non-letal dosages in laboratory animals (Bertazzoli et al. 1982).

Chemical transformations carried out directly on doxorubicin and dauno-rubicin included side-chain periodate oxidation of the corresponding 13-

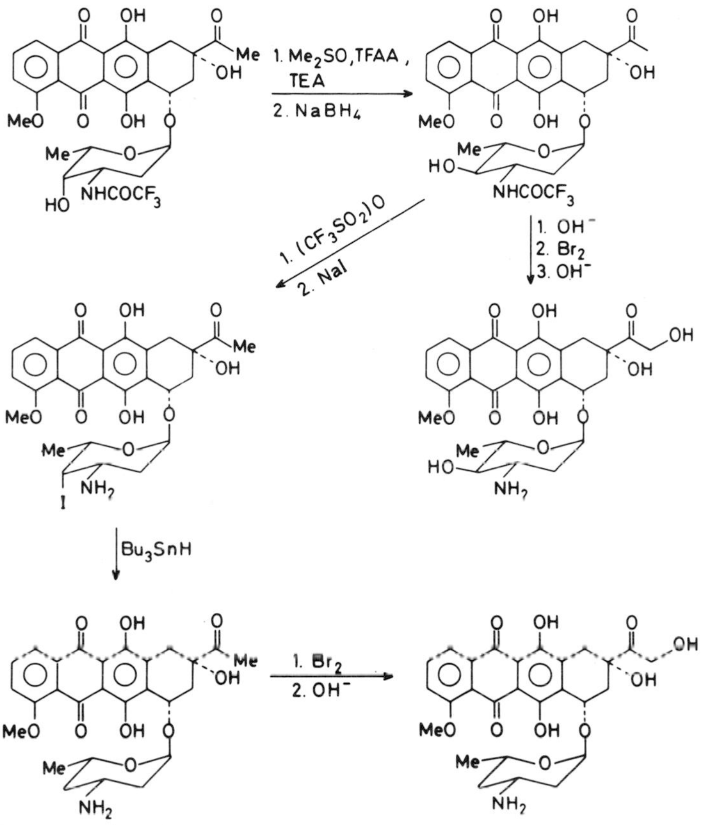

Fig. 4. Direct conversion of biosynthetic daunorubicin to 4'-epi and 4'-deoxy doxorubicin.

Table I

Activity of 4'-epidoxorubicin (epirubicin) as a single agent in different tumor diseases (Ganzina 1983).

Tumor Disease	Total Evaluable Cases	Complete+ Partial Remissions	Response Rate (%)
Breast carcinoma	133	40	30
Malignant melanoma	84	8	9
Advanced colorectal ca.	88	11[a]	16
Soft tissue sarcomas	43	8	21
Non small cell lung ca.	83	10[b]	12
Advanced gastric ca.	33	8	24
Head and neck	30	5	16
Non Hodgkin lymphoma	21	16[c]	76

(a) Mostly confined to rectum metastases. (b) Including minor responses. (c) Including drug combinations.

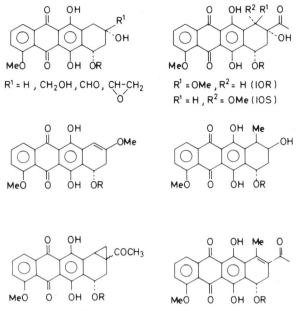

$R^1 = H$, CH_2OH , CHO , $CH-CH_2$
                                  O

$R^1 = OMe$, $R^2 = H$ (IOR)
$R^1 = H$, $R^2 = OMe$ (IOS)

Fig. 5. Semisynthetic analogues of daunorubicin modified on ring A.

dihydroderivatives, and reactions starting from N-trifluoroacetyl-9,10-an-hydrodaunorubicin to give the compounds presented in Fig. 5. Of the compounds, only 9-deacetyldaunorubicin, 9-deacetyl-9-hydroxymethyldauno-rubicin and 10(R)-methoxydaunorubicin displays antitumor activity in the P388 system comparable to that of the parent compound. Reduced activity was also exhibited by 8(R)-methoxydaunorubicin, a compound obtained by partial synthesis starting from daunomycinone (Penco *et al.* 1980).

Total synthesis of the daunomycinone system has received the attention of different researchers (Arcamone 1981). In our laboratory, this approach has resulted in highly potent analogues such as the 4-demethoxy analogues of daunorubicin and doxorubicin (Arcamone 1981). The new compound, 4-demethoxydaunorubicin, is presently undergoing extended clinical trials both in parenteral and oral formulation (Varini *et al.* 1981, Lambertenghi *et al.* 1982). Interestingly, the enantiomeric form of 4-demethoxydaunorubicin was com-pletely devoid of any biological activity (Arcamone *et al.* 1982).

Although the most promising second-generation antitumor anthracyclines are originated by semisynthesis or total synthesis, the search for new biosynthe-

R = COCH$_3$ (carminomycin)[a]
R = CHOHCH$_3$ (13-dihydrocarminomycin)[b]
R = CH$_2$CH$_3$ (13-deoxycarminomycin)[c]

R = CH$_2$OH (baumycins A1 and A2)[d]
R = CO$_2$H (baumycins B1 and B2)[d]

Fig. 6. The carminomycins and the baumycins (a) from *Actinomadura carminata*. (b) from *S. peucetius* strain 441 F$_1$. (c) from *S. peucetius var. carminatus*. (d) from *S. coeruleorubidus* (also N-acetyl and N-formyl daunorubicin and 13-dihydrodaunorubicin).

From Micromonospora n. sp. :

From S. peucetius var. aureus :

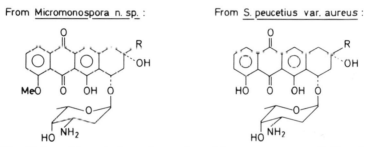

Fig. 7. The 11-deoxy biosynthetic analogues from *Micromonospora n.sp.* (left) and from *S. peucetius var. aureus* (right).

α - rhodomycinone (R = OH)
δ - rhodomycinone (R = CO$_2$Me)

α - citromycinone (R' = OH)
δ - citromycinone (R' = H)

H$_2$, Pd ‖(R=OH)

(R' = OH)

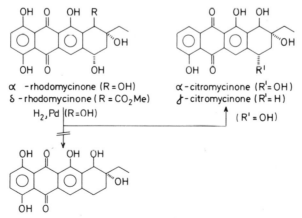

Fig. 8. 6-deoxyanthracyclinones from *S. purpurascens* (Brockmann & Niemeyer 1968).

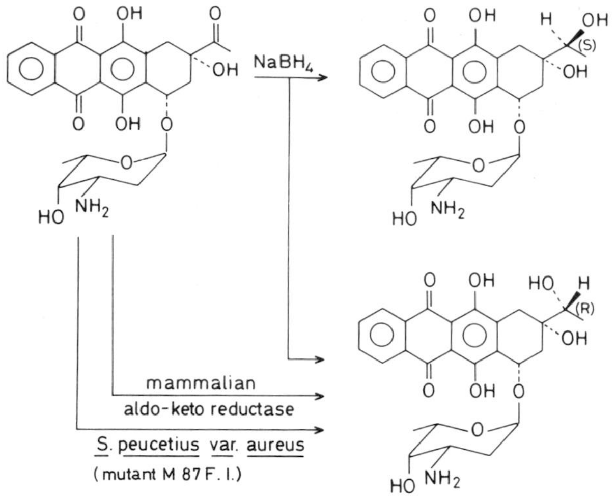

Fig. 9. Chemical and biological reduction of 4-demethoxydaunorubicin.

tic products should be considered as a major line of investigation, expecially when aimed towards the discovery of novel structural types.

Well-known biosynthetic daunorubicin analogues are carminomycin and the baumycins. In our laboratory, 13-dihydrocarminomycin (Cassinelli *et al.* 1978), 13-deoxocarminomycin and the 11-deoxy analogues (Arcamone *et al.* 1980, Cassinelli *et al.* 1982) were obtained from mutant strains of *S. peucetius* (Fig. 6, 7). From a different mutant we have isolated a rhodomycin complex consisting of 3 major components that were identified as β-rhodomycin I, β-rhodomycin and γ-rhodomycin I (synonym iremycin). Because of their particular interest, the 11-deoxy analogues were also prepared by total synthesis (Umezawa *et al.* 1980, Penco *et al.* 1983). The biological activity of the 11-deoxy analogues and the rare occurrence (Brockmann & Niemeyer 1968) of 6-deoxy anthracyclines (the only known biosynthetic anthracyclinones bearing a 6-deoxy group are those presented in Fig. 8) have prompted the total synthesis of new, daunorubicin related, 6-deoxy glycosides (Penco *et al.* 1983).

Biotransformation of antitumor anthracyclines in microbial cultures has been investigated by us, expecially in connection with studies of metabolism of anthracyclines in clinical patients. The presence of daunorubicinol, the main daunorubicin metabolite in man and in laboratory animals, in *S. peucetius* cultures has already been mentioned. More recently, we found that *S. peucetius var. aureus* was able to reduce the C-13 carbonyl of 4-demethoxydaunorubicin (idarubicin) to give the corresponding 13-dihydroderivative, idarubicinol, in good yields (Cassinelli *et al.* 1983). The reduction was stereoselective and the compound was found undistinguishable from a sample of idarubicinol isolated from human urine extracts by selective HPLC analysis (C-18 reverse-phase column). Both compounds had the same retention time (35 min) which corresponded to that exhibited by the minor component of the epimeric mixture resulting from the sodium borohydride reduction of idarubicin (Fig. 9). Absolute stereochemistry of both semisynthetic 13-dihydro derivatives was determined upon proton NMR analysis of the 9,13-O-isopropylidene derivatives of the corresponding aglycones. The metabolite identified as 4-demethoxy-13(R)dihydrodaunorubicin, idarubicinol, exhibits noticeable antitumor activity in standard experimental murine system, and is apparently responsible for the prolonged plasma levels of radioactivity after administration of radioactive idarubicin (Cassinelli *et al.* 1983).

REFERENCES

Arcamone, F. (1981) Doxorubicin, Anticancer Antibiotics. Medicinal Chemistry, a Series of Monographs. ed. deStevens, G., Vol. 17, Academic Press, New York.

Arcamone, F., Cassinelli, G., Di Matteo, F., Forenza, S., Ripamonti, M. C., Rivola, G., McCabe, T. & Clardy, J. (1980) The structures of novel antracycline antitumor antibiotics from *Micromonospora peucetica. J. Am. Chem. Soc. 102,* 1462–1463.

Arcamone, F., Cassinelli, G. & Penco, S. (1982) Recent developments in the chemistry of doxorubicin-related anthracycline glycosides. In: *Anthracycline Antibiotics,* ed. El Khadem, H. S., pp 59–74. Academic Press, New York.

Arcamone, F., Franceschi, G. & Penco, S. (1974) Process for the preparation of adriamycin and adriamycinone and adriamycin derivatives. U.S. Patent 3,803,124 (April 9, 1974).

Bertazzoli, C., Sammartini, Y., Balconi, F., Rovero, C., Nasini, A., Dell'Oro, I., Antongiovanni, V., Tosana, M. G. & Lux, B. (1982) Experimental Toxicology of 4'-Deoxydoxorubicin. Proc. Int. Cancer Congress, Sept. 8–15, 1982, Seattle, USA, Abs. n. 2325, p 407.

Brockmann, H. (1963) Anthracyclinone und Anthracycline. In: *Fortschritte der Chemie Organischer Naturstoffe,* vol. 21, pp 121–182. Springer Verlag, Wien.

Brockmann, H. & Niemeyer, J. (1968) α_2-Rhodomycinon, α-citromycinon, γ-cytromycinon. *Chem. Ber. 101,* 1341–1348.

Carter, S. K. (1975) Adriamycin. A review. *J. Nat. Cancer Inst. 55,* 1265–1274.

Casazza, A. (1982) Antitumor Activity of Anthracyclines: Experimental Studies. In: *Anthracycline Antibiotics in Cancer Therapy,* eds. Muggia, F. M., Young, C. W. & Carter, S. K., pp 13–29. Martinus Nijhoff Publishers, The Hague, Boston, London.

Cassinelli, G., Grein, A., Masi, P., Suarato, A., Bernardi, L., Arcamone, F., Di Marco, A., Casazza, A., Pratesi, G. & Soranzo, C. (1978) Preparation and biological evaluation of 4-O-demethyldaunorubicin (carminomycin I) and of its 13-dihydroderivative. *J. Antibiotics 31,* 178–184.

Cassinelli, G., Grein, A., Merli, S., Penco, S., Rivola, G., Vigevani, A., Zini, P. & Arcamone, F.

(1983) 4-Demetossi-13-(R)-diidrodaunorubicina, nuova antraciclina antitumorale ottenuta per biotrasformazione della 4-demetossidaunorubicina. II Convegno Nazionale Sostanze Organiche Naturali nell'Industria Chimica. Struttura e Sintesi. Pisa 26–28 maggio 1983.

Cassinelli, G., Rivola, G., Ruggieri, D., Arcamone, F., Grein, A., Merli, S., Spalla, C., Casazza, A., Di Marco, A. & Pratesi, G. (1982) New Anthracycline Glycosides. 4-O-Demethyl-11-deoxydoxorubicin and Analogues from *Streptomyces peucetius var. aureus. J. Antibiotics 35,* 176–183.

Cassinelli, G., Ruggieri, D. & Arcamone, F. (1979) Synthesis and antitumor activity of 4'-O-methyldaunorubicin, 4'-O-methyladriamycin, and their 4'-epi analogues. *J. Med. Chem. 22,* 121–123.

Ganzina, F. (1983) 4'-Epi-Doxorubicin: A Preliminary Overview of Clinical Data. *Cancer Treat. Rev. 10,* 1–22.

Giuliani, F. C., Zirvi, K. A., Kaplan, N. O. & Goldin, A. (1981) Chemotherapy of Human Colorectal Tumor Xenografts in Athymic Mice with Clinically Active Drugs: 5-Fluorouracil and 1,3-bis-(2-Chloroethyl)-1-Nitrosourea (BCNU) Comparison with Doxorubicin Derivatives: 4'-Deoxydoxorubicin and 4'-O-Methyldoxorubicin. *Int. J. Cancer 27,* 5–13.

Lambertenghi-Delliers, G., Pogliani, E., Maiolo, A. T. & Polli, E. E. (1982) 4-Demethoxydaunorubicin (IMI 30) in the Treatment of Adult Acute Leukemia. 3rd Int. Symp. on Therapy of Acute Leukemias, Rome, December 11–14, 1982.

Penco, S., Angelucci, F., Arcamone, F., Ballabio, M., Barchielli, G., Franceschi, G., Suarato, A. & Vanotti, E. (1983) Regiospecific Total Synthesis of 6-Deoxyanthracyclines: 4-Demethoxy-6-Deoxy daunorubicin. *J. Org. Chem. 48,* 405–406.

Penco, S., Angelucci, F., Ballabio, M., Barchielli, G., Suarato, A., Vanotti, E., Vigevani, A. & Arcamone, F. (1983) Synthesis and Ring A Conformations of New Anthracyclines. The 9th Int. Congress of Heterocyclic Chemistry, Aug. 21–26, 1983, Tokyo (Japan).

Penco, S., Angelucci, F., Ballabio, M., Vigevani, A. & Arcamone, F. (1980) Stereospecific Epoxidation of Anthracyclinones: a Route to 8(R)-Methoxydaunomycinone. *Tetrahedron Lett. 21,* 2253–2256.

Praga, C., International Medical Director of Farmitalia Carlo Erba, Milan, Italy, 1982, personal communication.

Suarato, A., Penco, S., Vigevani, A. & Arcamone, F. (1981) Anthracycline chemistry: direct conversion of daunorubicin into the L-arabino, L-ribo, and L-xylo analogues, and selective deoxygenation at C-4'. *Carbohyd. Res. 98,* C1–C3.

Umezawa, H., Takahashi, Y., Naganawa, H., Tatsuta, K. & Takeuchi, T. (1980) Synthesis of 4-Demethoxy-11-Deoxy Analogs of Daunomycin and Adriamycin. *J. Antibiotics 33,* 1581–1585.

Varini, M., Kaplan, S., Togni, P. & Cavalli, F. (1981) Phase I Trial of 4'-Demethoxydaunorubicin (IMI 30 – NSC 256439). 7th An. Meeting European Society for Medical Oncology, Lausanne, Oct. 28–31, 1981, Abs. n. 05-0374.

DISCUSSION

PORTOGHESE: Is intercalation important for the action of adriamycin?

ARCAMONE: I have not taken into consideration the modes of action because of time, but we consider that DNA intercalation is the main mechanism of action. We have collected a number of data concerning the stability of the complex between different analogues and double-stranded DNA, and we have found a fairly good correlation between the value of the stability constant and the potency, which does not mean anti-tumour activity. Adriamycin for example has a stability constant with native DNA in the order of 10^7. When the value of the stability constant is lower, you may have an anti-tumour effect, but higher doses of the compounds are needed.

PORTOGHESE: I think I recall some chronicle on experiments in which they covalently bound adriamycin to some macromolecules, and the compound was still anti-tumour active.

ARCAMONE: Yes, in my opinion, this means that when adriamycin is bound covalently to the macromolecules, it is no longer adriamycin, and the polymer is no longer the same polymer. You have synthetized a new compound which may have biological activity *per se*. In a recent paper, it was described that an inactive analogue became active after coupling with a polymer. So, we may conclude that if one makes a covalent linkage between adriamycin and any polymer, a new product is obtained, which may be active, but irrespective of the mechanism of action of adriamycin.

RAZDAN: Would you like to comment on the cardiotoxicity of some of the new analogues, which you have on the market, compared to adriamycin?

ARCAMONE: The cardiotoxicity of the new analogues is lower than that of adriamycin, at least in rats, mice, and in rabbits. Actually, adriamycin is one of the most cardiotoxic compounds we know within this series.

RAZDAN: Has it been shown which part of the molecule of adriamycin is responsible for the cardiotoxicity?

ARCAMONE: There are different opinions on that, and there have been a number of publications. Some publications say that DNA can also be inhibited in the heart. There is some evidence that radicals generated from the quinone units are involved in the cardiotoxicity. I am not convinced, because in this case any quinone should be cardiotoxic. Another theory is that the calcium channel can be inhibited by this compound. This phenomenon has been observed, but in very simple systems that have nothing to do with the heart, but such a mechanism still is a possibility.

LAZDUNSKI: I don't think there is any good evidence that the compound is active at the cell surface or on specific channels. The cardiotoxic effect probably is linked to the entry of the compound into the cell. The distribution has been studied, and unfortunately, the compound is everywhere inside the cell. Everywhere means that it is also accumulated in larger amount in the sarcoplasmic reticulum. This is a general pertubation, which may perturb the accumulation and the release of calcium in and from the sarcoplasmic reticulum. I personally believe that the cardiotoxicity is more likely to be the result of the interaction with the DNA.

ARCAMONE: Some pathologists involved in the animal toxicity studies have also noticed alterations of the sarcoplasmic reticulum.

LAZDUNSKI: This raises the question: what happens in cellular systems, which are relatively similar, like the skeletal muscle system and the smooth muscle system. What kind of alterations are observed? Do these compounds produce muscular weakness?

ARCAMONE: Yes, they do, but at higher doses, and the mechanism might be different. The higher toxic effects are cumulative and progressive. If you treat a rabbit for 6 weeks with 3 injections per week, and you analyze the heart after the 6 weeks, you observe alterations. If you then leave the animal for 1–2 months, and then make histologic examinations, the heart is in a much worse state. On the other hand, the muscular weakness is an acute effect.

CASSADY: There are some recent reports that, subsequent to intercalation, there are specific double-strand breaks in DNA, that appear to be mediated by enzymatic responses. I was just wondering whether the people at Farmitalia had an opinion on how this may relate to the mechanism of action of these compounds?

ARCAMONE: Breaks in DNA have been observed by our biologists looking at the effects of the drugs in cell culture. However, you may also have inhibition of cell growth without the breaks. So, the relevance of this effect for the anti-tumour effect still has to be established.

IV. Natural Products as Experimental Tools and Leads in Drug Design

Natural Toxins and Drug Development

Bernhard Witkop & Arnold Brossi

NATURAL PRODUCTS AS LEAD SUBSTANCES

Natural products from plants and animals historically and factually have been the most important source of lead substances that either directly, or indirectly after chemical modification or total synthesis, became useful therapeutic agents (König 1980).

Synthetic strategies and a better understanding of the parameters that govern the relation between structure and activity, such as the Hansch model (partition coefficient of a drug between water and octanol) (Seydel & Schaper 1979), the measurement of electronic factors (Hammett parameters ρ and σ) (Craig 1971), steric effects (Taft parameters), or the Topliss scheme (lipophilicity *versus* electronic factors, Topliss 1972), have all become meaningful steps in a more systematic approach to drugs that has reduced significantly the serendipity factor in medicinal research.

OPENING UP NEW SOURCES: MARINE BIOTOPES, AMPHIBIAN ALKALOIDS, FRESH-WATER ALGAE, MUSHROOMS AND INSECTS

Paul Scheuer has been pioneering the chemical approach to marine ecology (Scheuer 1978, 1982). A direct outcome of his efforts is the impressive structure of palytoxin (Moore & Bartolini 1981, Shimizu 1983), the most potent marine toxin known, the most complicated natural product, 64 chiral centers and 7 double bonds allowing geometric isomerism, ever elucidated by methods excluding x-ray crystallography, and the most active coronary vasoconstrictor (Kaul *et al.* 1974), presumably by interaction with Ca^{++} channels (Reuter 1983). The didemnins, cyclic depsipeptides, isolated from tunicates (Rinehart jr. *et al.*

National Institutes of Health National Institute of Arthritis, Diabetes, and Digestive and Kidney Diseases Bethesda, Maryland, 20205 U.S.A.

NATURAL PRODUCTS AND DRUG DEVELOPMENT, Alfred Benzon Symposium 20.

Editors: P. Krogsgaard-Larsen, S. Brøgger Christensen, H. Kofod, Munksgaard, Copenhagen 1984.

1983, 1982) possess strong antiviral and antineoplastic activities (Canonico *et al.*
1982). Continued interest in other active cyclopeptides, such as the immunosuppressive cyclosporin A from the fungus *Trichoderma polysporum* (Borel
1980), has recently been traced back to the stimulus derived from the first highly-
active cyclopeptides, the ama- and phallo-toxins from *Amanita* mushrooms
(Witkop 1983). Sea anemones have given us potent cardiotonic (Norton 1981),
and cardiotoxic marine peptides (Alsen 1983), the first time since William
Withering's introduction of fox-glove principles, the digitalis glycosides, that
natural products with such strong cardiotropic action have been discovered. As
all life originated probably from the sea, so living processes are illuminated by
products from the sea.

Batrachotoxins, histrionicotoxins, pumiliotoxins, completely novel, unsuspected and unpredictable structures, have given new leads and impetus to
synthetic organic chemistry, neurophysiology, pharmacology and to comparative evolutionary herpetology (Daly 1982, Witkop & Gössinger 1983, Myers &
Daly 1983).

South American hylid frogs belonging to the genus *Phyllomedusa,* have
yielded the heptapeptide *dermorphin,* a novel opioid peptide, which, surprisingly
enough, contains a D-alanine residue in its sequence: H-Tyr-D-Ala-Phe-Gly-
Tyr-Pro-Ser-NH$_2$. By intracerebroventricular injection 10 ng dermorphin had
one thousand times the analgesic effect of morphine at the same dosage
(Montecucchi *et al.* 1981). We must not forget at this junction that morphine, the
oldest analgesic natural product, has been modified to advantage recently,
especially in the promising series of 6-ketomorphinans (Schmidhammer *et al.*
1983).

Urotensin I, a straight-chain peptide of 38 amino acids, isolated from the
urophysis, a special neurosecretary system of unclear function in many fish,
produces a sustained hypotension in most mammalian species (MacCannel &
Lederis 1983).

An African frog, *Kassina senegalensis,* has provided us with a novel natural
representative of the family of antiserotinergic drugs, a harmane derivative
resulting from the condensation of tryptophan with a metabolite of arginine
(Aizawa 1982).

Dihydroadaline, derived from adaline (Gössinger & Witkop 1980), the toxin
of the lady bug, has high affinity to muscarinic acetylcholine receptors
(Burgermeister *et al.* 1978). A related homologous tropane, anatoxin-a, the
"very fast death factor" (VFDF) from the fresh-water bluegreen alga, *Anabaena*

Flos-Aquae (Carmichael & Gorham 1978), turned out to be the strongest agonist known for the nicotinic acetylcholine receptor (Spivak *et al.* 1980).

TOXINS AND THE CONCEPT OF SPECIFIC RECEPTORS

More and more we associate natural products with the receptors to which they bind, may they be neuronal, hormonal or endocrine, a viewpoint which was emphasized at the International Congress on Medicinal Plant Research, Natural Products as Medicinal Agents (Witkop 1981). On a more sophisticated level we now profit from, and return to, the pioneering thoughts of Paul Ehrlich (Witkop 1981, 1982). We are able to admire the growth of Ehrlich's ideas on the amboceptor, which we now call immunoglobulins, for which he prophetically postulated 2 binding sites, one for complement, the other for antigen molecules, bold eidetic concepts that were impressively vindicated by modern Röntgen-ray crystallography. In a similar way, the stepwise progression of more and more valid representations for the nicotinic acetylcholine receptor (nAchR) are equally impressive and help to understand the importance of 2 natural products, one the strongest agonist in this system, anatoxin-a from algae, the other histrionicotoxin from frogs, a special blocker of ion transport.

ANATOXINS AND OTHER SEMIRIGID AGONISTS AND THEIR INTERACTION WITH NICOTINIC ACETYLCHOLINE RECEPTORS

Anatoxin-a, as the natural (+)-enantiomer, is about 2.5 times more potent than racemic synthetic (+)-anatoxin-a (Spivak *et al.* 1983), and about 30 times more

Table I

Potency ratios for pairs of agonists tested at frog rectus abdominis muscles

Drug Pair	No. of frogs	Potency ratio	95% confidence interval
Natural vs. (±)-AnTX-a	7	2.5	2.2–2.9
Synthetic (+)-AnTXa vs. Carb	7	12	
(−)-Cytisine vs. (±)-AnTX-a	6	0.088	0.075–0.104
TMA vs. Carb	5	0.20	0.17–0.23
(+)-Muscarone vs. Carb	8	0.77	0.67–0.90
Arecoline methiodide vs. Carb	8	1.3	1.2–1.4
(−)-Ferruginine vs. Carb	8	0.2	
(−)-Ferruginine methiodide vs. Carb	8	3.3	2.7–4.0
(−)-Norferruginine vs. Carb	7	0.1–0.2	
Arecolone methiodide vs. Carb	9	8.6	7.5–10.0

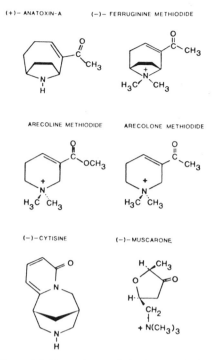

Fig. 1. Structures of the cyclic semi-rigid agonists studied. These projections were drawn to show the family resemblance among the top 4 agonists and the similar placement of the carbonyl and amine groups in the bottom 2 agonists. Although (−)-muscarone is depicted, racemic muscarone was used. In addition to these cyclic agonists, tetramethylammonium was also tested.

active than carbachol (Table I, Fig. 1). In addition, anatoxin-a, not being an ester, is, therefore, not a substrate of choline esterase. The stereoselectivity of the AChR for AnTX-a supports the view that the AChR does recognize chirality and more than 2 points on the agonist molecule. The high (>1000:1) stereoselectivity of the AChR for the moderately potent agonist, *trans*-3-acetoxy-1-methylthiane (Lambrecht 1981), studied on the *rectus abdominis* muscle of the frog *R. temporaria* also supports this view. Stereoselectivity by the nicotinic AChR has not been widely appreciated, partly because few optically active nicotinic agonists are known, and fewer of their enantiomeric pairs have been tested. The stereoselectivity of nicotinic receptors for the enantiomers of one agonist, nicotine, was found to vary considerably between various preparations (Barlow & Hamilton 1965, Abood *et al.* 1983). Another pair, (+)- and (−)-muscarone, does show little difference in nicotinic activity between enantiomers (Gyrmek & Unna 1958, 1960, Waser 1961), but this result can be explained by the following hypothesis. We propose that the AChR donates a hydrogen bond to the agonist (Beers & Reich 1970) and recognizes a plane defined by the hydrogen bond acceptor (*i.e.,* the carbonyl group and its 2 substituents). The anionic site of the AChR is positioned out of this plane, off the C=O axis. These conditions suffice to establish chirality at the recognition site, and, furthermore, help to explain the effect that quaternization has on agonist potency. The muscarone enantiomers are nearly equipotent because the quaternary nitrogen lies *on* the carbonyl plane (data from Pauling & Petcher 1972), so that the methyl groups, which, like ACh, probably bear the positive charge (Pullman *et al.* 1971), can project on either side of this plane, regardless of the enantiomer. This hypothesis explains the function of quaternization as a forced displacement of a methyl group out of the carbonyl plane. Although 3-acetylpyridine methiodide is a quaternary amine, the N-methyl group of this feeble agonist lies on the carbonyl plane. Arecoline (Meyer & Oelszner 1971, Burgen 1964) and arecolone (our results) are weaker than their N-methyl derivatives because steric crowding enforces the equatorial conformation, in which the methyl group is approximately on the carbonyl plane. In polycyclic agonists, such as AnTX-a, cytisine and nicotine, quaternization is unnecessary because the ring systems themselves separate the cationic regions from the carbonyl plane. N-methylation of nicotine, for example, enhances potency by only 1.8-fold (Barlow *et al.* 1969), and successive methylation of (−)-cytisine leads to incremental decreases in potency (Barlow & McLeod 1969). However, the activity of (−)-ferruginine methiodide did not fit this hypothesis. It is not clear why N-methylation so markedly enhanced its activity.

Two of the agonists, arecoline methiodide and (−)-ferruginine methiodide, have not been tested previously for nicotinic activity. Arecolone methiodide in particular may have future usefulness because it is very potent (Table 1), while being chemically stable and simpler than bicyclic agonists. Our finding of a potency ratio of 1.3 for arecoline methiodide to Carb agrees with the ratio of 1.4 found previously (Burgen 1964). From our results one can calculate a potency ratio fo cytisine to TMA of 5.5. By multiplying previous values for equipotent molar ratios involving cytisine, β-pyridylmethyltrimethylammonium, m-hydroxyphenylpropyltrimethylammonium, and TMA (Barlow *et al.* 1969, Barlow & McLeod 1969, Barlow 1976), one can compute a similar potency ratio of 5.3 as obtained by Barlow and co-workers. We found muscarone to be relatively weak, 0.8 times the potency of Carb. This contrasts with the reports that muscarone is twice as potent as ACh (Waser 1958). In the previous studies, however, no anticholinesterase agent was used, which can easily account for the discrepancy (we find ACh + 10 μM neostigmine to be about equipotent with (+)-AnTX-a in contracture experiments).

Conformation	Steric Energy Keal	Dihedral Angle C=C–C=0	Non-bonded Distance Between N and O of (O van der Waals Radius)
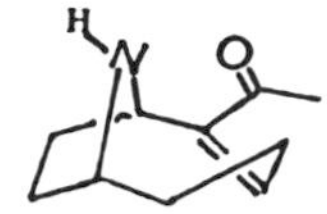 H-Anti-S-trans	ANAT 01　25.03	173.57	5.134
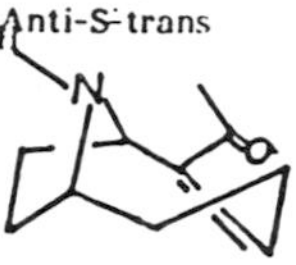 H-Anti-S-cis	ANAT 03　25.53	-8.78	6.257
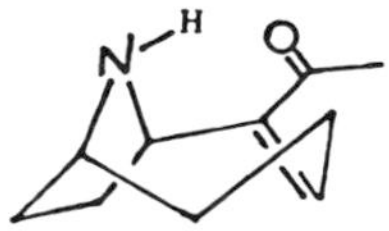 H-Syn-S-trans	ANAT 02　26.43	173.22	5.116
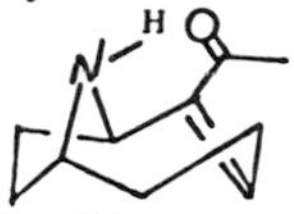 H-Syn-S-trans	ANAT 12　27.30	-171.89	5.126
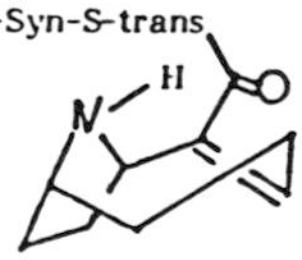 H-Syn-S-cis	ANAT 02A　26.12	-13.38	6.228
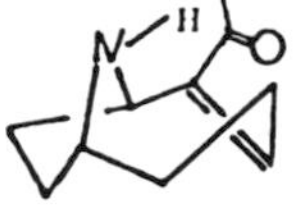 H-Syn-S-cis	ANAT 12A　27.65	21.30	6.366

Fig. 2. Preliminary results by Tamara Gund on (+)-anatoxin-a indicate that the 7-membered ring prefers the boat conformation. The lowest energy conformer (ANAT 01) is a boat with the amine hydrogen *anti* to the acetyl, and the carbonyl in the *s-trans* conformation. The boat conformation is presumably favored because of cross-ring repulsions in the chair. The energy difference between the s-*trans* and the s-*cis* enone isomers is only about 0.5 Kcal, with the *trans* being lower in energy. The C=C–C=O dihedral angle for the *cis* and *trans* isomers, and non-bonded distance value for minimized structures according to Beers and Reich's distance hypothesis are listed. The Dreiding model predictions that the *s-trans* does not have the proper distance for nicotinic activity (range 5.12–5.13 Å), but the s-*cis* fits the models very well (6.23–6.26 A.), can be concluded from the data.

MOLECULAR MODELING OF AGONIST AND RECEPTOR

Because L(+)-muscarine from the mushroom *Amanita muscaria* is a cholinergic agonist, the completely flexible natural agonist, acetylcholine, is presumed to assume a skewed (quasi-cyclic *cis* or gauche) rather than the extended conformation when binding to the nAChR, a view too simplistic to accomodate more recent advances. A semi-rigid agonist, such as anatoxin-a, still permits a large number of possible discrete conformations, 6 of which are presented in Fig. 2 and characterized by their energy content, as a function of steric arrangement of the dihedral angle of the conjugated carbonyl and the non-bonded distance between nitrogen and oxygen atoms (Gund unpublished, Gund *et al.* 1980). The lowest energy conformer (ANAT 01) is a boat with the amine hydrogen *anti* to the acetyl, and the carbonyl in the *s-trans* conformation. The boat conformation is presumably favored because of cross-ring repulsions in the chair. The energy difference between the *s-trans* and the *s-cis* enone isomers is only about 0.5 Kcal, with the trans being lower in energy. Dreiding model predictions show that the *s-trans* does not have the proper distance for nicotinic activity (Range 5.12–5.13 Å), but the *s-cis* fits the models of Beer and Reich very well (6.23–6.26).

Attempts to model the binding site of the receptor are facilitate by the very recent knowledge of the complete amino acid sequences of the α- (Noda *et al.* 1982), β- (Noda *et al.* 1983a), γ- (Claudio *et al.* 1983), and δ- (Noda *et al.* 1983) subunits of the nAChR of *Torpedo californica* and their structural homology (Noda *et al.* 1983b). Changeux views the AcCh binding site within 1–209 of the α-subunit on the synaptic side of the membrane facing the synaptic cleft (Devillers-Thiery *et al.* 1983). This long hydrophilic sequence should carry the AcCh binding site and the glycosylated residues that determine the interaction with monoclonal antibodies against the receptor at, or close to, the transmitter-binding region (James *et al.* 1982).

Kosower has developed a structural model of the acetylcholine receptor (AChR) on the basis of the complete amino-acid sequences of all the protein subunits of the AChR (Fig. 3). Single-group rotation (SGR) theory was used to select ion "channel elements". These "elements" are α-helical sequences of 24 amino acids in which + (lys) and − (glu or asp) side chains occupy one side and hydrophobic side chains the other. The AChR has 5 subunits, 2 α- and one each of β-, γ- and δ-subunits. Two channel elements were identified in each α-subunit, and one channel element in each of the other subunits, for a total of 7 elements around the ion channel. One of the 2 acetylcholine binding sites was located at the entry to the ion channel. Single-group rotation of a bound acetylcholine and

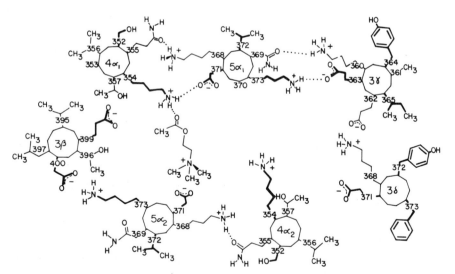

Fig. 3. Model of the acetylcholine/AChR ion channel in the open conformation according to Kosower.

its associated lysine from an initially *closed (Fig. 3)* conformation gave an *open* conformation, with a space just large enough for a hydrated Na$^+$ ion *(Fig. 4)*

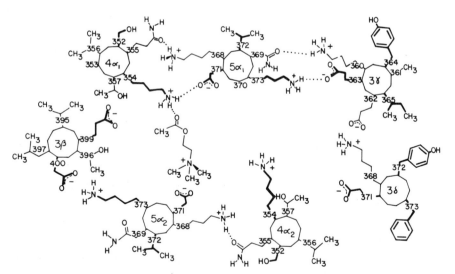

Fig. 4. Model of the acetylcholine/AChR ion channel in the closed conformation according to Kosower.

(Kosower 1983a,b). The binding site has been computer-modeled, using crystallographic data for α-helices of polypeptides, acetylcholine, d-tubocurarine and anatoxin-a (Kosower & Petsko, unpublished). The ion channel "core" of the AChR is surrounded by 17 hydrophobic helices. The structural model of the AChR has a mass distribution (extracellular, bilayer and intracellular) (Kosower 1983c) which is consistent with that obtained by analysis of electron micrographic images of organized AChR layers (Kistler 1982).

The hydrophobic helices have been the only transmembrane elements recognized by those who reported the sequences (Numa 1982, 1983a,b, Changeux 1983, Claudio 1983), and by themselves do not account for the binding of agonists, the gating of the ion channel, or for the passage of ions through the cell membrane. A strong homology between the AChR subunits sequences has been noted, but homology in function is not clear (Numa 1983b).

The bond lengths and angles of anatoxin-a are deducible from those published for N-acetylanatoxin-a (Huber 1972) and are being fitted to the computer-drawn receptor sites developed by E. M. Kosower.

HISTRIONICOTOXINS AND THE NICOTINIC ACETYLCHOLINE RECEPTOR (nAChR) IONOPHORE

While the recognition site of the AChR discriminates between optical antipodes, especially in the case of anatoxin-a, the ionophore fails to make a different response to natural $(-)$-perhydrohistrionicotoxin and its unnatural $(+)$-antipode or their depentyl analogs, respectively (Takahashi et al. 1982).

This lack of discrimination may reflect on the architecture of the ionophore, no longer considered a separate entity from the nAChR but an integral part, so that attempts to fractionate the ionophore as a discrete protein subunit on the basis of binding to histrionicotoxin now possess only historical interest (Eldefrawi et al. 1978). Our understanding of ion channels has been greatly helped by developments in the area of channel-forming peptides, such as gramicidin (Sarges & Witkop 1964, 1965, Urry et al. 1982), or alamethicin (Fox & Richards 1982).

New simplified N-benzyl-spiropiperidine analogs of HTX (Fig. 5) were prepared; they affect the excitable membrane by suppressing sodium and potassium conductances and block neuromuscular transmission by interacting with the ionic channel of the nAChR. The voltage- and concentration-dependent decrease of the peak EPC amplitude and marked shortening of τ_{EPC}

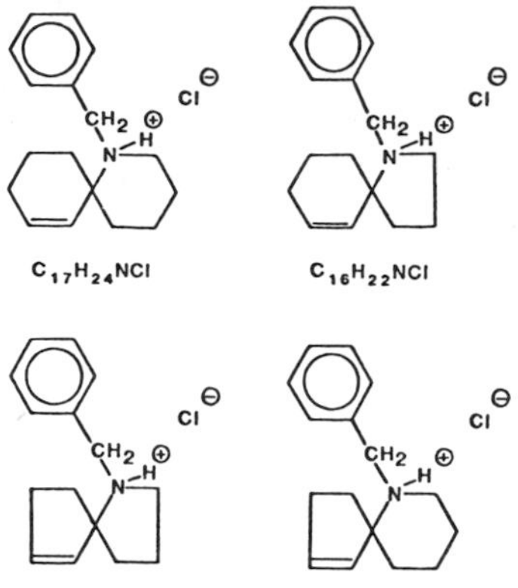

Fig. 5. N-Benzyl intermediates in the synthesis for the spiropiperidine system of histrionicotoxin as inhibitors of sodium and potassium conductances in the ion channel of the AcChR (Maleque 1983).

and τ_1 suggest that the analogs interact with the ionic channel in open conformation in contrast to HTX which interacts both in closed and open conformation (Maleque *et al.* 1983).

STRUCTURE ACTIVITY STUDIES OF HISTRIONICOTOXINS: THE PROSTHETIC CORE?

Further simplification of the histrionicotoxins would lead to unalkylated or

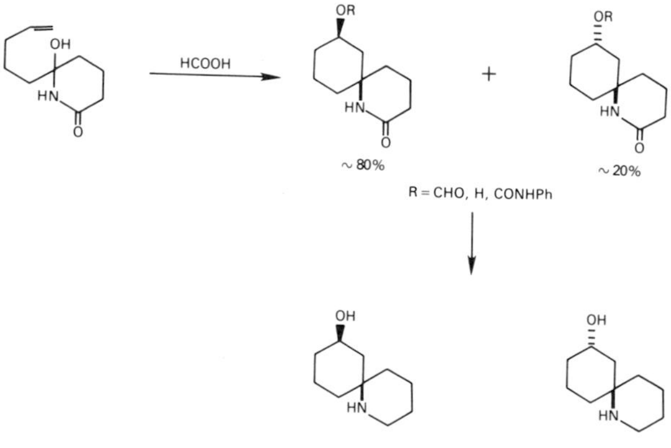

Fig. 6. Approach to "naked" spiropiperidines present in the histrionicotoxins by the cyclization method of Godleski (1981).

"naked" spiropiperidines of the type first prepared by E. Gössinger *et al.*
(Gössinger *et al.* 1975), and later by S. A. Goldeski (Goldleski *et al.* 1981). A
more recent approach to these structures yielded both the (natural) *cis*- as well as
the *trans*-esters, separable through their phenylisocyanate derivatives. The
chemistry of these spiropiperidine alcohols and ketones and the attachment of
ω-pentenyl side-chains (*Figs. 6–8*) was explored in depth (Gessner *et al.*, in

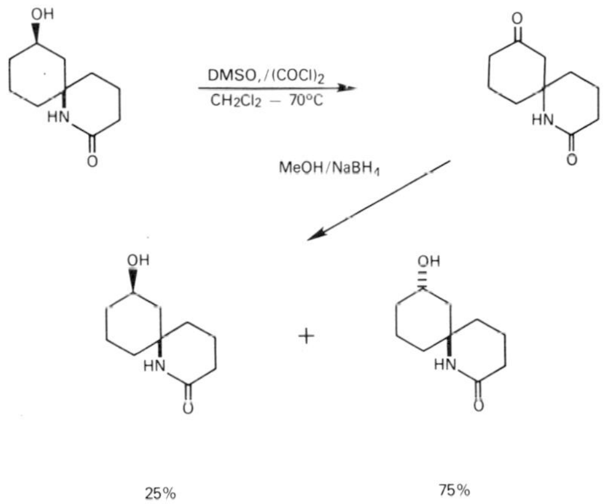

Fig. 7. Separation and resolution of diastereoisomeric spiropiperidines via sodium borohydride
reduction of ketones having only one chiral center (Gessner 1983).

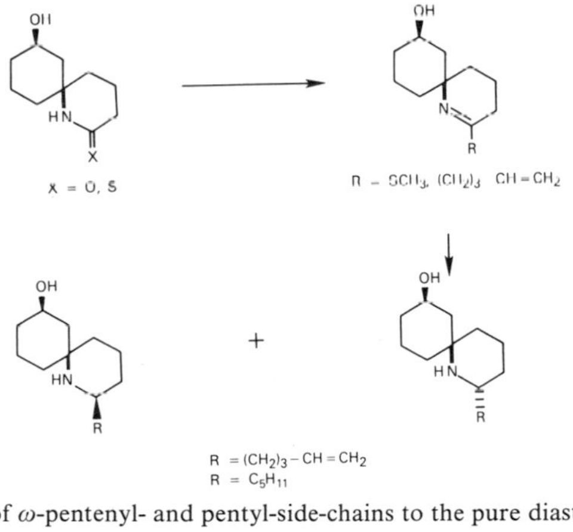

Fig. 8. Attachment of ω-pentenyl- and pentyl-side-chains to the pure diastereoisomers of "naked"
cyclohexanolspiropiperidines *via* alkylmercaptoimines (Gessner 1983).

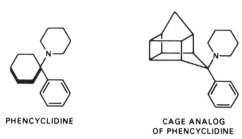

PHENCYCLIDINE   CAGE ANALOG
                            OF PHENCYCLIDINE

Fig. 9. Phencyclidine competes with the histrionicotoxins for potassium channels especially in the brain. Some cage analogs are even more effective.

preparation). Their evaluation for electrophysiological activity is in progress.

In this context phencyclidine may be considered as a further simplification of the histrionicotoxin molecule, comparable in its competitive and selective effects on certain potassium channels (Albuquerque *et al.* 1980) especially in the central nervous system (Vignon *et al.* 1982, Blaustein & Ickowica 1983) with pronounced behavioral effects. Attempts to improve the potency of phencyclidine, remarkable as it is, focus on cage analogs (Fig. 9) of this unique molecule (Witkop 1982, Kloog *et al.* 1979).

Photo-activated phencyclidine has been used for labelling its receptors (Blaustein & Ickowicz 1983, Oswald & Changeux 1981). We have studied the photochemistry of phencyclidines and found a surprising mode of cleavage that so far has not been taken into consideration in photolabeling experiments (Yonemitsu, unpublished).

MOLECULAR UNDERSTANDING OF DISEASES PRESAGES TREATMENT
Our increased understanding and awareness of the molecular events of nervous transmission and muscle action eventually will translate into new therapeutic approaches. We suspect that small, but important, differences in cholinergic channel properties are at the root of *myasthenia gravis,* presumably an autoimmune disorder affecting one or more components of the postsynaptic membrane, now being studied by monoclonal antibodies (Gomez & Richman 1983, Albuquerque *et al.* 1981). Other diseases, such as Alzheimer's disease, communication diseases in children, or muscular dystrophy, with a more genetic etiology, are believed to be connected with biochemical defects of nAChRs (or muscarinic AcChRs) in the central nervous system, or with reduced levels of enzymes involved in the biosynthesis and breakdown of acetylcholine (Davies

1983). Here, the availability and administration of centrally active sitedirected agonists of the anatoxin-a type is a challenge to the clinician and psychiatrist. Attempts to improve sleeping patterns and memory with cholinergic drugs, with simpler agonists and precursors, such as pilocarpine, physostigmine or choline, have been under clinical trial for a number of years. The elevation of these studies to a higher level of understanding of agonists would be desirable.

REFERENCES

Abood, L. G., Grassi, S. & Costanza, M. (1983) *FEBS Letters 157,* 147–149.

Akizawa, T., Yamasaki, K., Yasuhara, T. & Nakajima, T. (1982) *Biomed. Res. 3,* 232.

Albuquerque, E. X., Tsai, M.-C., Aronstam, R., Witkop, B., Eldefrawi, A. R. & Eldefrawi, M. E. (1980) *Proc. Nat. Acad. Sci. USA 77,* 1224–1228.

Albuquerque, E. X., Warnick, J. E., Mayer, R. F., Eldefrawi, A. T. & Eldefrawi, M. E. (1981) *Annals of the N. Y. Acad. Sci.,* 496–518.

Alsen, C. (1983) *Federation Proceedings 42,* 101–108.

Barlow, R. B. & Hamilton, J. T. (1965) The stereospecificity of nicotine. *Br. J. Pharmacol. 25,* 206–212.

Barlow, R. B. & McLeod, L. J. (1969) Some studies on cytisine and its methylated derivatives. *Br. J. Pharmacol. 35,* 161–174.

Barlow, R. B., Thompson, G. M. & Scott, N. C. (1969) The affinity and activity of compounds related to nicotine on the rectus abdominis muscle of the frog (*Rana pipiens*). *Br. J. Pharmacol. 37,* 555–584.

Barlow, R. B. (1976) The effects of pH on the activity of coryneine and related phenolic quaternary ammonium salts on the frog rectus preparation. *Br. J. Pharmacol. 57,* 517–520.

Beers, W. H. & Reich, E. (1970) Structure and activity of acetylcholine. *Nature (Lond.) 228,* 917–922.

Blaustein, M. P. & Ickowicz, R. K. (1983) *Proc. Nat. Acad. Sci. USA 80,* 3855–3859.

Cf. Borel, F. (1980) *Trends in Pharmacological Research,* 146.

Burgen, A. S. V. (1964) The comparative activity of arecoline and arecoline N-methosalt. *J. Pharm. Pharmacol. 16,* 638.

Burgermeister, W., Klein, W. L., Nirenberg, M. & Witkop, B. (1978) *Molec. Pharmacol. 14,* 751.

Canonico, P. G., Pannier, W. L., Huggins, J. W. & Rinehart, K. L. (1982) Antimicrobial agents and chemotherapy, S., 696.

Carmichael, W. W. & Gorham, P. H. (1978) *Mitteilungen Internat. Verein für Immologie 21,* 285–295.

Claudio, T., Ballivet, M., Patrick, J. & Heinemann, S. (1983) Nucleotide and deduced amino acid sequences of *Torpedo californica* acetylcholine receptor γ-subunit. *Proc. Nat. Acad. Sci. USA 88,* 1111–1115.

Daly, J. W. (1982) In: *Progress in the Chemistry of Natural Products, Vol. 41,* eds. Herz, W., Grisebach, H. & Kirby, G. W., pp. 205–340, Springer-Verlag Wien, New York.

Davies, P. (1983) The neurochemistry of Alzheimer's disease and senile dementia. *Medicinal Research Reviews 3,* 221–236.

Devillers-Thiery, A., Giraudat, J., Bentaboulet, M. & Changeux, J.-P. (1983) Complete mRNA coding sequence of the acetylcholine binding α-subunit from *Torpedo Marmorata* acetylcholine receptor. A model for the transmembrane organization of the polypeptide chain. *Proc. Nat. Acad. Sci. USA 80,* 2067–2071.

Eldefrawi, M. E., Eldefrawi, A. T., Mansour, N. A., Daly, J. W., Witkop, B. & Albuquerque, E. X. (1978) Acetylcholine receptor and ionic channel of *Torpedo* electroplax: Binding of per-hydrohistrionicotoxin to membrane and solubilized preparations. *Biochemistry 17,* 5474–5483.

Fox, R. O. & Richards, F. M. (1982) *Nature 300,* 325–329.

Gessner, W., Witkop, B., Takahashi, K., Albuquerque, E. X. & Bross, A., (in preparation.)

Godleski, S. A., Meinhart, J. D., Miller, J. D., Wallendael, S. V. (1981) *Tetrahedron Letters,* 2247.

Gomez, C. M. & Richman, D. P. (1983) Anti-acetylcholine receptor antibodies directed against the α-bungarotoxin binding site induce a unique form of experimental myasthenia. *Proc. Nat. Acad. Sci. USA 80,* 4089–4093.

Gössinger, E. & Witkop, B. (1980) *Monatshefte für Chemie, 111,* 803–811.

Gund, T., unpublished; *cf.,* Gund, T., Andose, J. D., Rhodes, J. B. & Smith, G. M. (1980) Three-dimensional molecular modeling and drug design. *Science 208,* 1425–1431.

Gyrmek, L. & Unna, K. R. (1960) Spectrum of action of muscarone and its derivatives. *J. Pharmacol. Exp. Ther. 128,* 30–36.

Gyrmek, L. & Unna, K. R. (1958) Relation of structure of synthetic muscarines and muscarones to their pharmacological action. *Proc. Soc. Exp. Biol. Med. 98,* 882–885.

Huber, C. S. (1972) *Acta Cryst. B28,* 2577–2582.

Cf. James, R. W., Kato, A. C., Rey, M.-J. & Fulpius, B. W. (1980) *FEBS Letters 120,* 145–148; (1982) *Trends in Pharmacological Science,* 315–316.

Kaul, P. N., Farmer, M. R. & Cierezko, L. C. (1974) *West Pharmacol. Soc. 17,* 249–301.

Kistler, J., Stroud, R. M., Klymkowsky, M. W., LaLancette, R. & Fairclough, R. H. (1982) Structure and function of an acetylcholine receptor. *Biophys. J. 37,* 371–383.

König, H. (1980) Pharmaceutical chemistry today – Changes, problems and opportunities. *Angew. Chemie (Internat. Ed.) 19,* 749–761.

Cf. Kloog, Y., Gabrialevitz, A. & Kalir, A. (1979) *Biochem. Pharmacol. 28,* 1447–1450.

Kosower, E. M. (1983a) Partial tertiary structure assignment for the acetylcholine receptor on the basis of the hydrophobicity of amino acid sequences and channel location using single group rotation theory. *Biochem. Biophys. Res. Commun. 111,* 1022–1026.

Kosower, E. M. (1983b) Partial tertiary structure assignments for the beta-, gamma- and delta-subunits of the acetylcholine receptor on the basis of the hydrophobicity of amino acid sequences and channel location using single group rotation theory. *FEBS Letters 155,* 245–247.

Kosower, E. M. (1983c) A molecular model for the bilayer helices of the acetylcholine receptor including an acetylcholine binding site. *FEBS Letters, 157,* 144–146.

Lambrecht, G. (1981) Struktur und Konformations-wirkungs-beziehungen heterozyklischer Ace-tylcholin-Analoga. 12. Synthese und cholinerge Eigenschaften stereoisomerer 3-Acetoxythiacy-clohexane. *Arzneim. Forsch. 31,* 634–640.

MacCannell, K. L. & Lederis, K. (1983) *Federation Proc. 42,* 91–95.

Maleque, M., Albuquerque, E. X., Witkop, B. & Brossi (1983) *J. Pharmacol. Exp.* Therap., in press.

Meyer, F. P. & Oelszner, W. (1971) Charakterisierung cholinerger Pharmaka im Hinblick auf ihre Rezeptoreigenschaften. *Acta Biol. Med. Germ. 26,* 799–809.

Myers, C. W. & Daly, J. W. (1983) *Scientific American 248,* 120–133.

Montecucchi, P. C., de Castiglione, R., Piani, S., Gozzini, L. & Erspamer, V. (1981) *Int. J. Peptide Protein Res. 17,* 275–283.

Moore, R. E. & Bartolini, G. (1981) *J. Amer. Chem. Soc. 103*, 2491 & 5572; *cf.* Shimizu, Y. (1983) *Nature 302*, 212.

Noda, M., Takahashi, H., Tanabe, T., Toyosato, M., Furutani, Y., Hirose, T., Asai, M., Inayama, S., Miyata, T. & Numa, S. (1982) Primary structure of α-subunit precursor of *Torpedo californica* acetylcholine receptor deduced from cDNA sequence. *Nature 299*, 793–797.

Noda, M., Takahashi, H., Tanabe, T., Toyosato, M., Kikyotani, S., Hirose, T., Asai, M., Takashima, H., Inayama, S., Miyata, T. & Numa, S. (1983a) Primary structures of β- and δ-subunit precursors of *Torpedo californica* acetylcholine receptor deduced from cDNA sequences. *Nature 301*, 251–255.

Noda, M., Takahashi, H., Tanabe, T., Toyosato, M., Kikyotani, S., Furutani, Y., Hirose, T., Takashima, H., Inayama, S., Miyata, T. & Numa, S. (1983b) Structural homology of *Torpedo californica* acetylcholine receptor subunits. *Nature 302*, 528–532.

Norton, T. R. (1981) Cardiotonic polypeptides from *anthopleura xanthogrammica* and *A. elegantissima. Federation Proc. 40*, 21–25.

Oswald, R. & Changeux, J.-P. (1981) *Proc. Nat. Acad. Sci. USA 78*, 3925–3929.

Pauling, P. & Petcher, T. J. (1972) Muscarone: an enigma resolved? *Nature (Lond.) 236*, 112–113.

Pullman, B., Courriere, Ph. & Coubeils, J. L. (1971) Quantum mechanical study of the conformational and electronic properties of acetylcholine and its agonists muscarine and nicotine. *Mol. Pharmacol. 7*, 397–405.

Cf., Reuter, H. (1983) Calcium channel modulation by neurotransmitters, enzymes and drugs. *Nature 301*, 569–574.

Rinehart, K. L., Jr., Cook, J. C., Jr., Pandey, R. C., Gaudioso, L. A., Meng, H., Moore, M. L., Gloer, J. B., Wilson, G. R., Gutowsky, R. E., Zierath, P. D. & Shield, L. S. (1982) *Pure Appl. Chem. 54*, 2409.

Rinehart, K. L., Jr., Gloer, J. B., Wilson, G. R., Hughes, R. G., Jr., Li, L. H., Renis, H. E. & McGovren, J. P. (1983) *Fed. Proc. 42*, 87–90.

Sarges, R. & Witkop, B. (1964) *J. Amer. Chem. Soc. 86*, 1862; (1965) J. Amer. Chem. Soc. 87, 2011.

Scheuer, P. J. (1978) Marine natural products, chemical and biological perspectives. Academic Press, New York.

Scheuer, P. J. (1982) Marine ecology: some chemical aspects. *Naturwiss. 69*, 528–533.

Schmidhammer, H., Jacobson, A. E., Brossi, A. (1983) *Medicinal Research Reviews 3*, 1–20.

Cf, Seydel, J. K. & Schaper, K. J. (1979) Chemische Struktur und biologische Aktivität von Wirkstoffen. In: Methoden der QSWA, Verlag Chemie, Weinheim- New York.

Shimizu, Y. (1983) *Nature 302*, 212.

Spivak, C. E., Witkop, B. & Albuquerque, E. X. (1980) *Molec. Pharmacol. 18*, 384–394.

Spivak, C. E., Waters, J., Witkop, B. & Albuquerque, E. X. (1983) *Mol. Pharmacol. 23*, 337–343.

Takahashi, K., Witkop, B., Brossi, A., Maleque, M. A. & Albuquerque, E. X. (1982) *Helv. Chim. Acta 65*, 252–261.

Topliss, J. G. (1972) *J. Med. Chem. 15*, 1006–1011.

Urry, D. W., Prasad, K. U. & Trapane, T. L. (1982) *Proc. Natl. Acad. Sci. USA 79*, 390–394.

Vignon, J., Vincent, J.-P., Bidard, J.-N., Kamenka, J.-M., Geneste, P., Monier, S. & Lazdunski, M. (1982) *Europ. J. Pharmacol. 81*, 531–542.

Waser, P. G. (1958) Struktur und Wirkung des Muscarins, des Muscarons und ihrer Stereoisomeren. *Experientia 14*, 356–358.

Waser, P. (1961) Strukturabhängigkeit der Wirkung muscarin-ähnlicher Verbindungen. *Experientia 17*, 300–302.

Witkop, B. (1981) Natural products, receptors and ligands. In: *Planta Medica, Special Volume,* eds. Beal, J. L., Reinhard, E., pp. 151–184, Hippokrates Verlag, Stuttgart.

Witkop, B. (1981) *Naturw. Rundsch. 34,* 361–379.

Witkop, B. (1982) In: Technology, science and society in the time of Alfred Nobel, eds. Bernhard, C. G., Crawford, E., Söbom, P., pp. 146–166, Pergamon Press, Oxford.

Cf., Witkop, B. (1982) *Heterocycles 17,* 431–445.

Witkop, B. & Gössinger, E. (1983) In: *The Alkaloids,* Vol. 21, ed. Brossi, A., pp. 139–253, Academic Press, New York.

Witkop, B. (1983) *Naturw. Rundschau 36,* 261–275.

Yonemitsu, O. & Witkop, B., unpublished.

DISCUSSION

NAKANISHI: What are your comments on the disagreement between the computer-derived most stable conformation of anatoxin, and the conformation in solution.

WITKOP: These are questions which are as much on our minds, as they are on yours. What we have to do is to co-ordinate the originally independent computer modelling research groups. It has only been within the last few days that they have started to co-ordinate their computer programmes. I think they have to iron-out some of the guiding parameters. As matters stand right now, anatoxin fits very well the open channel conformation of Kosoner in the computer model, and attempts are in progress for the closed conformation.

KROGSGAARD-LARSEN: Did I understand you correctly that the neurotransmitter recognition site and the ion channel function reside in the same biomolecule?

WITKOP: Earlier, we believed in the possibility that we have 2 different molecules. Professor Albuquerque and his group and we tried to separate the part of the acetylcholine receptor molecule that recognizes and binds to, say, bungarotoxin, and the other moiety that binds to histrionicotoxin. Such separation apparently was achieved using detergents, but I think what we did was to rip apart the entire molecule. Now it is fully established that both the receptor site and ion transport sites are part of the same molecule composed of 5 subunits.

LAZDUNSKI: Anatoxin apparently differs from other agonists. Is this compound unique in terms of desensitization?

WITKOP: Yes.

LAZDUNSKI: There is deactivation and then desensitization?

WITKOP: Yes.

DAVIES: Are there any specific monoclonal antibodies made against the receptor?

WITKOP: The monoclonal antibody approach is extremely important when it comes to a better understanding of *myastenia gravis.* In fact most progress has been achieved using the monoclonal antibody technique. The sequencing was also performed using related techniques of "genetic engineering".

KROGSGAARD-LARSEN: From your studies on the natural cholinergic toxins, are there any indications that the peripheral and the central muscarinic receptors have different properties?

WITKOP: That is a very valid question. We are slowly waking-up to the 2 worlds, the world of peripheral action and the world of central action. We face this especially with the neural peptides. We all know that insulin is so important in the pancreas, but all of a sudden claims turn up for potential importance in brain, too. The same situation exists for somatostatin and, of course, for acetylcholine. We know very little about acetylcholine receptors in the brain. Most of them have been considered to be of a muscarinic nature. Now, more and more people think the nicotinic acetylcholine receptors in the brain are also important. These aspects have become very timely in diseases like the Alzheimers disease, where something may be wrong with the acetylcholine system(s) in the CNS.

Natural Toxins and Their Analogues that Activate and Block the Ionic Channel of the Nicotinic Acetylcholine Receptor

Edson X. Albuquerque[1] & Charles E. Spivak[1,2]

INTRODUCTION

The nicotinic acetylcholine receptor (AChR) and its ionic channel, found at the peripheral synapse, are major focal points for research in our laboratories. We have introduced a variety of natural toxins and their synthetic analogues which activate or block the AChR, thus, revealing various states of this complex glycoprotein.

The actions of this receptor may be briefly summarized as follows: the AChR is an intrinsic glycoprotein, with molecular weight of about 250,000 (e.g., Reynolds & Karlin 1978, Martinez-Carrion et al. 1975). It spans the post-synaptic membrane like a "grommet" bearing carbohydrate filaments which wave in the synaptic gap. It extends from about 50 Å on the extracellular side to a cytoplasmatic tail of 15 Å (Klymkowsky et al. 1980, Ross et al. 1977). When a nerve impulse reaches the presynaptic nerve terminal, 6,000–10,000 molecules of the neurotransmitter acetylcholine (ACh) (Albuquerque et al. 1974, Fertuck & Salpeter 1974, Kuffler & Yoshikami 1975) are released in "quanta", diffusing through a synaptic gap of 400–600 Å to high-density patches of AChRs. Upon colliding with these AChRs brief electrical transients appear across the membrane. The binding of ACh to a recognition site on the AChR causes the ionic channel formed by the AChR protein to open, thereby allowing cationic currents (carried chiefly by sodium under normal conditions) to flow down their

[1]Department of Pharmacology & Experimental Therapeutics, University of Maryland School of Medicine, Baltimore, MD 21201, [2]Addiction Research Center, National Institute on Drug Abuse, Baltimore, MD 21224, U.S.A.

NATURAL PRODUCTS AND DRUG DEVELOPMENT, Alfred Benzon Symposium 20.
Editors: P. Krogsgaard-Larsen, S. Brøgger Christensen, H. Kofod, Munksgaard, Copenhagen 1984.

respective electrochemical potential gradients. The channel spontaneously closes after a few milliseconds have elapsed and is ready to be reactivated. Prolonged exposure to ACh or to other agonists produces a state(s), termed desensitization, in which the channel will not readily reopen.

MODE OF ACTION OF NOVEL AGONISTS:

Anatoxin-a

Certain specific natural products affect these processes in at least 4 major and sometimes overlapping ways. They may, 1) as agonists, mimic the action of the natural neurotransmitter, ACh, 2) block this action by competing with ACh, 3) block the AChR by binding at some other site(s) such that ACh still binds, but the ionic channel fails to open, or 4) behave as though they physically occlude (completely or partially) the channel once it has opened. Other mechanisms are likely to exist but are less readily defined by experimental probes currently available.

One of the most potent of the nicotinic agonists tested in frog muscle is an alkaloid obtained from some strains of the fresh-water cyanophyte *Anabaena flos-aquae* (Lyngh.) de Bréb. This alkaloid, anatoxin-a (AnTX-a, Fig. 1 Witkop & Brossi, this volume), has been extracted from algal cultures (Carmichael *et al.* 1975, Devlin *et al.* 1977), and synthesized from cocaine (Campbell *et al.* 1977), and from simpler starting materials (Bates & Rapoport 1979, Campbell *et al.* 1979). Despite this toxin's apparent structural dissimilarity to the natural transmitter, its physiological effects are nearly identical with those of ACh. Its overall potency, determined by contracture of the frog's *rectus abdominis* muscle, is about equivalent with that of ACh (plus 10 μ M neostigmine to inactivate acetylcholinesterase) and 30 times as potent as the commonly used agonist carbamylcholine (Spivak *et al.* 1979, Spivak *et al.* 1983). A more direct measure of this potency, achieved using intracellular recordings of the membrane depolarization produced by the toxin in muscle fibers, confirmed the high potency (Spivak *et al.* 1979). In addition, comparisons of natural, (+)-AnTX-a with the racemic mixture revealed marked stereoselectivity of the recognition site. The natural toxin was 2.1 to 3.1 (99% confidence interval) more potent than the racemic mixture, suggesting that (−)-AnTX-a is inert, or may even antagonize (+)-AnTX-a (Spivak *et al.* 1983). At the channel level, agonist potency depends on how frequently the channels open, the lifetime of the open channel (τ), and the conductance of the channel (γ). In other words, potency depends on the total electric charge that traverses the muscle membrane. To evaluate the channel properties the techniques of noise or fluctuation analysis and patch clamp were used. Briefly stated, in the fluctuation-analysis technique, negative feedback is used to maintain cells at a constant potential (voltage clamp) by 2 intracellular microelectrodes, one for recording membrane potential and one for injecting current. The application of the agonist (by micro-iontophoresis) not only increases this current, since the ion channels are opening, but also causes it to fluctuate due to the random opening and closing of individual channels. Fourier analysis of this fluctuating current yields estimates of channel lifetime and conductance (Anderson & Stevens 1973).

Using fluctuation analysis, AnTX-a was found to be unique among all the agonists studied so far, in that the channel lifetime it induces at 22° C (1.4 ± 0.1

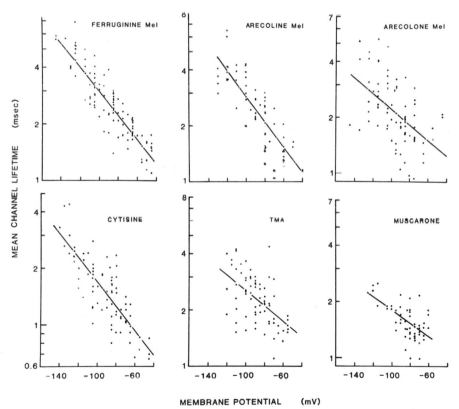

Fig. 1. *Mean channel lifetimes plotted as functions of membrane potential.* In these semi-logarithmic graphs each point represents an estimate obtained from a single spectrum. Regression lines are shown. (From Spivak *et al.* 1983, with permission from Molecular Pharmacology).

msec; n=9) is indistinguishable from that induced by the natural transmitter, ACh (1.4±0.3 msec; n=16) at −80 mV (uncertainties are standard errors). The channel conductance induced by AnTX-a (15.4±0.8 pS; n=16) is slightly less than that produced by ACh (17.9±0.9 pS; n=8) (Spivak et al. 1980). When the desensitization initiated by AnTX-a was compared to that induced by ACh, no difference was seen (Spivak et al. 1980). Thus, despite the fact that AnTX-a is a secondary amine and a bicyclic, conjugated ketone and that ACh a quaternary amine and an aliphatic ester, these 2 compounds are seen by the AChR to be nearly identical.

Structure activity relationship of agonists
Which structural elements of the nearly rigid agonist (+)-AnTX-a endow it with its high potency and similarity to ACh? According to Bates and Rapoport (1979), reduction of the double bond raises LD_{50} by about 10-fold. It may be that this double bond, being conjugated with the exocyclic carbonyl, locks the carbonyl in a co-planar conformation that is most suitable for activating the AChR. In considering the structure of AnTX-a, its similarity to arecoline, the active principle from betel nut, *Areca catechu,* was evident (Fig. 1, Witkop & Brossi, this volume). Though arecoline is known for its muscarinic effects and is a feeble nicotinic agonist (Meyer & Oelzner, 1971, Burgen 1964), its methiodide salt is 1.3 times more potent than carbamylcholine (Burgen 1964, Spivak et al. 1983), or about 1/20 as potent as (+)-AnTX-a at the nicotinic AChR. Simply changing this methyl ester to a methyl ketone to yield arecolone methiodide increased agonist potency by 6.6-fold. This new, semi-rigid nicotinic agonist modelled on AnTX-a is, then, among the most potent of the nicotinic agonists known. Another analogue, (−)-ferruginine, bears an even stronger structural resemblance to (+)-AnTX-a (Fig. 1, Witkop & Brossi, this volume). Natural, (+)-ferruginine is derived from the Australian plant *Darlingia ferruginea* (Bick et al. 1979). We tested the enantiomer, which has the same stereochemistry as (+)-AnTX-a. Though (+)-AnTX-a and nor-(−)-ferruginine differ in structure by a single methylene group, nor-(−)-ferruginine is only about 1/300 as potent as (+)-AnTX-a (Spivak & Albuquerque, unpublished results). (−)-Ferruginine itself (the tertiary amine) is even weaker, about 1/750 as potent as (+)-AnTX-a, but (−)-ferruginine methiodide is much more potent, being 1/9 as potent as (+)-AnTX-a (Spivak et al. 1983). To clarify this rather bewildering pattern of structure and activity, we investigated other semi-rigid agonists (Fig. 1, Witkop & Brossi, this volume). (−)-Cytisine is the active principle from *Laburnum*

anagyroides, and muscarone (we used a racemic mixture) is the oxidation product of muscarine, a toxic principle from the mushroom *Amanita muscaria.* Tetramethylammonium was compared to the other agonists because it is the simplest agonist and is completely rigid.

Relative potencies and channel effects of the agonists at the neuromuscular synapse
Relative potencies of all these agonists are shown in Table 1. At this point some correlation of structure with potency may be discerned (Spivak & Albuquerque 1982, Spivak *et al.* 1983, Witkop & Brossi, this volume). As mentioned above, small changes in structure produce marked changes in potency. Structure and potency, however, are both rather superficial levels of detail. Greater refinements in structure of these and other agonists are being approached by computer modelling (T. Gund, unpublished results). These calculations will yield information on conformation energies, charge distributions, van der Waals surfaces and electrostatic field potential contours.

We have achieved greater refinements in the actions of these agonists by studying the channel properties they induce. Our intent was to determine how these channel properties contribute to potency as well as to find correlations of

Table I

Potencies of agonists relative to (+)-AnTX-a.

Potencies, defined as the reciprocals of the equipotent molar ratios, were estimated using contracture of the rectus abdominis muscle from the frog *Rana pipiens. Data are from Spivak et al.* (1980, 1983).

Drug	Relative potency×100
(+)-AnTX-a	100
Arecolone Methiodide	29
(−)-Ferruginine methiodide	11
Arecoline methiodide	4.3
(−)-Cytisine	3.5
Carbamylcholine	3.3
(±)-Muscarone iodide	2.6
Tetramethylammonium iodide	0.67
Arecolone	0.57
nor-(−)-Ferruginine	0.3
(−)-Ferruginine	0.13
3-Acetylpyridine methiodide	0.07
Arecoline	0.03[a]

[a] Burgen, 1964.

these fundamental measurements with structure. First noise analysis was used to determine channel lifetimes (Fig. 1) and conductances. Lifetimes were exponential functions of membrane potential, as expected (Anderson & Stevens 1973, Magleby & Stevens 1972), and the regression lines shown in Fig. 1 yielded estimates of the mean channel lifetimes at -90 mV. These values are shown with the estimated channel conductances, in Table II. Addressing the first of our objectives, we wished to know to what extent these channel properties contribute to potency. The potency depends upon how much charge crosses a membrane treated with an agonist. This value is the product of channel opening frequency, the current and the lifetime of the open channels. Whereas fluctuation analysis gives no direct information on opening frequency, it does yield reliable estimates of the other 2. When mean channel lifetime and current (at -90 mV) are multiplied together to estimate the charge per channel and plotted against potency, one finds no correlation (Fig. 2). We conclude that, despite these variations in open channel properties, the frequency at which they are induced to open by the various agonists is predominant in determining potency. It is noteworthy, too, that though we see differences in τ, these result from only small changes in the activation energies for channel closure. There is evidence from the photo-isomerizable agonist, *trans*-bis-Q, that channel closure necessarily follows the unbinding of one agonist molecule from its recognition site (Sheridan & Lester 1982). This finding suggests that channel lifetime is governed by the lifetime of the proper agonist-receptor bond. Reinforcement for this view was obtained by Trautmann and Feltz (1980), who provided evidence

Table II

Average channel lifetime (τ) and conductance (γ) obtained by Fourier analysis of endplate current fluctuations.

Sartorius muscle fibers from the frog *Rana pipiens* were voltage clamped at 10°C. The τ values were estimated from the linear regression of ln τ on membrane potential. Uncertainties shown are standard errors. (From Spivak *et al.* 1983).

Agonist	τ at -90 mV msec	γ pS	Number of spectra
($-$)-Cytisine	1.45±0.04	11.2±0.5	80
(±)-Muscarone	1.68±0.05	11.8±0.5	53
Arecolone	2.02±0.08	10.4±0.3	77
Arecoline MeI	2.48±0.08	15.1±0.5	69
Tetramethylammonium	2.33±0.07	13.1±0.4	75
($-$)-Ferruginine methiodide	2.61±0.05	16.5±0.4	99
Acetylcholine	4.4 ±0.3	10.1±0.8	22

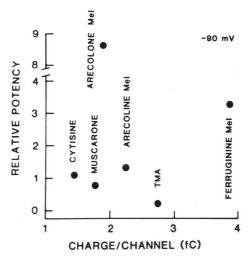

Fig. 2. *Relative potencies and mean charge admitted* (−90 mV) *per open channel plotted as a scattergram.* No correlation can be seen. (From Spivak *et al.* 1983, with permission from Molecular Pharmacology).

that when the AChR is occupied by 2 different agonists, the channel lifetime is the same as if only the agonist that produces the shorter channel lifetime were present. It seems hopeful, then, that the studies with rigid or semi-rigid agonists, both by molecular modelling and by correlation with channel lifetime, can reveal the forces and geometry required to hold the agonist in its activated (open channel) conformation. The variations in γ seen with various agonists (Spivak *et al.* 1983, Colquhoun 1979), as determined by fluctuation analysis, are harder to visualize uniquely at the molecular level. It is possible that only one conductance state exists, but that this state flickers (open to closed) so rapidly that the electronic filtering required by the technique averages amplitudes to a lower level.

To confirm that the channel properties induced by these agonists as inferred by fluctuation analysis is a true reflection of the channel properties, we are retesting the agonists by the "patch clamp" technique. This method, introduced by Neher and Sakmann (1976), permits one to record the rectangular pulse of current (about 2 p Amp amplitude) that flows when a single AChR ion channel opens. The method consists of preparing micropipettes whose tips, about 1 μm in internal diameter, are heat-polished to prevent impalement of the cell and coated with Sylgard to diminish capacitance and conductance across the glass shank. When these pipettes are carefully pressed against a clean (i.e., no collagen

membrane) cell surface and a slight suction applied, a seal of high (around 10 G
Ω) resistance forms such that the noise level of the background current is far less
than the current traversing a single ion channel. An example (Fig. 3) confirms
that one of our agonists, ferruginine methiodide, does indeed induce shorter
channel lifetimes than does ACh.

Mixed effects of drugs are so pervasive that they can be assumed to exist until
disproved. Agonists are no exception: they block their own action by
"desensitization", a term that itself encompasses 2 (perhaps more) kinetically
identifiable states (Sakmann et al. 1980, Feltz & Trautmann 1982). In addition,
one agonist, decamethonium, may terminate its own action by occluding the ion
channel it opened (Adams & Sakmann 1978, Milne & Byrne 1981).

In considering some of the agonists of the (+)-AnTX-a series, we see that 3-
carbonylpiperdidinium-like compounds tend to be active. The fact that 3-
acetylpyridine methiodide is an agonist (though a very weak one, Table 1), in
itself suggests that pyridostigmine (Fig. 5) may also behave as an agonist. This
agent, a well-known, reversible antagonist of acetylcholinesterase, is widely used
in the treatment of *myasthenia gravis*. We have recently confirmed this
prediction (Akaike et al. 1983). When patch-clamp pipettes contained pyridostigmine (100–200 μ M) as the only agonist, single-channel current pulses were
seen (Fig. 4). To prove that these currents were arising through the AChR

ACETYLCHOLINE

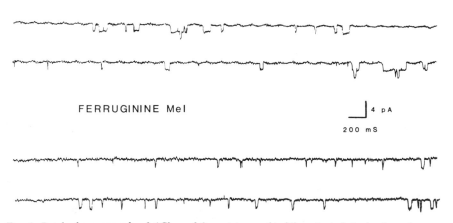

Fig. 3. Patch clamp records of ACh- and ferruginine methiodide-activated single channel currents
obtained from a rat myoball. The channels induced by ferruginine have clearly shorter lifetimes than
those induced by ACh, confirming the data obtained from fluctuation analysis.

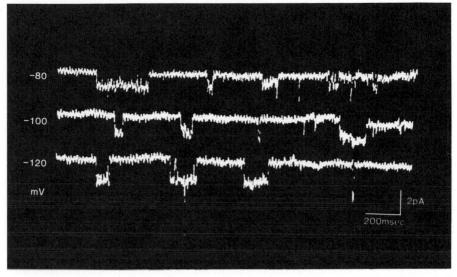

Fig. 4 Patch clamp records of single channel currents induced by pyridostigmine (100 μM). The patch of membrane from which this recording was made remained attached to the cell and the intrapipette potentials (with reference to the bath) are shown.

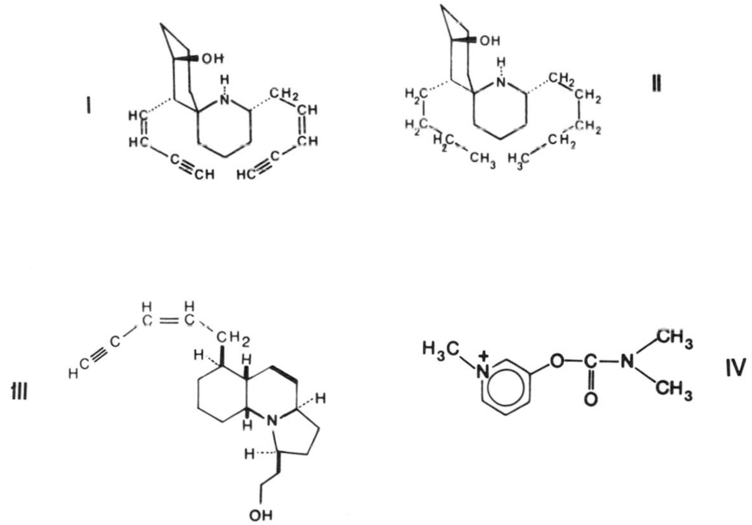

Fig. 5. Structures of 4 compounds that block the AChR non-competitively. Compounds I-IV all come from *Dendrobates histrionicus.* They are (I) histrionicotoxin, (II) perhydrohistrionicotoxin and (III) gephyrotoxin. Compound IV is pyridostigmine, a clinically used antagonist of acetylcholinesterase, now shown to have direct agonist as well as antagonist actions at the AChR as well.

channel, we pretreated the preparation (rat "myoballs", rounded myotubes grown in tissue culture) with α-bungarotoxin, which selectively and irreversibly blocks the recognition site of the AChR. The subsequent test showed no channel currents. Binding studies also confirmed that pyridostigmine bound to the recognition site of the AChR. Concentrations $>30 \mu M$ could partially inhibit the binding of 10 nM ACh or 5 nM α-bungarotoxin (Pascuzzo et al. 1983). The channel currents induced by pyridostigmine alone were of low frequency. This finding may explain the low potency of this compound, which had not been known previously to be an agonist[1]. The single-channel conductance induced by pyridostigmine was low, 12 pS, compared to that induced by ACh, 20 pS.

Further investigation into the action of pyridostigmine revealed that the drug was able to augment neuromuscular transmission at relatively low concentrations (10–100 μM) due to inhibition of acetylcholinesterase. Higher concentrations ($\geqslant 100\,\mu M$), however, block the AChR by a non-competitive mechanism(s) (Pascuzzo et al. 1983). The evidence for this action follows. Endplate current and miniature endplate current amplitudes were reduced, especially at the membrane potentials more negative than -100 mV. Addition of pyridostigmine to patch pipettes (with acetylcholine) caused "flickering" of channel currents followed by an increase in the number of channel currents of abnormally low amplitude (perhaps these were channels activated by pyridostigmine), and a gradual reduction in the frequency of channel opening until, at high pyridostigmine concentrations, it ceased altogether. Micro-iontophoretic application of acetylcholine to the neuromuscular junction in the presence of pyridostigmine, suggested that the blockade deepened when acetylcholine was applied simultaneously, a characteristic of drugs that behave as if they enhance desensitization. Binding experiments showed that, as other non-competitive blockers of the AChR do, pyridostigmine could block (at millimolar concentrations) the binding of [3H]-phencylidine and [3H]-perhydrohistrionicotoxin,

---

[1]One must consider, however, that receptors on cultured muscle fibers are different from those found at endplates of mature muscles. d-Tubocurarine, the classical competitive antagonist, acts as an agonist at the AChRs of rat myotubes (Trautmann 1982, Ziskind & Dennis 1978). However, we have been able to demonstrate that pyridostigmine activates the ACh receptor ion channels macromolecule in innervated single fibers of the interosseal muscle of frog toe. When a gigaohm seal was achieved with a micropipette at the perisynaptic region of these fibers, pyridostigmine (100–200 μM) evoked the appearance of low-conductance channels (about 1.48 pA and -100 mV, inside out condition), and low-frequency channels with similar characteristics to that observed in myoballs. These channel openings were not detected after either myoball or muscle fiber was treated with α-brungarotoxin (Akaike & Albuquerque, unpublished results).

agents that only block the AChR at a non-recognition site(s). Thus, this drug, so well known for its clinical blockade of acetylcholinesterase, has subclinical, direct and conflicting effects on the AChR.

Blockade of the AChR by a non-competitive mechanism was recognized (Albuquerque *et al.* 1973, 1974) in studies of an exotic family of alkaloids (Fig. 5) extracted from the skin of the arrow-poison frog, *Dendrobates histrionicus* (Daly *et al.* 1971). At that time, it seemed a reasonable possibility that the protein that recognizes ACh and the one that composes the ionic channel were separate but linked (Albuquerque *et al.* 1973a, b). It was proposed that the histrionicotoxins could, therefore, be markers useful in the separation, purification and characterization of these 2 entities (Eldefrawi *et al.* 1978, Eldefrawi *et al.* 1977). Though this notion of separate proteins was later disproved, the histrionicotoxins retained prominance as labels for identifying, even defining, the channel components of the AChR biochemically (e.g., Sobel *et al.* 1978, Elliott *et al.* 1979). Confidence in the histrionicotoxins as probes of channel components rested on binding studies that showed that the toxin binding site was distinct from the ACh recognition site (Elliott & Raftery 1977, Kato & Changeux 1976, Burgermeister *et al.* 1977, Elliott & Raftery 1979, Eldefrawi & Eldefrawi 1979, Eldefrawi *et al.* 1980), and on ample electrophysiological results that the toxins altered and blocked the AChR's ionic channel (Albuquerque *et al.* 1973a, b, 1974, Lapa *et al.* 1975, Kato & Changeux 1976, Albuquerque & Oliveira 1979, Spivak *et al.* 1982).

NATURAL TOXINS THAT ARE NON-COMPETITIVE BLOCKERS OF THE AChR:
Kinetic considerations
The numerous electrophysiological actions of the histionicotoxins, reviewed (Albuquerque *et al.* 1980), and extended (Spivak *et al.* 1982) elsewhere, are summarized in Table III. Some results are shown graphically in Fig. 6. Two or more binding sites for the toxins seem needed to account for the diversity of effects, especially the apparent dissociation of peak amplitude and decay-time constants (Table III, item 7). One sufficient scheme (below) requires that the AChR assume 2 conformations when the toxin is bound. In one conformation the channel can open, though with altered kinetics (hence the shortening of the epc decay); in the other the channel is immobilized in the closed conformation. It may be that in the "immobilized" conformation the gate, activated by the agonist, is still free to open but that another segment of the AChR protein moves

Table III

*The Electrophysiological Actions of the Histrionicotoxins (A), Depentylhistrionicotoxin (B), Gephyro-
toxin (C) and Meproadifen (D) on Endplate Currents (epcs) and Single Channel Currents.*

Observation	Interpretation
1. Decreases peak epc amplitude when epcs are triggered singly. Equilibrium is approached slowly (>1 hour). (A–D).	Blocks AChR ionic channel in its resting conformation.
2. a. Trains of epcs further decrease peak amplitude. (A,B,D).	Activation of the channel by the agonsts renders more AChRs vulnerable to blockade. Behaves like accelerated "desensitization".
b. Responses to trains of acetylcholine pulses applied by microiontophoresis fade much more rapidly if drug is present. (A,D).	
3. After a step hyperpolarization (from a holding potential of −50 mV) peak amplitudes diminish with time; the greater the step, the faster they diminish. Activation of the AChRs by agonists is not required. (A,B,D).	Either binding of the toxin is voltage dependent or transition of the toxin occupied receptor from unblocked to blocked conformation is voltage dependent.
4. Time constants for decays of epcs are shortened. (A–C).	Either the toxins occlude the open channel or they allosterically increase the rate constant for channel closure.
5. As toxin concentration increases time constants for epc decays decrease to a limiting value (ca. 1 msec). (A).	Simple occlusion of the open channel is excluded.
6. Voltage sensitivity for the decay time constants of the epcs is less in the presence of the toxins than under control condition. (A–C).	The toxins alter the dipole moment of the gate that closes the channel or modifies the electric field sensed by gate.

7. In contrast to the effect of the toxins on peak amplitudes the time constants of epc decays:
   a. Reach equilibrium faster (10 min <equilibrium time <1 hr) (A,D).
   b. Are unaltered by trains of epcs. (A,D).
	A single binding site for the toxins or a single conformation of the AChR that alters both peak amplitude and time constant for decay is excluded.

Observation	Interpretation
8. In patch clamp and fluctuation analysis they shortened channel lifetime and did not alter channel conductance (A–C).	Interpretation 4.
9. Increase channel opening frequency, followed by decrease and cessation of activity of channel openings, maintain unaltered channel lifetime and cause no change in channel conductance (D).	Interpretation 2. A single binding site is most likely.
10. No change in channel opening frequency but shortening of channel lifetime and maintain unaltered channel conductance (C).	Interpretation 4.

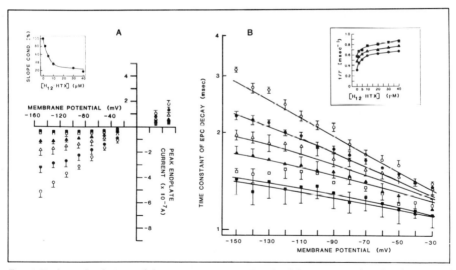

Fig. 6. Peak amplitude (A) and decay-time constants (B) of endplate currents plotted as functions of membrane potential under control condition (O) and in the presence of 2 (●), 5 (△), 30 (□) and 40 (■) μM perhydrohistironicotoxin. Data were obtained from frog sartorius muscles. Bars represent standard errors of at least 9 fibers from at least 3 muscles. The *inset* in B shows reciprocals of decay time constants plotted as a function of concentration and obtained at −50 mV (■), −80mV (▲) and −150 mV (●). (From Spivak *et al.* 1982 with permission from Molecular Pharmacology).

in, relieving strain caused by the bound toxin, to occlude the channel. Movement of this secondary gate could have different kinetics and voltage sensitivity than the normal gate, accounting for observations 4 and 6 in Table III. The scheme is as follows:

$$
\begin{array}{ccccccc}
R & \xrightarrow{\quad A \quad} & A_2R & \underset{\beta}{\overset{\alpha}{\rightleftharpoons}} & A_2R^* \\
T \updownarrow & & T \updownarrow & & T \updownarrow \\
RT & \xrightarrow{\quad A \quad} & A_2RT & \underset{\beta'}{\overset{\alpha'}{\rightleftharpoons}} & A_2R^*T & \text{Scheme I} \\
\updownarrow & & \updownarrow & & \updownarrow \\
\bar{R}T & \xrightarrow{\quad A \quad} & A_2\bar{R}T & \longrightarrow & A_2\bar{R}^*T
\end{array}
$$

In this scheme the AChR is represented by R when it is in its closed state, R* in its open channel state and $\bar{R}$ when it is blocked by the toxin; A represents the agonist and T the toxin. In the absence of histrionicotoxin, the channel is activated through the sequence shown in the top row. When the toxin is added some AChRs are converted to RT, an altered form of AChR that may still activate, but with altered kinetics (second row). To this point, the model (first 2 rows above) described endplate current decays obtained with 5 concentrations of perhydrohistrionicotoxin at membrane potentials ranging from -30 to -150 mV (Spivak et al. 1982, Fig. 6). The third row of the scheme may account for the closed channel blockade ($\bar{R}T$) and the use-dependent effect ($A_2RT \rightarrow A_2\bar{R}T$ and $A_2R^*T \rightarrow A_2\bar{R}^*T$). The use-dependent effect would arise from a favored pathway, $A_2RT \rightarrow A_2\bar{R}T$ or perhaps via $A_2R^*T \rightarrow A_2\bar{R}^*T \rightarrow A_2\bar{R}T$. The observed voltage dependence (Table III, obs. 3) may reside in the transition $R \rightarrow \bar{R}$ in its various forms. Channel closure from the A_2R^*T state could proceed via A_2RT or via $A_2\bar{R}^*T$.

The histrionicotoxins possess allenic and acetylenic bonds and a spiro linkage (Fig. 5). In addition, they have 4 chiral centers to which are attached the major structural groups of the molecule (Daly et al. 1971). Inversion of even a single chiral center could produce drastically different effects. Recently, the enantiomer of natural, $(-)$-perhydrohistrionicotoxin has been synthesized (Takahashi et al. 1982). When we compared both enantiomers carefully in frog sartorius muscles, we found no difference in their blockade of peak amplitude or shortening of the time constant for epc decay (Spivak et al. 1982, Spivak, Maleque & Albuquerque, unpublished observations). On the other hand action potentials in muscle were

Table IV

Effects of (+)- and (−)-H₁₂-HTX on muscle action potentials at incubation times ≥ 60 min.

Muscles were glycerol shocked to abolish the twitch. A current passing microelectrode held membrane potentials at − 100 mV before and between action potentials. Trains of 10 action potentials were elicited at 1 Hz. Means ± SE are shown with numbers of fibers in parentheses.

Action Potential	Condition	Threshold mV	Maximum Rate of Rise V/S	Overshoot mV	Maximum Rate of Fall V/S
Single	Control	48.6±0.5 (26)	363± 8 (26)	43±1 (26)	132±4 (25)
	(−)-H₁₂-HTX	57.8±1.0 (18)	195±21 (18)[a]	40±4 (18)	77±8 (18)
	(+)-H₁₂-HTX	58.2±1.2 (14)	125±14 (14)[a]	35±3 (14)	60±6 (14)
First of train	Control	48.5±0.5 (26)	361± 9 (26)	40±1 (25)	122±4 (25)
	(−)-H₁₂-HTX	58.3±1.1 (14)	177±20 (14)[a]	36±4 (14)	66±7 (14)[a]
	(+)-H₁₂-HTX	60.1±1.0 (14)	113±14 (13)[a]	32±3 (14)	44±4 (13)[a]
Last of train	Control	48.3±0.5 (26)	354± 8 (26)	40±2 (26)	102±5 (26)
	(−)-H₁₂-HTX	59.2±1.1 (13)	112±14 (14)[a]	28±4 (14)[b]	24±3 (14)[a]
	(+)-H₁₂-HTX	61.3±0.9 (14)	45± 7 (14)[a]	16±3 (14)[b]	7±2 (14)[a]

[a] The effects of the 2 enantiomers differ from each other at the P<0.02 level (2-sided Student's t test).
[b] The effects of the 2 enantiomers differ from each other at the P<0.05 level.

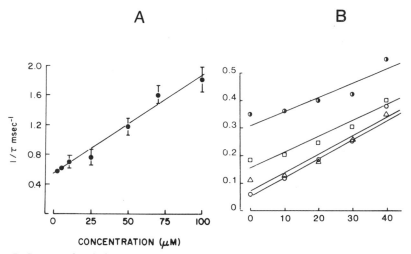

Fig. 7. Reciprocals of the time constants for the decay of epcs obtained in the presence of depentylperhydrohistrionicotoxin (A) and gephyrotoxin (B) plotted as functions of drug concentration. Unlike perhydrohistrionicotoxin (Fig. 6, inset B), these drugs produce linear plots suggesting occlusion of the open channel as the mechanism for blockade. Membrane potentials in B are −150 mV (○), −90 mV (△), −50 mV (□) and +50 mV (●). The temperature in A was 22° C and the temperature in B was 10°C.

slightly, but consistently, more affected (maximum rates of rise and fall were depressed and overshoot was decreased) by (+)- than by (−)-perhydrohistrionicotoxin (see below and Table IV). This finding ruled out the possibility that the toxins were producing all their effects via bulk lipid. We conclude that either the site on the AChR that binds the histrionicotoxins is symmetrical or that hydrophobic interactions overwhelm stereochemical ones (Spivak & Albuquerque 1982).

Alterations in the degree of saturation of the hydrocarbon chains in the histrionicotoxins does alter potency somewhat. Isotetrahydrohistrionicotoxin was most potent and octahydrohistrionicotoxin was least potent of 4 compared by recording endplate currents (Spivak et al. 1982).

When the n-pentyl chain was removed from perhydrohistrionicotoxin, the resulting alkaloid ("depentylperhydrohistrionicotoxin") retained activity as an AChR blocker. Like the parent compound, perhydrohistrionicotoxin (Spivak et al. 1982), the depentyl analogue blocked the peak amplitude of epcs by about 50% at 5 μM and also produced the voltage dependence in the extent of the blockade (Maleque et al. 1984). It is noteworthy that similar natural products, cis- and trans-2-methyl-6-undecyl piperidine, constituents of fire-ant venom, are also potent, non-competitive and practically irreversible blockers of the AChR (Yeh *et al.* 1975). Depentylperhydrohistrionicotoxin shortened the time constants for epc decay and channel lifetime, but, unlike its parent compound, this time constant approached no limiting value, at least up to concentrations that produced complete blockade of the AChR. In contrast to histrionicotoxins (Fig. 6), plots of the reciprocal of the time constants versus toxin concentration were linear (Fig. 7), suggesting that this toxin behaves as an open channel occluding agent (Spivak & Albuquerque 1982).

When both alkyl chains are removed from histrionicotoxins, the resulting compound still blocks the peak amplitude of epc, but potency is markedly reduced to about 0.01 to 0.02 that of the depentyl- and perhydrohistrionicotoxins (Spivak *et al.* 1982). This finding reinforces the view that hydroprobicity plays a large role in non-competitive blockade of the AChR.

The histrionicotoxins also affect the voltage sensitive Na and K channels of the electrically excitable membranes of skeletal muscle. To be evident, these effects require higher (70 μM) concentrations than do effects of the AChR, and are enhanced during trains of repetitive stimuli as shown in Table IV (Spivak *et al.* 1982). Generally, the toxins slow the rate of rise and fall of the action potential and decrease the overshoot. In relatively high concentrations, the toxins have a local anesthetic-like property, i.e., they partially decrease both sodium and potassium conductance. A surface charge effect is a perennial possibility supported by the observation that perhydrohistrionicotoxin raises threshold (Table IV). However, this is insufficient to explain the other effects because, whereas (+)- and (−)-perhydrohistrionicotoxin raise threshold indistinguishably, in other measurements the (+)-enantiomer was somewhat more effective (Table IV).

Besides the histrionicotoxins, the skin of *Dendrobates histionicus* yields another alkaloid, gephyrotoxin (Daly *et al.* 1977). Like the histrionicotoxins it contains a piperidine ring and a 5-membered hydrocarbon (vinylacetylene) chain (Fig. 5). Also like the histrionicotoxins it blocks the AChR, though it takes a higher concentration than depentyl- or perhydrohistrionicotoxin, about 30 μM, to block peak amplitudes of the epc by about 50% (Souccar *et al.* 1984a). Binding studies showed that gephyrotoxin's actions are non-competitive with respect to agonists (Souccar *et al.* 1984b). As was found with (+)- and (−)-perhydrohistrionicotoxin the 2 enantiomers of gephyrotoxin were not discerned by the AChR (Souccar *et al.* 1984b). Gephyrotoxin behaved as if it enhanced desensitization, as do the histrionicotoxins, but differed in a number of other actions. It showed no voltage dependence and, whereas it shortened the time constant for epc decay, this shortening did not approach a limiting value and behaved instead as an open channel blocker (Fig. 7, Souccar *et al.* 1984a).

The AChR is a chemical transducer that converts the chemical potential of an agonist into an electrical signal. Despite all that has been learned in recent years of the structural and behavioral characteristics of the AChR, molecular mechanisms remain obscure. Chemical tools, obtained from and frequently modelled on, natural products from diverse organisms, such as algae and amphibia, highlight aspects of the AChR's actions that will help to elucidate its mechanisms.

ACKNOWLEDGEMENTS

The authors are indebted to Ms. Mabel Alice Zelle for the computer analysis of the data. This work was supported, in part, by a grant from the National Institutes of Health, NS-12063, the United States Army contracts DAMD 17-81-C1279 and DAAG 29-81-K0161.

REFERENCES

Adams, P. R. & Sakmann, B. (1978) Decamethonium both opens and blocks endplate channels. *Proc. Natl. Acad. Sci. USA 75,* 2994–2998.

Akaike, A., Ikeda, S. R., Brookes, N., Pascuzzo, G. J., Rickett, D. L. & Albuquerque, E. X. (1983) The nature of the interaction of pyridostigmine with the nicotinic receptor-ionic channel complex. II. Patch clamp studies. (in press).

Albuquerque, E. X., Adler, M., Spivak, C. E. & Aguayo, L. (1980) Mechanism of nicotinic channel activation and blockade. *Ann. N. Y. Acad. Sci. 358,* 204–238.

Albuquerque, E. X., Barnard, E. A., Chiu, T. H., Lapa, A. J., Dolly, J. O., Jansson, S.-E., Daly, J. & Witkop, B. (1973) Acetylcholine receptor and ion conductance modulator sites at the murine neuromuscular junction: evidence from specific toxin reactions. *Proc. Natl. Acad. Sci. USA 70,* 949–953.

Albuquerque, E. X., Kuba, K. & Daly, J. (1974) Effect of histrionicotoxin on the ionic conductance modulator of the cholinergic receptor: a quantitative analysis of the endplate current. *J. Pharmacol. Exp. Ther. 189,* 513–524.

Albuquerque, E. X., Kuba, K., Lapa, A. J., Daly, J. W. & Witkop, B. (1973) Acetylcholine receptor and ionic conductance modulator of innervated and denervated muscle membranes. Effect of histrionicotoxins. In: *Exploratory Concepts in Muscular Dystrophy, Vol. II.,* ed. Milhorat, A. T., pp 585–600, Excerpta Medica, Amsterdam.

Albuquerque, E. X. & Oliveira, A. C. (1979) Physiological studies on the ionic channel of nicotinic neuromuscular synapses. In: *Advances Cytopharmacol. Vol. 3,* ed. Ceccarelli, B. and Clementi, F., pp. 197–211. Raven Press, New York.

Anderson, C. R. & Stevens, C. F. (1973) Voltage clamp analysis of acetylcholine produced endplate current fluctuations at frog neuromuscular junction. *J. Physiol. (Lond.) 235,* 655–691.

Bates, H. A. & Rapoport, H. (1979) Synthesis of anatoxin-a via intramolecular cyclization of iminium salts. *J. Am. Chem. Soc. 101,* 1259–1265.

Bick, I. R. C., Gillard, J. W. & Leow, H.-M. (1979) Alkaloids of *Darlingia ferruginea. Aust. J. Chem. 32,* 2537–2543.

Burgen, A. S. V. (1964) The comparative activity of arecoline and arecoline N-metho salt. *J. Pharm. Pharmacol. 16,* 638.

Burgermeister, W., Catterall, W. A. & Witkop, B. (1977) Histrionicotoxin enhances agonist-induced desensitization of acetylcholine receptor. *Proc. Natl. Acad. Sci. USA 74,* 5754–5758.

Campbell, H. F., Edwards, O. E., Elder, J. W. & Kolt, R. J. (1979) Total synthesis of dl-anatoxin-a and dl-isoanatoxin-a. *Pol. J. Chem. 53,* 27–37.

Campbell, H. F., Edwards, O. E. & Kolt, R. (1977) Synthesis of nor-anatoxin-a and anatoxin-a. *Can. J. Chem. 55,* 1372–1379.

Carmichael, W. W., Biggs, D. F. & Gorham, P. R. (1975) Toxicology and pharmacological action of anabaena flos-aquae toxin. *Science 187,* 542–544.

Colquhoun, D. (1979) The link between drug binding and response: theories and observations. In: *The Receptors,* Vol. 1. ed: O'Brien, R. D., chap. 3, pp. 93–142, Plenum Press, New York.

Daly, J. W., Witkop, B., Tokuyama, T., Nishikawa, T. & Karle, I. L. (1977) Gephyrotoxins, histrionicotoxins and pumiliotoxins from the neotropical frog *Dendrobates histrionicus. Helv. Chim. Acta 60,* 1128–1140.

Daly, J. W., Karle, I., Myers, C., W., Tokuyama, T., Waters, J. A. & Witkop, B. (1971). Histrionicotoxins: Roentgen-ray analysis of the novel allenic and acetylenic spiroalkaloids isolated from a Colombian frog, *Dendrobates histrionicus. Proc. Natl. Acad. Sci. USA 68,* 1870–1875.

Devlin, J. P., Edwards, E. O., Gorham, P. R., Hunter, N. R., Pike, R. K. & Stavric, B. (1977) Anatoxin-a, a toxic alkaloid from *Anabaena flos-aquae* NRC-44h. *Can. J. Chem. 55,* 1367–1371.

Eldefrawi, M. E., Aronstam, R. S., Bakry, N. M., Eldefrawi, A. T. & Albuquerque, E. X. (1980) Activation, inactivation and desensitization of acetylcholine receptor channel complex detected by binding of perhydrohistrionicotoxin. *Proc. Natl. Acad. Sci. USA 77,* 2309–2313.

Eldefrawi, M. E. & Eldefrawi, A. T. (1979) Biochemical studies on the ionic channel of *Torpedo* acetylcholine receptor. In: *Advances in Cytopharmacology* Vol. 3., eds: Ceccarelli, B. & Clementi, F., pp. 213–223, Raven Press, New York.

Eldefrawi, A. T., Eldefrawi, M. E., Albuquerque, E. X., Oliveira, A. C., Mansour, N., Adler, M., Daly, J. W., Brown, G. B., Burgermeister, W. & Witkop, B. (1977) Perhydrohistrionicotoxin – potential ligand for ion conductance modulator of acetylcholine receptor. *Proc. Natl. Acad. Sci. USA 74,* 2172–2176.

Eldefrawi, M. E., Eldefrawi, A. T., Mansour, N. A., Daly, J. W., Witkop, B. & Albuquerque, E. X. (1978) Acetylcholine receptor and ionic channel of *Torpedo* electroplax: binding of perhydrohistrionicotoxin to membrane and solubilized preparations. *Biochemistry 17,* 5474–5484.

Elliott, J., Dunn, S. M. J., Blanchard, S. G. & Raftery, M. A. (1979) Specific blinding of perhydrohistrionicotoxin to *Torpedo* acetylcholine receptor. *Proc. Natl. Acad. Sci. USA 76,* 2576–2579.

Elliott, J. & Raftery, M. A. (1977) Interactions of perhydrohistrionicotoxin with postsynaptic membranes. *Biochem. Biophys. Res. Commun. 77,* 1347–1353.

Elliott, J. & Raftery, M. A. (1979) Binding of perhydrohistrionicotoxin to intact and detergent-solubilized membranes enriched in nicotinic acetylcholine receptor. *Biochemistry 18,* 1868–1874.

Feltz, A. & Trautmann, A. (1982) Desensitization at the frog neuromuscular junction: a biphasic process. *J. Physiol (Lond.) 322,* 257–272.

Fertuck, H. C. & Salpeter, M. M. (1974) Localization of acetylcholine receptor by ^{125}I-labeled α-bungarotoxin binding at mouse motor endplate. *Proc. Natl. Acad. Sci. USA 71,* 1376–1378.

Kato, G. & Changeux, J.-P. (1976) Studies on the effect of histrionicotoxin on the monocellular electroplax from *Electrophorus electricus* and on the binding of ^{3}H-acetylcholine to membrane fragments from *Torpedo marmorata.* Mol. Pharmacol. 12, 92–100.

Klymkowsky, M. W. & Stroud, R. M. (1979) Immunospecific identification and three-dimensional structure of a membrane-bound acetylcholine receptor from *Torpedo californica. J. Mol. Biol. 128,* 319–334.

Krouse, M. E., Nass, M. M., Nerbonne, J. M., Lester, H. A., Wassermann, N. H. & Erlanger, B. F. (1980) Agonist-receptor interaction is only a small component in the synaptic delay of nicotinic transmission. In: *Neurotransmitter and Hormone Receptors in Insects.* eds: Satelle, D. B., Hall, L. M. & Hildebrand, J. G., pp. 17–26, Elsevier North Holland, New York.

Kuffler, S. W. & Hoshikami, D. (1975) The number of transmitter molecules in a quantum: An estimate from iontophoretic application of acetylcholine at the neuromuscular synapse. *J. Physiol. 251,* 465–482.

Lapa, A. J., Albuquerque, E. X., Sarvey, J. M., Daly, J. & Witkop, B. (1975) Effects of histrionicotoxin on the chemosensitive and electrical properties of skeletal muscle. *Exp. Neurol. 47,* 558–580.

Magleby, K. L. & Stevens, C. F. (1972) The effect of voltage on the time course of end-plate currents. *J. Physiol. (Lond.) 223,* 151–171.

Maleque, M. A., Takahashi, K., Witkop, B., Brossi, A. & Albuquerque, E. X. (1984) A study of the novel analogue depentylperhydrohistrionicotoxin with the nicotinic receptor-ion channel. (submitted).

Martinez-Carrion, M., Sator, V. & Raftery, M. A. (1975) The molecular weight of an acetylcholine receptor isolated from *Torpedo californica. Biochem. Biophys. Res. Commun. 65,* 129–137.

Meyer, F. P. & Oelszner, W. (1971) Charakterisierung cholinerger pharmaka im Hinblick auf ihre Rezeptoreigenschaften. *Acta biol. med. Germ. 26,* 799–809.

Milne, R. J. & Byrne, J. H. (1981) Effects of hexamethonium and decamethonium on end-plate current parameters. *Mol. Pharmacol. 19,* 276–281.

Neher, E. & Sakmann, B. (1976) Single channel currents recorded from membrane of denervated frog muscle fibers. *Nature 260,* 799–801.

Pascuzzo, G. J., Akaike, A., Maleque, M. A., Aronstam, R. S., Rickett, D. L. & Albuquerque, E. X. (1983) The nature of the interactions of pyridostigmine with the nicotinic acetylcholine receptor-ionic channel complex. I. Agonist, desensitizing and binding properties. (in press).

Reynolds, J. A. & Karlin, A. (1978) Molecular weight in detergent solution of acetylcholine receptor from *Torpedo californica. Biochem. 17,* 2035–2038.

Ross, M. J., Klymkowsky, M. W., Agard, D. A. & Stroud, R. M. (1977) Structural studies of a membrane-bound acetylcholine receptor from *Torpedo californica. J. Mol. Biol. 116,* 635–659.

Sakmann, B., Patlak, J. & Neher, E. (1980) Single acetylcholine-activated channels show burst-kinetics in presence of desensitizing concentrations of agonists. *Nature 286,* 71–73.

Sheridan, R. E. & Lester, H. A. (1982) Functional stoichiometry at the nicotinic receptor. *J. Gen. Physiol. 80,* 499–515.

Sobel, A., Heidmann, T., Hofler, J. & Changeux, J.-P. (1978) Distinct protein components from *Torpedo marmorata* membranes carry the acetylcholine receptor site and the binding site for local anesthetics and histrionicotoxin. *Proc. Natl. Acad. Sci. USA. 75,* 510–514.

Souccar, C., Varanda, W. A., Daly, J. W. & Albuquerque, E. X. (1984a) Interactions of gephyrotoxin with the acetylcholine receptor-ionic channel complex. I. Blockade of the ion channel. (in press).

Souccar, C., Varanda, W. A., Daly, J. W. & Albuquerque, E. X. (1984b) Interactions of gephyrotoxin with the acetylcholione receptor-ionic channel complex. II. Enhancement of desensitization. (in press).

Spivak, C. E. & Albuquerque, E. X. (1982) The dynamic properties of the nicotinic acetylcholine receptor ionic channel complex: activation and blockade. In: *Progress in Cholinergic Biology: Model Cholinergic Synapses.* eds: Hanin, I. & Goldberg, A. M., pp. 323–357, Raven Press, New York.

Spivak, C. E., Maleque, M. A. & Albuquerque, E. X. (1982) Actions of (+)-vs. (−)-per-hydrohistrionicotoxin at the frog neuromuscular junction. *Pharmacologist 24,* 103.

Spivak, C. E., Maleque, M. A., Oliveira, A. C., Masukawa, L. M., Tokuyama, T., Daly, J. W. & Albuquerque, E. X. (1982) Actions of the histrionicotoxins at the ion channel of the nicotinic acetylcholine receptor and at the voltage sensitive ion channels of muscle membranes. *Mol. Pharmacol. 21,* 351–361.

Spivak, C. E., Waters, J., Witkop, B. & Albuquerque, E. X. (1983) Potencies and channel properties induced by semirigid agonists at frog nicotinic acetylcholine receptors. *Mol. Pharmacol. 23,* 337–343.

Spivak, C. E., Witkop, B. & Albuquerque, E. X. (1980) Anatoxin-a: a novel, potent agonist at the nicotinic receptor. *Mol Pharmacol 18,* 384–394.

Takahashi, K., Witkop, B., Brossi, A., Maleque, M. A. & Albuquerque, E X, (1982) Total synthesis and electrophysiological properties of natural (−)-perhydrohistrionicotoxin, its unnatural (+)-antipode and their 2-depentyl analogs. *Helv. Chim. Acta 65,* 252–261.

Trautmann, A. (1982) Curare can open and block ionic channels associated with cholinergic receptors. *Nature 298,* 272–275.

Trautmann, A. & Feltz, A. (1980) Open time of channels activated by binding of two distinct agonists. *Nature 286,* 291–293.

Yeh, J. Z., Narahashi, T. & Almon, R. R. (1975) Characterization of neuromuscular blocking action of piperidine derivatives. *J. Pharmacol. Exp. Ther. 194,* 373–383.

Ziskind, L. & Dennis, M. J. (1978) Depolarising effect of curare on embryonic rat muscles. *Nature 276,* 622–623.

DISCUSSION

NAKANISHI: What are the biological effects of simple acetylcholine analogues in which the 2 methylene groups have been replaced by cyclopropane, cyclobutane, or cyclopentane, and with cis- or trans-orientation of the functional groups?

ALBUQUERQUE: I have not studied these compounds.

WITKOP: There is a group in Japan, as well as in Uppsala (Richard Dahlbom), who have synthesized such compounds.

ALBUQUERQUE: I don't know if they have done these types of biochemical experiments.

PORTOGHESE: The synthesis and effects of the *cis*- and *trans*-cyclopropane analogues of acetylcholine were published quite a number of years ago (1). It was found that the *trans*-isomer was as active as acetylcholine, whereas the *cis*-form was not.

LAZDUNSKI: What is the difference between anatoxin and carbamoylcholine or acetylcholine in binding experiments?

ALBUQUERQUE: The electrophysiological experiments using anatoxin show that this is a very potent agonist, certainly more potent than carbamylcholine (Spivak *et al.* 1980, p. 321).

KROGSGAARD-LARSEN: Is it likely that these different agonists may differ substantially in the receptor occupancy time, and is it possible that one could correlate the receptor frequency with the receptor occupancy time?

ALBUQUERQUE: In 1973 we measured the receptor occupancy in preparations, where one can calculate almost precisely the density of the receptor (2,3).

LAZDUNSKI: There is a very important natural compound which is classical in this field, but which you have not talked about, namely curare. Could you tell us how you see the mechanism of action of curare in the light of your studies of cholinergic agonists?

ALBUQUERQUE: The reason why I did not mention curare is that this compound has a rather complex action on the nicotinic receptor at the neuromuscular synapse. The agent is an antagonist of the acetylcholine receptor and also a blocker of the associated ionic channels. The difficulty with studies of curare on this kind of channel is that you have to be very careful about what preparation is used. If you use for example, a denervated preparation or a neuroblast, then curare is no longer a blocker; it appears to interact with the nicotinic receptor as an agonist. But as mentioned above, in the mature muscle curare is not only an agonist but also a non-competitive blocker of the ACh receptor. Apparently, α-bungarotixin is the most reliable antagonist of the acetylcholine receptor.

LAZDUNSKI: Is it possible that molecules like curare, which are considered as antagonists, are in fact agonists which open the channel, but with such a low frequency of opening that when one looks at the macroscopic properties of the system, it looks like an antagonist molecule? It is a fundamental point in pharmacology to differentiate between agonists and antagonists.

(1) Armstrong, P. D., Cannon, J. G. & Long, J. P. (1968) Nature 220, 65–66.

(2) Albuquerque, E. X., Barnard, E. A., Jansson, S. & Wieckowski, J. (1973) Life Sciences 12, 545–52;

(3) Albuquerque, E. X., Barnard, E. A., Porter, C. W. & Warnick J. E. (1974) Proc. Natl. Acad. Sci. USA 71, 2818–22.

Natural Toxins as Pharmacological Tools to Study the Molecular Aspects of Electrical Excitability in Nerve, Skeletal Muscle and Cardiac Cells

Michel Lazdunski

The purpose of this chapter is to summarize the recent developments in the molecular analysis of the fast sodium channel and of the calcium-dependent K^+ channel using biochemical approaches. A particular emphasis will be put on the different natural toxins that can now be used to analyse the properties of these channels.

THE FAST SODIUM CHANNEL

The fast Na^+ channel is the channel which is responsible for the fast rising phase of the action potential in nerve, muscle and cardiac cells. There are now several different classes of neurotoxins that have been found to interact with the fast Na^+ channel.

(a) Tetrodotoxin (TTX) and saxitoxin (STX)

These 2 toxins are probably the most widely used tools both by electro-physiologists and by biochemists to study the Na^+ channel. Both toxins have been obtained in a tritiated form (Ritchie & Rogart 1977, Chicheportiche *et al.* 1980) and both of them have been used for the biochemical titration of Na^+ channels in different preparations of excitable membranes. The main properties of this association are the following: [³H]STX and [³H]TTX derivatives form

Centre de Biochimie du CNRS, Faculté des Sciences Parc Valrose, 06034 Nice Cedex, France

NATURAL PRODUCTS AND DRUG DEVELOPMENT, Alfred Benzon Symposium 20.
Editors: P. Krogsgaard-Larsen, S. Brøgger Christensen, H. Kofod, Munksgaard, Copenhagen 1984.

with the Na$^+$ channel a complex that has a dissociation constant near 1–5 nM. However low-affinity binding-sites for TTX derivatives have also been found in different excitable cells (mammalian cardiac cells in culture, mammalian muscle cells in culture several neuronal cell lines, etc.) (Lombet *et al.* 1982, Renaud *et al.* 1983, Frelin *et al.* 1983); in this case the dissociation constant is near 1 μM (Lombet *et al.* 1982). The physiological expression of low-affinity binding sites for TTX as Na$^+$ channels is under the control of innervation.

The [^{3}H]STX and [^{3}H]TTX binding component of the Na$^+$ channel can be solubilized from the membrane and it can be extensively purified (Norman *et al.* 1983, Barhanin *et al.* 1983b, Agnew *et al.* 1978, Barchi *et al.* 1980, Hartshorne *et al.* 1981, Moore *et al.* 1982). The final steps of the purification lead to the enrichment in the preparation of a single polypeptide component with a MW of near 260,000. Antibodies against this polypeptide immunoprecipitate the [^{3}H]STX binding activity (Moore *et al.* 1982). Affinity labelling with TTX derivatives also specifically labels a polypeptide band at MW 270,000 (Lombet *et al.* 1983).

(b) Veratridine, batrachotoxin, aconitine, grayanotoxin

All these lipid-soluble toxins stabilize an open form of the Na$^+$ channel, and have been extensively investigated using ^{22}Na$^+$ flux studies in a variety of excitable cells in culture (neuroblastoma, skeletal muscle cells, cardiac cells) (Lazdunski & Renaud 1982, Catterall 1980, Lazdunski *et al.* 1980). The most active of all these compounds is batrachotoxin; less active compounds like veratridine and other veratrum alkaloids have a similar type of action.

An interesting aspect of the action of the lipid-soluble toxins is that they not only change the gating properties of the Na$^+$ channel, they also change the selectivity of the channel (Frelin *et al.* 1981b). In contrast to the open form of the Na$^+$ channel obtained by electrical stimulation which is very selective for Na$^+$ *versus* most other monovalent inorganic or organic cations except Li$^+$, the open form of the Na$^+$ channel obtained by treatment with veratridine, batrachotoxin or the other analogous toxins loses much of its ionic specificity; its selectivity resembles that of the nicotinic receptor channel after activation by acetylcholine. The results of this large change of selectivity after toxin treatment is that K$^+$ rapidly leaks out of the cell through the Na$^+$ channel (the ratio being the entry of 2 Na$^+$ ions for the efflux of one K$^+$ ion) (Jacques *et al.* 1980a). The toxin-induced K$^+$ efflux significantly decreases the internal concentration of K$^+$

(Jacques *et al.* 1980a) and is largely responsible for the toxicity of these compounds.

The target site of lipid-soluble toxins is distinct from the common TTX/STX receptor. The site of action of lipid-soluble toxins that stabilize the open form of the Na^+ channel is the same as that recognized by local anaesthetics on the same channel (Frelin *et al.* 1981a).

Finally, although lipid-soluble toxins have always been considered to be specific for the Na^+ channel, it is important to underline that very recent results show that they are also active on slow Ca^{2+} channels in neuroblastoma cells. However, whereas veratridine and batrachotoxin activate the Na^+ channel, they block Ca^{2+} channel activity. Na^+ channel activation and Ca^{2+} channel blockade occur in the same toxin concentration range (Romey & Lazdunski 1982). The action of veratridine and batrachotoxin on both Na^+ and Ca^{2+} channels may suggest that these channels have some structural analogies.

(c) Scorpion toxins (North American and North African) and sea anemone toxins
These toxins are polypeptides (Fig. 1). They are miniproteins highly cross-linked with disulfide bridges (Lazdunski & Renaud 1982, Catterall 1980).

Detailed voltage-clamp studies have been carried out to determine the mechanism of action of these toxins on a wide range of excitable tissues (heart cells, myelinated and non-myelinated nerves, neuroblastoma cells ...) (Mozhayeva *et al.* 1980, Romey *et al.* 1975, Romey *et al.* 1976b). They have all shown that these toxins are very specific for the Na^+ channel and that they specifically slow-down the inactivation step (closing of the channel) without altering activation (opening of the channel), the result being, of course, the production of long-lasting action potentials and the release of neurotransmitters from nerve terminals (Romey *et al.* 1976b, Romey *et al.* 1976a, Abita *et al.* 1977). The toxins have been radiolabelled to a very high specific radioactivity and their interaction with their specific binding-sites has been analysed at the molecular level.

The main properties of the interaction of these toxins with rat brain synaptosomes are the following:
(i) Scorpion toxins (from the scorpion *Androctonus australis Hector* or *Leiurus quinquestriatus*) have the highest affinity for Na^+ channels ($K_d = 1$ nM), but their binding properties are voltage-dependent. These toxins bind to the Na^+ channel in polarized but not in depolarized membranes (Ray *et al.* 1978, Rochat *et al.* 1979, Vincent *et al.* 1980).
(ii) Even the most active sea anemone toxins (*Anemonia sulcata* toxin V for

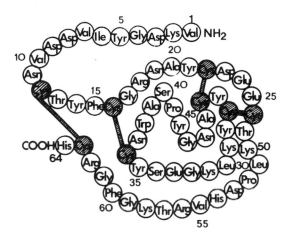

Toxin II from scorpion venom (Androctonus australis Hector)

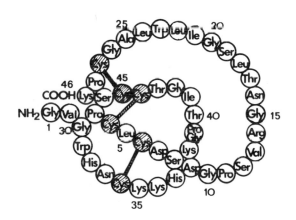

Toxin V from sea anemone (Anemonia sulcata)

Fig. 1. Structures of toxin II from the scorpion Androctonus australis Hector and of Toxin V from the sea anemone Anemonia sulcata.

example) bind to Na^+ channels in synaptosomes with a lower affinity than the scorpion toxins; the dissociation constant of the toxin-receptor complex in the case of toxin V is of the order of 200 nM. However, the binding properties of the radiolabelled sea anemone toxins to Na^+ channels in synaptosomes is not significantly voltage-dependent (Vincent *et al.* 1980).

(iii) Sea anemone toxins are useful tools to detect differences between Na^+ channels from different excitable tissues. They are more efficient than scorpion toxins on Na^+ channels of rat muscle cells and rat cardiac cells in culture. Dissociation constants found for *Anemonia sulcata* toxin V are 2 nM for rat muscle cells and for rat cardiac cells, *i.e.*, 2 orders of magnitude lower than those found for rat brain synaptosomes. The increase of affinity found for cardiac cells and muscle cells in culture is accompanied by the appearance of a voltage-dependence of anemone toxin binding. For example, while the K_d is 2 nM for ATX_V binding to polarized rat muscle cells in culture, it becomes $K_d = 100$ nM after membrane depolarization.

An interesting observation is that high affinity for sea anemone toxins is observed for cells which have a low affinity ($K_d \simeq 1 \mu M$) for TTX. This series of polypeptide toxins interact with the external face of the Na^+ channel.

The analysis of structure-function relationships of *Anemonia sulcata* toxin II (Barhanin *et al.* 1981) has shown that there are 2 important elements in the active site of the toxin. The first is Arg_{14}; this residue is essential for the binding activity and its chemical modification prevents binding of the toxin to its receptor on the Na^+ channel. The second element of the active site is made up of the 3 negatively charged carboxylates in the sequence. Chemical modification of these carboxylates does not prevent toxin binding to its receptor (Barhanin *et al.* 1981), but it suppresses the effect of the toxin on Na^+ channel inactivation. In other words, this chemical modification transforms the sea anemone toxin into an antagonist devoid of toxic activity although retaining its binding activity.

(d) Scorpion toxins from Central and South America

Prototypes of toxins of these kinds are extracted from *Centruroides suffusus suffusus* and *Tityus serrulatus* venoms (*Centruroides* scorpions are also found in some parts of the United States). These toxic compounds once again are miniproteins with a molecular weight of the order of 7,000 daltons. Their sequences are not yet entirely known and it is not yet possible to know the differences which separate these toxins from those of the previous series.

We have found that *Centruroides suffusus suffusus* toxin and *Tityus γ* toxin both block the Na^+ current in skeletal muscle cells (Jaimovich *et al.* 1982), and more recent results indicate that they are active on all kinds of excitable tissues at very low concentrations (Wheeler *et al.* 1982, Barhanin *et al.* 1982). These toxins can be prepared in the radiolabelled form using [125]iodine. The main properties of their interaction with the Na^+ channel are the following:

(i) They bind to a toxin binding-site at the surface of the Na^+ channel that is distinct from all toxin binding-sites described to date.

(ii) Their affinity for the Na^+ channel is very high. The interaction between the channel and *Centruroides suffusus suffusus* toxin II has a dissociation constant $K_d = 0.4$–0.7 nM (Wheeler *et al.* 1982, Barhanin *et al.* 1982); the interaction with *Tityus serrulatus serrulatus* γ toxin has a dissociation constant of 2–5×10^{-12} M *i.e.* about 3 orders of magnitude lower than that found for TTX.

(iii) Their binding to Na^+ channels is not voltage-dependent. Because of their very high affinity for the Na^+ channel (particularly for *Tityus* γ toxin) and because of this voltage-independent interaction, these toxins will probably turn out to be the most useful of all, both for analysing the structure of the channel and for all problems involving its localization.

The protein component of the Na^+ channel that binds *Tityus* γ toxin has now been identified. Affinity labelling experiments have identified a polypeptide with a molecular weight of 266–277,000 as the receptor of the toxin γ (Barhanin *et al.* 1983a). This molecular weight is similar to that found for the TTX-binding component (see above). Indeed, radiation-inactivation experiments show that binding activities for labelled TTX and for labelled *Centruroides* and *Tityus* γ toxin disappear in parallel (Barhanin *et al.* 1983a), indicating an identical molecular weight of 266,000 for both receptors. The most probable conclusion is that the polypeptide with a molecular weight of 260–270,000 has both the TTX and *Centruroides/Tityus* binding sites in its sequence.

Stoichiometry determinations in synaptosomes indicate that sites on the Na^+ channel are in the proportion 2:1:1 for sea anemone toxin, *Tityus* γ toxin and TTX respectively.

(e) Pyrethroids

Pyrethroids are derivatives of chrysanthemic acid that are now extensively used as insecticides. These molecules transform fast Na^+ channels into slower ones (Vijverberg *et al.* 1983, Jacques *et al.* 1980). We have studied their mechanism of action on neuroblastoma cells (Jacques *et al.* 1980). They stimulate $^{22}Na^+$ entry through the Na^+ channel of these cells and do so by acting on a site that is distinct from all other toxin sites discussed till now. They work in synergy with both lipid-soluble toxins and polypeptide toxins that slow down Na^+ channel inactivation (like *Androctonus australis Hector* toxin II or sea anemone toxins). Some pyrethroids are inactive on the Na^+ channel, but their lack of activity does

Table I

A summary of the different classes of toxins acting on the Na⁺ channel

Toxin	Physiological effect
Tetrodotoxin (TTX) Saxitoxin (STX)	block Na$^+$ currents
Lipid-soluble molecules Veratridine Batrachotoxin (BTX) Aconitine Grayanotoxins (GTXs)	cause persistent activation of Na$^+$ channels
North America or North Africa Scorpion toxins (ScTXs) *Androctonus australis Hector* (Toxin II) *Leiurus quinquestriatus* Buthus eupeus	specifically slow down Na$^+$ current inactivation
Polypeptide toxins from sea anemone (ATXs) *Anemonia sulcata* (Toxin II and V) *Anthopleura xanthogrammica* (Toxin I and II)	
Central or South America scorpion toxins *Centruroides suffusus suffusus* (Css$_{II}$) *Tityus serrulatus (Tityus γ)*	block the early Na$^+$ current and create a new type of channel activated at lower potentials
Pyrethroids	modify the closing of fast Na$^+$ channels

not mean that they lack the property of recognition of the channel; they work as antagonists against the effects of active pyrethroids.

The previous discussion shows the large variety of actions exerted by different classes of toxins on the Na$^+$ channel. Table I provides a summary of the most important classes of toxins oriented against the Na$^+$ channel.

An important problem is to determine whether or not excitable cells are the only type of cells containing Na$^+$ channels. We have shown that Na$^+$ channels are also present in non-impulsive cells including fibroblasts (Romey *et al.* 1979, Pouysségur *et al.* 1980, Frelin *et al.* 1982). These Na$^+$ channels have all the neurotoxin binding-sites found for functional Na$^+$ channels. However, Na$^+$ channels in fibroblasts and other non-impulsive cells (Romey *et al.* 1979, Pouysségur *et al.* 1980, Frelin *et al.* 1982) are not physiologically expressed. We have called these Na$^+$ channels silent Na$^+$ channels. Silent Na$^+$ channels cannot be activated electrically but they can be activated chemically using lipid-soluble toxins or mixtures of these toxins and sea anemone toxins (Romey *et al.* 1979, Pouysségur *et al.* 1980, Frelin *et al.* 1982). Under these conditions, when one measures $^{22}Na^+$ fluxes through Na^+ channels the non-impulsive cells start to generate electrical signals.

THE Ca^{2+}-DEPENDENT K^+ CHANNEL
This channel has attracted a lot of interest during the past few years; it links Ca^{2+} metabolism to membrane polarization and is responsible for the repetitive electrical activity of many excitable cells (Meech 1978).

Apamin, a bee venom polypeptide of 18 amino-acids with 2 disulfide bridges (Fig. 2), blocks the Ca^{2+}-dependent K^+ channel in nerve and muscle cells at very low concentrations Hugues *et al.* 1982a, Hugues *et al.* 1982b, Hugues *et al.* 1982c). The toxin can be prepared in a highly radioactive state. The dissociation constant for the apamin-receptor complex is $1.5-2.2 \times 10^{-12}$ M in neuroblatoma cells. Once bound to its receptor site, the toxin dissociates only very slowly ($t^{1/2}=1$ h at 0°C for neuroblastoma cell membranes). The number of Ca^{2+}-dependent K^+ channels in neuroblastoma cells appears to be at most 20% of the number of fast Na^+ channels. The Ca^{2+}-dependent K^+ channels is detectable only once the neuroblastoma cells are morphologically differentiated suggesting that these channels may be preferentially located in dendrites.

Affinity labeling of the Ca^{2+}-dependent K^+ channel with apamin (Hugues *et al.* 1982d) indicates that the receptor of this toxin is a polypeptide with a molecular weight of near 30,000. The total MW of the Ca^{2+}-dependent K^+ channel determined by this laboratory in collaboration with Dr. Ellory (Cambridge) is 250,000.

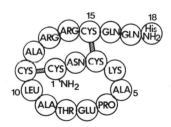

Fig. 2. The structure of apamin, a bee venom toxin.

ARE THESE DIFFERENT TOXINS SUSCEPTIBLE OF PHARMACOLOGICAL
APPLICATION?
Ionic channels and singularly Na^+ channels are the target for a number of useful
drugs like local anesthetics, antiarhythmic drugs, anti-convulsive drugs, etc. A
better knowledge of their structure and mechanism through the use of natural
neurotoxins could certainly help in the devising of new drugs with more
interesting properties than those which already exist. Of course, it is also
possible that some of the toxins could be interesting pharmacological agents by
themselves. The best candidates for such a role appear to be the sea anemone
toxins. These polypeptide toxins are the strongest cardiotonic molecules known
(Lazdunski & Renaud 1982). They slow down the closing of the Na^+ channel in
cardiac cells, thereby producing a massive entry of Na^+ and an indirect
activation of the Na^+/Ca^{2+} exchange system. The indirect stimulation of Ca^{2+}
entry is responsible for the inotropic effect of the molecule (Romey et al. 1980).
The most active of the sea anemone toxins, like toxin V from *Anemonia sulcata,*
are cardiotonic at concentrations as low as $10^{-10}-10^{-9}$ M.

ACKNOWLEDGEMENTS
The author is very grateful to the following members of this laboratory who have
participated during the last few years in the work described in this paper: Dr. J.
Barhanin, Dr. R. Chicheportiche, Dr. M. Fosset, Dr. C. Frelin, Dr. M. Hugues,
Dr. Y. Jacques, Dr. E. Jaimovich, P. Léopold, Dr. A. Lombet, Dr. G. Ponzio,
Dr. J. F. Renaud, Dr. G. Romey, A. and E. Schmid, Dr. H. Schweitz, Dr. P.
Vigne, Dr. J. P. Vincent and Dr. K. P. Wheeler.

This work was supported by the Centre National de la Recherche Scientifique
(ATP 133), the Délégation Générale à la Recherche Scientifique et Technique
(grant 81.E.0575) and by the Institut National de la Santé et de la Recherche
Médicale (CRL 80.30.10 and Action Concertée 79.7.1003).

REFERENCES
Abita, J. P., Chicheportiche, R., Schweitz, H. & Lazdunski, M. (1977) *Biochemistry 16,* 1838–
    1844.
Agnew, W. S., Levinson, S. R., Brabson, J. S. & Raftery, M. A. (1978) *Proc. Natl. Acad. Sci.
    USA 75,* 2606–2610.

Barchi, R. L., Cohen, S. A. & Murphy, L. E. (1980) *Proc. Natl. Acad. Sci. USA 77*, 1306–1310.

Barhanin, J., Giglio, J. R., Léopold, P., Schmid, A., Sampaio, S. V. & Lazdunski, M. (1982) *J. Biol. Chem. 257*, 12553–12558.

Barhanin, J., Hugues, M., Schweitz, H., Vincent, J. P. & Lazdunski, M. (1981) *J. Biol. Chem. 256*, 5764–5769.

Barhanin, J., Pauron, D., Lombet, A., Norman, R. I., Vijverberg, H. P. M., Giglio, J. R. & Lazdunski, M. (1983b) *EMBO Journal 2*, 915–920.

Barhanin, J., Schmid, A., Lombet, A., Wheeler, K. P., Lazdunski, M. & Ellory, J. C. (1983a) *J. Biol. Chem. 258*, 700–702.

Catterall, W. A. (1980) *Ann. Rev. Pharmacol. Toxicol. 20*, 15–43.

Chicheportiche, R., Balerna, M., Lombet, A., Romey, G. & Lazdunski, M. (1980) *Eur. J. Biochem. 104*, 617–625.

Frelin, C., Lombet, A., Vigne, P., Romey, G. & Lazdunski, M. (1982) *Biochem. Biophys. Res. Commun. 107*, 202–208.

Frelin, C., Vigne, P. & Lazdunski, M. (1981b) *Eur. J. Biochem. 119*, 437–442.

Frelin, C., Vigne, P. & Lazdunski, M. (1983) *J. Biol. Chem. 258*, 6272–6276.

Frelin, C., Vigne, P., Ponzio, G., Romey, G., Tourneur, Y., Husson, H. P. & Lazdunski, M. (1981a) *Mol. Pharmacol. 20*, 107–112.

Hartshorne, R. P. & Catterall, W. A. (1981) *Proc. Natl. Acad. Sci. USA 78*, 4620–4624.

Hugues, M., Duval, D., Schmid, H., Kitabgi, P., Lazdunski, M. & Vincent, J. P. (1982b) *Life Sci 31*, 437–443.

Hugues, M., Romey, G., Duval, D., Vincent, J. P. & Lazdunski, M. (1982a) *Proc. Natl. Acad. Sci. USA 79*, 1308–1312.

Hugues, M., Schmid, H. & Lazdunski, M. (1982d) *Biochem. Biophys. Res. Commun. 107*, 1577–1582.

Hugues, M., Schmid, H., Romey, G., Duval, D., Frelin, C. & Lazdunski, M. (1982c) *EMBO Journal 9*, 1039–1042.

Jacques, Y., Romey, G., Cavey, M. T., Kartalovski, B. & Lazdunski, M. (1980b) *Biochim. Biophys. Acta 600*, 882–897.

Jacques, Y., Romey, G. & Lazdunski, M. (1980a) *Eur. J. Biochem. 111*, 265–273.

Jaimovich, E., Ildefonse, M., Barhanin, J., Rougier, O. & Lazdunski, M. (1982) *Proc. Natl. Acad. Sci. USA 79*, 3896–3900.

Lazdunski, M., Balerna, M., Barhanin, J., Chicheportiche, R., Fosset, M., Frelin, C., Jacques, Y., Lombet, A., Pouysségur, J., Renaud, J. F., Romey, G., Schweitz, H. & Vincent, J. P. (1980) *Ann. N.Y. Acad. Sci. 358*, 169–182.

Lazdunski, M. & Renaud, J. F. (1982) *Ann. Rev. Physiol. 44*, 463–473.

Lombet, A., Frelin, C., Renaud, J. F. & Lazdunski, M. (1982) *Eur. J. Biochem. 124*, 199–203.

Lombet, A., Norman, R. I. & Lazdunski, M. (1983) *Biochem. Biophys. Res. Commun. 114*, 126–130.

Meech, R. W. (1978) *Ann. Rev. Biophys. Bioeng. 7*, 1–18.

Moore, H. P. H., Fritz, L. C., Raftery, M. A. & Brockes, J. P. (1982) *Proc. Natl. Acad. Sci. USA 79*, 1673–1677.

Mozhayeva, G. N., Naumov, A. P., Nosyreva, E. D. & Grishin, E. V. (1980) *Biochim. Biophys. Acta 597*, 587–602.

Norman, R. I., Schmid, A., Lombet, A., Barhanin, J. & Lazdunski, M. (1983) *Proc. Natl. Acad. Sci. USA 80*, 4164–4168.

Pouysségur, J., Jacques, Y. & Lazdunski, M. (1980) *Nature 286*, 162–164.

Ray, R., Morrow, C. S. & Catterall (1978) *J. Biol. Chem. 253*, 7307–7313.

Renaud, J. F., Kazazoglou, T., Lombet, A., Chicheportiche, R., Jaimovich, E., Romey, G. & Lazdunski, M. (1983) *J. Biol. Chem. 258,* 8799–8805.

Ritchie, J. M. & Rogart, R. B. (1977) *Rev. Physiol. Biochem. Pharmacol. 79,* 1–50.

Rochat, H., Bernard, P. & Couraud, F. (1979) In: *Advances in Cytopharmacology* (eds. B. Ceccarelli & F. Clement) pp. 325–334. Raven Press, New York.

Romey, G., Abita, J. P., Chicheportiche, R., Rochat, H. & Lazdunski, M. (1976a) *Biochim. Biophys. Acta 448,* 607–619.

Romey, G., Abita, J. P., Schweitz, H., Wunderer, G. & Lazdunski, M. (1976b) *Proc. Natl. Acad. Sci. USA 73,* 4055–4059.

Romey, G., Chicheportiche, R., Lazdunski, M., Rochat, H., Miranda, F. & Lissitzky, M. (1975) *Biochem. Biophys. Res. Commun. 64,* 115–121.

Romey, G., Jacques, Y., Schweitz, H., Fosset, M. & Lazdunski, M. (1979) *Biochim. Biophys. Acta 556,* 344–353.

Romey, G. & Lazdunski, M. (1982) *Nature 297,* 79–80.

Romey, G., Renaud, J. F., Fosset, M. & Lazdunski, M. (1980) *J. Pharm. Exper. Ther. 213,* 607–615.

Vijverberg, H. P. M., van der Zalm, J. M. & van den Bercken, J. (1982) *Nature 295,* 601–603.

Vincent, J. P., Balerna, M., Barhanin, J., Fosset, M. & Lazdunski, M. (1980) *Proc. Natl. Acad. Sci. USA 77,* 1646–1650.

Wheeler, K. P., Barhanin, J. & Lazdunski, M. (1982) *Biochemistry 21,* 5628–5634.

DISCUSSION

ANAND: I was rather concerned by your observation of the action of pyrethroids on mammalian systems as this might affect their application as an insecticide. What kind of action did you observe? Do they depress or excite the cells or do they only possess high affinity?

LAZDUNSKI: The effects of pyrethroids on mammalian and insect cells are identical. They create repetitive activity, but the difference is that you have to use much higher concentrations in the mammalian system. Fortunately, the pyrethroids do not easily pass the blood-brain barrier and not many accidents have been reported. I don't think that we can find compounds, which are active in insects and completely inactive in mammals. In the case of pyrethroids there is a difference by a factor of 10^3–10^4 in the affinity, and I think that this is good enough to be safe.

DJERASSI· Concerning the last peptide neurotoxin that you mentioned, have you or others done any systematic modification of this relatively simple peptide in order to determine, which structural elements are essential for activity?

LAZDUNSKI: In 1975, we modified different amino-acid residues of the peptide. Residues in positions 13 and 14, which are arginine groups, are crucial for tivity. If you modify the other residues or the α-amino groups, you don't lose the activity, but if you make cumulative modifications you lose activity. Merrifield in the United States synthesized compounds which were modified at the arginine residues. He replaced arginine residues by other residues devoid of positively charged groups, and he lost activity.

DJERASSI: Attempts to reduce the size of the peptide without loss of activity would, in my opinion, be an obvious approach?

LAZDUNSKI: The most obvious for me, may be to gain more information on the three-dimensional structure of the peptide. We have tried, and are still trying, to crystallize many of the toxins for X-ray crystallography. In the case of pamine, all attempts so far have failed.

DJERASSI: In my opinion, the simplest way of attacking your structure activity problem is to accept that the arginines are essential and that the disulphide bridges are indispensable. Keeping these structural parameters intact, you can systematically reduce the size of the molecule in order to find the minimum size of the molecule required for activity. This approach may simplify your subsequent conformational studies. Your proposal involves many complicated chemical problems, but it certainly is worthwhile trying.

DAVIES: Is the peptide active as a monomer?

LAZDUNSKI: It forms dimers or higher polymers in solution, but I would tend to believe that at the concentration at which it is active (10^{-11} M) it exists predominantly as a monomer.

NAKANISHI: A general question about the hydrophobicity and hydrophilicity of the sodium channel. First of all, the pK value of the carboxylate group of critical importance is 6.2. Is this correct? Some of the active toxins are hydrophobic and some are hydrophilic. Are they interacting with the inside and/or outside of the membrane?

LAZDUNSKI: There are 2 kinds of toxins, the lipid soluble toxins and all of the hydrophilic toxins including tetrodotoxin. They can all be active from the outside of the membrane. The lipid-soluble toxins, but not tetrodotoxin, are also active when applied to the inside of the membrane as shown by many people including Dr. Albuquerque. A pK of 6.2 for a carboxylate group is not unusual in systems. There are frequent examples of that in enzymes' active sites.

Structure-Activity Studies in Cardiac Glycosides

Thomas R. Watson, H. T. Andrew Cheung & Richard E. Thomas

A very broad range of drugs produces therapeutically beneficial effects on the heart and blood vessels. Of these, the cardiac glycosides form a particular group which has, as its principal pharmacological activity, the ability to alter the cardiovascular function through increasing the force of myocardial contraction. All of the beneficial effects produced by the use of these drugs in the treatment of congestive heart disease, increased cardiac output, decreased heart size, blood volume and venous pressure, diuresis and reduction of edema, can be explained on the basis of an increase in the force of contraction, i.e., a positive inotropic effect. The other categories of drugs which act upon the heart do so by other mechanisms which reduce its workload by reducing the blood load, i.e., by reducing blood volume and pressure. This may be achieved by using diuretics and anti-hypertensive agents, by correcting arrythmias, and by preventing and treating atherosclerosis.

The most commonly used glycoside, digoxin (from _Digitalis lanata Ehrh._) is responsible for one of the highest rates of drug-induced death, and one of the highest rates of drug-induced hospital admission. The therapeutic effects of digoxin in man are associated with plasma concentrations of the order of $1-2\times10^{-9}$M (ca. $1-2\,\mu g/mL$), and toxic effects are shown by concentrations only twice as high. It is this very low therapeutic ratio which has stimulated much research to identify the relationship between the cardiotonic and cardiotoxic effects and to improve the therapeutic ratio; to identify the digitalis receptor and to map its topography; and to design drugs which might be as effective as the natural products but which act with a much higher margin of safety.

Pharmacy Department, The University of Sydney, Australia.

NATURAL PRODUCTS AND DRUG DEVELOPMENT, Alfred Benzon Symposium 20.
Editors: P. Krogsgaard-Larsen, S. Brøgger Christensen, H. Kofod, Munksgaard, Copenhagen 1984.

THE DIGITALIS RECEPTOR

There is convincing evidence that the digitalis glycosides do not penetrate the cell membrane, e.g., a digitoxin-albumin conjugate shows positive inotropic activity, and the majority of those working in this field accept that a Mg^{2+}-dependent membrane-bound Na^+, K^+-ATPase is the digitalis receptor. A principal function of this enzyme is to act as a pump to maintain the high K^+/Na^+ ratio that is characteristic of the intracellular fluid. This activity is specifically inhibited by cardiac glycosides. The enzyme consists of two polypeptide sub-units which exert the catalytic action, and an associated glycoprotein which is essential for activity. This system, the Na^+, K^+-pump, extends through the cell membrane from the external to the internal surface. The cardiac glycosides bind to the external surface of the enzyme and the catalytic site for the reaction, $ATP \rightarrow ADP + Pi$, is located on the inner surface. The model, which at this stage best explains the action of the pump, is that the binding of various ligands induces conformational changes in the enzyme which result in Na^+ ions being pumped out of, and K^+ ions being pumped into the cell. The binding of cardiac glycosides to the enzyme appears to inhibit these conformational changes, thereby closing the ion transport channels, and thus, reducing the activity of the pump. That in turn, by a mechanism as yet not clearly defined, mediates the contractility of the heart muscle. This general mechanism was first suggested in 1961 (Repke 1963), and over the intervening years has stimulated much research effort to identify the actual mechanism which results in an increase in the force of contraction.

STRUCTURE ACTIVITY STUDIES

The general structure of most of the known naturally ocurring cardiac glycosides is shown in Fig. 1. The number of hexose units may vary from 1 to 4, and compounds are known in which oxygen functional groups are located at one or more of the steroidal carbon atoms, and olefinic bonds are occasionally found at C4, C5 or C8.

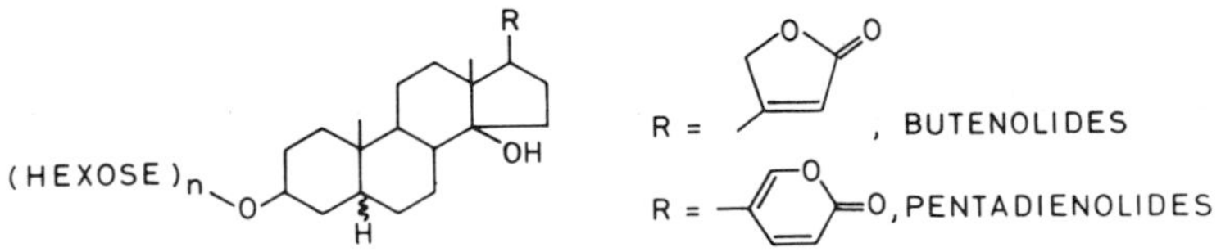

Fig. 1. General structure of the cardiac glycosides.

The early studies of the biological activity of the cardiac glycosides were designed to determine whether the toxicity of these compounds was an extension of the tonic effects, or whether these effects could be separated, i.e., did different mechanisms operate? Most of thsoe studies did not provide information which can be interpreted in terms of the mechanism of action of these compounds, as they simply measured toxicity in whole animals. Thus, although the cat toxicity studies (Chen 1963, Tamm 1963, Guntert & Linde 1981) give some indications of the relative toxicity of these compounds, those data do not allow for the varying pharmacokinetic factors, or the more recently identified differing rates of onset and reversal of inotropy, which exist between compounds of different chemical structure.

More recently, a number of *in vitro* test systems which avoid the pharma-cokinetic effects have been used for comparing the relative potency of these compounds. Isolated guinea-pig left-atrium has been used to measure inotropy (Brown & Thomas 1983), and purified preparations of Na^+, K^+-ATPase to measure relative potency, in terms of the inhibition of the enzyme activity (I_{50}), and the affinlty of the compounds for the receptor as measured by the equilibrium dissociation constants (K_D) (Yoda 1974, Wallick *et al.* 1974, Rohrer *et al.* 1979). The whole-animal toxicity experiments showed that most glycosides were more potent (toxic) than their respective aglycones, but the number and structure of carbohydrate units did not appear to have a marked effect. It was also shown that any modification of the lactone side-chain (at C17β) abolished activity, e.g., by epimerisation, saturation of the olefinic bond(s), or the formation of the isolactone (saturation and bonding to the C14β-OH). These studies also identified the need for the β-hydroxy group at C14, and the consequent cis C/D ring junction. As most of the known compounds at that time were of the 5β-H steroid structure it was assumed that that configuration was also essential for activity.

The importance of the lactone has been investigated (Thomas *et al.* 1974, Rohrer *et al.* 1979) using compounds in which the C17β-lactone of digitoxigenin has been replaced by α, β-unsaturated functional groups which are isosteric with the butenolide. Some of these compounds have been shown to possess positive inotropic activity on isolated guina-pig left-atrium. This activity has been correlated (Smith *et al.* 1982) with the ability of the side-chain ($-CH=CH-CR=A$, where R is alkyl, and A is a hetero atom) to polarise in the vicinity of the receptor to a form in which the hetero atom is negative with respect to the β-carbon (C20). The ^{13}C-nmr chemical shifts of the β-carbon were used as a measure of the polarisation. The acrylonitrile analogue was the most active compound with a potency relative to digitoxigenin of 0.7:1. The methylacrylate ester analogue had a relative potency of 0.3, and the corresponding acid, and amide were essentially inactive.

On the basis of this, and similar studies using glycosides rather than aglycones, and many C17 analogues with structurally different groups, a model of the cardiac glycoside receptor composed of 4 binding regions was proposed (Thomas *et al.* 1974b). In that model, the receptor lies within a cleft, and the principal binding interaction involves a redistribution of charge in the receptor induced by polarisation of the side chain of the steroid. This interaction is envisaged as locating the cardiac glycoside at the appropriate binding region of Na^+, K^+-ATPase which then allows the other parts of the glycoside molecule to bind to the appropriate sites, viz., the steroid binding area for the surface of the steroid (hydrophobic bonding), and H-bonding sites for functional groups on the β-face, and the sugarbinding area. Other modifications of the side chain including the compound Actodigin® (Ayerst) in which the C17 butenolide of digitoxigenin β-D-glucoside is linked to the steroid through C22 rather than C20 as in the normal cardenolides, have been investigated. (Fullerton *et al.* 1980, Rohrer *et al.* 1979). Actodigin® was reported to have a substantially improved therapeutic ratio, (Mendez *et al.* 1974), but it has the low potency, rapid onset, and reversal of activity which is typical of the aglycones.

The introduction of oxygen functional groups $(-OH, =O$ or $-O-)$, or unsaturation at almost any part of the steroid tends to reduce potency. For example, the equilibrium dissociation constants (K_D) for digitoxin, digoxin (12β-hydroxydigitoxin) and gitoxin (16β-hydroxydigitoxin), are 1.1, 3.6 and 17.8 ($\times 10^{-9}$M; beef-heart Na^+, K^+-ATPase) respectively, indicating a decrease in potency with hydroxy group substitution in two positions of the steroid.

Compounds of both 5α-H and 5β-H steroids appear to be bound comparably to the receptor, as highly potent aglycones and glycosides of both series are known. Digitoxigenin 18 and uzarigenin 12 have very similar K_D values (10.3 and 14.3×10^{-9}M (beef heart) respectively), and the corresponding constants for the glycosides digitoxigenin-α-L-rhamnoside (5.2×10^{-9}M) and uzarigenin-α-L-rhamnoside (6.8×10^{-9}M), are also of the same order of magnitude. (Inotropic activity, ΔF_{75}, guinea-pig left atria; digitoxigen-α-L-rhamnoside 6.3×10^{-8}M, uzarigenin-α-L-rhamnoside, 15×10^{-8}M).

The changes in the equilibrium dissociation constants illustrated by these few examples (for others, Brown *et al.* 1983) provide support for the hypothesis that

Table I

	COMPOUND	STRUCTURE	RELATIVE INOTROPIC ACTIVITY (a)
1	GOMPHOSIDE		23
2	EPI-GOMPHOSIDE		0·2
3	4'-HYDROXY GOMPHOSIDE		1
4	DIDEHYDRO GOMPHOSIDE		2·5
5	GOMPHOGENIN-β-D-4',6'-DIDEOXY-ALTROSIDE		12
6	GOMPHOGENIN-β-D-4',6'-DIDEOXY-ALLOSIDE		12
7	GOMPHOGENIN-β-D-4',6'-DIDEOXY-MANNOSIDE		0·3
8	GOMPHOGENIN		0·05

(a) ΔF_{75}; GUINEA PIG LEFT ATRIA. DIGITOXIGENIN = 1

the steroid part of the molecule is bound to the receptor by hydrophobic forces, and the introduction of polar functional groups inhibits effective hydrophobic binding, or destabilises the complex.

WATSON ET AL.

Table II

COMPOUND	STRUCTURE	RELATIVE INOTROPIC ACTIVITY[a]
9 ASCLEPOSIDE UZARIGENIN-β-D-6'-DEOXYALLOSIDE		3
10 UZARIGENIN-α-L-RHAMNOSIDE		9[b]
11 UZARIGENIN-β-D-GLUCOSIDE		0·5[b]
12 UZARIGENIN		1·2[b]

(a) ΔF_{75}; GUINEA PIG LEFT ATRIA. DIGITOXIGENIN = 1

(b) BROWN et al. 1983

The glycosides are more potent than their aglycones, and as the potency of the aglycones is modified by substitution of polar functional groups in the steroid, similarly, variations to the structure (and number) of the carbohydrate moiety(s) alters the potency of the glycosides. The effect is clearly shown by the compounds listed in Tables I, II and III. The most active compounds are those which have one 6-deoxy-sugar attached to the aglycone (either 5α-H, or 5β-H) by either an α-or β-glycosidic link, ie. the α-L-rhammosides, the α-L-thevetoside, the β-D-digitoxoside and the β-D-4,6-dideoxyalloside (gomphoside). This implies that a hydrophobic binding site for the sugar assists the binding of the glycoside to the receptor, and hence, increases the inotropic effect. This hypothesis is supported by the observation (Tables II, III) that those glycosides with a 6-hydroxymethyl group in the carbohydrate are generally less potent, e.g., the β-D-glucosides and β-D-galactoside. This effect may be due to the 6-hydroxymethyl inhibiting the binding at the hydrophobic site.

Table III

	COMPOUND	STRUCTURE	RELATIVE INOTROPIC ACTIVITY (a)
13	NERIIFOLIN DIGITOXIGENIN-α-L-THEVETOSIDE		27
14	DIGITOXIGENIN-α-L-RHAMNOSIDE		22
15	DIGITOXIGENIN-β-D-DIGITOXOSIDE		15
16	DIGITOXIGENIN-β-D-GLUCOSIDE		3
17	DIGITOXIGENIN-β-D-GALACTOSIDE		1
18	DIGITOXIGENIN		1

(a) ΔF_{75} ; GUINEA PIG LEFT ATRIA. (BROWN et al. 1983)

DIGITOXIGENIN = 1

If the hydroxy groups of the sugars are esterified or blocked by other groups (e.g., cyclic ketal formation), the activity of the derivative is reduced in comparison with the underivatised glycoside. Epimerisation of sugar hydroxy groups also has a marked effect on the activity of the compounds (e.g., Table III, digitoxigenin-β-D-glucoside 16, and β-D-galactoside 17). These observations have stimulated much research to identify the position, and configuration of the carbohydrate hydroxy group(s) that are involved in binding with a hydrogen-donor binding site on the receptor.

A study of the rates of association and dissociation of cardiac glycosides with different sugars, with Na⁺, K⁺-ATPase (Yoda 1974) led to the suggestion that only the equatorial 3′-hydroxy group, and possibly the axial 3′-hydroxy and - methoxy groups could bind to the sugar-specific site on the enzyme, but other hydroxy groups at 2′, and 4′ could not.

The difference in activity between digitoxigenin-β-D-glucoside, and digitoxigenin-β-D-galactoside has been attributed (Brown & Thomas 1983) to the difference in configuration at 4′, where the 4′-hydroxy group of the glucoside is equatorial, and that of the galactoside is axial. They also point out that the 4′-hydroxy group of the rhamnosides and thevetosides is equatorial, and that this equatorial hydroxy group is common to all of the potent glycosides which were tested, regardless of the stereochemistry of the glycosidic linkage. Also, thevetose has an equatorial 3-methyl ether which does not appear to reduce the potency of the glycoside neriifolin, 13. However, acetylation of the axial 2′-hydroxy group of digitoxigenin-α-L-rhamnoside 14, reduces activity markedly, and appears to destabilise the complex, or inhibit its formation.

The results which have been published relate to glycosides in which the sugar is joined to the aglycone by single bonds between C3-O-C1′, and the conclusions drawn with respect to the interaction of the carbohydrate functional groups with the receptor have neglected the conformational freedom of the sugar moiety. The restriction to rotation can be significantly higher than the activation energy of complex formation, ca. 20 Kcal/mol (Yoda 1973), and this may be an important factor in determining the difference in activity between glycosides with different sugars.

CARDIAC GLYCOSIDES OF THE ASCLEPIADACEAE

Many of the cardiac glycosides isolated from species of the Asclepiadaceae have an unusual glycoside linkage in which the carbohydrate is doubly linked through oxygen atoms at C2α and C3β of the steroid. All of the known aglycones of this type of cardiac glycoside are 5α-H steroids except those of the affinosides (Abe & Yamauchi 1982) which are of the 5β-H series. The absolute configuration of gomphoside from *Asclepias fruticosa* L. (renamed recently as *Gomphocarpus physocarpus*), and a number of related glycosides has been established (Cheung & Watson 1980).

Tables I, II, III give the partial structures and inotropic potencies relative to digitoxigenin, of a number of cardiac glycosides which have gomphogenin 8, uzarigenin 12, or digitoxigenin 18, as the aglycone. From these data the variation of the potentiation of the inotropic activity of the aglycones, by formation of glycosides is strikingly illustrated by gomphoside, which is 450 times more potent than gomphogenin, neriifolin is 27 times more potent than digitoxigenin, but digitoxigenin-β-D-galactoside and its aglycone are equipotent.

As gomphoside has a rigid structure, and is one of the most potent cardiac glycosides known, it is a useful model for the investigation of the structure-activity requirements in the carbohydrate part of these compounds. Modification of the 2'- and 3'-hydroxy groups of gomphoside by acetylation, or the formation of the 2', 3'-isopropylidene derivative reduces the activity by 1–2 orders of magnitude. Epimerisation of the 3'β-OH group to form 3'-*epi*gomphoside 2, or oxidation to 3'-didehydrogomphoside 4 reduces activity markedly. Reduction of gomphoside opens the dioxan ring to produce the two glycosides 5, and 6, which have the same relative activity. As these compounds differ only in the configuration at 2', the inference is that the configuration at 2' is not important for activity. Reduction of 3'-*epi*gomphoside 2, forms 7 which is substantially less active than either gomphoside, or the 3'-epimeric isomer 5. This is further evidence of the importance of the 3'-(axial) hydroxy group.

Ascleposide 9, is the 6-deoxyalloside of uzarigenin. Its inotropic activity is about one order of magnitude less than that of gomphoside, and 4'-hydroxy-gomphoside 3, is slightly less active than ascleposide. The difference between these two compounds (9 and 3) is the extra oxygen atom at C2, C2' in the rigid structure of 3, but both have hydroxy groups in the same position and configuration.

Thus, the apparent structural features, of those glycosides related to gomphoside, which influence potency are: (1) the 4'6'-dideoxyhexose; (2) the 3'(axial) hydroxy group; (3) the configuration of the hydroxy group at 2' does not affect the activity; (4) most derivatives of the 2' and 3' hydroxy groups reduce activity; and (5) the presence of a 4'-(equatorial)hydroxy group reduces activity.

These observations indicate that gomphoside binds to the receptor through the 3'-(axial) hydroxy, and the 5'(equatorial) methyl groups. However, the digitoxigenin derived glycosides, neriifolin 13, digitoxigenin-α-L-rhamnoside 14, and digitoxigenin-β-D-digitoxoside 15, are highly potent compounds of comparable activity with gomphoside, but the uzarigenin glycosides, ascleposide 9, and uzarigenin-α-L-rhamnoside 10, are significantly less potent. All of these glycosides have freely rotating sugars.

Calculations, using x-ray crystallographic data, of the potential energy of the

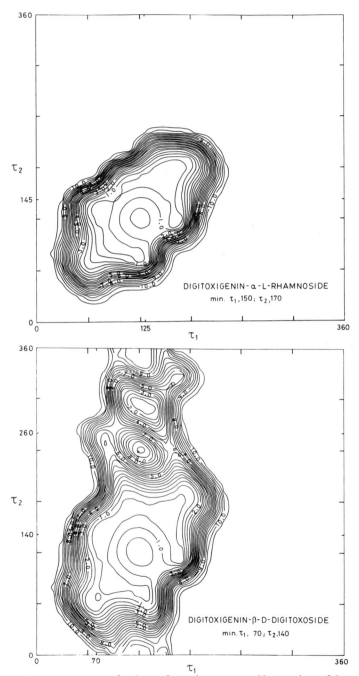

Fig. 2. Potential energy contours for the conformations generated by rotations of the carbohydrate about the 2 torsion angles τ_1 (C2, C3-0,C1′) and τ_2 (C3, O-C1′, C2′).

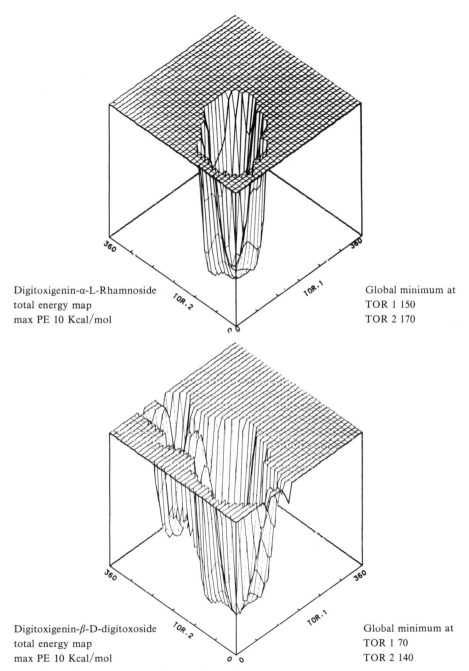

Digitoxigenin-α-L-Rhamnoside
total energy map
max PE 10 Kcal/mol

Global minimum at
TOR 1 150
TOR 2 170

Digitoxigenin-β-D-digitoxoside
total energy map
max PE 10 Kcal/mol

Global minimum at
TOR 1 70
TOR 2 140

Fig. 3. Three-dimensional maps of the conformational potential energy of the carbohydrate rotated about the 2 torsion angles τ_1 (C2, C3–O, C1′) and τ_2 (C3, O-C1′, C2′).

conformations of the glycosides, which are due to the rotation of the sugar about the C3-O-C1' bonds relative to the steroid, result in contour maps which show those torsion angles which define the conformational minima (Fig. 2). The three-dimensional plot (Fig. 3) shows more strikingly the relationship between potential energy and the torsion angles (τ_1 and τ_2). Using this data, and with the aid of a computer-graphics system, we are investigating the relationship between conformation of the sugar (in both 5α-H, and 5β-H steroid series) and inotropic activity relative to the apparently effective complexation with the receptor of the conformationally rigid gomphoside.

The conformational potential energy contour map of digitoxigenin-α-L-rhamnoside 14, (Fig. 2) shows the presence of a broad energy minimum in the region [$\tau_1 = 125° \pm 45°$, $\tau_2 = 145° \pm 55°$]. If this molecule is superimposed on a molecule of gomphoside, such that the lactone, and the D, C and B rings are totally coincident, (Fig. 4) then the conformation of the rhamnose in which the 3'-hydroxy and the 5'-methyl groups of both molecules are very nearly coincident, lies within the region of minimum conformational energy of the glycoside.

Thus, the binding of digitoxigenin-α-L-rhamnoside to the same sugar-binding sites as gomphoside is highly favourable, and the potencies are comparable.

The conformational energy map for neriifolin is very similar to that of digitoxigenin-a-L-rhamnoside even though thevetose has a 3'-methoxy group, and the configuration of the 2'-hydroxy group is equatorial rather than axial. This is further evidence against the involvement of the 2' hydroxy group in binding, and apparently the methyl ether does not inhibit binding with the receptor.

The proposed active conformation for digitoxigenin-β-D-digitoxoside 15 [$\tau_1 = 70°$, $\tau_2 = 260°$] in which the 3'-hydroxy and 5'-methyl groups of the

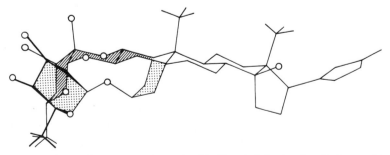

Fig. 4. The superimposed structures of gomphoside (I) and digitoxigenin-α-L-rhamnoside.

digitoxose lie closely to the corresponding groups of gomphoside when the two molecules are superimposed, is located at the side of the potential energy 'well'approximately 3 Kcal mol^{-1} above the minimum. (Fig. 2, 3). This is not a preferred conformation for the glycoside in the unbound form. Thus, it can be argued that, although digitoxigenin β-D-digitoxoside can bind effectively to the binding sites for gomphoside in this conformation, it is less likely to bind to the receptor than the α-L-rhamnoside. Consequently, it is less active (ca. 40%) than the α-L-rhamnoside.

For those glycosides of either the 5α-H or 5β-H steroid series which have lower activity it is possible that the conformational energy is such that only one binding group can interact with the receptor in a conformation that is close to the preferred conformation, and that interaction may involve the methyl or any hydroxy group in the carbohydrate. Such binding would be less than optimal in comparison with that of the highly potent glycosides, and consequently the pharmacological response is reduced.

A complicating factor in this hypothesis that at present has not been evaluated is the effect of the C2-hydroxy group of gomphogenin on the activity of those analogues of gomphoside which have a singly-bonded sugar moiety, e.g., 5, 6 and 7. The relative potency of gomphogenin is 1/24 of that of uzarigenin, and that of 7 is of the same order of magnitude as digitoxigenin. However, the relative inotropic potencies of 5 and 6 are 12-times greater than that of digitoxigenin; 10-times greater than uzarigenin. The fact that in both of these compounds the configuration of the 3'-hydroxy and the 5'-methyl is the same as they are in gomphoside does not account for their equal activity, as the conformations that would enable both to bind to the receptor similarly to gomphoside differ markedly in potential energy, [$\tau_1 = 90°$, $\tau_2 = 250°$, P.E., $5 = 8$ Kcal mol^{-1}, P.E., $6 = 1000$ Kcal mol^{-1}]. This difference is due to the different configurations of the C2'-hydroxy group and its steric interaction with the C2-hydroxy group of the steroid. Further investigation of the preferred conformations of these compounds is in progress.

CONCLUSION

This brief survey of structure-activity studies in cardiac glycosides shows that considerable progress has been made in recent years towards identifying those features of the molecular structure which are important for the production of positive inotropic activity. However, none of the compounds designed as a result of these studies has been shown to be significantly better, or safer than the natural products which have been used in one form or another virtually for centuries.

It appears from our studies with the conformationally rigid glycosides that the problem of designing a drug which could be synthesised readily, and would replace the existing compounds in use in medicine, is more complex than might have been envisaged.

ACKNOWLEDGEMENTS

The authors wish to acknowledge the substantial contributions to this work made by Mr. Francis Chiu, Dr. R. Wells and Ms. K. Williams.

REFERENCES

Abe, F. & Yamauchi, T. (1982) Affinoside and companion glycosides from the stem and bark of *Anodendron affine* (Anodendron II). *Chem. Pharm. Bull 30*, 1183–1193.

Bossaller, C. & Schmoldt, A. (1979) Dehydro-digitoxosides of digitoxigenin and digoxigenin:binding to beef heart (Na^+K^+-ATPase) in relation to unchanged digitoxosides. *Naunyn-Schmiedeberg's Arch. Pharmacol. 306*, 11–15.

Brown, L. (1981) *Synthesis and Biological Activity of Some Digitalis Analogues.* PhD. Thesis. University of Sydney, NSW. Australia.

Brown, L., Erdmann, E. & Thomas, R. (1983) Digitalis structure-activity relationship analysis; conclusions from indirect binding studies with cardiac Na^+, K^+-ATPase. *Biochem. Pharmac. 32*, (in press).

Brown, L. & Thomas, R. (1983) Comparison of the inotropic effects of some 5α-cardenolides on guinea pig left atria. *Arzneimittel-Forschung 33* (in press).

Cheung, H. T. A. & Watson, T. R. (1980) Stereochemistry of the hexosulose of cardenolides of the Asclepiadaceae. *J. Chem. Soc. Perkin Trans. 1*, 2162–2168.

Chen, K. K. (1963) New aspects of cardiac glycosides. In: *Proceedings of the First International Pharmacological Meeting, Stockholm, 1961.* Vol. 3. pp. 27–45, eds. Wilbrandt, W. and Lindgren, P., Pergamon Press, Oxford.

Guntert, T. W. & Linde, H. H. A. (1981) *Handbook of Experimental Pharmacology. 56/1*, pp. 13–24. ed. Greef, K., Springer Verlag, Berlin, Heidelberg, N.Y.

Mendez, R., Pastelin, G. & Kabela, E. (1974) The influence of the position of attachment of the lactone ring to the steroid nucleus on the action of cardiac glycosides. *J. Pharmacol. Exp. Ther. 188*, 189–197.

Repke, K. H. R., (1963) Metabolism of cardiac glycosides. In: *Proceedings of the First International Pharmacological Meeting, Stockholm, 1961.* Vol. 3. pp. 47–73, eds. Wilbrandt, W. & Lindgren P. Pergamon Press, Oxford.

Rohrer, D. C., Fullerton, D. S., Yoshioka, K., From, A. H. L. & Ahmed, K. (1979) Functional receptor mapping for modified cardenolides. In: *Computer Assisted Drug Design.* pp. 259–279, eds. Olson, E. C. & Christoffersen, R. E., A. C. S. Symposium Series 112. American Chemical Society, Washington, D. C.

Smith, P., Brown, L., Boutagy, J. & Thomas, R. (1982) Cardenolide analogues 14. Synthesis and biological activity of glucosides of $C17\beta$-modified derivatives of digitoxigenin. *J. Med. Chem. 25,* 1222–1226.

Tamm, C. (1963) The stereochemistry of the glycosides in relation to biological activity. In: *Proceedings of the First International Pharmacological Meeting, Stockholm 1961.* Vol. 3. 11–26. eds. Wilbrandt, W. & Lindgren, P., Pergamon Press, Oxford.

Thomas, R., Boutagy, J. & Gelbart, A. (1974a) Synthesis and biological activity of semisynthetic digitalis analogues. *J. Pharm. Sci. 63,* 1649–1683.

Thomas, R., Boutagy, J. & Gelbart, A. (1974b) Cardenolide Analogues V. Cardiotonic activity of semisynthetic analogues of digitoxigenin. *J. Pharmacol. Exp. Ther. 191,* 219–231.

Thomas, R. Brown, L., Boutagy, J. & Gelbart, A. (1980) The dose response information for structure-activity relationship studies. *Circ. Res. (Suppl.). 46,* I 167–172.

Van Winkel, W. B., Allen, J. C. & Schwartz, A. (1972) The nature of the transport ATP'ase-digitalis complex III. Rapid binding studies and effects of ligands on the formation and stability of magnesium plus phosphate-induced glycoside-enzyme complex. *Arch. Biochem. Biophys. 151,* 85–92.

Wallick, E. T., Dowd, F., Allen, J. C. & Schwartz, A. (1974) The nature of transport adenosine triphosphatase-digitalis complex VII. Characteristics of ouabagenin-Na^+, K^+-adenosine triphosphatase interaction. *J. Pharmacol. Exp. Ther. 189,* 434–444.

Yoda, A. (1973) Structure-activity relationships of cardiotonic steroids for the inhibition of Na^+, K^+-ATPase. 1. Dissociation rate constants of various enzyme cardiac glycoside complexes formed in the presence of magnesium and phosphate. *Mol. Pharmacol. 9,* 51–60.

Yoda, A. (1974) Association and dissociation rate constants of the complexes between various cardiac monoglycosides and Na^+, K^+-ATPase, *N. Y. Acad. Sci. 242,* 598–616.

DISCUSSION

ALBUQUERQUE: You said that gomphoside is much more potent than the digitalis glycosides. Is the binding site of gomphoside the same as that of digitalis? Did you have the opportunity to correlate the potency of these drugs with their toxicity? What is the therapeutic index for gomphoside?

WATSON: The binding sites for gomphoside are the same as for the digitalis glycosides, i.e., cardenolide and a sugar-binding site. As far as therapeutic ratio is concerned, unfortunately gomphoside is no better than the digitalis glycosides, so that gomphoside itself is not a useful drug.

LAZDUNSKI: You have presented a number of derivatives which are of great interest for people like us who look at the receptor. There are 2 systems in the cardiac membrane, which are responsible for the inotropic effect and for the cardiotoxic effect of these componds. The first one is the one that you have described, i.e., the sodium-posassium ATPase. The other system is known as the sodium-calcium exchange. We have studied in cardiac cells in culture the binding of digitalis compounds and the inhibition of potassium influx, the accumulation of sodium, and the entry of calcium under the influence of these compounds. What we see with ouabain or with the derivatives is that if we follow ouabain binding, or if we follow the ouabain inhibition of potassium entry, if we follow ouabain-induced sodium accumulation, we get the same dissociation constant for ouabain, which is normal. Now, sodium has accumulated inside the cell, and this accumulation will trigger the sodium-calcium exchange system, and calcium in turn will increase in concentration inside the cell. If in the same cell, and one does the dose-response curve for the ouabain-dependent sodium accumulation and for the ouabain-dependent calcium entry, one finds that they are superimposable. The inotropic effect itself is due to the sodium-potassium ATPase: sodium accumulates inside the cell, triggers the sodium-calcium exchange, and internal calcium increases to provoke stronger contractions. The toxic effect, such as arythmia, is also due to the inhibition of the sodium-potassium ATPase; when a very large number of pumps are inhibited the membrane will depolarize. Then the cardiotoxic effect and the cardiotonic effect are due to the inhibition of exactly the same system. The cardiotoxic effect is due to direct inhibition of the pump, the cardiotonic effect is due to the partial inhibition of the pumps which triggers an activation of the sodium/calcium exchange system. For all these reasons, I believe that compounds more potent in cardiotonicity will automatically become more potent in cardiotoxicity.

WATSON: I agree with this view, which is consistent with our findings.

KUTNEY: After my lecture a few of you asked privately, what about the situation of plant tissue culture in commercial applications. The first commercial application will, in fact, be in *Digitalis lanata*. Plant tissue cultures of this plant are now being used in Germany to optimize the commercial production of appropriate 12-hydroxy compounds, because the enzymic systems of the plant have that capability, whereas the fungi and bacteria, which many people have tried over the years, do not.

WATSON: Thank you for that information.

WAGNER: As far as I understood it, you have used an *in vitro* system for testing the positive inotropic effect?

WATSON: Yes.

WAGNER: My question is, do you think that this test system is also appropriate for screening plant extracts? In many plant extracts you have a lot of substances, which have been shown to possess positive inotropic effect.

WATSON: The system probably is more complex than is necessary for screening.

WAGNER: I do not mean cardiac glycosides, I mean screening of plant extracts for other substances. There are a lot of compounds which have positive inotropic effects.

WATSON: Yes, certainly, the system would be appropriate for such purposes.

ATTA-UR-RAHMAN: I was wondering if you have looked at the possibility of using high resolution NMR to study the conformation that these molecules adopt in solution, and see whether they can provide some information about the topography of the receptor sites.

WATSON: We have not done that, but it certainly could be done. The conformation in solution is not necessarily that important as far as the binding is concerned, because the binding site may be a hydrophobic region, and when the drug-receptor complex is formed, the water molecules have been squeezed out, if you like. So, the conformation of these compounds in solution is not necessarily indicative of the conformation in which they will bind.

ATTA-UR-RAHMAN: The second question I wanted to ask was whether any studies have been done on the plant extract themselves?

WATSON: Initially, we studied the plant extracts. That is how we came across the active compounds. The extracts were infused into guinea-pigs, in which the activity of the heart was monitored.

Current Status of Gossypol, Zoapatanol and Other Plant-Derived Fertility Regulating Agents

Harry H. S. Fong

A number of plant derived, non-steroidal compounds including gossypol, zoapatanol, trichosanthin, vasicine, yuanhuacine, and derivatives of the latter, are being evaluated as potential fertility-regulating agents. The possibility that such compounds could be developed as clinically useful agents has been discussed (Farnsworth *et al.* 1983). The most promising substances for fertility regulation in the male and in the female may be gossypol and zoapatanol, respectively.

GOSSYPOL

Gossypol is a polyphenolic bis-sesquiterpene derived primarily from *Gossypium* species (cotton) of the Malvaceae. Typically, the optically inactive form of gossypol is isolated from this source. However, (+)-gossypol has been obtained from a related plant, *Thespesia populnea* Soland. ex. Correa (Malvaceae) in good yield (King & de Silva 1968). The existence of gossypol in enantiomeric forms is due to the atropisomerism resulting from restricted rotation about the naphthyl-naphthyl bond (Fig. 1). Since most studies reported in the literature have utilized optically inactive gossypol, the term "gossypol", therefore, refers to this entity, unless otherwise noted.

The clinical effects of gossypol, and results of studies on its antifertility effects in various animal species have been reviewed extensively (Farnsworth & Waller 1982, Kalla 1982, Lei 1982, Liu *et al.* 1981, Prasad & Diczfalusy 1982, Qian 1981, Xue 1981, Zatuchni & Osborne 1981, Zhou & Lei 1981). Although no reports have been published indicating that gossypol actually produces infertility in

World Health Organization, Collaborating Center for Traditional Medicine, College of Pharmacy, Health Sciences Center, University of Illinois at Chicago, Illinois 60612, U.S.A.

NATURAL PRODUCTS AND DRUG DEVELOPMENT, Alfred Benzon Symposium 20.
Editors: P. Krogsgaard-Larsen, S. Brøgger Christensen, H. Kofod, Munksgaard, Copenhagen 1984.

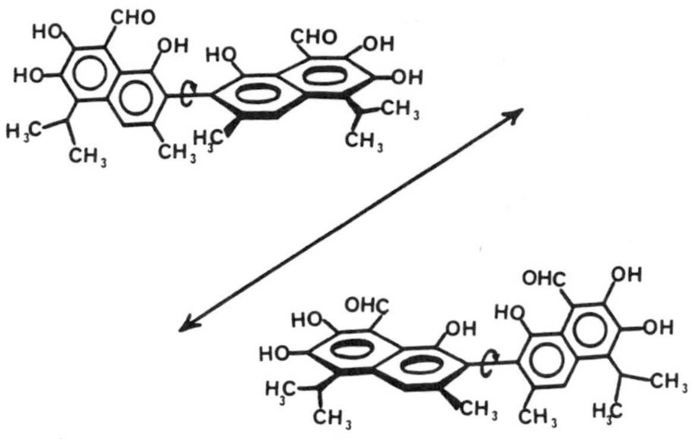

Fig. 1. Atropisomers of gossypol

humans, the decreased sperm counts reported in Chinese men using gossypol (Anon. 1978, Liu *et al.* 1981), and the antifertility effects demonstrated in rats (Chang *et al.* 1980, Hadley *et al.* 1981) and hamsters (Chang *et al.* 1980, Waller *et al.* 1983) argue for pursuing the development of gossypol as a potentially useful clinical agent. This paper will, thus, concentrate on reviewing recent studies concerning the chemistry and biology of gossypol as related to such potential development. Specifically to be discussed are gossypol stability studies; comparative antifertility effects of (±)- and (+)-gossypol; searches for (−)-gossypol by resolution of (±)-gossypol into its enantiomers, and by phyto-chemical studies of Malvaceous plants; and synthesis of gossypol analogues/derivatives.

Stability studies

Despite extensive chemical and biological studies of gossypol, little is known concerning its stability, particularly under common laboratory conditions. Our interest in conducting such a study was prompted by the need we felt for such information to assist in our biological and chemical studies of this compound. The WHO Special Programme of Research in Human Reproduction, and the Center for Population Research, NIH (USA), both recognized the value such information could have for biologists choosing solvents for gossypol, for use in their antifertility studies, and for chemists engaged in the separation of gossypol optical isomers and in the synthesis of gossypol analogues. A collaborative program was, thus, established between WHO and NIH, for expanded studies to be carried out on the stability of gossypol in various organic solvents, in aqueous buffers, in other solutions suitable for administration to animals, and in tablet form, by research groups in Beijing, Chicago, and London, and at NIH. These studies are still in progress.

Our initial study concerned the stability of (±)-gossypol, of its acetic acid complex, and of (+)-gossypol. Each was stored neat (in the solid state) and dissolved in various organic solvents; the complex was also stored suspended in an aqueous medium. All were stored under laboratory working conditions: at room temperature (25°C) and exposed to 12 h of fluorescent light (50–55 foot candles)/day. The results, reported in terms of half-lives, are shown in Table I. All 3 forms of gossypol were very stable when stored neat, as was (±)-gossypol acetic acid when suspended in a steroid suspending vehicle (Worthley & Schott

Table I

Stability of (±)-gossypol acetic acid, (±)-gossypol, and (+)-gossypol at 25°C and 50–55 foot candles of light[a]

Solvent	Half-Life (Days)		
	(±)-Gossypol[b] Acetic Acid	(±)-Gossypol[b]	(+)-Gossypol[b]
Neat	(112)[c]	(112)[d]	(112)[d]
Steroid Suspending Vehicle (SSV)	(253)[c]	–[e]	–[e]
Benzene	60.1	75.2	50.1
Chloroform	60.1	37.6	33.4
Dimethylsulfoxide	60.1	33.4	15.0
t-Butanol	60.1	30.1	10.1
Methylene chloride	32.0	–[e]	–[e]
Diethyl ether	15.0	23.1	15.8
2-Propanol	10.0	1.4, (13.0)[f]	0.9, (10.0)[f]
Acetone	7.5	4.4	5.4
Ethyl acetate	7.5	4.2	3.3
Acetonitrile	4.1	2.8, (16.7)[f]	7.2
Ethanol	3.1, (20)[f]	0.9, (13.1)[f]	1.0, (15.8)[f]
Methanol	1.7	0.9	11.4
Pyridine	0[g]	0[g]	0[g]

[a] Approximately 12 h laboratory fluorescent light/day
[b] Concentration=0.05–0.10 mg/ml
[c] No signs of decomposition when analyzed on this day
[d] Only minor decomposition found by this day
[e] Not tested
[f] Biphasic degradation
[g] Compound was very unstable in this solvent; less than 40% of sample was detectable at time 0 (Sample preparation time was less than 15 min)

1966). Stability of all 3 forms was also quite good in benzene, as was that of the gossypol-acetic acid complex in chloroform, *t*-butanol, and dimethylsulfoxide. (±)-Gossypol was also reasonable stable in the same solvents. Stability of all 3 forms in the more polar solvents, especially the lower alcohols, was very poor. The alkaline solvent, pyridine, destroyed all 3 forms of gossypol virtually on contact, supporting the finding of Lee *et al.* (1982) that gossypol decomposed faster at pH 8.5 than at pH 7.0.

Nomeir & Abou-Donia (1982) have reported on the stability of gossypol (acetic acid) dissolved in 5 of the solvents which we had employed (methanol, ethanol, chloroform, acetonitrile, and acetone), and stored at 5 different temperatures (37, 22, 5, −10, and −80°C). Stability was very high at temperatures below freezing and poor to moderate at the higher temperatures employed. In their experiment, the materials were stored in continuous darkness (Nomeir & Abou-Donia, personal communication).

Antifertility effects of gossypol isomers

Most studies concerning the biological effects of gossypol have employed (±)-gossypol. However, (+)-gossypol has been studied by 2 groups, and shown to be devoid of antifertility effects in male rats (Wang *et al.* 1979), and in male hamsters (Waller *et al.* 1983). In our study, (±)-gossypol, administered at a dose of 40 mg/kg/day for 7 weeks completely inhibited fertility in male hamsters; (+)-gossypol, however, similarly administered at a dose of 40 mg/kg/day [twice the dose of this isomer that treatment with (±)-gossypol had provided] was ineffective. These results suggested that male fertility might be inhibited by (−)-gossypol in an enantioselective manner; the importance of obtaining and biologically evaluating (−)-gossypol is obvious.

The search for (−)-gossypol

To date, (−)-gossypol has not been reported from nature, nor has it been synthesized. A number of laboratories around the world, however, have been attempting to obtain it, either (a) by resolution of the racemic mixture by various means and/or (b) by phytochemical investigation of plants in taxa of the Malvaceae.

With respect to (a), one approach involves the use of a chiral stationary phase for HPLC separation of the enantiomers (Pirkle *et al.* 1981, Pirkle & Schreiner 1981), a technique which has been used successfully to separate the enantiomers of other binaphthols. Alternatively, resolution may be attempted by the use of chiral amines and amino acids; gossypol is known to bind to proteins and amino acids (Markman & Rzhekhin 1969), and to form derivatives with amines (Adams *et al.* 1960). Successful separation of the optical isomers has been achieved at the Institute of Materia Medica, Chinese Academy of Medical Sciences, Beijing (Si *et al.* 1983); details of the separation procedure(s) employed, however, remain to be published.

With respect to (b), other Malvaceous plants are being investigated for the presence of ($-$)-gossypol. To date, some 20 species representing 10 of the 85 genera of the Malvaceae have been investigated at the Royal Danish School of Pharmacy by Jaroszewski, J., (personal communication) for the presence of ($-$)-gossypol. This enantiomer has so far not been found in the plants examined. Jolad *et al.* (1975) had reported the occurrence of gossypol in *Montezuma speciosissima* Sesse & Moc. (Malvaceae), but not the optical rotation of the isolate. We recently isolated gossypol from this plant and found it to be the ($+$)-isomer.

A report has appeared in the literature indicating the presence of gossypol in rubber seed meal [*Hevea brasiliensis* Muell. Arg. (Euphorbiaceae)] (Abdullah & Hutagalung 1981), although the authors themselves had stated that their finding should be considered tentative. Subsequent analyses (HPLC and UV) of this plant material by Jaroszewski (personal communication) and by ourselves have failed to confirm the presence of gossypol.

Synthesis of gossypol analogues/derivatives
The synthesis of analogues/derivatives that might be more effective and/or less toxic, is a logical extension of the current studies on gossypol. In a study of 18 gossypol derivatives substituted with various groups at the hydroxyl and/or aldehyde functions, only the derivative containing an N,N-diethylethylimino group at each of the aldehyde functions **2** (Fig. 2) showed activity (Wang *et al.*

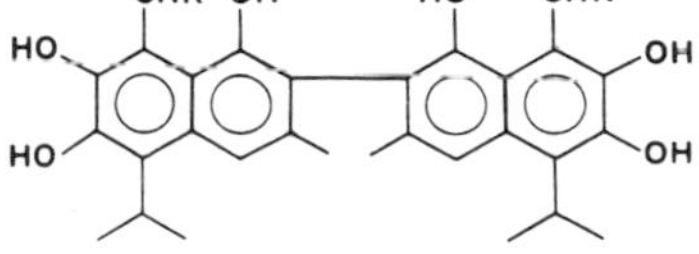

$$(2)\ R = NCH_2CH_2N \begin{smallmatrix} C_2H_5 \\ C_2H_5 \end{smallmatrix}$$

Fig. 2. A biologically active gossypol derivative

1979); however, a higher dose than that required for gossypol was needed, and weight loss occurred in the treated rats. Currently a number of research groups are engaged in synthesizing and/or testing other gossypol analogues/derivatives, under the sponsorship of WHO, NIH and other agencies.

ZOAPATANOL

Tea prepared from the leaves of *Montanoa tomentosa* Cerv. (Compositae), the zoapatle plant, reportedly has been used in Mexico for over 400 years to induce menses and labor, and to terminate early pregnancy (Levine *et al.* 1979). Recently, a tea prepared from this plant produced significant cervical dilatation and menstrual-like cramps, although not abortion, in six women dosed briefly during the first trimester of pregnancy (Landgren *et al.* 1979). Investigation of this plant has led to the isolation of a number of compounds, including the oxepane diterpenoids, zoapatanol 3 and montanol 4 (Levine *et al.* 1979, Kanojia *et al.* 1982), and the kaurene diterpene, kaura-9(11)-16-dien-19-oic acid (kauradienoic acid, grandiflorenic acid 5) (Caballero & Walls 1970) (Fig. 3). The latter has been reported to produce contraction of the guinea-pig uterus *in vitro* (Lozoya *et al.* 1983), while the first 2 were reported to produce contractions in rabbit uteri *in situ* (Wachter & Kanojia 1978), zoapatanol being effective at a lower dose than that required for montanol. Zoapatanol, but not montanol, effectively interrupted pregnancy in the 22-day pregnant guinea-pig assay (Hahn *et al.* 1981), as evidenced by a high percentage of non-viable implants in the

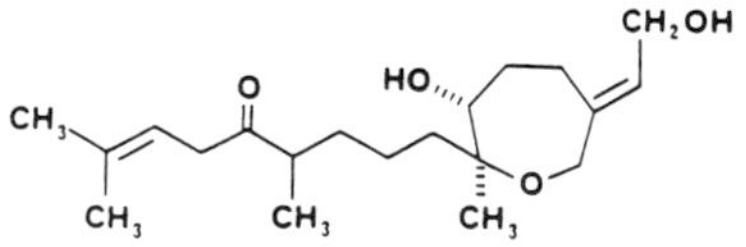

(3) Zoapatanol

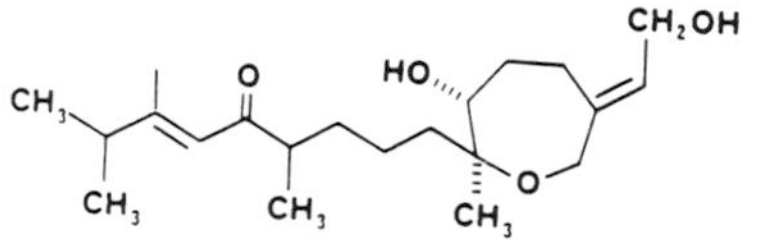

(4) Montanol

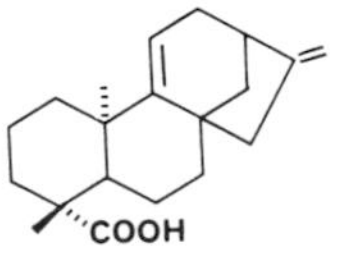

(5) Kauradienoic (Grandiflorenic) Acid

Fig. 3. Biologically active principles from *Montanoa tomentosa*

treated animals. Such observations argue for continuing the investigation of this plant's constituents, particularly zoapatanol and derivatives thereof, with a view toward developing a clinically useful agent. A number of reviews have already been published concerning folkloric uses, biological effects, and clinical evaluation of the tea and/or isolates, extracts, and fractions of *M. tomentosa* (Farnsworth *et al.* 1983, Gallegos 1983, Hahn *et al.* 1980, Levine *et al.* 1981). This paper therefore will concentrate on reviewing recent studies concerning the stability of zoapatanol; synthesis of zoapatanol analogues/derivatives; and phytochemical investigation of *Montanoa* species and subspecies.

Stability studies
We have studied the stability of zoapatanol stored at 3 different temperatures (5,25 and 55°C), in the neat state (oil), in alcoholic solution, and in aqueous solution. The alcoholic solution was an ethanol extract of the leaves of *M. tomentosa* Cerv. spp. *tomentosa*. The aqueous solution was a tea prepared by

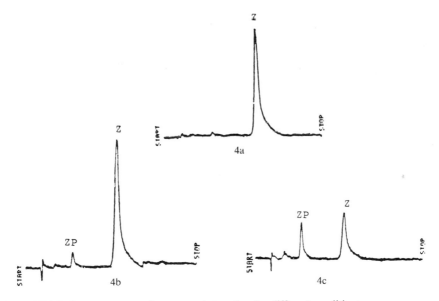

Fig. 4. HPLC chromatograms of zoapatanol stored under different conditions
4a = Chromatogram of zoapatanol stored in benzene at − 10°C for 26 days
4b = Chromatogam of zoapatanol stored neat at − 10°C for 18 days
4c = Chromatogram of zoapatanol stored at 25°C and exposed to fluorescent light for 3 days
Z = Zoapatanol peak
ZP = Zoapatanol decomposition/conversion product peak

boiling the leaves for 15 min; the trace quantity of zoapatanol in the tea, however, necessitated adding a known amount to the tea to permit quantitation of zoapatanol for the duration of the study. At an elevated temperature (55°C), zoaptanol was more stable in the ethanol extract than either in the tea or as the oil, with half-lives of 75, 15 and 8.4 h, respectively. The stability was the same for both the neat and alcoholic sample (half-life=151 h) at 25°C. At this temperature, the half-life of zoapatanol in the tea was 75 h. At 5°C, the oil was most stable, followed by the ethanol and tea samples, with projected half-lives of 1 504, 430, and 115 h, respectively.

In Fig. 4 are shown the chromatograms of samples of zoapatanol stored under other conditions. The single peak representing zoaptanol (Fig. 4a) indicates the stability of this compound when stored at -10°C in benzene for 26 days. A decomposition/conversion product can be noted, however, in the zoapatanol sample stored neat at -10°C for 18 days (Fig. 4b). More of this decomposition/conversion product formed when neat zoapatanol was stored in the light at 25°C for 72 h (Fig. 4c).

Zoapatanol analogues/derivatives

A large number of oxepane derivatives of the 4 structural types shown in Fig. 5, having a variety of substituents (e. g., hydroxy, alkyl, alkoxy, phenoxy, heterocycloalkoxy, oxo, thioxo, hydroxyimino, alkoxyimino, halo, amino, and alkylamino) present at one or more of the indicated (R) positions have been prepared from zoapatanol or montanol (Kanojia *et al.* 1978). They have been reported to induce uterine contractions at doses ranging from 0.25–100 mg/kg, and to interrupt pregnancy at doses ranging from 2.5–400 mg/kg, the actual dosage employed depending on the species of animal being treated. By way of comparison, the parent zoapatanol induced uterine contractions (rabbit, *in situ*) at doses of 1–4 mg/kg. i.v. (Wachter & Kanojia 1978), and interrupted pregnancy at doses of 25–85 mg/kg i.p. (Hahn *et al.* 1981).

Total synthesis of a 3,6-oxido analogue 6 (Fig. 5) of zoapatanol 2 possessing uteroevacuant activity (no supporting data published), has been reported (Chen & Hajos 1980, Hajos 1981). Water soluble calcium (Morita & Shirasaka 1982a), and basic amino acid (Morita & Shirasaka 1982b) salts of this compound have been prepared, suggesting that this compound may be of particular interest as a potential antifertility agent.

With a view toward determining the importance of the ethano bridge in compounds like 6 for biological activity, Wani *et al.* (1983) synthesized a series

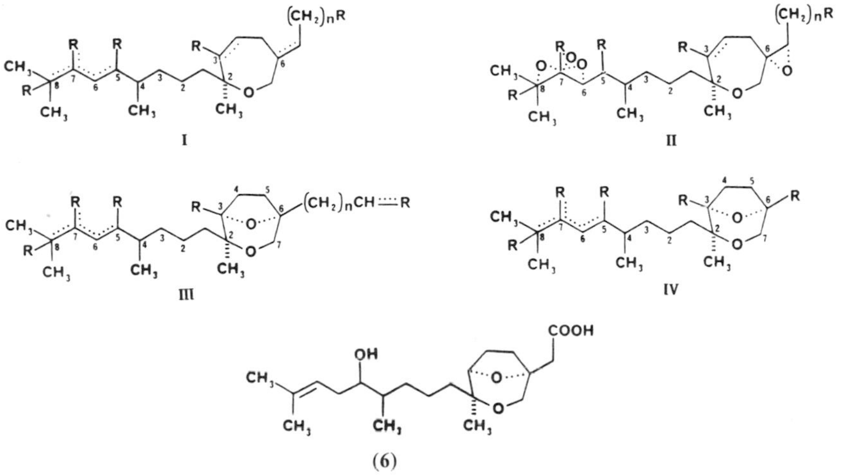

Fig. 5. Oxepane and oxido-oxepane derivatives of zoapatanol
I–II   = Structural types of active oxepane derivatives
III–IV = Structural types of active oxido-oxepane derivatives
– –   = Positions of possible unsaturation
R   = Substituent positions
(6)   = 1RS,4SR,5RS-4-(4,8-Dimethyl-5-hydroxy-7-nonen-1-yl)-4-methyl-3,8-dioxabicyclo
          [3.2.1]octane-1-acetic acid

of 1,4-dioxane analogues (**7, 8, 10 & 11**, Fig. 6). They postulated that these simpler structures might possess similar properties; atomic scale models had shown that the steric relationship of the substituents originally present at C-2 and C-6 of the oxido ring were preserved following removal of the ethano bridge. Unfortunately, none of the 4 compounds interrupted pregnancy in the guinea-pig at the doses employed. Jiang *et al.* (1983) has also synthesized 1,4-dioxane analogues (**7 & 9**, Fig. 6), but by a different route; no biological testing was reported.

Phytochemical investigation of Montanoa species
Zoapatanol can now be obtained by total synthesis (Chen & Rowland 1980, Kane & Doyle 1981a, b, Nicolaou *et al.* 1980). Nevertheless, the wide interest in this plant-derived compound, and in derivatives prepared from it, argue for investigations aimed at identifying its most abundant natural source(s). Consequently, 7 *Montanoa* species or subspecies were cultivated at the University of Illinois Pharmacognosy and Horticulture Field Station. The dried

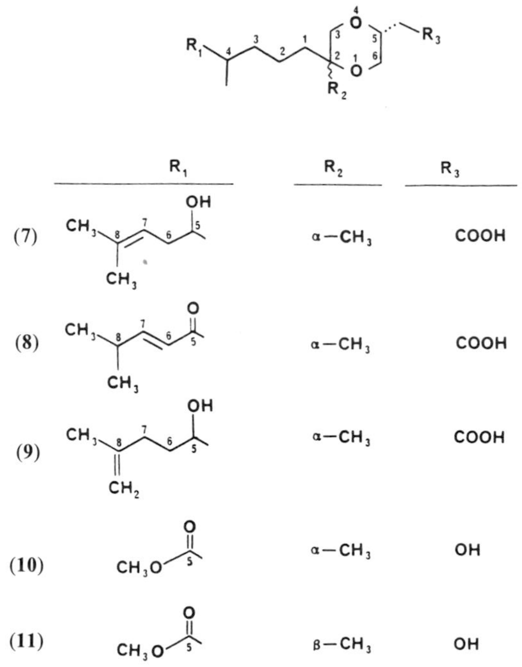

Fig. 6. 1,4-Dioxane analogues of zoapatanol

leaves were extracted with ethyl acetate, and these extracts analyzed by HPLC for zoapatanol content. The highest concentrations of zoapatanol were found in *M. leucantha* (Lag.) Blake spp. *leucantha* (*ca.* 0.04%) and *M. tomentosa* Cerv. ssp. *microcephala* (Sch.-Bip.) Funk (0.03%). Concentrations of *ca.* 0.01–0.02% zoapatanol were found in *M. leucantha* (Lag.) Blake ssp. *arborescens* (DC.) Funk *M. tomentosa* Cerv. ssp. *tomentosa,* and *M. tomentosa* Cerv. ssp. *xanthiifolia* (Sch.-Bip.) Funk. *M. mollisima* Brong. ex. Groenl. contained <0.01% zoapatanol, and none was detected in *M. laskowskii* McVaugh.

Although specific searches for zoapatanol and/or analogues thereof in *Montanoa* species have not previously been reported in the literature, a number of phytochemical isolation studies on such species have been carried out. To date, these studies have resulted in the isolation of a total of 16 kaurene diterpenes and 10 germacranolide sesquiterpenes (structural types I–II and III–IV, respectively, shown in Fig. 7) from 4 *Montanoa* species: *M. tomentosa* Cerv. (Caballero *et al.* 1970, Geissman & Griffin 1971, Lozoya *et al.* 1983, Quijano *et al.* 1982); *M. pteropoda* Blake (Bohlmann & Le Van 1978); *M.*

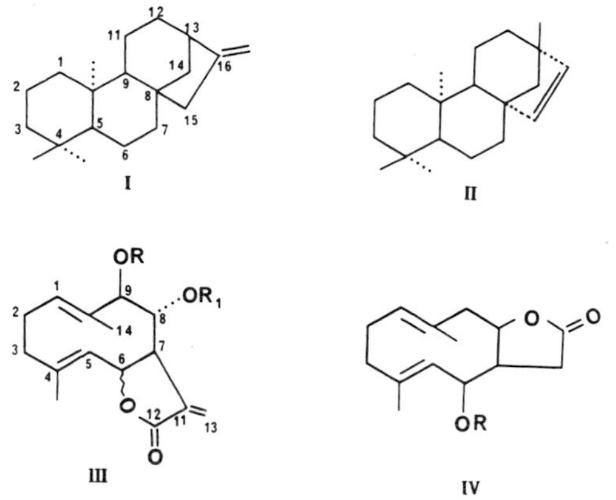

R=Ac or Angelate (expoxyangelate)
R₁=Ac or Angelate (expoxyangelate)

Fig. 7. Structural types of kaurene diterpenes and germacranolide sesquiterpenes from Montanoa species

I & II   = Kaurene diterpenes
III & IV = Germacranolide sesquiterpenes

hibiscifolia (Benth.) Sch.-Bip. (Herz *et al.* 1980); and *M. frutescens* (Mairet) Hemsl. (Quijano *et al.* 1979). Three of these isolates (tomentosin, zoapatlin, and monoginoic acid) reportedly are not responsible for the biological activity of zoapatle (Kanojia *et al.* 1982), but no data were presented. Kauradienoic acid (grandiflorenic acid) (5) has been reported to exert a uterotonic effect *in vitro* (guinea-pig) (Lozoya *et al.* 1983). Further study of this compound, as well as testing of the other isolates would seem worthwhile if sufficient quantities could be obtained.

SUMMARY

Active investigations are currently in progress to develop plant-derived compounds such as gossypol and zoapatanol, for fertility regulation in the human male and female, respectively. Despite obvious differences between these compounds and their respective usages, similarities in the research approaches concerning them exist and have been presented: (a) determinations of their stability under various conditions so that further biological and chemical investigations of these compounds might be facilitated; (b) attempts to synthesize more potent and/or less toxic analogues/derivaties of each; and (c) phytochemical investigations aimed at finding more abundant natural sources (HPR Projects 77918c, 82027).

ACKNOWLEDGEMENTS

The author wishes to thank Dr. A. S. Bingel for her interest, helpful discussions, suggestions, and assistance in the preparation of the manuscript. The assistance of Drs. G. A. Cordell, A. T. Elvin, N. R. Farnsworth, D. D. Soejarto and D. P. Waller is also acknowledged. He is also grateful to Ms. D. Guilty for typing the manuscript.

Research support was furnished, in part, by the Special Programme of Research, Development and Research Training, World Health Organization (HPR Projects 77918c, 82027).

REFERENCES

Abdullah, A. B. & Hutagalung (1981) Gossypol in rubber seed meal. *Pertanika 4(1),* 96–98.

Adams, R., Geissman, T. A. & J. D. Edwards (1960) Gossypol, a pigment of cottonseed. *Chem. Rev. 60,* 555–574.

Anon. (1978) Gossypol- A new antifertility agent for males. *Chinese Med. J. 4,* 417–428.

Bohlmann, F. & Le Van, N. (1978) New kaurenoic acid derivatives and germacranolides from *Montanoa pteropoda. Phytochemistry 17,* 1957–1960.

Caballero, Y. & Walls, F. (1970) Natural products from zoapatle. *Bol. Inst. Quim. Univ. Nacl. Auton Mexico 22,* 79–102.

Chang, M. C., Gu, Z. & Saksena, S. K. (1980) Effects of gossypol on the fertility of male rats, hamsters and rabbits. *Contraception 21,* 461–469.

Chen, R. H. K. & Hajos, Z. G. (1980) Total synthesis of 1RS, 4SR, 5RS-4-(4,8-dimethyl-5-hydroxy-7-nonen-1-yl)-4-methyl-3,8-dioxabicyclo-[3.2.1]-octane-1-acetic acid *United States patent* 4,215,048. Through *Chem. Abstr.* (1981) 94:84184Q.

Chen, R. & Rowland, D. A. (1980) Total synthesis of (±)-zoapatanol. *J. Amer. Chem. Soc. 102,* 6609–6611.

Farnsworth, N. R. & Waller, D. P. (1982) Current status of plant products reported to inhibit sperm. *Res. Front. Fetil. Regulation 2(1),* 1–16.

Farnsworth, N. R., Fong, H. H. S. & Diczfalusy, E. (1983) New fertility regulating agents of plant origin. In: *Proc. Internat. Symposium on Research of the Regulation of Human Fertility, Stockholm, Sweden, Feb. 1983,* ed. Diczfalusy, E. (In Press).

Gallegos, A. J. (1983) The zoapatle I – A traditional remedy from Mexico emerges to modern times. *Contraception 27,* 211–225.

Geissman, T. A. & Griffin, T. S. (1971) Sesquiterpene lactones. Tomentosin from *Montanoa tomentosa* Cerv. *Rev. Latinoamer. Quim. 2,* 81–83.

Hadley, M. A., Young, C. L. & Dym, M. (1981) Effects of gossypol on the reproductive system of male rats. *J. Androl. 2,* 190–199.

Hahn, D. W., McGuire, J. L. & Chang, M. C. (1980) Contragestational agents. In: *Research*

Frontiers in Fertility Regulation, eds. Zatuchni, G. I., Labbok, M. H. & Sciarra, J. J., pp. 362–374. Harper, New York.

Hahn, D. W., Ericson, E. W., Lai, M. T. & Probst, A. (1981) Antifertility activity of *Montanoa tomentosa* (zoapatle). *Contraception 23,* 133–140.

Hajos, Z. (1981) Total synthesis of 1RS,4SR,5RS-4-(4,8-dimethyl)-5-hydroxy-7-nonen-1-yl)-4-methyl-3,8-dioxabicyclo-[3.2.1]-octane-1-acetic acid and related compounds. *United States patent* 4, 284,565.

Herz, W., Govindan, S. V. & Blount, J. F. (1980) *trans, trans-*Germacra-1(10),4-dien-*cis-*6,12-olides from *Montanoa hibiscifolia. J. Org. Chem. 45,* 1113–1116.

Jiang, J. B., Urbanski, M. J. & Hajos, Z. G. (1983) Total synthesis of dioxane analogues related to zoapatanol. *J. Org. Chem. 48,* 2001–2005.

Jolad, S. D., Wiedhopf, R. M. & Cole, J. R. (1975) Tumor-inhibitory agent from *Montezuma speciosissima* (Malvaceae). *J. Pharm. Sci. 64,* 1889–1890.

Kalla, N. R. (1982) Gossypol – The male antifertility agent. *IRCS J. Med. Sci. 10,* 766–769.

Kane, V. V. & Doyle, D. L. (1981a) Total synthesis of (±)-zoapatanol: A stereospecific synthesis of a key intermediate. *Tetrahedron Lett. 22,* 3027–3030.

Kane, V. V. & Doyle, D. L. (1981b) Total synthesis of (±)-zoapatanol. *Tetrahedron Lett. 22,* 3031–3034.

Kanojia, R. M., Wachter, M. P. & Chen, R. H. K. (1978) Oxepanes. *United States patent* 4, 102,895.

Kanojia, R. M., Wachter, M. P., Levine, S. D., Adams, R. E., Chen, R., Chin, E., Cotter, M. L., Hirsch, A. F., Huettemann, R., Kane, V. V., Ostrowski, P., Shaw, C. I., Mateos, J. L., Noriega, L., Guzman, A., Mijarez, A. & Tovar, L. (1982) Isolation and structural elucidation of zoapatanol and montanol, novel oxepane diterpenoids from the Mexican plant zoapatle *(Montanoa tomentosa). J. Org. Chem. 47,* 1310–1319.

King, T. J. & de Silva, L. B. (1968) Optically active gossypol from *Thespesia populnea. Tetrahedron Lett. 1968,* 261–263.

Landgren, B. M., Aedo, A. R., Hagenfeldt, K. & Diczfalusy, E. (1979) Clinical effects of orally administered extracts of *Montanoa tomentosa* in early human pregnancy. *Amer. J. Obst. Gynecol. 135,* 480–484.

Lee, C. Y., Moon, Y. S., Duleba, A. & Chan, A. F. (1982) The instability of gossypol. *Contraceptive Delivery System 3(3/4),* 274.

Lei, H.-P. (1982) Review and prospects of gossypol research. *Acta Pharm. Sinica 17,* 1–4.

Levine, S. D., Hahn, D. W., Cotter, M. L., Greenslade, F. C., Kanojia, R. M., Pasquale, S. A., Wachter, M. & McGuire, J. L. (1981) The Mexican plant, zoapatle *(Montanoa tomentosa)* in reproductive medicine, past, present and future. *J. Reprod. Med. 26,* 524–528.

Levine, S. D., Adams, R. E., Chen, R., Cotter, M. L., Hirsch, A. F., Kane, V. V., Kanojia, R. M., Shaw, C., Wachter, M. P., Chin, E., Huettemann, R., Ostrowski, P., Mateos, J. L., Noriega, L., Guzman, A., Mijarez, A. & Tovar, L. (1979) Zoapatanol and montanol, novel oxepane diterpenoids, from the Mexican plant zoapatle *(Montanoa tomentosa). J. Amer. Chem. Soc. 101,* 3404–3405.

Liu, Z.-Q., Liu, G.-Z., Hei, L.-S., Zhang, R.-A. & Yu, C.-Z. (1981) Clinical trial of gossypol as a male antifertility agent. In: *Recent Advances in Fertility Regulation,* eds. Chang, C. F., Griffin, D. & Woolman, A., pp. 160–163. Atar S. A., Geneva.

Lozoya, X., Enríquez, R. G., Bejar, E., Estrada, A. V., Girón, H., Ponce-Monter, H. & Gallegos, A. J. (1983) The zoapatle V – The effect of kauradienoic acid upon uterine contractility. *Contraception 27,* 267–279.

Markman, A. L. & Rzhekhin, V. P. (1969) *Gossypol and Its Derivatives,* pp. 79–84, Israel Program for Scientific Translation, Jerusalem.

Morita, Y. & Shirasaka, T. (1982a) Method for the preparation of the calcium salt of 3,8-dioxabi-cyclo-[3.2.1]-octane-1-acetic acid. *Japanese patent* 82-126491.

Morita, Y. & Shirasaka, T. (1982b) The basic amino acid salt of 3,8-dioxabicyclo-[3.2.1]-octane-1-acetic acid derivative. *Japanese patent* 82-123185.

Nicolaou, K. C., Claremon, D. A. & Barnette, W. E. (1980) Total synthesis of ($\pm$)-zoapatanol. *J. Amer. Chem. Soc. 102,* 6611–6612.

Nomeir, A. A. & Abou-Donia, M. B. (1982) Gossypol: High-performance liquid chromatographic analysis and stability in various solvents. *J. Amer. Oil Chem. Soc. 59,* 546–549.

Pirkle, W. H. & Schreiner, J. L. (1981) Chiral high-pressure liquid chromatographic stationary phases. 4. Separation of the enantiomers of bi-naphthols and analogues. *J. Org. Chem. 46,* 4988–4991.

Pirkle, W. H., Finn, J. M., Schreiner, J. L. & Hamper, B. C. (1981) A widely useful chiral stationary phase for the high-performance liquid chromatography separation of enantiomers. *J. Amer. Chem. Soc. 103,* 3964–3966.

Prasad, M. R. N. & Diczfalusy, E. (1982) Gossypol. *Int. J. Androl. Suppl. 5,* 53–70.

Qian, S.-Z. (1981) Effect of gossypol on potassium and prostaglandin metabolism and mechanism of action of gossypol. In: *Recent Advances in Fertility Regulation,* eds. Chang, C.-F., Griffin, D. & Woolman, A. pp. 152–159. Atar S. A., Geneva.

Quijano, L., Calderón, J. S., Gómez, G. & Ríos, T. (1979) Montafrusin, a new germacrolide from *Montanoa frutescens. Phytochemistry 18,* 843–845.

Quijano, L., Calderón, J. S., Gómez, F. & Ríos, T. (1982) Zoapatanolide A and B, two new heliangolides from *Montanoa tomentosa. Phytochemistry 21,* 2041–2044.

Si, Y.-K., Huang, L. & Zhou, J. (1983) Separation of (-)-gossypol from its racemic form. *Ke Kue Tong Bao* 1983, 640.

Wachter, M. P. & Kanojia, R. M. (1978) Purification of utero-evacuant extracts from plant substances. *United States patent* 4,086,358.

Waller, D. P., Bunyapraphatsara, N., Martin, A., Vournazos, C. J., Ahmed, M. S., Soejarto, D. D., Cordell, G. A., Fong, H. H. S., Russell, L. D. & Malone, J. P. (1983) Effect of (+)-gossypol on fertility in male hamsters. *J. Androl. 4,* 276–279.

Wang, Y., Luo, Y. & Tang, X. (1979) Studies on the antifertility actions of cotton seed meal and gossypol. *Acta Pharm. Sinica 11,* 662–669.

Wani, M. C., Vishnuvajjala, B. R., Swain, Jr., W. E., Rector, D. H., Cook, C. E., Petrow, V., Reel, J. R., Allen, K. M. & Levine, S. G. (1983) Synthesis and biological activity of zoapatanol analogues. *J. Med. Chem. 26,* 426–430.

Worthley, E. G. & Schott, C. D. (1966) Pharmacotoxic evaluation of nine vehicles administered intraperitoneally to mice. *Lloydia 29,* 123–129.

Xue, S. P. (1981) Studies on the antifertility effect of gossypol, a new contraceptive for males. In: *Recent Advances in Fertility Regulation,* eds. Chang, C. F., Griffin, D. & Woolman, A., pp. 122–146. Atar S. A., Geneva.

Zatuchni, G. I. & Osborn, C. K. (1981) Gossypol: A possible male antifertility agent. *Res. Front. Fertil. Regulation 1(4),* 1–15.

Zhou, L.-F. & Lei, H.-P. (1981) Recovery of fertility in rats after gossypol treatment. In: *Recent Advances in Fertility Regulation,* eds. Chang, C. F., Griffin, D. & Woolman, A., pp. 147–151. Atar S. A., Geneva.

DISCUSSION

JAROSZEWSKI: Dr. Fong may have left us with the impression that the cotton plants contain only racemic gossypol as opposed to *Thespesia populnea* which contains (+)-gossypol. This is not quite true. In fact, all known gossypol sources contain (+)-gossypol, but its enantiomeric purity varies very much. For *T. populnea,* the enantiomeric excess of (+)-gossypol is 80–100%, for the cotton plant perhaps 20%, depending on the variety and plant part. Whether (+)- or (±)-gossypol is isolated, depends on the isolation procedure employed. Thus, from the cotton plant gossypol is usually obtained by treatment of an ether extract of the plant material with acetic acid, which results in precipitation of the well-known acetic acid complex with (±)-gossypol. (±)-Gossypol does not form the complex with acetic acid and remains in the solution. The isolation procedure employed originally for *T. populnea* does not involve formation of the acetic acid complex and, thus, (+)-gossypol was obtained. Incidentally, it would be very interesting to know what sort of regulatory mechanisms determine the optical purity of gossypol present in a given plant. Since (+)-gossypol does not racemize readily, it appears that both (+) gossypol and (±) gossypol are produced enzymatically, but what factors determine their ratio?

FONG: Dr. Jaroszewski's comments on gossypol occurrence are correct and appreciated. I have no information to offer on the question of enzymatic control of optical purity.

WITKOP: I think that in the area of control of population growth nobody probably comes from an area more interested in this problem than Dr. Huang. Would you kindly enlighten us on the attempted resolution of gossypol?

HUANG LIANG: In the literature, many attempts on the resolution of gossypol 1 by physical and memical methods have been made but with no successful results. The tautomerism, possibly between 3 forms of the substituted naphthalene moiety of gossypol, the aldehyde 2, cyclic hemiacetal 3 and the enol 4, which eventually would give 6 tautomeric forms of gossypol, 3 with 2 identical halves, and 3 unsymmetrical forms, might be the cause of the trouble in the resolution. When we carried out the condensation of racemic gossypol with optically active amine, (+)-1-phenyl-2-propylamine, the product showed 2 sports on TLC. Fractional crystallization or chromatographic separation gave unsatisfactory results. The resolution has finally been achieved by acetylation of the condensation product by which the tautomerism could be blocked. From the acetates, 5 compounds have been separated. The postulated structures have been based upon mass spectroscopy and nmr data. Two main products, being disastereoisomers **5**, were hydrolyzed to give a pair of enatiomors, (+)- and (−)- gossypol. Their CD curves being mirror images to each other were shown in Fig. 1. However, one question remains to be solved. From the literature, specific relation of natural (+)-gossypol has been reported by Fong to be +340 and by King to be +450. Our absolute values of (+) and (−) forms coincide with the former. Right now we are repeating the process to check the optical purity of the product and also to obtain more samples for biological tests.

RAZDAN: During the last 3 years we have been working on analogues of gossypol. We have had no problem in reacting the compound as an acetic-acid complex which confirms what you just said, Dr. Huang Liang, that it is quite stable. Unfortunately, we have not been able to come up with any compound more potent than gossypol. We have also made the hexa-acetate, which was found to be inactive, which I find very surprising. We are continuing this work.

RAPOPORT: How easy is it to racemize gossypol?

FONG: It is not easy. The energy barrier to rotation of the atropisomers has been calculated to be greater than 80 Kcal/mole.

JAROSZEWSKI: A very brief answer to Professor Rapoport's question: (+)-gossypol can be boiled in toluene (117°C) without racemization, but appears to racemize (or decompose?) on a brief heating in ethylene glycol at 190°C (1).

DJERASSI: The key question, I think, really is not to get a more potent compound, because there is nothing wrong with the potency or activity of gossypol. The problem is with the side-effects and particularly the hypokalemic effects. I would like to pose the question whether the hypokalemic activity is associated with one antipode or the other. I want to ask you: I know that nothing has been done with (−)-gossypol, what about the plus antipode. Have you examined the hypokalemic activity in animals of the (+)-antipode and compared it with that of the racemic compound?

FONG: No, we have not done such comparative studies.

DJERASSI: I think, the key problem is going to be whether the (+)- and (−)-antipodes really have different activity.

FONG: As I understand it, the hypokalemic effect was a problem only in a couple of provinces in China, where hypokalemia occurs due to dietary deficiency of potassium. When calcium supplements were given along with gossypol, the incidence of gossypol-induced hypokalemia was zero (2). Further, hypokalemia has not been observed in clinical studies outside China (3).

HUANG LIANG: It is very hard to study the hypokalemia experimentally, because no animal model of hypokalemia is available. You have to observe it in man.

WALL: I would like to ask either Dr. Huang or Dr. Fong on the subject of the safety of gossypol. The structure worries me a little bit.

LAZDUNSKI: As a biologist I would like to ask the question: Does one know how it works? What is its effect on the sperm?

HUANG LIANG: It has been used in men in about 9,000 cases.

LAZDUNSKI: What is the mechanism of action?

HUANG LIANG: A lot of people are working on the mechanism. It has been reported that gossypol acts selectively on specific isoenzyme LDHX. The action is assumed to be very specific for the testicles and also for the sperm. But right now I start to doubt it. As to Dr. Wall's question, it is true that over approximately the past 40 years, most of the reports were concerned with the toxicity of gossypol, but the dose we use now really is very low, at 20 mg/day.

FONG: The mechanism of action is unknown. A number of theories have been proposed. One involves inhibition of mitochondrial energy-producing enzyme, but the data are inconclusive. There have been theories about effects on prostaglandin synthesis, as well as on membrane cation transfer enzymes. The effects on sperm during and after maturation are far from being fully elucidated.

HUANG LIANG: Concerning the physical disposition, the concentration of gossypol in the testicles really is low.

ANAND: I have a question for Dr. Fong and Dr. Farnsworth about zoapatanol. Based on the available data, zoapatanol does not appear very promising as an abortifacient, while the decoction used as tea was supposed to be active in clinical cases. What could be the reason – have we missed the avtive compound?

FONG: There are no clinical data on zoapatanol. The only clinical studies reported to date were on a tea preparation (4), the dose of which may have been inadequate. Until we have some clinical data on zoapatanol, we cannot draw any conclusions about its effectiveness.

ANAND: Some clinical data on zoapatanol are available in some reports.

DJERASSI: If we are going to have a long discussion on gossypol and zoapatanol, why don't we focus on the important aspects, and not on the trivial aspects of these 2 compounds. In the context of zoapatanol, I would say perhaps the most telling aspect for me is that the pharmaceutical companies are not working very actively in the field anymore. That must mean something. Scientifically, the most important aspect of gossypol is that it really represents the only significant advance in relation to male contraception during the last 20 years. The importance of resolving gossypol lies, of course, in the possibility that one antipode is better than the other in terms of activity or, even more importantly, in terms of side-effects. That question can now be solved in China, and I am glad it is in China, because it is a Chinese discovery originally. The other reason why it is so important to know whether the configuration is an essential structural parameter is that if this should be the case, then it is almost certain that most of the simplification experiments are not going to work, because a dimeric structure will be required. My own guess is that you will require the dimer, and, therefore, structural manipulations have to be done in a more subtle manner. I agree entirely with Dr. Huang that one has to be very much aware of the tautomeric problems in addition to the configurational aspects. From a clinical point of view, the irony is that while in China more than 8000 people have taken gossypol, some of them have been taking it since 1972, not a single man has been subjected to gossypol in the United States. I think it is an ironic situation, and probably one that will not change for a while. What we really have to be interested in is fertility control in humans and not just in rodents. In the field of male contraception we are faced with long-term effects (ranging over 40–50 years), much more than in the field of female contraception (ca. 20–30 years).

(1) Dechary, J. M. & Pradel, P. (1971) *J. Amer. Oil Chem. Soc. 48*, 563–564.
(2) Qian, S.-Z. (1981) (see ref. p. 368).
(3) Prasad, M. R. N. & Diczfalusy, E. (1982) (see ref. p. 368).
(4) Landgren, B. M. *et al.* (1979) (see ref. p. 367).

Antihepatotoxic Principles in Oriental Medicinal Plants

Hiroshi Hikino

In advanced nations, infectious diseases are now almost under control due to sanitation improvements and the development of antibiotics and vaccines. One of the infectious diseases which still cannot be controlled is viral hepatitis, which can lead to chronic hepatitis and eventually, liver cirrhosis.

Further, in view of the special position of the liver in the cardiovascular system, slow blood flow in the liver, and the role of the liver to catch and treat foreign substances positively, not only microbes such as viruses and bacilli, but also chemicals ingested, reach this organ, and sometimes induce morbid changes. Such chemicals are, for example, ethyl alcohol, toxins in food, peroxidized edible oil and pharmaceuticals (certain antibiotics, chemotherapeutics, CNS-active drugs, etc).

Western medicine has found no clear and definite treatment, however, there are a number of traditional herbal drugs which are reputed to be effective for liver disorders in the Orient. Thus, we turn to Oriental medicines for possibly promising hepato-protective drugs.

For confirmation of liver-protective activity and clarification of active principles of those drugs, it is essential that suitable assay methods are available. The magnitude of the liver-protective activity can be evaluated by morphological examinations and by determination of hepatic functions and the survival rate.

Studies of liver lesions and potentially protective drugs have, so far, been conducted by *in vivo* assay methods mainly using rats. However, it is very difficult to perform such *in vivo* experiments utilizing rats for activity-directed guidance of fractionation of extracts of crude drugs, primarily because they are costly in animals, require a lot of sample, and give marked variation and rather poor reproducibility of results.

Department of Natural Products Chemistry, Pharmaceutical Institute, Tohoku University, Japan

NATURAL PRODUCTS AND DRUG DEVELOPMENT, Alfred Benzon Symposium 20.
Editors: P. Krogsgaard-Larsen, S. Brøgger Christensen, H. Kofod, Munksgaard, Copenhagen 1984.

As larger variation in results has been observed with mice than with rats, a screen employing mice was thought to be impractical. Although the D-galactosamine (GalN)-induced liver damage model cannot be prepared with mice, but still requires rats, the carbon tetrachloride (CCl_4)-induced liver damage model can now, in fact, also be prepared with mice if suitable strains are selected. Thus, a number of Oriental medicines were screened with mice of a suitable strain (Kiso *et al.* 1982a).

Using the CCL_4-induced liver damage model in mice, we isolated desoxy-podophyllotoxin from *Thujopsis dolabrata* leaves as the liver-protective principle (Hikino *et al.* 1979). Desoxypodophyllotoxin was also revealed to exhibit a protective action against GalN-induced liver damage (Kiso *et al.* 1982b). Further, in order to clarify the relationship between the chemical structures and the liver-protective actions, effects of desoxypodophyllotoxin and its 6 analogs on CCl_4-induced liver lesion in mice and on GalN-induced liver lesion in rats were investigated, indicating that these analogs have liver-protective actions in general, and that certain structural features are important for the revelation of the activity (Kiso *et al.* 1982c).

The CCl_4-induced liver damage model in mice represents a substantial improvement compared with utilizing rats, but some problems still remain in regard to cost, sample size and variation and reproducibility of the results.

ASSAY METHODS FOR ANTI-HEPATOTOXIC ACTIVITY USING CARBON TE-TRACHLORIDE- AND D-GALACTOSAMINE-INDUCED CYTOTOXICITY IN PRI-MARY CULTURED HEPATOCYTES

In order to devise simple and reliable methods which are appropriate for screening of anti-hepatotoxic constituents in the plant kingdom, the possibility was investigated of using primary cultured hepatocytes instead of whole animals.

Hepatocytes of high viability can now be isolated in a good yield by the recirculating perfusion method (Berry & Friend 1969, Seglen 1976), and maintained in a good viability for several days under certain conditions (Tanaka *et al.* 1978, Kato *et al.* 1979).

The basic idea was to culture isolated hepatocytes with a hepatotoxin and a sample, and to determine the anti-hepatotoxic effect of the sample by measuring the level of GPT released from primary cultured hepatocytes into the culture medium.

Because experimental liver lesion models can be produced by various hepatotoxins, among which the best studied are CCl4 and GalN, the damage to liver cells by these 2 hepatotoxins was examined to assess the utility of the assay methods.

When devising the assay method using CCl4-induced cytotoxicity, it was found that rat hepatocytes pre-incubated for 1.5 h were more sensitive to CCl4, than those pre-incubated for 24 h, but it was alleged that, immediately after perfusion, isolated hepatocytes suffered from membrane damage which was recovered after incubation for over 24 h. Because similar anti-hepatotoxicity was observed with hepatocytes pre-incubated for 1.5 and 24 h (Table I), 24 h-pre-incubated hepatocytes, whose membrane functions were more fully restored, have been used. Thus, by testing several conditions, a satisfactory assay method was achieved which consisted of pre-incubation of isolated rat hepatocytes for 24 h, addition of CCl4 and a sample, and determination of the GPT level in the culture medium at 60 min thereafter. Although mice can equally be employed, the number of cells obtainable from a mouse is much less than that from a rat (Kiso *et al.* 1983a).

In testing the assay method utilizing GalN-induced cytotoxicity, it was found that GalN challenge caused marked increase of the GPT level with rat hepatocytes pre-incubated for 1.5 h, but produced only slight increase of the transaminase level in those pre-incubated for 24 h. While, lesser increase of the GPT level was observed by treatment with GalN in cultured-mouse hepatocytes. Thus, the satisfactory assay procedure was found to consist of pre-incubation of isolated rat hepatocytes for 1.5 h, addition of GalN and a sample, and determination of the GPT level in the medium at 30 h thereafter (Kiso *et al.* 1983b).

Because anti-hepatotoxic effects are evaluated by measurement of the transaminase activity in these assay methods, enzyme inhibitory effects of test samples should be checked separately. When enzyme inhibitory effects of test samples are too intense to determine anti-hepatotoxic effects, other evaluation methods can be adopted.

Although the damage to the cells is likely to be the result of mechanisms similar to those responsible for the toxicity of CCl4 and GalN in the intact animals, *in vitro* experiments may still carry the risk of creating experimental systems which do not reflect events which occur in the intact animal. Thus, to evaluate the procedures using CCl4 and GalN-intoxicated hepatocytes *in vitro,* natural products of known anti-hepatotoxic activity *in vivo,* were screened by

Table I

Effect of known hepatoprotective natural products on carbon tetrachloride- and galactosamine-induced cytotoxicity in primary cultured rat hepatocytes

Substance	Dose (mg/ml)	GPT (%) CCl_4[a'] (1.5 h†)	CCl_4[a] (24 h††)	GalN[b] (1.5 h†)
Control	–	100±2	100±0	100±3
Cynarin	0.01	101±6	100±3	95±2
	0.1	101±5	112±2	84±4
	1.0	100±2	84±4	48±2**
Desoxypodophyllotoxin	0.01	97±2	85±0**	93±3
	0.1	82±2*	73±1**	50±2**
	1.0	49±2**	33±1**	92±5
Glycyrrhetinic acid	0.01	97±3	91±1**	102±7
	0.1	49±1**	39±1**	58±6*
	1.0	15±0**	9±1**	27±1**
Glycyrrhizin	0.01	93±3	92±2	103+6
	0.1	88±1*	85±2*	100±5
	1.0	40±1**	30±1**	24±1**
Methionine	0.01	98±1	90±3	106±2
	0.1	93±2	94±3	113±1
	1.0	98±3	111±4	122±5
Picroside I	0.01	101±3	88±1**	96±5
	0.1	97±2	88±3*	122±2
	1.0	85±3	92±1*	111±2
Picroside II	0.01	97±3	106±4	103±4
	0.1	103±1	103±5	101±3
	1.0	89±1*	96±3	78±1*
Silybin	0.01	94±2	86±3*	106±5
	0.1	91±2	72±2**	103±3
	1.0	29±1**	21±1**	66±2**

[a'], [a] After pre-incubation (1.5† or 24 h††), the cells were exposed to the medium (1.0 ml) containing 10 mM CCl_4/ethanol (0.01 ml) and a sample in dimethylsulfoxide (DMSO, 0.01 ml). At 60 min after the CCl_4 challenge, GPT value in the medium was measured.

[b] After pre-culture (1.5 h†), the cells were exposed to the medium (1.0 ml) containing 0.5 mM GalN and a sample in DMSO (0.01 ml). At 30 h after the GalN challenge, GPT value in the medium was determined.

n=3 (dishes). Significantly different from the control, $p<0.01$* or $p<0.001$**.

these methods. It was found that most of the natural products tested exhibited significant anti-hepatotoxic activity (Table I), demonstrating that *in vivo* assay methods can be satisfactorily replaced by these *in vitro* assay methods (Kiso *et al.* 1983a, Kiso *et al.* 1983b).

The assay methods, thus developed, offer many excellent advantages: numerous samples may be evaluated at one time at low cost, a small sample size is required, there is little variation and good reproducibility of results. These assay methods have proved to be extremely useful for the primary evaluation of extracts, fractions and constituents of crude drugs for liver-protective activity. Comparison of costs and sample sizes required for the *in vivo* and *in vitro* assay methods is shown in Table II.

Although the *in vitro* assay methods are excellent in many respects, they may possibly give results discrepant with those obtained by *in vivo* assay methods, particularly in cases where substances which exhibit anti-hepatotoxic activity only after they have been affected metabolism *in vivo*, would produce negative responses, while substances which are easily converted into inactive metabolites *in vivo*, would still give positive responses with *in vitro* assay.

Though it is known that viruses, chemicals and other factors cause liver disorders, the types of the morbid change they produce in the liver are much less than the number of causes: thus, they have something in common, to one degree or another. Therefore, it is believed that the assay methods, thus devised, using primary cultured rat hepatocytes *in vitro*, are useful for primary detection (but not final confirmation) of anti-hepatotoxic activity of materials of plant origin.

DETECTION OF ANTI-HEPATOTOXIC ACTIVITY OF CRUDE DRUGS AND CLARIFICATION OF THEIR ACTIVE PRINCIPLES

A number of Oriental drugs were screened by these assay methods, and it was found that some exhibited significant anti-hepatotoxic activity. A search for the anti-hepatotoxic principles in the active drugs was carried out and the

Table II
Cost and sample size for assay of 400 samples

Assay method	Cost	Sample size
Rat *in vivo*	$2000 (133)	200 mg/rat (200)
Mouse *in vivo*	$ 330 (22)	20 mg/mouse (20)
Rat *in vitro*	$ 15 (1)	1 mg/dish (1)

Table III

Effect of constituents of Curcuma *rhizomes and their analogs on carbon tetrachloride- and galacto-samine-induced cytotoxicity in primary cultured rat hepatocytes*

Substance	Dose (mg/ml)	GPT (%) CCl$_4$[a]	GalN[b]
Control	–	100±1	100±1
Curcumin	0.01	92±3	100±3
	0.1	42±5**	89±1*
	1.0	20±5**	44±1**
p-Coumaroylferuloylmethane	0.01	88±4	106±2
	0.1	37±4**	90±1*
	1.0	17±1**	53±1**
Di-*p*-coumaroylmethane	0.01	88±1	104±1
	0.1	62±1**	85±1*
	1.0	35±2**	66±1**
Control	–	100±1	100±2
Cinnamic acid	0.01	94±2	102±4
	0.1	94±2	95±3
	1.0	98±1	77±2**
p-Coumaric acid	0.01	92±3	103±1
	0.1	95±3	105±2
	1.0	94±1	86±3
O-Methyl-*p*-coumaric acid	0.01	97±2	89±2*
	0.1	100±2	86±2*
	1.0	95±2	72±2**
Caffeic acid	0.01	88±2	98±5
	0.1	69±1**	58±1**
	1.0	51±2**	18±1**
Ferulic acid	0.01	80±3*	97±7
	0.1	88±2*	103±6
	1.0	88±4	96±8
O-Methylferulic acid	0.01	94±2	88±4
	0.1	79±1**	95±2
	1.0	103±3	74±2**
Sinapic acid	0.01	99±1	97±1
	0.1	107±2	94±2
	1.0	102±3	89±2*
O-Methylsinapic acid	0.01	99±2	90±2
	0.1	101±2	87±2*

Table III

Effect of constituents of Curcuma *rhizomes and their analogs on carbon tetrachloride- and galacto-samine-induced cytotoxicity in primary cultured rat hepatocytes*

Substance	Dose (mg/ml)	GPT (%) CCl$_4$[a]	GalN[b]
	1.0	101±5	73±1**
Protocatechuic acid	0.01	97±3	97±4
	0.1	103±1	81±3*
	1.0	97±4	74±3*

[a,b] Experimental conditions were the same as those given in the legend to Table I.
n=3 (dishes). Significantly different from the control, $p<0.01$* or $p<0.001$**.

anti-hepatotoxic effects of the active principles evaluated. Some of the results are described below.

Anti-hepatotoxic principles of Curcuma longa rhizomes
Because an extract of the rhizomes of *Curcuma longa* (Zingiberaceae) exhibited intense preventive activity against CCl$_4$-induced liver damage *in vivo*, the extract was fractionated by monitoring the activity to allow the curcuminoids shown by the *in vitro* assay methods to exert significant anti-hepatotoxic action (Table III).

It was quite possible, however, that the curcuminoids are cleaved *in vivo* to cinnamic acid derivatives, which in turn exhibit anti-hepatotoxic activity. Consequently, the anti-hepatotoxic effects of some analogs of ferulic acid and *p*-coumaric acid, probable metabolites of the curcuminoids, were also assayed, revealing that only caffeic acid showed a significant effect, while remaining analogs elicited no significant activity (Table III). Because none of the curcuminoids above assayed, gave any caffeic acid, it was concluded that the curcuminoids exhibit anti-hepatotoxic activity *per se* (Kiso *et al.* 1983c).

Anti-hepatotoxic principles of Atractylodes rhizomes
As extracts of certain samples of the rhizomes of *Atractylodes* (Compositae) showed anti-hepatotoxic activity by *in vitro* assay, the main sesquiterpenoid constituents were screened to indicate that atractylon, β-eudesmol and hinesol elicited significant anti-hepatotoxic actions (Table IV).

Although it was probable that these sesquiterpenoids exhibited their anti-hepatotoxic effect after metabolic degradation to furnish active metabolites *in vivo*, atractylenolide II and III, which are auto-oxidation products of atractylon

Table IV

Effect of constituents of Atractylodes *rhizomes on carbon tetrachloride- and galactosamine-induced cytotoxicity in primary cultured rat hepatocytes*

Substance	Dose (mg/ml)	GPT (%) CCl$_4$[a]	GalN[b]
Control	–	100±4	100±2
Atractylon	0.01	67±3*	99±1
	0.1	53±6*	92±2
	1.0	25±2**	84±1*
Atractylenolide I	1.0	68±7	107±2
Atractylenolide II	1.0	74±1*	94±5
Atractylenolide III	1.0	103±5	97±4
β-Eudesmol	0.01	83±6	104±2
	0.1	70±4*	94±1
	1.0	53±2**	79±1**
Hinesol	0.01	79±6	101±1
	0.1	62±3*	99±1
	1.0	31±1**	73±2**

[a,b] Experimental conditions were the same as those given in the legend to Table I.
n=3 (dishes). Significantly different from the control, $p<0.01$* or $p<0.001$**.

in vitro and possible *in vivo* metabolites of atractylon, showed no or only weak anti-hepatotoxic activity, and the metabolic mixtures of these sesquiterpenoids obtained by treatment with microsomes disclosed no significant activity, demonstrating that atractylon, β-eudesmol and hinesol are effective *per se* (Kiso *et al.* 1983d).

Anti-hepatotoxic principles of Artemisia capillaris buds

In order to understand the anti-hepatotoxic activity of the ears of *Artemisia capillaris* (Compositae), some samples collected in the crude drug market were screened using the CCl$_4$-induced liver-damage model in mice, showing that the activity of the ears varied markedly depending on lots. Because this remarkable variation was thought to be due to difference in dates and locations of collection, the ears of this plant were harvested periodically during the season when they are possibly collected for preparation of the crude drug, and screened for anti-hepatotoxic activity. The results indicated that this plant gives the strongest activity and consequently the most effective drug preparations when in bud in

Table V

Effect of constituents of Artemisia capillaris *buds and their analogs on carbon tetrachloride- and galactosamine-induced cytotoxicity in primary cultured rat hepatocytes*

Substance	Dose (mg/ml)	GPT (%) CCl$_4$[a]	GalN[b]
Control	–	100±1	100±3
Capillarisin	0.1	85±4	47±2**
	0.3	40±1**	5±1**
	1.0	20±1**	3±2**
4'-Methylcapillarisin	0.1	88±2*	82±1*
	0.3	77±2**	79±1*
	1.0	68±4*	85±2*
7-Methylcapillarisin	0.1	82±1**	
	0.3	91±2	
	1.0	68±1**	
Arcapillin	0.1	92±3	78±6
	0.3	87±1**	61±2**
	1.0	39±1**	46±1**
Cirsilineol	0.1	94±4	89±4
	0.3	95±1	86±3
	1.0	80±7	79±3
Cirsimaritin	0.1	90±1*	88±5
	0.3	89±4	83±9
	1.0	80±8	78±2*
Eupatolitin	0.1	99±2	
	0.3	80±1**	
	1.0	86±4	
Isorhamnetin	0.1	71±2**	105±2
	0.3	65±2**	96±4
	1.0	48±1**	100±2
Quercetin	0.1	86±1**	80±3
	0.3	70±1**	83±2
	1.0	46±2**	69±3*
Rhamnocitrin	0.1	90±2	
	0.3	93±5	
	1.0	92±3	
Cacticin (isorhamnetin-3-galactoside)	0.1	104±1	26±1**
	0.3	102±0	41±2**
	1.0	105±1	28±2**

Table V

Effect of constituents of Artemisia capillaris *buds and their analogs on carbon tetrachloride- and galactosamine-induced cytotoxicity in primary cultured rat hepatocytes*

Substance	Dose (mg/ml)	GPT (%)	
		$CCl_4^{a)}$	$GalN^{b)}$
Isorhamnetin-3-glucoside	0.1	104±1	48±4**
	0.3	103±1	45±4**
	1.0	104±0	34±1**
Hyperin	0.1	107±0	23±0**
(quercetin-3-galactoside)	0.3	105±2	37±2**
	1.0	100±2	73±3*
Control	–	100±2	100±1
Umbelliferone	0.1	98±3	63±2**
	0.3	94±0	48±3**
	1.0	22±0**	23±1**
Methylumbelliferone	0.1	105±2	84±1**
	0.3	98±1	87±2*
	1.0	73±1**	71±1**
Esculetin	0.1	108±1	82+1**
	0.3	116±6	68±1**
	1.0	15±1**	21±1**
6-Methylesculetin	0.1	87±3	90±5
	0.3	80±3*	84±3*
	1.0	29±2**	41±3**
7-Methylesculetin	0.1	101±0	48±0**
	0.3	101±2	46±1**
	1.0	85±1*	31±2**
6,7-Dimethylesculetin	0.1	95±1	72±5*
	0.3	94±2	68±6*
	1.0	32±1**	36±2**
Esculin	0.1	106±3	94±3
	0.3	95±3	84±1**
	1.0	33±1**	12±0**
7-Methylesculin	0.1	103±1	70±3**
	0.3	95±3	91±4
	1.0	84±5	70±1**

[a,b)] Experimental conditions were the same as those given in the legend to Table I.

n=3 (dishes). Significantly different from the control, $p<0.01$* or $p<0.001$**.

September. The extract of the buds was then fractionated by monitoring the activity to yield various flavonoids and a coumarin (6,7-dimethylesculetin). Anti-hepatotoxic activity of these constituents and their analogs was measured by the *in vitro* assay methods (Table V).

Although of the components of *Artemisia capillaris* buds, capillarisin has the most intense anti-hepatotoxic activity, its content was about one-tenth of that of dimethylesculetin, demonstrating that the latter represents the anti-hepatotoxic activity of the crude drug (Kiso *et al.* 1983e).

Anti-hepatotoxic principles of Schizandra chinensis fruits

From the fruits of *Schizandra chinensis* (Schizandraceae), more than 30 lignans having the dibenzocyclooctane skeleton have been isolated (Ikeya *et al.* 1982) and some of them were reported to suppress CCl_4-, GalN-, orotic acid and α-naphtylisothiocyanate-induced liver damage *in vivo,* utilizing mice and rats (Bao *et al.* 1979, Maeda *et al.* 1982). However, a broader evaluation of the anti-hepatotoxic effects of the *Schizandra* lignans has not been performed due to lack of materials.

Our *in vitro* assay methods enabled 22 *Schizandra* lignans to be evaluated for their anti-hepatotoxic effects (Table VI). Most lignans were effective, among which certain congeners exhibited prominent activity.

Although the anti-hepatotoxic effects of the lignans were dose-dependent in the CCl_4-induced cytotoxicity assay, the inhibitory actions of most lignans were diminished at a higher dose in the GalN-induced cytotoxicity assay. This was explained by the fact that, in addition to anti-hepatotoxic activity, simultaneous hepatotoxic activity was elicited by these lignans with longer treatment at higher doses (Table VI), which in turn led to cancellation of the anti-hepatotoxic effect.

The anti-hepatotoxic effects, thus estimated by the *in vitro* assay methods, were compared with those evaluated by the *in vivo* assay methods to reveal that both sets of effects are in general accord, providing support for the utility of the *in vitro* assay methods for screening anti-hepatotoxic activity.

The structure-activity relationship of these lignans suggested that the methylenedioxy group of the dibenzocyclooctane skeleton may play an important part in anti-hepatotoxic activity (Hikino *et al.* unpublished).

MECHANISM OF ANTI-HEPATOTOXIC ACTIVITY OF ACTIVE PRINCIPLES

It is now generally recognized that in the case of CCl_4-induced liver lesion, CCl_4

Table VI

Effect of constituents of Schizandra chinensis *fruits on carbon tetrachloride- and galactosamine-induced cytotoxicity in primary cultured rat hepatocytes*

Substance	Dose (mg/kg)	CCl$_4$[a] (%)	GPT (%) GalN($\pm$)[b] (%)	GalN($-$)[c] IU/l
Control	–	100±2	100±1	30±2
(±)-Deoxyschizandrin	0.01	105±3	76±2**	28±2
	0.1	76±1**	45±3**	26±1
	1.0	57±1**	92±5	176±5**
(±)-Gomisin K₃	0.01	102±4		
	0.1	86±1*		
	1.0	51±2**		
Deoxygomisin A	0.01	80±5	45±1**	
	0.1	40⊥4**	42⊥2**	
	1.0	24±3**	94±5	
Gomisin J	0.01	86±3	88±1**	28±2
	0.1	50±0**	68±6*	86±3**
	1.0	29±0**	74±2**	87±0**
Dimethylgomisin J	0.01	83±6	73⊥3*	28±2
	0.1	83±2*	47±2**	25±3
	1.0	86±2*	97±3	94±5**
Gomisin N	0.01	92±1	44±1**	22±1
	0.1	88±4	83±2*	40±4
	1.0	19±2**	105±2	126±4**
( )-Gomisin L₁ methylether	0.01	28±2**		
	0.1	24±1**		
	1.0	11±1**		
Wuweizisu C	0.01	39±4**	42±3**	
	0.1	21±1**	42±2**	
	1.0	12±2**	84±2**	
Schizandrin	0.01	103±1	84±2**	27±1
	0.1	110±2	81±2**	28±1
	1.0	90±4	96±2	129±1**
Gomisin H	0.01	92±1	90±4	28±2
	0.1	95±3	89±3	25±2
	1.0	88±3	47±5**	42±1*
Gomisin A	0.01	105±1	57±2**	24±0
	0.1	113±0	23±2**	19±1
	1.0	35±2**	85±1**	113±6**

Table VI

Effect of constituents of Schizandra chinensis *fruits on carbon tetrachloride- and galactosamine-induced cytotoxicity in primary cultured rat hepatocytes*

Substance	Dose (mg/kg)	CCl$_4$[a] (%)	GPT (%) GalN(+)[b] (%)	GalN(−)[c] IU/l
Gomisin O	0.01	75±4*	62±0**	
	0.1	50±2**	36±2**	
	1.0	27±1**	82±2**	
Angeloylgomisin Q	0.01	101±6	83±5	
	0.1	105±6	72±2**	
	1.0	89±1*	96±4	
Gomisin Q	0.01	108±4	82±2**	
	0.1	107±4	78±4*	
	1.0	104±3	65±1**	
Gomisin B	0.01	99±1	68±2**	27±0
	0.1	88±3	22±2**	19±2
	1.0	4±0**	49±2**	63±2**
Deangeloylgomisin B	0.01	111±6	73±2**	23±2
	0.1	32±4**	64±2**	22±1
	1.0	7±1**	32±2**	23±3
Gomisin C	0.01	98±2	49±3**	19±2
	0.1	93±1	30±3**	30±4
	1.0	11±0**	79±4*	107±2**
Gomisin F	0.01	75±4*	82±4*	22±2
	0.1	83±6	53±2**	22±2
	1.0	82±4	72±3**	113±4**
Deangeloylgomisin F	0.01	101±2	83±4	28±1
	0.1	78±4**	74±2**	22±1
	1.0	67±3**	57±3**	36±1
Gomisin G	0.01	95±2	84±1**	25±2
	0.1	90±1	51±3**	23±2
	1.0	80±1**	82±2*	114±2**
Schisantherin D	0.01	10±1**	49±3**	
	0.1	33±2**	59+2**	
	1.0	16±1**	62±2**	
Gomisin D	0.01	99±1	53±3**	24±2
	0.1	96±3	26±3**	20±1
	1.0	42±0**	81±3*	116±5**
Acetylbinankadsurin A	0.01	103±1	63±3**	26±2
	0.1	97±3	61±3**	36±3
	1.0	95±2	89±1**	123±2**

[a,b] Experimental conditions were the same as those given in the legend to Table I.

[c] An experiment was conducted similarly to b) with sample but without GalN.

n=3 (dishes). Significantly different from the control, p<0.01* or p<0.001**.

is first metabolized by drug-metabolizing enzymes represented by cytochrome P-450 in the liver endoplasmic reticulum to highly reactive CCl_3 radical which induces peroxidation of polyunsaturated fatty acids in the endoplasmic reticulum, leading to liver lesion (Chart 1). Although generation of free radical and formation of lipid peroxides were observed in CCl_4-induced cytotoxicity using primary cultured hepatocytes, the intensity of the signals for the generated free radicals and the amounts of the formed peroxides were found to be rather small and, therefore, inhibitory effects of test samples cannot be evaluated with great precision. Then, the effects were alternatively determined in the *in vitro* systems using rat-liver microsomes. Some of the results are presented below.

Mechanism of anti-hepatotoxic activity of glycyrrhizin and glycyrrhetinic acid
One of the representative hepato-protective substances, glycyrrhizin, and its aglycone, glycyrrhetinic acid, (Table I) were studied. Although glycyrrhizin showed no significant activity, glycyrrhetinic acid exhibited apparent activity in inhibition of free-radical generation and disclosed suppression of lipid peroxide formation by CCl_4, similar to that of the reference vitamin E, in the *in vitro* assays utilizing rat-liver microsomes. To our surprise, however, although vitamin E showed an intense inhibitory action on peroxide formation by auto-oxidation of linoleic acid *in vitro*, glycyrrhizin and glycyrrhetinic acid exerted essentially no such actions.

These data indicate that the inhibitory action on free-radical generation and the anti-oxidative action, play an important part in the anti-hepatotoxic activity of glycyrrhetinic acid by a mechanism different from that of vitamin E. Glycyrrhizin may elicit its anti-hepatotoxic activity after hydrolysis to its aglycone (Kiso *et al.* unpublished).

Mechanism of anti-hepatotoxic activity of atractylon
Although atractylon, a constituent of *Atractylodes* rhizomes, showed suppressive activity in CCl_4-induced cytotoxicity using primary cultured hepatocytes (Table IV), it generated free radical *per se* and apparently increased the free-radical generation by CCl_4 in the *in vitro* system with rat-liver microsomes. In order to classify the increased free radical, similar experiments were carried out, but with $^{13}CCl_4$. As a result it was found that the increased free radical was composed of those from $^{13}CCl_4$ and from atractylon.

Combined evidence points to there being "bad" free radical and "good" free radical for cytotoxicity, and free radical is not always connected with liver

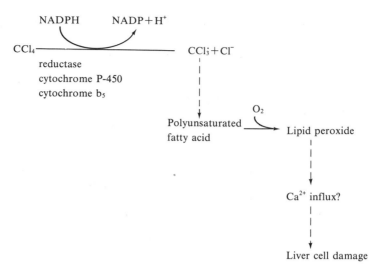

Chart 1
Scheme of mechanism for CCl₄-induced liver-cell damage

damage (Kiso *et al.* unpublished). The mechanism by which substances such as atractylon appear to generate free radical with liver microsomes but, alternatively, suppress CCl₄-induced cytotoxicity, is of considerable interest.

REFERENCES

Bao, T.-T., Xu, G.-F., Liu, G.-T., Sun, R.-H. & Song, Z.-Y. (1979) A comparison of the pharmacological actions of seven constituents isolated from Fructus Schizandrae. *Yao Hsueh Hsueh Pao* *14,* 1–7.

Berry, M. N. & Friend, D. S. (1969) High-yield preparation of isolated rat liver parenchymal cells. *J. Cell Biol. 43,* 506–520.

Hikino, H., Sugai, T., Konno, C., Hashimoto, I., Terasaki, S. & Hirono, I. (1979) Liver-protective principle of *Thujopsis dolabrata* leaves. *Planta medica 36,* 156–163.

Ikeya, Y., Taguchi, H. & Yosioka, I. (1982) The constituents of *Schizandra chinensis* Baill. XII. Isolation and structure of a new lignan, gomisin R, the absolute structure of wuweizisu C and isolation of schisantherin D. *Chem. Pharm. Bull. 30,* 3207–3211 and references cited therein.

Kato, S., Aoyama, K., Nakamura, T. & Ichihara, A. (1979) Biochemical studies on liver functions in primary cultured hepatocytes of adult rats. III. Changes of enzyme activities on cell membranes during culture. *J. Biochem. 86,* 1419–1425.

Kiso, Y., Konno, C., Hikino, H., Hashimoto, I., Yagi, Y. & Wakasa, H. (1982b) Protective action of desoxypodophyllotoxin on D-galactosamine-induced liver lesion in rats. *Chem. Pharm. Bull. 30,* 3817–3821.

Kiso, Y., Konno, C., Hikino, H., Yagi, Y. & Hashimoto, I. (1982c) Liver-protective actions of desoxypodophyllotoxin and its analogs. *J. Pharm. Dyn. 5,* 638–641.

Kiso, Y., Ogasawara, S., Hirota, K., Watanabe, N., Oshima, Y., Konno, C. & Hikino, H. (1983e) Antihepatotoxic principles of *Artemisia capillaris* buds. *Planta medica in press.*

Kiso, Y., Suzuki, Y., Konno, C., Hikino, H., Hashimoto, I. & Yagi, Y. (1982a) Application of carbon tetrachloride-induced liver lesion in mice for screening of liver protective crude drugs. *Shoyakugaku Zasshi 36,* 238–244.

Kiso, Y., Suzuki, Y., Watanabe, N., Oshima, Y. & Hikino, H. (1983c) Antihepatotoxic principles of *Curcuma longa* rhizomes. *Planta medica* in press.

Kiso, Y., Tohkin, M. & Hikino, H. (1983a) Assay method for antihepatotoxic activity using carbon tetrachloride-induced cytotoxicity in primary cultured hepatocytes, *Planta medica 49,* 222–225.

Kiso, Y., Tohkin, M. & Hikino, H. (1983b) Assay method for antihepatotoxic activity using galactosamine-induced cytotoxicity in primary cultured hepatocytes. *J. Nat. Prod.* in press.

Kiso, Y., Tohkin, M. & Hikino, H. (1983d) Antihepatotoxic principles of *Atractylodes* rhizomes. *J. Nat. Prod.* in press.

Maeda, S., Sudo, K., Miyamoto, Y., Takeda, S., Shinbo, M., Aburada, M., Ikeya, Y., Taguchi, H. & Harada, M. (1982) Pharmacological studies on Schizandra fruits. II. Effects of constituents of Schizandra fruits on drug-induced hepatic damage in rats. *Yakugaku Zasshi 102,* 579–588.

Seglen, P. O. (1976) Preparation of isolated rat liver cells. *Methods Cell Biol. 13,* 29–83.

Tanaka, K., Sato, M., Tomita, Y. & Ichihara, A. (1978) Biochemical studies on liver functions in primary cultured hepatocytes of adult rats. I. Hormonal effects on cell viability and protein synthesis. *J. Biochem. 84,* 937–946.

DISCUSSION

WITKOP: You have tried to compress a monograph into a brief talk and I must compliment you. You have been addressing one of the most important problems in long-range toxicity of drugs. It is very difficult to comment on your talk primarily because the number of mechanisms involved in the phenomonon of hepatotoxicity is very large.

WAGNER: I agree with Dr. Hikino that there is a great need for simple screening tests, but the main problem is that there are numerous liver diseases, which cannot all be covered by one test. Therefore, I strongly recommend to include some other liver-damaging agents, such as the pyrrolizidine alkaloids or phalloidin and by this enlarge the spectrum of damaging agents.

HIKINO: We have already devised the other *in vitro* cytotoxicity model systems induced by peroxides (ADP^{3-}, cumene hydroperoxide, etc.), employing primary cultured rat hepatocytes and found that they are useful for evaluation of anti-hepatotoxic activity. Phalloidin has been shown by Russo et al. (1) to be hepatotoxic against primary cultured rat hepatocytes, although application to assessment of anti-hepatotoxic activity docs not seem to have been attempted. We have also observed that pyrrolizidine alkaloids exhibit significant cytotoxic action on primary cultured rat hepatocytes. We wish to evaluate effects of a number of plant constituents on those *in vitro* liver lesion models.

LAZDUNSKI: I can see the advantages of using liver cells in culture, but there is a disadvantage in using such cultured cells, it is known that they rapidly lose their differentiation ability. Many other cells can be kept in primary culture without loss of their differentiation state. Did you try to see whether the natural compounds included in your studies, have an effect on the differentiation state of the liver cell? Would they prevent them from de-differentiating?

WITKOP: This question probably is impossible to answer, but the test *per se* may look promising enough for pharmaceutical companies to look at it very seriously.

---

(1) Russo, M. A., Kane, A. B. & Farber, J. L. (1982) *Am. J. Pathol. 109*, 133–144.

Immunostimulants of Fungi and Higher Plants

Hildebert Wagner

INTRODUCTION

Apart from bacterial, viral and tumour antigens which specifically influence the immune system and lead to the formation of specific antibodies, there are many material and immaterial factors in our environment, which unspecifically influence our immune system. These influences can be positive or negative. Negative factors, such as drugs, alcohol, pesticides or physical and psychological stress, may suppress our immune system and lead to a reduced resistance against infection or tumour. These factors may also induce allergies and autoimmune diseases.

However, other agents may also enhance the non-specific resistance of the host to those diseases mentioned above. For a long time these influences were neither understood nor could they be put on a rational basis. If we want to utilize the positive effects and develop drugs which can be used as immunostimulants in a prophylactic or therapeutic way, these compounds must be chemically well-defined and the mechanisms of their actions must be known. The following discussion will be restricted to immunostimulating agents.

DEFINITION AND FUNCTION OF IMMUNOSTIMULANTS

Immunostimulants are compounds, leading predominantly to a nonspecific stimulation of the immune system. Such compounds are also called mitogens. Non-specific immunostimulants do not affect immunological memory cells, and, as their pharmacological efficacy fades comparatively quickly, they have to be administered either in intervals or continously. This kind of acquired immunity has been denoted "paramunity". (Mayr *et al.* 1979, Stickl & Mayr

Institut für Pharmazeutische Biologie der Universität München, 8000 München 2, West Germany.

NATURAL PRODUCTS AND DRUG DEVELOPMENT, Alfred Benzon Symposium 20.
Editors: P. Krogsgaard-Larsen, S. Brøgger Christensen, H. Kofod, Munksgaard, Copenhagen 1984.

1979). Non-specific stimulating agents primarily influence the cellular immune system, i.e., components of the mononuclear-phagocyte system such as macrophages and granulocytes, and in the second place the lymphocytes. (Waksman 1980, Lohmann-Matthes 1981). These agents, generally, not only interact with one but with more types of immune competent cells, due to the narrow linkage between the unspecific and specific immune system. This is one handicap in developing effective immunostimulating agents without any side and cascade effects. As in some cases immunostimulants may also stimulate T-suppressor cells, and, thereby, reduce the immune resistance, the terms immunomodulators or immunoregulators very often seem to be more appropriate. In this context, the term immunoadjuvant has also to be mentioned. Immunoadjuvants are substances that enhance the immune response without acting as antigens or mitogens themselves. Prototypes are some plant fatty oils with or without added Mycobacteria (complete or incomplete Freund's adjuvant) (Freund 1956). Which kinds of strategies are available for developing immunostimulating drugs?

PROTOTYPE AND POTENTIAL IMMUNOSTIMULANTS

A variety of natural and synthetic products are available which can be regarded as model-compounds for the development of such agents. The lipopolysaccharides of gram-negative bacteria, the endotoxins, represent the prototype of an active high molecular weight compound. Meanwhile, however, it could be corroborated that a low molecular weight subunit of cell-wall peptidoglycan, a muramyl dipeptide (MDP), is responsible for the increase in non-specific resistance, the stimulatory effect on bone marrow and the adjuvant effect. This would mean that the lipopolysaccharides as components of the outer membrane, are responsible for the O-orR-antigenicity and production of antibodies only. The naturally-occurring aristolochic acid of Aristolochia (Kluthe et al. 1982) and the synthetic levamisol are prominent representatives of the low molecular weight series. A great number of compounds with potential immunostimulating activity have been found in both classes of compounds, but only a few of them have reached the state of preclinical trial.

Low molecular-weight compounds
In the class of low molecular-weight compounds, terpenoids such as sesquiterpenlactons (Hall et al. 1979), and phorbolesters (Abb et al. 1972), alcaloids such as cepharanthine from *Stephania cepharantha* (Kasajima 1974, Sugiyoshi 1976),

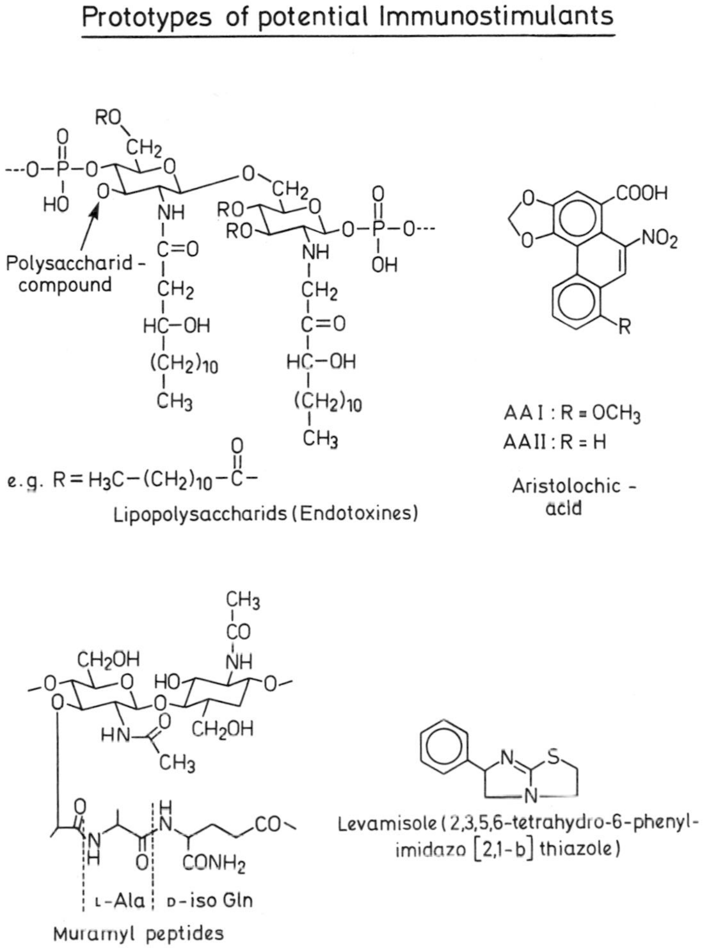

Prototypes of potential Immunostimulants

Fig. 1. Prototypes of high- and low-molecular weight compounds with immunostimulating activity

or phenolic and chinoid compounds such as Cleistanthin from *Cleistanthus collinus* (Rao & Nair 1970), and lipids such as ubiquinones (Block *et al.* 1978, Mayer *et al.* 1980), and lysolecithin (Munder *et al.* 1980) are predominating. Their exact mode of action is unknown. The activities reported in the literature range from a stimulation of the phagocytosis and interferon production to a specific stimulation of natural killer cells or other cytotoxic effector cells.

High molecular-weight compounds
In the class of high molecular-weight compounds with immunostimulating

Table I

Medicinal plants frequently used for "Reizkörpertherapie" and "Umstimmungstherapie" (immuno-
stimulation) (according to Rote Liste® 1983) List of registered drugs in the Federal Republic of
Germany issued by the Federal Association of the Pharmaceutical Industry e.V., Frankfurt am
Main, FRG

Chamomilla recutita*	Cynanchum vincetoxicum (Vincetoxicum)
Achyrocline saturoides*	Echinacea purpurea, angustifolia*
Aconitum napellus	Eupatorium cannabium, perfoliatum*
Althaea officinalis	Euphrasia officinalis
Aristolochia clematitis	Gelsemium sempervirens
Arnica montana*	Marrubium vulgare
Baptisia tinctoria	Pneumus boldus
Bryonia dioica	Phytolacca americana
Calendula officinalis*	Scrophularia nodosa
Carex flav./elong./vesic	Thuja occidentalis
Centaurium minus*	Viscum album

*) Compositae family

activity, glycoproteins, polysaccharides, nucleoproteins and proteins are among the more privileged compounds. The lectins are well-known T-lymphocyte mitogens. However, they will not attain therapeutic importance due to their various side effects. Some polysaccharides from fungi, mushrooms, algae and lichens, such as the glucans *Lentinan, Schizophyllan, Pachymaran* or *Zymosan* merit attention. Their molecular weights range between 20,000 and 1 million. The sugar chains primarily contain $1 \rightarrow 3$ and $1 \rightarrow 6$, occasionally also $1 \rightarrow 4$ and $1 \rightarrow 2$ linkages. It is remarkable that most of them show anti-tumour activity, which is mainly due to a stimulation of phagozytosis, T-helper cells and interferon production. (Wagner & Proksch 1983).

In our approach to immunostimulating agents from higher plants, we have concentrated our interests in plants which have been used for a long time empirically for the so-called "Reiz- or Umstimmungstherapie" (shock therapy or a therapy of general reorientation of the organism as a whole).

POLYSACCHARIDES FROM MEDICINAL PLANTS

In Table I are listed those plants, the extracts of which have been used empirically as immunostimulants. The active principles of all of them are unknown, with one exception (Aristolochia). None of these plants contains a conspicuous class of chemical constituents. It is, however, remarkable that a

$$[^\beta\!\!\rightarrow\!\!4)\text{-Xyl p-}(1^{\underline{\beta}}\!\!\rightarrow\!\!4)\text{-Xyl p-}(1^{\underline{\beta}}\!\!\rightarrow\!\!4)\text{-Xyl p-}(1^{\underline{\beta}}\!\!\rightarrow\!\!4)\text{-Xyl p-}(1^{\underline{\beta}}\!\!\rightarrow]_n$$

$$\begin{array}{c} \downarrow \\ 2 \\ \uparrow \end{array}$$

$$\begin{bmatrix} \rightarrow 3)\text{-4-O-Methyl-GluA p-}(1^{\underline{\alpha}}\!\!\rightarrow \\ \rightarrow 6)\text{-Gal p-}(1^{\underline{\alpha}}\!\!\rightarrow \\ \rightarrow 5)\text{-Ara f-}(1^{\underline{\alpha}}\!\!\rightarrow \\ \text{Ara f-}(1^{\underline{\alpha}}\!\!\rightarrow \\ \rightarrow 4)\text{-Xyl p-}(1^{\underline{\beta}}\!\!\rightarrow \\ \text{Xyl p-}(1^{\underline{\beta}}\!\!\rightarrow \\ \rightarrow 3)\text{-Glu p-}(1^{\underline{\alpha}}\!\!\rightarrow \end{bmatrix}$$

$$[^\alpha\!\!\rightarrow\!\!4)\text{-Gal p-}(1^{\underline{\alpha}}\!\!\rightarrow\!\!2)\text{-Rha p-}(1^{\underline{\alpha}}\!\!\rightarrow\!\!2)\text{-Rha p-}(1^{\underline{\alpha}}\!\!\rightarrow\!\!4)\text{-Gal p-}(1^{\underline{\alpha}}\!\!\rightarrow]_n$$

$$\begin{array}{c} \downarrow \\ 4 \\ \uparrow \end{array}$$

$$\begin{bmatrix} \rightarrow 3)\text{-Glu A p-}(1^{\underline{\beta}}\!\!\rightarrow \\ \rightarrow 5)\text{-Ara f -}(1^{\underline{\alpha}}\!\!\rightarrow \\ \rightarrow 4)\text{-Gal p -}(1^{\underline{\alpha}}\!\!\rightarrow \\ \rightarrow 3)\text{-Glu p -}(1^{\underline{\beta}}\!\!\rightarrow \\ \rightarrow 4)\text{-Xyl f -}(1^{\underline{\beta}}\!\!\rightarrow \\ \text{Gal p -}(1^{\underline{\beta}}\!\!\rightarrow \\ \rightarrow 2)\text{-Rha p -}(1^{\underline{\alpha}}\!\!\rightarrow \end{bmatrix}$$

Fig. 2 and Fig. 3. Structural proposals for polysaccharide I and II of *Echinacea purpurea*

great percentage of the plants belong to the Compositae family. As we had no chemical guide line, we used for immunological screening the granulocyte *in vitro* test (Brandt 1967), and the *in vivo* carbon-clearance test (Biozzi *et al.* 1953). Both allow the functional state and the efficiency of the mononuclear phagocyte system to be measured. Using these test systems, we found strong enhancement of phagocytosis in all water extracts of the investigated plants. Fractionation and immunological monitoring revealed polysaccharides as active principles. As far as *Echinacea purpurea* is concerned, we succeeded in assigning activity to 2 chemically defined polysaccharides (Proksch 1982).

One of them could be shown to be a heteroxylan with a $1 \rightarrow 4$ linked xylose backbone and a mean m.w. of 35,000. The heteroxylan contains rhamnose, arabinose, xylose, galactose, glucose and 4-0-methylglucuronic acid as sugar components in a molar ratio of 0.3:1:4.9:0.9:0.4:0.9. Branching occurs at each fifth sugar unit. Side chains are connected to the main chain at C-2-OH of the xylose units. Glucuronic acid units appear to be situated directly in the vicinity of the main chain. The glycosidic bonds in the side chains are mainly $1 \rightarrow 3$ and

Table II

Immunostimulating polysaccharides from fungi, lichens and algae

	Polysaccharides	type	linkage	M.W.
Fungi	Zymosan	glucan	$\beta1\rightarrow3$	50–120000
	Mannozym	mannan	$\beta1\rightarrow3$	5– 20000
			$\left.\begin{array}{l}\beta1\rightarrow3\\\beta1\rightarrow4\end{array}\right\}$	50– 65000
	Lentinan	glucans	$\beta1\rightarrow3$	ca 500000
	Pachyman		$\left.\begin{array}{l}\beta1\rightarrow2\\\beta1\rightarrow6\end{array}\right\}$	–1 Mill
	Pachymaran			
	Schizophyllan	glucan	$\left.\begin{array}{l}\beta1\rightarrow3\\\beta1\rightarrow6\end{array}\right\}$	ca 400000
	Krestin (PSK)	glucan	$\left.\begin{array}{l}\beta1\rightarrow4\\\beta1\rightarrow6\end{array}\right\}$	50–100000
			+coval. proteins	
Lichens			glucans	
Algae	Pustulan		$\beta1\rightarrow6$	
	Lichenan		$\beta1\rightarrow3$	
			$\beta1\rightarrow4$	100000–
	Isolichenan		$\alpha1\rightarrow3$	500000
			$\alpha1\rightarrow4$	
	Laminaran		$\beta1\rightarrow3$	
			$\beta1\rightarrow6$	

$1\rightarrow6$ acids and have α-configuration. The second polysaccharide is composed of rhamnose, arabinose, galactose and glucuronic acid in a molar ratio of 0.8:0.6:1.0:0.6. The main chain consists of rhamnose and galactose in a ratio of 1:1. The side chains are connected to the main chain via C-4-OH at each second rhamnose unit. Linkage between rhamnose units occurs via hydroxyl groups of C-1 and C-2, while galactose units are joined via C-1- and C-4-OH-groups. Arabinose, rhamnose, galactose and glucuronic acid are found in the side chains of this polysaccharide. The arabinorhamnogalactan has a mean m.w. of 450,000. In its structure the first polysaccharide resembles heteroxylans isolated from cell walls of grasses, bamboo, maize cobs, rye, wheat or beech wood. The backbone of the second polysaccharide is quite similar to the structures of some gums and mucilages.

   The separation of the different polysaccharide mixtures and the structure elucidation of pure polysaccharides from the other plants have not yet been completed, but we know the sugar composition, the m.w. ranges and the immunological activities of the main polysaccharides (Wagner *et al.* 1983).

Table III

Influence of plant polysaccharides on microphagocytosis (granulocyte-test according to Brandt 1967)

plant/extraction procedure	mean enhancement of phagocytosis %
Echinacea purpurea (1:1) (0,5 N NaOH/H$_2$O extract)	45[a]
Eupatorium cannab. (1:2) (0,5 N NaOH/H$_2$O extract)	22[b]
Eupatorium perfol. (1:0.5) (0,5 N NaOH/H$_2$O extract)	37[a]
Matricaria recutita (1:4) (H$_2$O-extract)	31[c]
Arnica montana (1:4) (H$_2$O-extract)	44[a]
Achyrocline saturoides (1.4) (H$_2$O-extract)	33[a]
Sabal serrulata (1:4) (H$_2$O-extract)	36[a]
Eleutherococcus senticosus (0,5 N NaOH/H$_2$O-extract	52[c]
Krestin (for comparison)	25[d]

*) The polysaccharide fractions were prepared from H$_2$O- or 0,5 N NaOH/H$_2$O-extract in a modified procedure according to Caldes *et al.* (1981). The precepitations were performed with different H$_2$O-MeOH-proportions (1:0.5/1:1/1:2/1:4)

a) test-dil. 0.001%; b) test-dil. 0.05%; c) test-dil. 0.01%; d) test-dil. 0.005%.

With some exceptions, all of them belong to the heteroxylan or arabino-rhamnan- and galactan series with varying amounts of glucuronic- or ga-lacturonic acid. The m.w. range between 25,000 and 500,000 or more. The linkages in the individual components are α- and β, with preferred $1 \rightarrow 3$, $1 \rightarrow 4$ and $1 \rightarrow 2$ linkages. All of them display, more or less, a high degree of branching with a complex net structure and are highly water soluble. When we investigated the immunological activities on the phagocytic immune system, all compounds displayed a high stimulatory activity on the granulocytes and the macrophages, which was in about the same order as that observed with aristolochic acid or muramylpeptides (Wagner *et al.* 1983, Tables III, IV). Comparing these activities with those of the glucans from fungi and algae, the same activity is noticed, although at much lower concentrations than those reported for the different glucans. Detailed studies on the mechanism of action have been performed with the Echinacea polysaccharides (Stimpel *et al.* 1983). 1 μg of the

Table IV

Carbon-clearance rate of plant polysaccharides in mice (conc. 10 mg/kg one day) (test according to Biozzi et al. 1953)

plant	regression-coefficients		RC_{tr}/RC_c
	control	treated	
Echinacea purp. 1:4	−0.0647	−0.1397	2.1681
(H₂O-extract MG≥5000)			
Echinacea purp. 1:1	−0.0612	−0.1323	2.2152
(NaOH-extract MG≥5000)			
Eupatorium cannab.	−0.0597	−0.1087	1.8193
Matricaria recutita	−0.0731	−0.1848	2.5268
Arnica montana	−0.0851	−0.2027	2.3841
Achyrocline saturoides	−0.0583	−0.1350	2.3136
Calendula offic.	−0.0615	−0.0792	1.2874
Sabal serrulata	−0.0731	0.02791	3.8163
Altheaea offic.	−0.0597	−0.1306	2.1870
Baptisia tinctoria	−0.0603	−0.0791	1.3105
Eleutherococcus senticosus	−0.0386	−0.1122	2.9040
Krestin*	−0.0467	0.0831	1.400

RC_{tr}/RC_c >1.0 stimulation; <1.0 suppression

* dose 60 mg/kg (Krestin=Protein covalent bound polysaccharide from Coriolus versicolor)

highly purified polysaccharide was able to stimulate macrophages to high cytotoxic activity against tumour target cells (P 815), as well *in vitro* as *in vivo* (^{51}Cr-release-assay). Moreover the increased state of activity of polysaccharide-stimulated macrophages could be demonstrated by measuring the chemoluminescence (Fig. 4). Furthermore, the polysaccharide was capable of stimulating bone-marrow macrophages to cytokine-production (IL-1, LAF). By using the T-lymphocyte transformation test and measuring the incorporation rate of ^{3}H-thymidin it was found that the polysaccharide had a much lower mitogenic effect on B-cells compared with that of a typical B-cell mitogene like lipopolysaccharide (LPS). The T-cell stimulation found with a rough polysaccharide fraction, however, could not be reproduced with a purified polysaccharide.

FUNCTION AND STRUCTURE-ACTIVITY RELATIONSHIPS OF POLYSACCHA-RIDES

It is too early to draw conclusions from the present results on structure/activity relationships, but it appears that the polysaccharides of high molecular weight and with a complex and anionic structure have a higher degree of binding

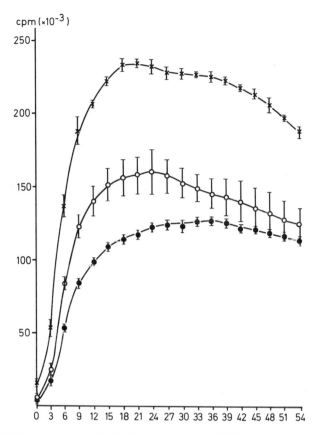

Fig. 4. Effect of Echinacea-polysaccharide I on the oxygen radical production by bone-marrow macrophages (chemoluminescence) (Stimpel *et al.* 1983)

•——• control

○——○ control+E.-polys. (0.2 mg/ml)

×——× 24 h with E.-polys. activated macrophages+luminol/zymosan

affinity to membranes of immunocompetent cells than simple glucans. This hypothesis is corroborated by the observation that certain polysaccharides of non-microbial origin, such as agar, plant gums, plant mucilage and other polysaccharides from plants, mentioned in this review, are capable of cross-reacting with anti-pneumococcal and other antisera. (Heidelberger 1960, 1982, Caldes *et al.* 1981). Immunologic active polysaccharides are those from cereals. Matricaria, Carthamus or Althaea may serve as an example. This means that there is a high degree of probability of a complex polysaccharide containing much more immuno-determinant regions in its molecule than simple glucan chains. This may also explain the pronounced effects that these complex poly-saccharides exert on unspecific stimulation.

The investigated polysaccharides are not the only immunologically active polysaccharides from higher plants. Similar or identical activities have been reported for polysaccharide mixtures or fractions of cereals, bamboo, sugar cane, *Astragalus* species, *Angelica acutiloba, Carthamus tinctorius, Eleuthero-coccus senticosus, Viscum album,* and others (Wagner *et al.* 1983).

The utilization of this class of compounds as immunostimulants is handi-capped by the difficulty in reproducing the isolation procedure and isolating chemically well-defined polysaccharides of constant activity. It can be assumed, however, that these compounds may soon serve as appropriate structure models for a kind of drug designing, i. e., the development of synthetic mitogens. It may also be possible to produce these, or similar polysaccharides, in tissue cultures under controlled conditions. This approach, however, requires more basic research on the mechanism of immunostimulation and the essential structural requirements for a potential mitogen.

The finding that extracellular and intramural polysaccharides from bacteria can cross react with polysaccharides from higher plants shows the similarity of the biosynthesis of cell wall polysaccharides in animals and plants. Therefore, it is not surprising that, e. g., arabinogalactans, hitherto considered as typical for the cell wall pattern of many plants, have been found also in bovine lung (Roy & Glaudemans 1978), and in the cell surface of trypanosomatid *Crithidia fasciculata* (Gottlieb 1978). *Vice versa* characteristic alginic acids enriched in uronic acids have been found in exine and intine layers of cyts of *Azotobacter vinelandii.* In this context it has to be mentioned that specific polysaccharides on the outer plasmalemma surface of plant protoplasts are discussed as receptors for the β-glycan elicitors of the phytoalexin response in fungal infection, which, e. g., have been shown to agglutinate potato-leaf protoplasts (Peters *et al.* 1978). The rejection mechanism against grafts, however, is not as specific in plants as it is in animals. This fact, once more, supports the hypothesis that these types of polysaccharides might be more appropriate unspecific immunostimulants than simple glucans.

Our last investigations on the possible toxicity, carcinogenicity or mutageni-city of these polysaccharides have shown no negative result. As polysaccharides are easily biodegradable, a further requirement for a safe immunostimulant is fulfilled. Studies on the other requirements, set up by WHO for the development of an effective and safe immunostimulant: "no cascade effects, not too high and not too low stimulating activity and no allergic side effects", have to be carried out. Furthermore, it has to be investigated whether these polysaccharides are the only immunostimulating principles in these plants, and whether the immuno-stimulating effects can be expected also after oral administration.

REFERENCES

Abb, J., Bayliss, G. I. & Deinhardt, F. (1979) Lymphocyte Activation by the Tumorpromoting Agent 12-0-Tetradecanoyl-phorbol-13-acetate (TPA). *J. Immunol. 122*, 1639.

Belkin, M., Hardy, W. G., Perrault, A. & Sato, H. (1959) Swelling and Vacuolization Induced in Ascites Tumor cells by Polysaccharides from Higher Plants. *Cancer Res. 19*, 1050.

Biozzi, G., Benacerraf, B. & Halpern, B. N. (1953) Quantitative study of the granulopectic activity of the R.E.S. II. A study of the kinetics of the granulopectic activity of the R.E.S. in relation to the dose of carbon injected. Relationship between the weight of the organs and their activity. *Br. J. Exp. Pathol. 34*, 441.

Block, L. H., Georgopoulos, A., Mayer, P. & Drews, J. (1978) Nonspecific Resistance to Bacterial Infections, Enhancement by Ubiquinone-8. *J. Exp. Med. 148*, 1228.

Brandt, L. (1967) Studies on the phagocytic activity of neutrophilic leucocytes. *Scand. J. Haematol. Suppl. 2.*

Caldes, G., Prescott, B., Thomas, Ch.-A. & Baker, Ph. I. (1981) Characterization of a poly-saccharide from Carthamus tinctorius that cross reacts with Type III Pneumococcal poly-saccharide. *J. Gen. Appl. Microbiol. 27*, 157.

Chedid, L., Miescher, P. A. & Mueller-Eberhard, H. L. (1980) Immunstimulation. Springer-Verlag, Berlin-Heidelberg-New York.

Chen, L. J., Shen, M. L., Wang, M. Y., Zhai, S. K. & Lin, M. Z. (1981) Effect of Astragalus polysaccharides on phagocytic function in mice. *Chung-kuo Yao Li Hsueh, Pao, 2 (3)*, 200, C.A. 95, 185472.

Freund, J. (1956) The mode of action of immunologic adjuvant. *Adv. Tuberc. Res. 7*, 130.

Gottlieb, M. (1978) Polysaccharides of Crithidia fasciculata. Identification and partial Characteri-zation of a Cell Surface Constituent. *Biochim. Biophys. Acta, 541*, 444.

Hall, I. H., Lee, K. H., Starness, C. O., Sumida, Y., Wu, R. Y., Wadell, T. G., Cochran, J. W. & Gerhart, K. G. (1979) Anti-Inflammatory activity of Sesquiterpene Lactones and related compounds. *J. Pharm. Sci. 68*, 537.

Heidelberger, M. (1960) Structure and Immunological Specifity of Polysaccharides. *Fortschritte d. Chem. org. Naturst. 18*, 503.

Heidelberger, M. (1982) Cross-Reactions of Plant Polysaccharides in Antipneumococcal and Other Antisera, an Update. *Fortschritte d. Chem. org. Naturst. 42*, 288.

Ishizuka, M., Iinuma, H., Takenchi, T. & Umezawa, H. (1972) Effect of Diketocoriolin B on Antibody Formation. *J. Antibiotics 25*, 320.

Kasajima, T. (1974) Effect of cepharanthine in promoting antibody production. *Japan J. Reticulo-endothelial Soc. 14*, 1.

Kluthe, R., Vogt, A. & Batsford, Arzneim.-Forsch./Drug Res. *32*, 443 (1982) Doppelblindstudie zur Beeinflussung der Phagozytosefähigkeit von Granulozyten durch Aristolochiasäure.

Kumazawa, Y., Mizunoe, K. & Otsuka, Y. (1982) Immunostimulating polysaccharide separated from hot water extract of Angelica acutiloba Kitagawa (Yamato Tohki). *Immunology 47*, 75.

Lohmann-Matthes, M.-L. (1981) Der Makrophage. *Biologie in unserer Zeit 11*, 135.

Lutomski, I., Garecki, P. & Halasa, J. (1981) Immunologische Eigenschaften der Saponinfraktion aus Aralia mandshurica. *Planta med. 42*, 116.

Mayer, P., Hamberger, H. & Drews, J. (1980) Differential Effects of Ubiquinone Q7 and Ubiquinone Analogs on Macrophage Activation and Experimental Infections in Granulocytopenic Mice. *Infection 8*, 256.

Mayr, A., Raettig, H., Stickl, H. & Alexander, M. (1979) Paramunität, Paramunisierung, Paramunitätsinducer. *Fortschritt der Medizin 97*, 1205.

Munder, R. G., Modolell, M., Andreesen, R., Weltzien, H. U. & Westphal, O. (1980) In: *Immunstimulation*, eds. Chedid, L., Miescher, P. A., Mueller-Eberhard, H. J., p. 177. Springer-Verlag, Berlin-Heidelberg-New York.

Peters, B. M., Gribbs, D. N. & Stelzig, D. A. (1978) Agglutination of Plant Protoplasts by Fungal Cell Wall Glucans. *Science 201*, 364.

Proksch, A. (1982) Dissertation Universität München.

Rao, R. R. & Nair, T. B. (1970) Investigations on Induction of Neutrophilic Granulocytosis and Toxicity of Cleistanthin-CIBA GO, 4350 – A New Glycoside from Cleistanthus collinus (Roxb.). *Pharmacology 4*, 347.

Roy, N. & Glaudemans, C. P. J. (1978) On the structure of mammalian-lung galactan *Carbohydr. Res. 63*, 318.

Stickl, H. & Mayr, A. (1979) Über die Wirksamkeit eines neuen Paramunitätsinducers (PIND-AVI) für Mensch und Tier. *Fortschritte der Medizin 97*, 1781.

Stimpel, M., Lohmann-Matthes, M.-L., Proksch, A. & Wagner, H. (1983) Das immunologische Wirkprinzip von geeigneten Polysaccharid-Fraktionen aus Echinacea purpurea M. und ihre potentielle Verwendung in der prophylaktischen Therapie. *Dtsch. Med. Wochenschrift* (in press).

Sugiyoshi, K. (1976) Inhibitory effect of cepharanthine in histamine release from rat mast cells. *Allergy 25*, 685.

Wagner, H. & Proksch, A. (1983) Immunostimulants of Fungi and Higher Plants. In: *Progress in Medicinal and Economic Plant Research*, Vol. I, eds. Farnsworth, N., Hikino, H. & Wagner, H. Academic Press (London) in press.

Wagner, H., Proksch, A., Riess-Maurer, I., Vollmar, A., Odenthal, S., Stuppner, H., Jurcic, K., Le Turdu, M. & Heur, Y. H. Immunstimulierend wirkende Polysaccharide (Heteroglykane) aus höheren Pflanzen I. *Arzneim. Forsch. (Drug Res.)*, in press.

Waksman, B. H. (1980) Adjuvants and Immunregulation by Lymphoid Cells. In: *Immunstimulation*, eds. Chedid, L., Miescher, P. A. & Mueller-Eberhard, H. J., p. 5. Springer-Verlag Berlin-Heidelberg-New York.

DISCUSSION

WITKOP: Is it possible that in some diets, somewhere in the world, people regularly eat these polysaccharides and then maybe, there is an immuno-stimulating effect?

WAGNER: This idea is not absolutely new, and the food chemists have realized the possibility. For a long time nobody believed that oral substances could be of interest, because they are quickly degraded, etc. Investigations with Krestin have shown that a stimulation can take place in the intestine, even though the compounds are not absorbed.

ARCAMONE: My first question: has some of this plant polysaccharide been tested for the protection of mice, for example, from bacteria or viral infections? My second question: can you rule out the possibility that the observed activities are due, or partly due, to contamination of the original plant material with endotoxins originating in bacteria?

WAGNER: Concerning your last question: by a number of chemical and analytical procedures we have excluded the possibility of endotoxins (lipopoly-saccharides) in our active fractions. Concerning the first question: it has been established that some types of compounds are effective, prophylactically as well as therapeutically, but we do not know anything about the optimal doses, and we do not know anything about side-effects.

DAVIES: Do any of the polysaccharides have activity as adjuvants for known antigens?

WAGNER: Some of the polysaccharides have adjuvant activity. Some of these polysaccharides have the same activity as the muramyl peptide which, however, has side-effects.

ANAND: Polysaccharides are often associated with interferon inducers isolated from natural sources. Do these polysaccharides have interferon inducing activity *per se*?

26*

WAGNER: Some of the polysaccharides are reported to be typical interferon inducers, but not all.

ANAND: I suppose you made sure that your polysaccharides were totally free of nucleic acid?

WAGNER: Yes, they are absolutely free. They do not contain any nitrogen.

LAZDUNSKI: You described immunostimulation by your polysaccharide. You have also mentioned that lysolecithin esters are immunostimulants. Did you try to make hybrid molecules between your polysaccharide and lysolecithin and see whether you could improve your immunostimulating activity?

WAGNER: No, we have not done this, but of course if would be a good idea to do so.

CHRISTOPHERSEN: It is not clear to me whether your test system could also detect an immunosuppressive activity. In case it would, did you encounter any?

WAGNER: A test system to differentiate between immunostimulating and immunosuppressive activity has only recently been developed. One has to test both, as very often higher doses stimulate and lower doses suppress or vice versa. It is also necessary to differentiate between the different subpopulations of the T-lymphocytes.

Chemistry and Structure-Activity Relationship of the Histamine Secretagogue Thapsigargin and Related Compounds

S. Brøgger Christensen, Elsebeth Norup & Ulla Rasmussen

About 300 B.C. the father of botany, Theophrastos, described how the skin irritation provoked by application of the resin from an umbelliferous plant found in Cyrene (an ancient Greek colony on the peninsula west of Egypt) was used in medicine for the relief of rheumatic pains. The drug also was included in the famous work of Dioscorides: *Materia Medica* (approximately 50 A.D.). Ever since, advantage has been taken of this resin in traditional Arabian medicine. In 1673 Linnea in *Mantissa Plantarum* named the plant *Thapsia garganica*. Preparations of this plant have been described in several pharmacopoeias, the latest being the French pharmacopoeia of 1937. Except for some investigations late in the 19th century (Tschirch & Stock 1936), the first attempt to isolate the active principles was published in 1970 (Krogsgaard-Larsen & Sandberg 1970). In contrast to the linearly annulated coumarins found to be responsible for the photophytodermatitis provoked by a number of umbelliferous species (Murray *et al.* 1982), the 2 coumarins isolated from *T. garganica,* scopoletin and 6-methoxy-7-geranyloxycoumarin, were found to be inactive after application to the skin. No aromatic compound could be detected in the fraction containing the active principles. Using reversed phase chromatography and HPLC the 2 major skin-irritant constituents were finally separated and isolated in a pure state in 1978. The compounds were named thapsigargin **1** and thapsigargicin **2** (Rasmussen *et al.* 1978).

Departments of Chemistry BC and Pharmacognosy, Royal Danish School of Pharmacy, Copenhagen, Denmark.

NATURAL PRODUCTS AND DRUG DEVELOPMENT, Alfred Benzon Symposium 20.
Editors: P. Krogsgaard-Larsen, S. Brøgger Christensen, H. Kofod, Munksgaard, Copenhagen 1984.

After incubation with peritoneal rat mast cells, **1**, and **2** proved to be very potent non-cytotoxic histamine liberators. The mediator-releasing properties make **1** a potential tool for investigation of the pathogenesis of acute allergic reactions and generalized inflammatory responses, in which histamine secretion is centrally involved (Kazimierczak & Diamant 1978, Pepys & Edwards 1979, Pearce 1982).

1,2,6,8-11,17-21   4   5,16   3,7

CHEMICAL INVESTIGATIONS OF THAPSIGARGIN

Structural elucidation of thapsigargin

The non-crystalline nature of thapsigargin **1** prohibited a X-ray analysis and only a broad peak at m/z 650–652 was found in the FD-mass spectrum. IR-Spectroscopy, however, revealed the presence of a γ-lactone and a number of ester groups. After transesterification with methanol methyl acetate, methyl angelicate, methyl butyrate, and methyl octanoate were demonstrated in the reaction mixture by combined gas chromatography-mass spectroscopy (Christensen *et al.* 1980). In the EI-mass spectrum of **1**, a prominent peak was found at m/z 446.1944 ($C_{24}H_{30}O_8$). Assuming that this peak originates by elimination of octanoic and acetic acid, the molecular formula of **1** was estimated to $C_{34}H_{50}O_{12}$. Subtraction of the formulae of the known acyl groups leaves a C_{15}-nucleus strongly suggesting the compound to be a sesquiterpene lactone. Comparisons between the NMR-spectra of **1** and those of a number of model compounds, revealed pronounced similarities with the spectra of trilobolide **3** isolated from the umbelliferous plant *Laser trilobum* (L.) Borkh. (Holub *et al.* 1973). The absence of signals corresponding to those of the H(2) protons in **3** confirmed the skeleton of **1** to be that of a 2,3,7,8,10,11-oxygenated-$\Delta^{4(5)}$-C_6-guaianolide. Thionyl chloride promoted transformation into an epoxide **4** disclosed a vicinal dihydroxy moiety. The locations of the 4 acyl residues were established by spectroscopical investigations of partially hydrolyzed products (Christensen *et al.* 1980). The relative configurations at all the asymmetric centers except those bearing the 2 hydroxy groups were proven by a X-ray analysis of **4**. (Christensen *et al.* 1982). Nuclear Overhauser experiments and the resistance of **1** toward periodic acid compared to the lability of **5**, disclosed the relative configuration at the remaining 2 centres (Christensen & Schaumburg 1983). Application of a modification of Horeaus method indicated the absolute configuration shown in formula **1**. This conclusion is based on a HPLC separation and quantification of the epimeric 2-phenylbutanoates formed by reacting **6** with optical inactive 2-phenylbutyric anhydride.

According to Dreiding stereomodels only 2 low-energy conformations of **1** are possible. The weak couplings between H(8) and the 2 protons attached to C(9) together with the observed 1-, 2-, and 3- bond carbon-hydrogen coupling constants indicated the conformation depicted in Fig. 1 to be favored (Christensen & Schaumburg 1983).

Structural elucidation of sesquiterpene lactones related to thapsigargin

The potent biological effects of thapsigargin **1** prompted an investigation of other Thapsia species leading to isolation of trilobolide **3**, thapsivillosin F **7**, and a number of hexaoxygenated guaianolides only differing from **1** in the structures of the acyl residues. In all cases, the structures of the sesquiterpene nuclei are based on ^1H and ^{13}C NMR-spectroscopy (Rasmussen *et al.* 1981). CI- Mass spectroscopy has been found applicable for the location of non-isomeric acyl groups. The prominent peaks in the spectra of **1, 2, 8,** and **9** can be rationalized by the fragmentation pattern shown in Fig. 2. If this pattern is common for all

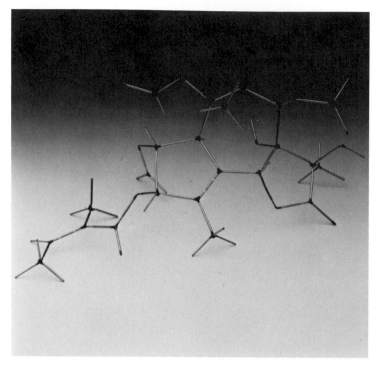

Fig. 1 Dreiding stereomodel of thapsigargin. For clarity the acetyl, butanoyl, octanoyl and angeloyl moieties have been exchanged with formyl groups. Reprinted with permission from Christensen & Schaumburg 1983. Copyright 1983 American Chemical Society.

the isolated hexaoxygenated guianolides the locations of the 4 acyl residues can be deduced by observing the following regularities: (i) the last 2 steps in the fragmentation pattern depicted to the left in Fig. 2, define the acyl residues attached to O(8) and O(3); (ii) the first acid to be eliminated has been esterized with either the allylic alcohol group at C(3) of the tertiary alcohol group at C(10); (iii) the remaining acyl residue must be attached to O(2), as NMR-spectroscopy proves C(7) and C(11) to bear free hydroxy groups.

The structures of thapsivillosin B **10**, thapsivillosin C, thapsivillosin E, thapsivillosin G, thapsivillosin I, and thapsivillosin J all are deducted from the CI-mass spectra (Christensen *et al.* unpublished). The locations of the acyl groups in thapsitranstagin **11** were established by NMR-spectroscopic investigations of partially hydrolyzed products. The structures of thapsivillosin A and thapsivillosin D are at the present under investigation.

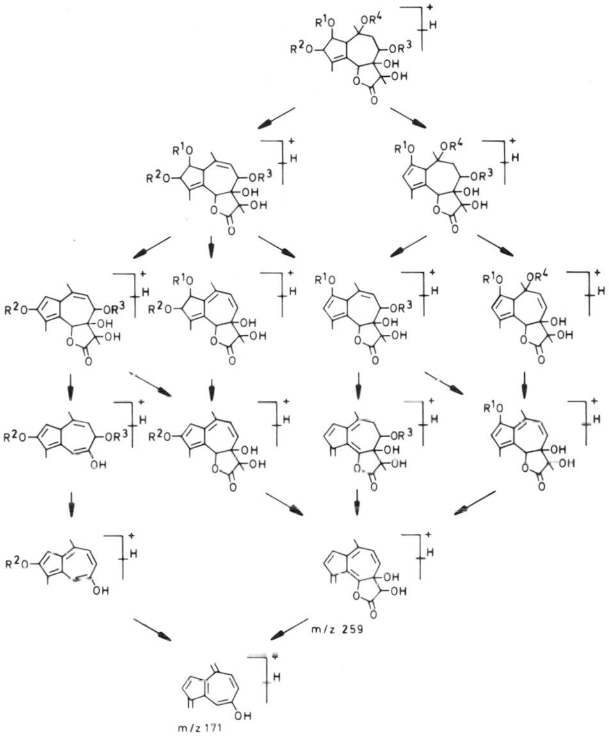

Fig. 2. Fragmentation pattern of tetra-acylated 2,3,7,8,10,11-hexaoxygenated-$\Delta^{4(5)}$-C$_6$-guaianolides observed in the chemical ionization mass spectra using isobutane as reagent gas. The double bonds in the fragments are tentatively located.

Some of the above-mentioned guaianolides are esters of butanoic, hexanoic, octanoic, 6-methyloctanoic, or 6-methylheptanoic acid. Although naturally occurring, none of these acids has previously been reported to be esterized with hydroxylated sesquiterpene lactones.

Chemistry of thapsigargin
In order to prepare derivatives for structure activity studies, and as a part of the structural elucidation, investigations of the chemistry of thapsigargin **1** have been initiated. As was described for trilobolide **3** (Holub *et al.* 1973) treatment of **1** with thionyl chloride in pyridine afforded formation of an epoxide **4**. Although this epoxide formation is easily rationalized, only one analogous thionyl chloride-promoted transformation of a vicinal diol into an epoxide has been

reported (Coxon *et al.* 1965). Attempts to convert the simple *trans*-dihydroxy-γ-lactones **12-15** into epoxide by thionyl chloride treatment in all cases yielded elimination and rearrangement products (Christensen & Pedersen, unpublished).

As in the case of other tertiary alcohols, the 2 tertiary hydroxy groups in **1** can only be acylated with difficulty. Acetylation of both hydroxy groups was accomplished using 4-dimethylaminopyridine as a catalyst (Hölfe *et al.* 1978), and acetic anhydride as a reagent (Christensen, unpublished). In contrast to the tetrasubstituted double bond in **3** (Holub *et al.* 1973), the corresponding double bond in **1** is not hydrogenated over platinum even after prolonged treatment. Under these conditions, the trisubstituted double bond in the angeloyl moiety is reduced, apparently stereoselectively, as only one doublet originating in the formed 2-methylbutanoate arises in the 270 MHz ¹H NMR-spectrum.

Selective hydrolysis of the butanoate is accomplished by dissolving **1** in a 0.25 M solution of sodium carbonate in aqueous methanol. Upon acidification, only **6** and **16** are isolable from the reaction mixture beside unreacted **1** (Christensen *et al.* 1982). Treatment of **1** with stronger bases leads to extensive degradation, whereas a number of partially hydrolyzed products have been isolated after potassium hydroxide promoted saponification of the epoxide **4**, in which the β-hydroxy-lactone function is masked. Five products **17–21** have been isolated after hydrolysis of **1** in a 10% solution of trifluoroacetic acid in aqueous methanol. All of these products are butanoates. The presence of the methoxy derivative **18** indicates the $A_{AL}1$ mechanism (March 1977) to be operating for the cleavage of the allylic ester. As has been observed for other lactones (Wolfrom & Wood 1951, Hulyalkar 1966) sodium borohydride reduces **1** to a mixture of the two semi-acetals **22** and **23**.

| 22,23 | 12,14 | 13,15 |

22 R = αOH   12 m = 2   13 m = 2
23 R = βOH   14 m = 3   15 m = 3

Labelling of thapsigargin
Acylation of **6** with vinylacetic anhydride in the presence of 4-dimethylamino-pyridine yields **9**, possessing a mono-, a tri-, and a tetrasubstituted double bond.

By taking advantage of the ability of hydridocarbonyltris (triphenylphosphine) rhodium (I) (O'Connor & Wilkinson 1968), selective to catalyze reduction of terminal double bonds deuterated **1** could be prepared by treatment of **9** with deuterium. Spectroscopic investigations revealed an average per molecule of 1 deuterium in the 4 position, 1 deuterium in the 3 position and 0.5 deuterium in the 2 position of the butyrate moiety (Christensen unpublished).

MAST CELL-MEDIATOR RELEASE

As the release of histamine and other mediators from tissue mast cells and circulating basophil leukocytes is centrally involved in the pathogenesis of acute allergic responses and generalized inflammatory responses (Kazimierczak & Diamant 1978, Pepys & Edwards 1979), a number of investigations have been made in order to understand the mechanism regulating the secretions. Most of the data obtained have been derived from studies on peritoneal rat mast cells, which are readily obtained and purified to homogeneity (Uvnäs & Thon 1959). It should be emphasized, however, that there are marked functional and morphological differences between mast cells from different species and even from various tissues within a given animal (Ennis & Pearce 1980, Pearce & Ennis 1980, Ennis 1982). Although it may not be possible to draw universally applicable conclusions, it is to be expected, that the broad mechanism of the secretion process is common.

The ultrastructural changes during mast cell-secretion are now well established (Anderson *et al.* 1973). In contrast, the sequence of biochemical events occurring between activation and the final secretory response, still remains to be elucidated, although a number of potential intermediate steps might have been discovered. Thus, an increased phospholipidmethylation and further metabolization (Axelrod & Hirata 1982), and an increased phosphatidylinositol turnover (Cockroft & Gomperts 1979), has been demonstrated in activated mast cells. Also the role of the cyclic nucleotides during secretion is debated, as is the role of calcium ions (Pearce 1982).

The number of agents, which activates mast cells, includes polycations as polylysine and compound 48/80, anaphylatoxins, calcium ionophores, a prominent example being A23187, the plasma substitute dextran, sodium fluoride and a diversity of drugs. Secretion may also be induced by antibodies to the IgE receptor molecule on the mast cell, or by lectins such as concanavalin A, which simulated the anaphylactic reaction by cross-binding the carbohydrate moieties in the Fc region of IgE antibodies fixed to the surface of the target cells (Kazimierczak & Diamant 1978, Pearce 1982, Lagunoff *et al.* 1983).

Histamine releasing properties of thapsigargin.

Peritoneal rat mast cells by incubation with thapsigargin **1** release histamine in the presence of calcium ions in a dose-dependent way (Fig. 3) (Rasmussen *et al.* 1978). Inhibition of the secretory action by pretreatment of the cells with antimycin A confirms the reaction to be dependent on endogenous ATP and consequently to be non-cytotoxic (Rasmussen *et al.* 1978). After incubation of the cells with **1** and calcium ions, a period of approximately 1 min precedes the histamine release. Cells pretreated with **1** in the absence of calcium ions, however, respond to the secretory action of the ions, whenever they are introduced. After dilution of the pretreated cells yielding a concentration of **1**, which was too low for triggering a release, the secretion induced by addition of calcium ions became dependent on the time of their addition. Half the optimal histamine release was found when calcium ions were introduced 15 min after dilution of the treated cells (Patkar *et al.* 1979). Thus, the secretory reaction induced by **1** and calcium ions may be divided into a two-step reaction, a calcium ion-independent activation and a calcium ion-dependent release. In contrast to the stimulatory step, the secretory step is markedly counteracted by hypertonicity of the incubation medium. Therefore, it seems likely that the uptake of calcium ions, generally believed to precede the secretion, is a passive transport (Diamant & Patkar 1980).

The few studies performed on the mechanism of the action of thapsigargin

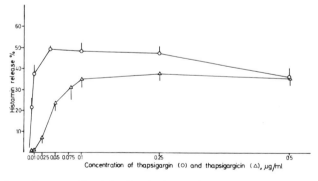

Fig. 3. Histamine release mediated by incubating peritoneal rat mast cells with increasing concentrations of thapsigargin **1** (o) and thapsigargicin **2** ($\triangle$) in a calcium chloride (10^{-3}M)-containing medium. (Rasmussen *et al.* 1978).

have led to the conclusion, that among various calcium- and energy- dependent histamine-releasing agents, thapsigargin most closely resembles the action of fluoride (Patkar *et al.* 1979).

Structure activity relationships for thapsigargin
The histamine-releasing activities of the acylated hexaoxygenated guaianolides (Table I) seem to reflect the lipophilicities of the attached acyl moieties, i.e., a more lipophilic side-chain yields a more potent secretagogue. In contrast, at least one of the 2 vicinal hydroxy groups is essential for activity, as transformation of thapsigargin **1** into an epoxide **4**, or a diacetate, abolished the histamine-releasing properties. The absence of activity of the model compounds **12–15** proves, that the presence of a α,β-dihydroxy-γ-lactone moiety is not sufficient for stimulatory effects. Neither of the inactive compounds shows antagonistic properties.

The activity of the mixture of the semi-acetals **22** and **23** shows that the γ-lactone carbonyl group is not essential for mast cell-activating properties.

The equipotence of **6** and **16** is surprising, as the 2 hydroxy groups are *trans* disposed in **6** and *cis* disposed in **16**. If, however, it is assumed that the

Table I
Relative histamine-releasing activity of thapsigargin related compounds.

Compound	0.1 μg/ml	1.0 μg/ml	2.5 μg/ml
1	100	100	
2	72±10		
3		76±3	94±1
4	3.2±0.1	2.2±0.1	3.0±0.1
5			83±8
6	4.5+0.1	95±3	
7		54±4	89±1
8		65±16	123±40
10	3.2±1	94±6	
11	18±2	85±11	
16	2.3±0.7	91±16	
19		27±3	13±9
20		60±4	71±10
22+23		110±22	93±15

The release are given as percentage of the maximum thapsigargin-mediated release. In no cases was histamine release observed in a calcium-ion-free incubation medium. The experiments were accomplished according to the method of Rasmussen *et al.* 1978.

24,25

26

27

24 R = H

25 R = (structure)

carboxylate **24** is the biologically active form, equipotence would be expected, because both **6** and **16** are converted into this ion. The presence of **24** in the incubation medium has proven by dissolving either **6** or **16** in the buffer (pH 7) used for the incubation studies, and in both cases demonstrating an acidic extract to contain **6** as well as **16**. Thapsigargin **1** must be exptected to form an analogous carboxylate ion **25** when dissolved in the incubation medium.

Comparisons between the activity of thapsigargin, other sesquiterpene lactones, and phorbols

A number of biological activities including cytotoxic (Lee *et al.* 1971, Rodriguez *et al.* 1976, Cassady & Suffness 1980), anti-inflammatory (Hall *et al.* 1979, 1980), anti-microbial (Rodriguez *et al.* 1976, Lee *et al.* 1977), and allergenic effects (Mitchell & Dupuis 1971, Towers 1977, Mitchell 1975), have been reported for other sesquiterpene lactones. The presence of an α,β-unsaturated carbonyl moiety is believed to be important for these effects. This structure is present in the angeloyl group of thapsigargin **1**. The histamine-releasing activity of dihydrothapsigargin **8**, and the inability of alantolactone **26** to stimulate mast cells, proves the α,β-unsaturated carbonyl moiety not to be essential for the activation mediated by **1**.

Another group of terpenes, the phorbols, are known as skin irritants. As the phorbols are co-carcinogenic (Hecker & Schmidt 1974), the ability of **1** and related compounds to activate ornithine decarboxylase and their affinity towards the phorbol receptor, have been investigated. None of the compounds **1, 2, 4**, or **5** showed any affinity for the receptor, or any ornitine decarboxylase activating effects (Fujiki, private communication), just as 12-0-tetradecanoyl-phorbol-13-acetate **27** does not induce a non-cytotoxic histamine secretion from mast cells (Christensen & Norup, unpublished). Thapsigargin **1** and thapsigargi-cin **2** have also been found unable to promote the morphological changes in epithelial-cell cultures, which are characteristic for the phorbols and other tumor promoters (Arenholt, private communication).

ACKNOWLEDGEMENTS

This project has been supported by grants from The Danish Medical Research Council, Bikubenfonden, and Ekspeditionssekretær, cand. jur. Torkil Steenbecks Legat. The authors wish to thank Mrs. A. Bing, and Mr. S. Stilling for skilful secretarial and technical assistance.

REFERENCES

Anderson, P., Slorach, S. A. & Uvnäs, B. (1973) Sequential exocytosis of storage granules during antigen-induced histamine release from sensitized rat mast cells *in vitro. Acta Physiol. Scand. 88,* 359–

Axelrod, J. & Hirata, F. (1982) Phospholipid methylation and the receptor-induced release of histamine from cells. *Trends Pharmacol. Sci. 3,* 156–8.

Cassady, J. M. & Suffness, M. (1980) Terpenoid Antitumor Agents. In: *Anticancer Agents Based on Natural Product Models,* eds. Cassady, J. M. & Douros, J. D., pp. 201–69. Academic Press, New York.

Christensen, S. B., Rasmussen, U. & Christophersen, C. (1980) Thapsigargin, Constitution of a Sesquiterpene Lactone Histamine Liberator from *Thapsia garganica. Tetrahedron Lett. 21,* 3829–30.

Christensen, S. B., Rasmussen, U., Larsen, I. K. & Christophersen, C. (1982) Thapsigargin and Thapsigargicin, Two Histamine Liberating Sesquiterpene Lactones from *Thapsia garganica. J. Org. Chem. 47,* 649–52.

Christensen, S. B. & Schaumburg, K. (1983) Stereochemistry and Carbon-13 Nuclear Magnetic Resonance Spectroscopy of the Histamine-Liberating Sesquiterpene Lactone Thapsigargin. *J. Org. Chem. 48,* 396–9.

Cockroft, S. & Gomperts, B. D. (1979) Evidence for a role of phosphatidylinositol turnover in stimulus-secretion Coupling. *Biochem. J. 178,* 681–7.

O'Connor, C. & Wilkinson, G. (1968) Selective homogeneous hydrogenation of alk-1-enes using hydridocarbonyltris (triphenylphosphine) rhodium (I) as catalyst. *J. Chem. Soc. (A)* 2665–71.

Coxon, I. M., Hartshorn, M. P. & Kirk, D. N. (1965) Acid-catalyzed reactions of 13,17a-Epoxy- and 17a,18-Epoxy-C-nor-D-homo-spirostans. *Tetrahedron 21,* 2489–99.

Diamant, B. & Patkar, S. A. (1980) The Influence of hypertonicity on histamine release from isolated rat mast cells. *Agents Action 10,* 140–4.

Ennis, M. (1982) Histamine release from human pulmonary mast cells. *Agents Action 12,* 60–3.

Ennis, M. & Pearce, F. L. (1980) Differential reactivity of isolated mast cells from the rat and guinea-pig. *Eur. J. Pharmacol. 66,* 339–45.

Hall, I. H., Lee, K. H., Starnes, C. O., Sumida, Y., Wu, R. Y., Waddell, T. G., Cochran, J. W. & Gerhart, K. G. (1979) Anti-inflammatory activity of sesquiterpene lactones and related compounds. *J. Pharm. Sci. 68,* 537–41.

Hall, I. H., Starnes, C. O., Lee, K. H. & Waddell, T. G. (1980) Mode of action of sesquiterpene lactones as anti-inflammatory agents. *J. Pharm. Sci. 69,* 537–43.

Hecker, E. & Schmidt, R. (1974) Phorbolesters - the irritants and co-carcinogens of *Croton tiglium* L. *Fortschr. Chem. Org. Naturst. 31,* 377–467.

Hölfe, G., Steglich, W. & Vorbrüggen, H. (1978) 4-Dialkylaminopyridine als Hochwirksame Acylierungskatalysatoren. *Angew. Chem. 90,* 602–615.

Holub, M., Samek, Z., de Groote, R., Herout, V. & Sorm, F. (1973) The structure of the Sesquiterpenic triester lactone trilobolide. *Collect. Czechslov. Chem. Commun. 38,* 1551–62.

Hulyalkar, R. K. (1966) Selective reduction of substituted aldono-lactones to aldose derivatives. *Can. J. Chem. 44,* 1594–6.

Kazimierczak, W. & Diamant, B. (1978) Mechanisms of histamine release in anaphylactic and anaphylactoid reactions. *Prog. Allergy 24,* 295–365.

Krogsgaard-Larsen, P. & Sandberg, F. (1969) Coumarins from *Thapsia garganica L.* The structure of a new coumarin. *Acta Chem. Scand. 24,* 1113–4.

Lagunoff, D., Martin, F. W. & Read, G. (1983) Agents that release histamine from mast cells. *Ann Rev. Pharmacol. Toxicol. 23,* 331–51.

Lee, K., Huang, E., Piantadosi, C., Pagano, J. S. & Geissmann, T. A. (1971) Cytotoxicity of sesquiterpene lactones. *Cancer Res. 31,* 1649–54.

Lee, K., Ibuka, T., Wu, R. & Geissmann, T. A. (1977) Structure-antimicrobial activity relationships among the sesquiterpene lactones and related compounds. *Phytochemistry 16,* 1177–81.

March, J. (1977) *Advanced Organic Chemistry,* pp. 349–53. McGraw-Hill, Tokyo.

Mitchell, J. C. & Dupuis, G. (1971) Allergic contact dermatitis from sesquiterpenoids of the compositae family of plants. *Br. J. Dermatol. 84,* 139–50.

Mitchell, J. C. (1975) Contact allergy from plants. *Recent Adv. Phytochem. 9,* 119–38.

Murray, R. D. H., Méndez, J. & Brown, S. A. (1982) *The Natural Coumarins,* pp. 291–311. John Wiley & Sons, New York.

Patkar, S. A., Rasmussen, U. & Diamant, B. (1979) On the mechanism of histamine release induced by thapsigargin from *Thapsia garganica. Agents Action 9,* 53–7.

Pearce, F. L. (1982) Calcium and histamine secretion from mast cells. *Prog. Med. Chem. 19,* 59–109.

Pearce, F. L. & Ennis, M. (1980) Isolation and some properties of mast cells from the mesentery of the rat and guinea-pig. *Agents Action 10,* 124–31.

Pepys, J. & Edwards, A. M. (1979) *The Mast Cell: Its Role in Health and Disease.* Pitman Medical, Turnbridge Wells.

Rasmussen, U., Christensen, S. B. & Sandberg, F. (1978) Thapsigargin and thapsigargicin, two new histamine liberators from *Thapsia garganica. L. Acta Pharm. Suec. 15,* 133–40.

Rasmussen, U., Christensen, S. B. & Sandberg, F. (1981) Phytochemistry of the genus thapsia. *Planta Med. 43,* 336–41.

Rodriguez, E., Towers, G. H. N. & Mitchell, J. C. (1976) Biological activities of sesquiterpene lactones. *Phytochemistry 15,* 1573–80.

Seyle, H. (1965) *The Mast Cells.* Butterworth, London.

Towers, G. H. N., Mitchell, J. C., Rodriguez, E., Bennett, F. D. & Rao, P. V. S. (1977) Biology and chemistry of *Parthenium hysterophorus* L., a problem weed in India. *J. Sci. Ind. Res. 36,* 672–84.

Tschirch, A. & Stock, E. (1936) *Die Harze* vol. 2, pp. 1540–2. Verlag von Gebrüder Borntraeger, Berlin.

Uvnäs, B. & Thon, I. (1959) Isolation of biologically intact mast cells. *Exp. Cell. Res. 18,* 512–20.

Wolfrom, M. L. & Wood, H. B. (1951) Sodium borohydride as a reducing agent for sugar lactones. *J. Am. Chem. Soc. 73,* 2933–4.

DISCUSSION

NAKANISHI: I think you can determine the absolute configuration by looking at the CD sign at around 225 nm, in particular if you compare with that of your di-hydro ester **8**, because there should be an excitation coupling of the double bond and the α-β-unsaturated ester function.

BRØGGER CHRISTENSEN: We will do this, because we are aware that the Horeau method is empirical. We chose it because it has been found safe on a very similar compound (1).

ATTA-UR-RAHMAN: Have you tried making the other possible vicinal diol by opening up the epoxide?

BRØGGER CHRISTENSEN: Attempts to open the epoxide yields cleavages at other places in the molecule before the epoxide opens.

KROGSGAARD-LARSEN: You showed a variety of compounds related to the natural products and some of them were inactive in the release experiments. Are some of these compounds antagonists?

BRØGGER CHRISTENSEN: The variety of natural products were all active. Some preliminary tests indicated, that the epoxide had some antagonistic activity. We have not been able to reproduce this later on.

LAZDUNSKI: What is the toxicity of the compound when you inject it *i.p.* or *i.v.*?

BRØGGER CHRISTENSEN: At i.p. injection on mice, the acute LD_{50} after 6h is 1.9 mg/kg. It is difficult to test, as further deaths occur within a short time.

LAZDUNSKI: Does the compound act on basophils, too?

BRØGGER CHRISTENSEN: Yes, it releases histamine from human basophils.

LAZDUNSKI: Does the molecule act from the outside or from the inside of the cell? That can be investigated easily, I think, as you can add the molecule, then wash, then add calcium ions.

418 DISCUSSION

BRØGGER CHRISTENSEN: The compound has been added to the cells, in a calcium-free medium, after some washings, calcium has been added, and activity was observed. This could indicate that the compound is acting from the inside, but it also could indicate that the compound in some way has activated the cells.

LAZDUNSKI: Have you looked by electron microscopy to what happened to the storage granules in the cell?

BRØGGER CHRISTENSEN: No, not by electron microscopy.

WAGNER: As the allergic reaction is concerned, the situation becomes more complicated because there are a lot of these sesquiterpene lactones which have immunostimulating effects. It would be of interest to eliminate the hydroxyl groups or to test the epoxide in order to see if the derivatives are non-allergenic.

(1) Herz W. & Kagan, M. B. (1967) *J. Org. Chem. 32,* 216–218.

V. CNS-Active Natural Products in Drug Development

Non-Equilibrium Opioid Receptor Antagonists

P. S. Portoghese* & A. E. Takemori[+]

Narcotic antagonists have been employed extensively as pharmacological tools for investigating opioid receptors. In this connection the agonists, naloxone **1** and naltrexone **2**, both of which are derived from the natural product, thebaine, have contributed immensely to the significant research advances in the mode of action of opioids.

1 $R = CH_2CH = CH_2$
2 $R = CH_2 - \triangleleft$

With the concept of multiple opioid receptors (Portoghese 1965, Martin 1967, Takemori *et al.* 1969), and the more recent pharmacological evidence (Iwamoto & Martin 1981) supporting this concept, the question of antagonist specificity has become very important in attempting to evaluate the selectivity of agonist ligands. The cross-reactivity of naloxone and naltrexone is an inherent limitation in this regard. This presentation describes an approach to the design of highly selective, if not specific, opioid antagonists. The basis for the design involves the concept of "receptor recognition amplification" through covalent binding. Such non-equilibrium antagonists are serving as valuable receptor probes and may have clinical utility as ultra-long acting narcotic antagonists.

Departments of Medicinal Chemistry* and Pharmacology[+], University of Minnesota, Minneapolis, Minnesota, 55455 U.S.A.

NATURAL PRODUCTS AND DRUG DEVELOPMENT, Alfred Benzon Symposium 20.
Editors: P. Krogsgaard-Larsen, S. Brøgger Christensen, H. Kofod, Munksgaard, Copenhagen 1984.

DESIGN RATIONALE

Our design rationale was based upon the principle of recognition-site-directed alkylation (Baker 1967). High receptor selectivity (recognition amplification) is attainable through this approach because 2 recognition steps are required. This is the primary recognition step, which is synonymous with receptor affinity, and a second step that involves proper alignment of the electrophile (of the receptor-bound ligand) with a neighboring nucleophile (Fig. 1). Thus, if different types of opioid receptors contain patterns of nucleophiles that differ, it is reasonable that the receptor type whose nucleophiles are most reactive and in closest proximity to the electrophilic center of the complexed ligand will be alkylated.

It is, in principle, possible to increase the selectivity of a non-equilibrium antagonist by increasing the selectivity of the first recognition step, or the second recognition step, or both. As different opioid receptor types and subtypes possess similar topography, it is the second recognition step which has greater capacity for conferring selectivity if one assumes that different receptor types possess significant differences in nucleophile density or distribution.

The task of designing specific or highly selective non-equilibrium ligands is difficult because the location and constitution of nucleophiles on opioid receptors are not known. Moreover, it is conceivable that a receptor nucleophile

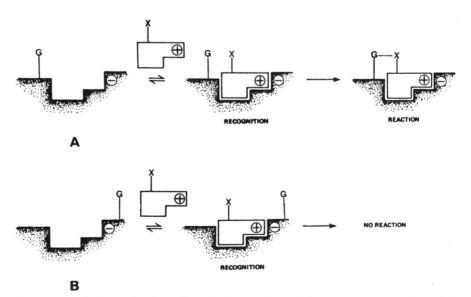

Fig. 1. Schematic illustration of an affinity label interacting with 2 receptor types (A and B). Only in receptor Type A are the electrophile X and nucleophile G within covalent bonding distance.

can be properly juxtaposed with an electrophile without forming a covalent bond due to low reactivity. Consequently, the approach we have taken was to first employ a highly reactive electrophilic group as a means of locating proximal nucleophiles on the receptors. Once located, then fine-tuning was accomplished by identical attachment of a less reactive electrophilic moiety to the ligand in order to increase selectivity.

This rationale led to the development of β-chlornaltrexamine (β-CNA) 3, a highly reactive non-equilibrium opioid antagonist (Portoghese *et al.* 1978). Due to the promiscuous nature of the electrophile (aziridinium ion) generated in β-CNA, the selectivity of this ligand is conferred largely from the first recognition step. Consequently, its order of irreversible blockage of different receptor types (*mu>kappa>delta*) presumably reflects the order of its equilibrium affinity for these receptors *in vitro* (Ward *et al.* 1982a). In mice, β-CNA produces ultralong narcotic antagonism (≥3 days) after a single i.c.v. dose (1.2 nmol) (Portoghese *et al.* 1978, Portoghese *et al.* 1979, Caruso *et al.* 1980). By comparison, the effect of the equilibrium ligand, naltrexone 2, lasts less than 2 h.

3

β-Chlornaltrexamine 3 has been employed as a pharmacological and biochemical tool in a variety of studies. Because β-CNA alkylates all types of opioid receptors, it has been employed in conjuction with protecting concentrations of type-selective opioid ligands *in vitro* in order to obtain a selectively blocked opioid receptor population (Ward *et al.* 1982b).

β-FUNALTREXAMINE (β-FNA), A *MU* OPIOID RECEPTOR NON-EQUILIBRIUM ANTAGONIST

As the data from our experiments with β-CNA 3 indicated that it alkylated multiple opioid receptor types without any significant irreversible binding to other classes of receptors (Caruso *et al.* 1979, Fantozzi *et al.* 1981), we focussed our attention on the development of ligands that contain electrophiles that are less reactive and more selective than the aziridinium ion. The fumaramate methyl ester group was one of several electrophilic moieties employed for this purpose (Portoghese *et al.* 1980). This ligand has been named *β*-funaltrexamine (*β*-FNA) **4**.

4

The pharmacological profile of *β*-FNA differs from that of *β*-CNA in several respects (Portoghese *et al.* 1980, Takemori *et al.* 1981). Unlike *β*-CNA, *β*-FNA behaves as an agonist when tested on the electrically stimulated guinea-pig ileum (GPI), and in this regard it is approximately five-times more potent than morphine. Analysis of the pA$_2$ value of naloxone versus *β*-FNA revealed that this agonism is probably mediated through *kappa* opioid receptors. Remarkably, thorough washing of the GPI removed the agonism, but the response of the muscle to morphine was irreversibly blocked. This morphine antagonism was found to be a time-dependent and concentration-dependent inhibition. Significantly, *β*-FNA does not irreversibly antagonize its own agonist effect, suggesting that its agonist and antagonist effects are mediated through different receptor systems.

The most important difference between *β*-FNA and *β*-CNA was the apparent specificity of *β*-FNA in non-equilibrium blockage of *mu* receptors in smooth muscle preparations (GPI and MVD) (Ward *et al.* 1982a, Ward *et al.* 1982b, Portoghese *et al.* 1980, Takemori *et al.* 1981). Thus, the activities of *kappa* agonists on the GPI and *delta* agonists on the MVD are unaffected by exposure to *β*-FNA. In fact, the specificity of *β*-FNA is exemplified by its ability to transform the GPI from a preparation which contains both *mu* and *kappa* receptors to one which is devoid of functional *mu* receptors but consists principally of *kappa* receptors (Ward *et al.* 1982b). Such a transformation was demonstrated by the change of pA$_2$ value of naloxone-morphine to that similar to naloxone-ethylketazocine after incubation of the GPI with *β*-FNA and washing. It is noteworthy that the depletion of functional *mu* receptors by *β*-FNA in the GPI is manifested as a parallel shift in the dose-response curve of morphine; no diminution of the maximum effect is observed because morphine apparently possesses full intrinsic activity at *kappa* receptors. On the other hand, since *β*-CNA is capable of alkylating both *mu* and kappa receptor systems they are both depleted, and this is characterized by a reduced maximal effect (Ward *et al.* 1982a, Caruso *et al.* 1979).

The prolonged blockage (3–4 days) of morphine analgesia by a single dose of *β*-FNA in mice (Ward *et al.* 1982c), rats (Messing *et al.* 1982), and monkeys (Aceto *et al.* to be published), is consistent with the *in vitro* results. That *β*-FNA acts in the brain has been demonstrated by the fact that parenteral administration antagonizes the effects of i.c.v. morphine (Messing *et al.* 1982). Another feature which is consistent with its *in vitro* specificity is the long-lasting *β*-FNA-induced antagonism of *mu* but not *kappa* agonists (Ward *et al.* 1982c).

ROLE OF C-6 STEREOCHEMISTRY IN NON-EQUILIBRIUM BLOCKAGE

The studies with *β*-FNA **4** *in vitro* and *in vivo* have emphasized the critical importance of the second recognition step (Fig. 1) leading to its covalent association with the *mu* opioid receptor system. Thus, in spite of the fact that *β*-FNA is a potent *kappa* agonist (Takemori *et al.* 1981), and presumably has high affinity (good primary recognition characteristics) for *kappa* receptors, no alkylation of these recognition sites occurs. The inertness of *kappa* receptors to *β*-FNA is most likely due to the absence of sufficiently reactive nucleophiles in proximity to the electrophilic carbon of *β*-FNA when it forms a complex with this receptor system.

Further evidence relating to the role of the second recognition step in the covalent binding of *β*-FNA to the *mu* receptor system was obtained from an investigation of the *β*-FNA epimer, α-FNA **5** (Sayre 1983a). As the 6α-fumaramate moiety is expected to be oriented differently from that in the 6*β* epimer, it was expected that α-FNA would be incapable of properly aligning its electrophile with the same nucleophile on the *mu* receptor system. This should be manifested by the inability of α-FNA to behave as a non-equilibrium antagonist

5

because of the high selectivity of the fumaramate moiety. Indeed it was found that α-FNA did not act as an irreversible antagonist of morphine on either the GPI or MVD. In fact, α-FNA was capable of protecting against the irreversible blockage by β-FNA. This suggested that a deficient second recognition step and not primary recognition is responsible for the inertness of α-FNA toward the *mu* receptor system.

In harmony with this concept, the chirality at C-6 becomes less important in the second recognition step as the ligand electrophile is made more reactive (Sayre *et al.* 1983a, Sayre *et al.* 1983c). This is because the ability to distinguish between different types of nucleophiles becomes less efficient as reactivity of the electrophile is increased. Thus, we have observed that among 3 epimeric pairs of compounds which contain electrophiles (fumaramate methyl ester, isothiocyanate, nitrogen mustard), the order of selectivity parallels their reactivity.

Two extreme cases illustrating this are presented in Figs. 2, 3. Although an array of nucleophiles are present (G^1-G^4), some within covalent bonding

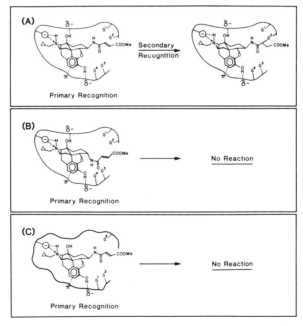

Fig. 2. A schematic illustration of recognition between (A) the fumaramate moiety of β-FNA **4** and a proximal nucleophile G^2. No reaction (no secondary recognition) takes place with α-FNA **5** at the same receptor type (B) or with β-FNA at a different receptor type (C) because an appropriate receptor nucleophile is not properly aligned with the electrophilic center.

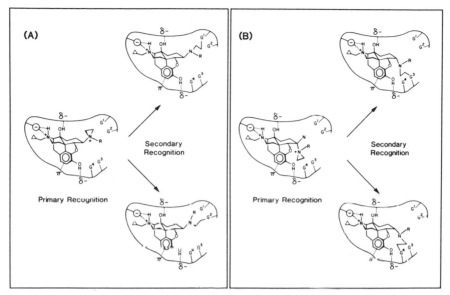

Fig. 3. A schematic illustration of the interaction of β-CNA (A) and its epimer α-CNA (B), at identical receptors. Note that different nucleophiles are alkylated due to the high reactivity of the aziridinium electrophile.

distance, the fumaramate moiety of β-FNA reacts only with one of these (Fig. 2A). Due to the epimeric relationship of the Michael acceptor group in α-FNA, this moiety projects into a receptor locus where the nucleophiles either are not properly aligned or are not of the right constitution to participate in conjugate addition (Fig. 2B). Similarly, β-FNA does not alkylate other opioid receptor types because the proper nucleophile is distal to the electrophilic center of the Michael acceptor (Fig. 2C). On the other hand, with an extremely reactive electrophile, there is minimal difference between receptor covalent binding capacity of the 2 epimers (α- and β-CNA) (Fig. 3). The aziridinium ion generated in the chlornaltrexamine epimers reacts with multiple electrophiles within covalent bonding distance of either the β-epimer (Fig. 3A), or α-epimer (Fig. 3B).

EVALUATION OF OPIOID RECEPTOR TYPE SELECTIVITY WITH β-FNA

As β-FNA **4** specifically blocks the effects mediated by *mu* opioid receptors, it has become a useful tool for evaluating the selectivity of opioid agonists.

Pretreatment of the GPI and MVD with 200 nM β-FNA for 30 min followed by thorough washing afforded preparations devoid of functional *mu* receptors (Ward *et al.* 1982b). This produced a GPI preparation that contained only functional *kappa* receptors. Employing this *kappa* preparation we have investigated a number of commonly employed opioids in order to evaluate their interaction at *mu* and *kappa* receptors (Table I) (Takemori & Portoghese, to be published). The IC_{50} ratio reflects the extent of the interaction at *mu* receptors. All of these ligands produced full dose-response curves on the treated GPI, indicating that they possess full intrinsic activity at *kappa* receptors. This included typical *mu* agonists (e.g., morphine, fentanyl) as well as the *delta* agonist, DADLE. The IC_{50} values of the typical *kappa* agonists, ethylketazocine and nalorphine, were unaffected by this treatment, suggesting their agonist effect is mediated predominantly via the *kappa* receptor. As most, if not all, of the ligands (Table I) clearly are capable of interacting with both *mu* and *kappa* receptors, this study indicates that even prototypical ligands are not specific for a single opioid receptor type. Moreover, the question of specificity and cross-selectivity can be addressed only if a specifically acting ligand such as β-FNA is employed. Therefore, without the availability of type-specific ligands as receptor probes, any conclusions derived from use of conventional protypical ligands may represent a closed circle of reasoning.

Table I

Effect of Agonist Ligands on the β-FNA-treated GPI

Compound	IC_{50} Ratio[a]
"Mu Ligands"	
Morphine	26.5
Fentanyl	25.4
Methadone	45.1
Etorphine	8.2
"Delta Ligands"	
DSLET	31.5
DADLE	87.4
"Kappa Ligands"	
Ethylketazocine	1.2
Nalorphine	1.3

[a] The IC_{50} determined on the treated (60 min incubation with 200 nM β-FNA followed by 20 washes) GPI divided by the IC_{50} in the identical untreated preparation.

DIFFERENT RECOGNITION SITES MEDIATE OPIOID AGONISM AND ANTA-GONISM

Recently, studies with β-FNA **4** and its N-methyl analogue, β-FOA **6**, have prompted us to question the belief that agonism and antagonism are mediated through identical receptor sites (Portoghese & Takemori 1983). Though each of these ligands differ only in the nature of the N-substituent, only β-FNA irreversibly blocks the agonist action of *mu* agonists (Portoghese *et al.* 1980). Thus, β-FOA is a reversibly acting *mu* agonist with no detectable irreversible activity. These results can be explained either by (a) the presence of distinct receptor sites for *mu* agonism and antagonism or (b) by a difference in the nature of the interaction of agonists and antagonists with a single receptor type.

6

In an effort to distinguish between these possibilities, we have evaluated the ability of opioid agonists and antagonists to protect against the irreversible antagonism of morphine's effects by β-FNA (20 nM for 30 min) in the GPI preparation (Portoghese & Takemori 1983).

Most of the agonists afforded relatively poorer protection of β-FNA antagonism than that exhibited by the antagonists (Table II). The capability of the compounds to protect against the irreversible antagonism of β-FNA did not correlate with their agonist activity (IC_{50}), but appeared to correspond to their antagonist potency (Ke). Thus, as protectors, the antagonists had a rank potency of nalorphine<naloxone<naltrexone<diprenorphine. Comparison of this protective ability of the ligands with their Ke values from the literature (Gyang & Kosterlitz 1966) revealed the same rank order.

The effectiveness of narcotic antagonists to protect *mu* receptors in the GPI preparation against irreversible blockage by β-FNA is in contrast to the relatively poor protection afforded by a variety of opioid agonists. The fact that a variety of agonists, including morphine, possess an antagonistic component (Gyang & Kosterlitz 1966, Kosterlitz & Watt 1968) in the GPI preparation and the apparent parallel relationship between this antagonism (Ke values) and their

Table II

Protection of the Irreversible β-FNA Antagonism by Various Opioid Agonists and Antagonists

Protector	N	Morphine IC$_{50}$ Ratio[a]±S.E.	IC$_{50}$ (nM)	Ke[b]
None	7	6.1±0.5		
Morphine (1 μM)	4	4.0±0.7	24	88
β-FOA (500 nM)	5	5.2±0.7	22	
RX 783006[c] (1μM)	4	2.3±0.6	28	
DAME[d] (1 μM)	4	3.1±0.1	21	
Etorphine (1 nM)	5	2.3±0.3	0.3	
Ethylketazocine (10 nM)	4	4.6±1.2	0.6	
Nalorphine (200 nM)	4	1.9±0.2	28	4.5
Nalorphine (1 μM)	4	1.4±0.3		
Naloxone (2 nM)	4	3.4±0.5		1.2
Naloxone (20 nM)	4	1.9±0.3		
Naloxone (200 nM)	4	1.1±0.2		
Naltrexone (2 nM)	4	2.4±0.6		0.38
Naltrexone (20 nM)	4	1.0±0.1		
Naltrexone (200 nM)	4	1.0±0.1		
Diprenorphine (3 nM)	4	1.8±0.2		0.13

[a] IC$_{50}$ after treatment/control IC$_{50}$; statistical analyses were determined by the method of D. J. Finney, *Statistical Methods in Biological Assay,* 2nd Ed., Hafner Publ. Co., New York, 1964.
[b] Ke (equilibrium constant) were taken from Kosterlitz & Watt.
[c] [D-Ala-^{2},MePhe^4,Gly-ol^5]enkephalin (B. K. Handa, A. C. Lane, J. A. H. Lord, B. A. Morgan, M. J. Rance & C. F. C. Smith, *Eur. J. Pharmacol., 70,* 531, 1981)
[d] [D-Ala^2,Met^5]enkephalinamide

ability to protect against β-FNA tend to suggest the presence of separate recognition sites for *mu* agonists and antagonists. As both β-FOA **6** and β-FNA **4** contain an identical electrophilic moiety at the C-6 position, the unreactivity of β-FOA at *mu* receptors is consistent with its interaction at a site which does not possess an accessible requisite nucleophile for covalent association. Moreover, the inability of β-FOA to protect against β-FNA-induced, irreversible antagonism strongly implicates separate sites for these ligands.

The presence of separate recognition sites for *mu* agonists and antagonists provides a reasonable basis for rationalizing the differential effects of various types of treatments on the binding of opioid agonists and antagonists. These include protein modifying reagents (Pasternak *et al.* 1975b), enzymatic treatments (Pasternak & Snyder 1975), heat (Creese *et al.* 1975), and exposure to various cations (Pert *et al.* 1973, Pasternak *et al.* 1975a), and GTP (Childers &

Snyder 1978). Also, separate agonist and antagonist sites have been postulated from *in vivo* data (Takemori 1974).

As β-FNA specifically and irreversibly antagonizes the effects of *mu* agonists without affecting *kappa* or *delta* opioid activity it appears likely that β-FNA interacts covalently with a site that is uniquely coupled to the *mu* receptor. A plausible functional role for this site is the regulation of *mu* receptors in response to endogenous *mu* ligands. Thus, the data suggest that naloxone and naltrexone may exert their antagonistic effect by interacting with a neighboring regulatory site *rho* which is allosterically coupled to the *mu* receptor.

A model consistent with this data is illustrated schematically in Fig. 4. We propose that a *mu* receptor subunit is associated with a regulatory subunit which contains a recognition site *rho* that is topographically similar, but not identical, with its neighboring *mu* receptor. Agonists have higher affinity for the *mu* receptor while antagonists possess higher affinity for the regulatory site *rho*. We envisage that occupation of the *rho* site triggers a vectorial (unidirectional) conformational change which results in a decrease in the affinity of the agonist binding site *mu*. The *rho* site becomes bound by an agonist only after its

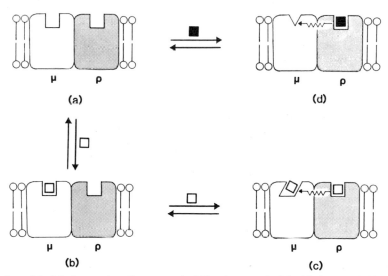

Fig. 4. A model of the interaction af a *mu* agonist (□) and antagonist (■) with the *mu* opioid receptor and a neighboring regulatory site *rho*. An agonist at low concentration binds seslectively to the *mu* receptor (b) and at higher concentrations to the *rho* regulatory site (c). The latter interaction triggers a vectorial decrease in the affinity of the *mu* receptor (symbolized by ↜ⱳⱳ⁻). The selective interaction of an antagonist at the *rho* site induces a vectorial loss of affinity of the *mu* receptor.

neighboring *mu* receptor is occupied, whereas narcotic antagonists interact selectively with the *rho* site. The vectorial change induced by antagonist is manifested by a considerably greater affinity loss at the *mu* receptor than the interaction of agonists with the *rho* site.

The presence of separate recognition sites for opioid agonists and antagonists suggest a number of intriguing possibilities which are outlined below. (1) The "purity" of the agonistic effect is determined by the relative affinity of a ligand for the *mu* and *rho* sites. This is consistent with the reported presence of antagonistic component in the GPI for all agonist ligands tested. It is conceivable that modulation of *mu* agonist binding by Na^+ and GTP resides in the vectorial coupling component of the complex. (2) Tolerance can be viewed as an increase in the number of *mu* receptor subunits that are functionally coupled with the regulatory subunit *rho*. This could be effected by agonist-induced increase of *rho* subunits or by a mobile receptor (Cuatrecasas & Hollenberg 1976) mechanism involving the association between monomeric *mu* and *rho* subunits. This would explain the increased sensitivity to narcotic antagonist by mice soon after they have been exposed to a *mu* agonist (Takemori *et al.* 1973).

DIFFERENTIATION BETWEEN MU OPIOID RECEPTOR SUBTYPES

Different receptor subtypes are expected to possess far fewer distinguishing features than receptor types. Therefore, the problem of developing non-equilibrium agents to distinguish between different receptor subtypes should be a more formidible task than achieving specificity among receptor types. Using a model based on the assumption that differences between opioid receptor subtypes become more evident as the distances from a central locus on the receptor is increased, we should in principle be able to take advantage of such differences in the design of subtype-selective non-equilibrium antagonists. The principle utilized in such design is schematically illustrated in Fig. 5, where it can be seen that while a nucleophile G proximal to both subtypes is the same, a distal nucleophile is different. Thus, one of our design strategies was to attack the electrophile at the terminus of an "extender" chain in an effort to reach into a locus where such differences might occur.

This approach led to the development of compounds that exhibit differential ability to irreversibly block the *mu* receptor system in the GPI and MVD (Sayre *et al.* 1983a, Sayre *et al.* 1983b). Thus, while the maleimide (**2**, Table III) does not block the effects of morphine in either preparation, the "extended" analogue,

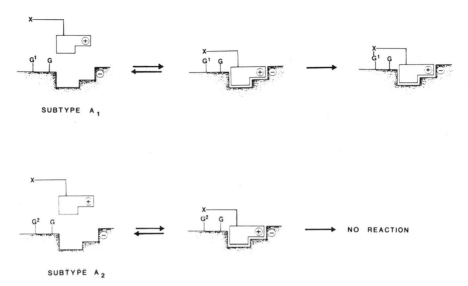

Fig. 5. Differentiation between receptor subtypes A_1 and A_2 by means of extending the electrophile X to different nucleophiles G^1 and G^2.

maleylacetamide (**3**, Table III) is a potent irreversible antagonist at *mu* receptors only in the MVD. This is in contrast to β-FNA (**1**, Table III) which does not distinguish between *mu* receptors in the MVD and GPI. It therefore appears that the *mu* receptor system in the GPI and MVD are different and can be classified as subtypes.

We have found that the iodoacetamide (**4**, Table III) also exhibits similar ability to block the *mu* receptor system in the MVD without affecting *mu* receptors in the GPI. Presumably, the nucleophile that is alkylated in this case is probably not identical to that alkylated by the maleylacetamide.

Interestingly, the allyl analogue of β-FNA (**5**, Table III) exhibits selectivity toward the GPI *mu* receptor system. The reason for this is not known, but one possible explanation is that β-FNA and its allyl analogue have different relative affinities (first recognition step) for the *mu* receptors in these preparations.

In light of our studies that suggest that agonists and antagonists bind to different recognition sites (Fig. 4), it is possible that the differences between the *mu* receptor system in the MVD and GPI does not arise from the *mu* receptor, but rather from differences between the regulatory (*rho*) sites that are coupled to the *mu* receptor.

Table III

Irreversible Antagonist Potency

| R' | R | IC$_{50}$ Ratio (treated/control)[a] | | | |
| | | GPI | | MVD | |
		M	EKC	M	DADLE
1 $\overset{H}{\underset{H}{NHCOC=CCOOMe}}$ (β-FNA)	CH$_2$–◁	12.0	1.1	10.6	1.1
2	CH$_2$–◁	1.3	1.4	0.8	1.1
3 NHCOCH$_2$N	CH$_2$–◁	3.3	1.0	30 (50%)[b]	1.8
4 NHCOCH$_2$I	CH$_2$–◁	2.1	1.2	20 (50%)[b]	1.8
5 $\overset{H}{\underset{H}{NHCOC=CCOOMe}}$	CH$_2$CH=CH$_2$	6.4	1.9	2.8	1.1

[a] Agonist (M=Morphine, EKC=ethylketazocine, or DADLE=[D-Ala^2, D-Leu^5]-enkephalin) IC$_{50}$ after incubation (30 min at 200 nM) and washing (20×) divided by control (untreated preparation) IC$_{50}$.

[b] IC$_{30}$ ratios were estimated because response was decreased to 50% of maximum after treatment.

REFERENCES

Aceto, M., Dewey, W., Takemori, A. E. & Portoghese, P. S. To be published.

Baker, B. R. (1967) *Design of Active-Site-Directed Irreversibly Enzyme Inhibitors,* John Wiley Sons, New York.

Caruso, T. P., Larson, D. L., Portoghese, P. S. & Takemori, A. E. (1980) Pharmacological studies with an alkylating narcotic agonist, chloroxymorphamine and antagonist, chlornaltrexamine. *J. Pharmacol. Exp. Ther. 213,* 539–544.

Caruso, T. P., Takemori, A. E., Larson, D. L. & Portoghese, P. S. (1979) Chloroxymorphamine, an opioid site-directed alkylating agent having narcotic agonist activity. *Science 204,* 316–318.

Childers, S. R. & Snyder, S. H. (1978) Guanine nucleotides differentiate agonist and antagonist interactions with opiate receptors. *Life Sci. 23,* 759–762.

Creese, I., Pasternak, G. W., Pert, C. B. & Snyder S. H. (1975) Discrimination by temperature of opiate agonist and antagonist receptor binding. *Life Sci. 16,* 1837–1842.

Cuatrecasas, P. & Hollenberg, M. D. (1976) Membrane receptors and hormone action. *Adv. Protein Chem. 30,* 251–451.

Fantozzi, R., Mullikan-Kilpatrick, D. & Blume, A. (1981) Irreversible inactivation of opiate receptors in neuroblastoma X glioma hybrid NG108–15 by chlornaltrexamine. *J. Mol. Pharmacol. 20,* 8–15.

Gyang, E. A. & Kosterlitz, H. W. (1966) Agonist and antagonist actions of morphine-like drugs on the guinea-pig-isolated ileum. *Br. J. Pharmacol. 27,* 514–527.

Iwamoto, E. T. & Martin, W. R. (1981) Multiple opioid receptors. *Med. Res. Rev. 1,* 411–436.

Kosterlitz, H. W. & Watt, A. J. (1968) Kinetic parameters of narcotic agonists and antagonists with particular reference to N-allylnoroxymorphone (naloxone). *Br. J. Pharmacol. 33,* 266–276.

Martin, W. R. (1967) Opioid antagonists. *Pharmacol. Rev. 19,* 464–521.

Messing, R. B., Portoghese, P. S., Takemori, A. E. & Sparber, S. B. (1982) Antagonism of morphine-induced behavioral suppression by opiate receptor alkylators. *Pharmac. Biochem. Behav. 16,* 621–626.

Pasternak, G. W., Snowman, A. M. & Snyder, S. H. (1975a) Selective Enhancement of [^{3}H]opiate agonist binding by bivalent cations. *Mol. Pharmacol. 11,* 735–744.

Pasternak, G. W. & Snyder, S. H. (1975) Opiate receptor binding: enzymatic treatments that discriminate between agonist and antagonist interactions. *Mol. Pharmacol. 11,* 478–484.

Pasternak, G. W., Wilson, H. A. & Snyder, S. H. (1975b) Differential effects of protein-modifying reagents on receptor binding of opiate agonists and antagonists. *Mol. Pharmacol. 11,* 340–351.

Pert, C. B., Pasternak, G. & Snyder, S. H. (1973) Opiate agonists and antagonists discriminated by receptor binding in brain. *Science 182,* 1359–1361.

Portoghese, P. S. (1965) A new concept on the mode of interaction of narcotic analgesics with receptors. *J. Med. Chem. 8,* 609–616.

Portoghese, P. S., Larson, D. L., Jiang, J. B., Caruso, T. P & Takemori, A. E. (1979) Synthesis and pharmacologic characterization of an alkylating analogue (chlornaltrexamine) of naltrexone with ultralong-lasting antagonist properties. *J. Med. Chem. 22,* 168–173.

Portoghese, P. S., Larson, D. L., Jiang, J. B. & Takemori, A. E. (1978) 6β-[N,N-Bis(2-chloroethyl)amino]-17-(cyclopropylmethyl)-4,5α-epoxy-3,14-dihydroxymorphinan (chlornaltrexamine), a potent opioid receptor alkylating agent with ultralong narcotic antagonist activity. *J. Med. Chem. 21,* 598.

Portoghese, P. S., Larson, D. L., Sayre, L. M., Fries, D. S. & Takemori, A. E. (1980) A novel opioid receptor site directed alkylating agent with irreversible narcotic antagonistic and reversible agonistic activites. *J. Med. Chem. 23,* 233–234.

Portoghese, P. S. & Takemori, A. E. (1983) Different receptor sites mediate opioid agonism and antagonism. *J. Med. Chem. 26,* 1341–1343.

Sayre, L. M., Larson, D. L., Fries, D. S., Takemori, A. E. & Portoghese, P. S. (1983a) The importance of carbon -6 chirality in conferring irreversible opioid antagonism to naltrexone-derived affinity labels. *J. Med. Chem. 26,* 1229–1235.

Sayre, L. M., Portoghese, P. S. & Takemori, A. E. (1983b) Difference between mu receptors in the guinea pig ileum & mouse vas deferens. *Eur. J. Pharmacol. 90,* 159–160.

α-chlornaltrexamine produces concurrent irreversible agonistic and irreversible antagonistic activities. *J. Med. Chem. 26,* 503–506.

Takemori, A. E. (1974) Biochemistry of drug dependence. *Ann. Rev. Biochem. 43,* 15–33.

Takemori, A. E., Kupferberg, H. J. & Miller, J. W. (1969) Quantitative studies on the antagonism by naloxone of some narcotic and narcotic-antagonist analgesics. *J. Pharmacol. Exp. Ther. 169,* 627–638.

Takemori, A. E., Larson, D. L. & Portoghese, P. S. (1981) The irreversible narcotic antagonistic and reversible agonistic properties of the fumarate methyl ester derivative of naltrexone. *Eur. J. Pharmacol. 70,* 445–451.

Takemori, A. E., Oka, T. & Nishiyama, N. (1973) Alteration of analgesic receptor antagonist interaction induced by morphine. *J. Pharmacol. Exp. Ther. 186,* 261–265.

Takemori, A. E. & Portoghese, P. S., (to be published).

Ward, S. J., Portoghese, P. S. & Takemori, A. E. (1982a) Pharmacological profiles of β-funaltrexamine (β-FNA) and β-chlornaltrexamine (β-CNA) on the mouse *vas deferens* preparation. *Eur. J. Pharmacol. 80,* 377–384.

Ward, S. J., Portoghese, P. S. & Takemori, A. E. (1982b) Improved assays for the assessment of κ- and δ- properties of opioid ligands. *Eur. J. Pharmacol. 85,* 163–170.

Ward, S. J., Portoghese, P. S. & Takemori, A. E. (1982c) Pharmacological characterization *in vivo* of the novel opiate, β-funaltrexamine. *J. Pharmacol. Exp. Ther. 220,* 494–498.

DISCUSSION

ALBUQUERQUE: We have observed that naltrexone and levallorphan in micromolar concentrations block and generate subconductance state of the ionic channel of the nicotinic acetylcholine receptor as detected by binding studies as well as by electrophysiological means. Thus, high concentrations of these compounds might also interact with the cholinergic system of the ileum.

PORTOGHESE: I think your point is very well taken. If we use very high concentrations or relatively high concentrations of naltrexone on the ileum we see an enhancement of the contractions which supports your point.

KROGSGAARD-LARSEN: Are you considering labelling these irreversible antagonists in order to map out the proteins with which they interact?

PORTOGHESE: We are doing that right now with [^{3}H]-β-FNA with a specific activity of 60 Ci/mM. I might add that we have evidence that the recognition site for the antagonist is not the same as the recognition site for the agonist. This may be an allosterically coupled system, because we have done protection experiments which suggest that agonists are extremely ineffective at protecting against the alkylation by β-FNA. Antagonists are very effective at protecting.

WALL: Have you tried to make other types of alkylating agents with various degrees of activity.

PORTOGHESE: We made numerous compounds and concluded that there is no relationship between reactivity and ability to alkylate the receptor. We interpret this as meaning that the second recognition step is very important.

LAZDUNSKI: Did you try to discriminate between all the effects which you have described using a binding assay?

PORTOGHESE: We have done binding experiments, in which the stereospecific binding is decreased considerably upon incubation with the alkylating agent, but we have not really gone into binding studies in any great depth.

LAZDUNSKI: The binding studies, of course, may tell a little more about the mechanism, because stability of your preparation for a longer period might be dubious.

PORTOGHESE: A limitation of binding studies is that you have destroyed the integrity of the system.

CASSADY: Do you have a feeling to what extent β-CNA actually reaches the receptor? Do you consider the bis-alkylating properties of β-CNA an important factor?

PORTOGHESE: Recent investigations have proven the same type of activity whether β-CNA is given subcutaneously or intraperitoneally. So, β-CNA does seem to reach the receptor. I do not know if β-CNA crosslinks with anything, but the monovalent analogue is also active.

Morphine and Related Opioid Analgesics

Henry Rapoport

The CNS-active opium poppy (*P. somniferum*) alkaloids have for millennia
served mankind as most efficacious pain killers. However, they have suffered
from a number of deleterious side effects, the major one being addiction. In
attempts to eliminate these side effects and increase analgesic potency,
thousands of derivatives of these natural products have been prepared. Many
synthetic analogues also have been made, incorporating various structural
features of the natural products.

Probably the most powerful analgesics that have resulted from these efforts
are the 6,14-ethenomorphinan type. These compounds are derived from
thebaine or oripavine, themselves convulsants, by an initial Diels-Alder
reaction. Etorphine, prepared by this route, is active at 10^{-9} molar, over 1000
times more active than morphine. Of equal interest is the fact that the 2 epimers
at C-19 differ in analgesic activity by a factor of 50.

In an effort to explain and understand both (1) the powerful potency and (2)
the difference between epimers, we have synthesized a number of structural
variants. By examining the analgesic activity of these compounds and the
epimeric differences, we have developed an hypothesis about the lipophilic and
hydrophilic regions of the active site in the receptor. These concepts have been
translated to a conformational hypothesis for enkephalin, man's natural
analgesic.

Recently (Loew & Berkowitz 1979) quantum mechanical calculations have
been carried out for conformational differences between the C-19 epimers for
various alkyl chain lengths. These calculations show that conformations with a
hydrogen bond between the C-6 methoxyl and the C-19 hydroxyl are lowest in
energy for both epimers, consistent with NMR and crystallographic results.
With the hydroxyl group thus fixed, the larger substituent will occupy one of 2
different areas, depending on whether the absolute stereochemistry is *R* or *S*.

Department of Chemistry, University of California, Berkeley, California 94720, U.S.A.

NATURAL PRODUCTS AND DRUG DEVELOPMENT, Alfred Benzon Symposium 20.
Editors: P. Krogsgaard-Larsen, S. Brøgger Christensen, H. Kofod, Munksgaard, Copenhagen 1984.

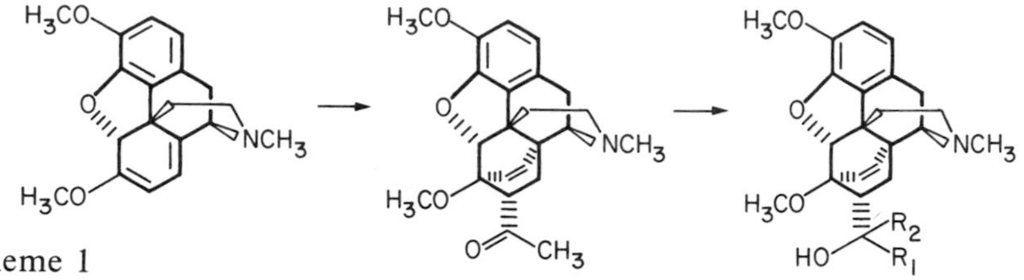

Scheme 1

The increased binding of the alkyl chain with a lipophilic site on the receptor might then account for an increase in the activity of one diastereomer relative to the other. This hypothesis is shown in Scheme 3.

To examine this hypothesis, we have prepared the epimeric alcohols where the C-6 methoxyl has been replaced by a hydrogen. In this way, intramolecular H-bonding will be eliminated as a factor in determining the active conformation of the alkyl chain. To effect these preparations, we required the diene, 6-demethoxythebaine as educt.

An effective procedure for the preparation of dienes from allylic alcohols has been recently developed using an arylsulfenyl chloride (Reich *et al.* 1978). With this work as a model, codeine was treated with 2,4-dinitrobenzenesulfenyl chloride, and the allylic sulfoxide, resulting from rearrangement of the sulfenate ester, was the product. Presumably, the trans relationship of the C-14 hydrogen and the sulfoxide prevented elimination. Attempted isomerization to the *cis*-sulfoxide with lithium diisopropylamide or potassium *tert*-butoxide proved unsuccessful.

Isocodeine, however, on reaction with the sulfenyl chloride underwent rearrangement to the *cis*-sulfoxide which readily eliminated. Thus, codeine was converted to isocodeine using N,N-dimethylformamide dineopentyl acetal and acetic acid in toluene, followed by methanolysis of the resulting isocodeine acetate, in an overall yield of 90%. Treatment of isocodeine with 2,4-

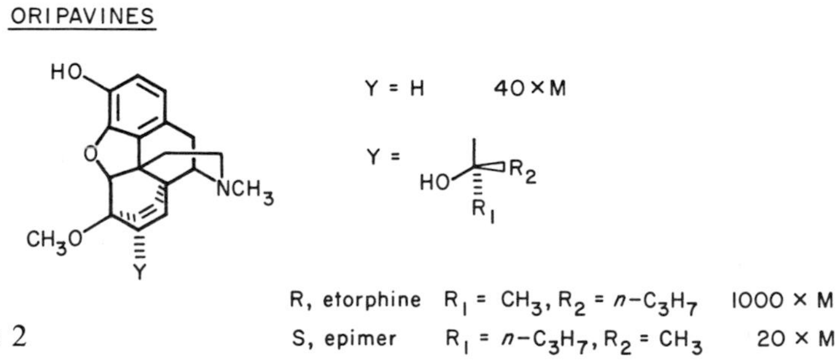

ORIPAVINES

Scheme 2

Y = H		$40 \times M$
R, etorphine	$R_1 = CH_3, R_2 = n-C_3H_7$	$1000 \times M$
S, epimer	$R_1 = n-C_3H_7, R_2 = CH_3$	$20 \times M$

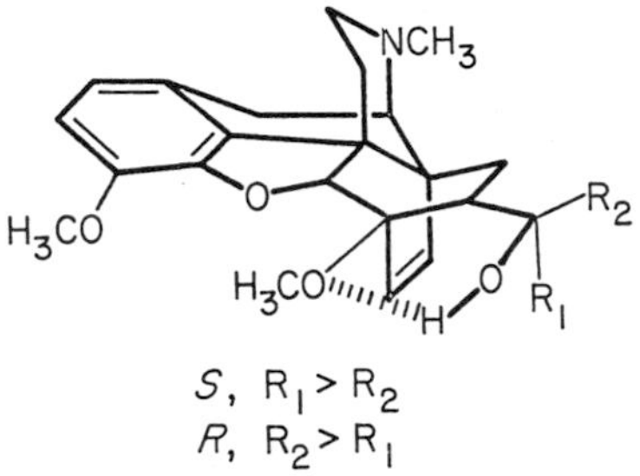

$$S, \; R_1 > R_2$$
$$R, \; R_2 > R_1$$

Scheme 3

dinitrobenzenesulfenyl chloride in dichloromethane afforded 6-demethoxythebaine in 61% yield. This sequence is shown in Scheme 4.

Reaction of 6-demethoxythebaine with methyl vinyl ketone afforded the adduct in 50% yield. HPLC analysis showed that the ketone was an 88:12 mixture of 6-demethoxy-7α-thevinone and a slightly less polar compound. The preparative separation of these compounds was very difficult; however, partial purification gave an enriched sample of the minor isomer. Computer subtraction of the NMR spectrum of the major isomer from that of the enriched sample gave a spectrum which indicates that the minor ketone is the 8α-regioisomeric adduct.

For the synthesis of the desired alcohols from the Diels-Alder adducts, 6-demethoxythevinone was treated with n-butyllithium to afford a mixture of tertiary alcohols and recovered ketone. HPLC analysis showed the mixture of alcohols had an R/S ratio of 12:1 and was obtained in 86% yield along with 14% recovered ketone. The crude product mixture was then treated with sodium borohydride in order to facilitate separation by forming the more polar secondary alcohol. Reduction gave a mixture of secondary and tertiary alcohols,

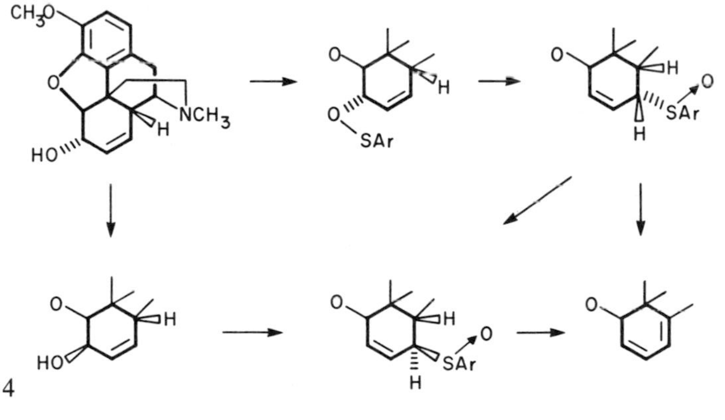

Scheme 4

from which chromatography on silica gel afforded the diastereomerically pure R and S alcohols. Assignment of the stereochemistry is based on the corres-pondence of the NMR signal of the carbinol methyl group of one diastereomer with that of (R)-propylthevinol at δ 0.97 (Fulmor *et al.*). The other diastereomer has a methyl signal at δ 1.07. Alternatively, methyllithium could be added to butyl ketone to give a mixture of R- and S-alcohols in which the S isomer predominated slightly.

Demethylation of the alcohols was attempted with potassium hydroxide in diethylene glycol and with diphenylphosphide anion in tetrahydrofuran; in each case there was extensive decomposition. The best demethylation was sodium propanethiolate in dimethylformamide (Michne 1978). By this procedure, the R-alcohol was demethylated in 69% yield and the S alcohol was demethylated in 52% yield to 19(R)-and 19(S)-*n*-butyl-6-demethoxy-7α-orvinol, respectively. These transformations are shown in Scheme 5.

The pharmacological activity of the diastereomeric phenolic tertiary alcohols was determined using the tail-flick method in Sprague-Dawley rats (Janssen *et al.* 1963). The standard compound used for control and comparison was 19(R)-*n*-propylorvinol (etorphine) which has been established to have 1000-times the analgesic effect of morphine.

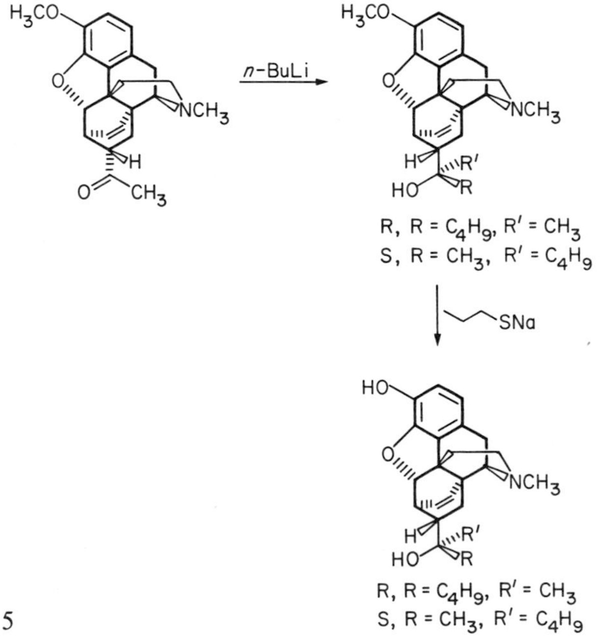

Scheme 5

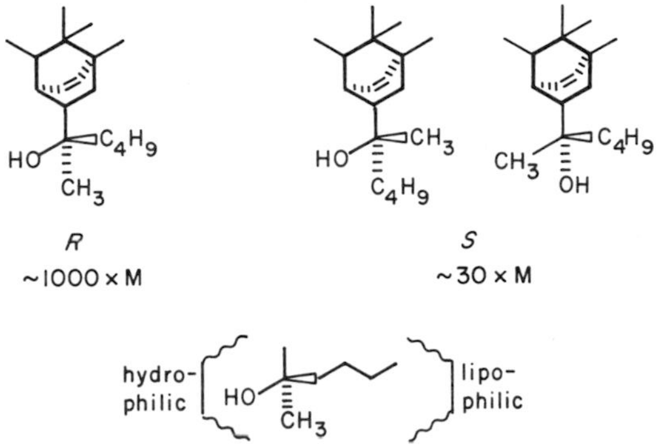

Scheme 6

The dose-response curve of the (R)-phenol corresponded fairly well to that of etorphine with a 50% response value (3.5×10^{-3} μmol/kg); the (S)-phenol gave 50% response values (1.5×10^{-1} μmol/kg) only 20–40-times that of morphine. An examination of the time-response data showed that peak activity occurred around 40 min after injection.

The analgesic activity of the R and S-phenols shows the hydrogen bond between the methoxy group and the tertiary alcohol is not necessary for the potent activity. Based on these results, the R configuration is necessary for maximum activity. This specificity for the R configuration in the 6-demethoxy series is quite interesting. As there are no intramolecular hydrogen-bonding constraints nor any apparent intramolecular steric interactions in either R or S-isomer there must be relatively free conformational mobility about the C7-C19 bond in both. Thus, the alkyl side chain of each carbinol is free to interact with a potential lipophilic binding site in the receptor. The fact that the R absolute configuration leads to much greater activity than the S, supports a second binding site hypothesis for this region of the receptor. These data and the resulting hypothesis are shown in Scheme 6.

To test this hypothesis we have considered the diastereomeric 19-deoxy derivatives, the 19-butyl-7α-orvinans, and the furans, the 6-demethoxy-19-butyl-6,20-epoxy-7α-orvinans. Both series still have the steric and lipophilic components of etorphine and the 6-demethoxy analogues, but would be unable to form a hydrogen bond to a second binding site in that region.

This series of compounds was synthesized by a route based on the conversion of a ketone into an epoxide. Rearrangement of this epoxide should produce an aldehyde which could be easily reduced to the desired primary alcohol. Following a method for the preparation of epoxides from sterically hindered ketones via thioanisole (Shanklin *et al.* 1973), the anion of thioanisole was formed using n-butyllithium and DABCO and was treated with thebuvinone. The mixture of diastereomeric adducts, purified by chromatography to thoroughly remove unreacted ketone, was treated first with trimethyloxonium tetrafluoroborate and then aqueous sodium hydroxide. Isolation afforded a 1.5/1 mixture of diastereomeric epoxides in 30–45% yield. Rearrangement of the epoxides with boron trifluoride etherate produced the aldehydes which were reduced with sodium borohydride to the primary alcohols. The mixture of alcohols was separated into the pure diastereomers by column chromatography affording the *R*-isomer in 42% yield and the *S*-isomer in 36% yield. The synthetic sequence is shown in Scheme 7.

The next target was to reduce the hydroxymethyl to a methyl group. For this purpose the mesylate was prepared and treated with lithium triethylboro-hydride. Butylthevinan could be isolated but the yields ranged from 0–80%. The accompanying product was shown to have ring closed to a tetrahydrofuran and to be the 6,20-epoxy derivative. Presumably furan ring-formation occurs by a mechanism in which the C-6 methoxy oxygen attacks the carbon bearing the mesyloxy group to form oxonium ion. Nucleophilic attack then removes the methyl group and gives furan.

The ratio of 19-deoxy derivative to 6,20-epoxy furan formed in the reduction reaction could be kept near 1/1 by the use of low temperatures in the preparation and reduction of the mesylate and by minimizing the residence times of the mesylate in tetrahydrofuran prior to addition to the reducing agent. The most consistent results were obtained with lithium aluminum hydride as reductant. Thus, the mesylate of each diastereomer was prepared using methanesulfonyl chloride, and the crude mesylate was dissolved in tetrahydrofuran and immediately added to a cold mixture of lithium aluminum hydride in tetrahydrofuran. The products were separated by preparative thin-layer

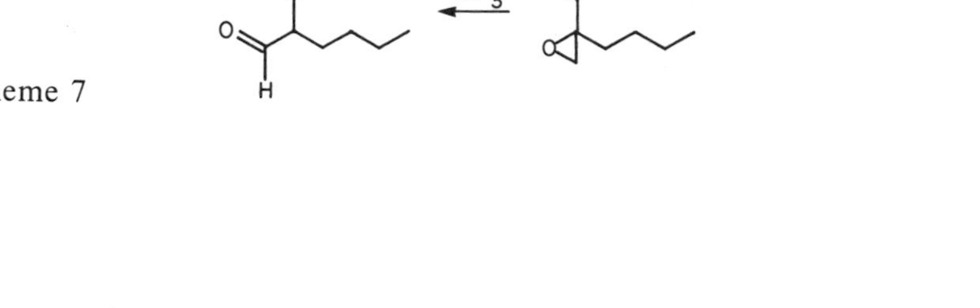

Scheme 7

chromatography. The process is illustrated in Scheme 8. Demethylation of the aromatic methyl esters to afford the phenols was accomplished using sodium propanethiolate in dimethylformamide. The crude products were purified by alumina chromatography to produce the phenols in 50–60% yield.

The analgesic activities of the R and S isomers of the 19-butylorvinans, the 6-demethoxy-19-butyl-6,20-epoxyorvinans, and the 19-butyl-20-hydroxyorvinans were determined using the tail-flick method in Sprague-Dawley rats. The values relative to morphine as are shown in Table I and were acquired by the up-down method using a cut-off level of 6 s (Dixon 1965). The analgesia of the phenols was antagonized by naloxone, indicating that the activity was produced through the opiate μ receptor.

Most earlier proposals concerning structure-activity relationships and opiate receptor modelling using etorphine and its analogues were based on the existence of an intramolecular hydrogen bond between the C-6 methoxy and the C-19 alcohol which would fix the position of the lipophilic side-chain in one region of space. Our results using the 6-demethoxyorvinols, show that an intramolecular hydrogen bond is not necessary for potent activity. There remains the possibility that an intermolecular hydrogen bond may assist in orienting the side chain to the lipophilic region of the receptor. Preparation of the 6,20-epoxyfuran allows an examination of this hypothesis. The butyl group in the rigid tetrahydrofurans is locked in the α or β stereochemistry. Previous models have placed the sidechain in the β position in order to achieve maximum activity. However, the S furan with the butyl group down in the α position, is the more active diastereomer.

Therefore, we propose that the lipophilic site of the opiate receptor which accommodates the side-chain is located below C-8 nearer to the 6,14-etheno

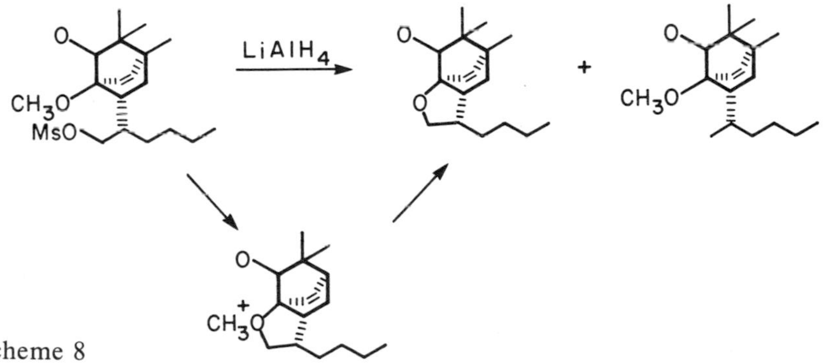

Scheme 8

Table I

Comparative Agonist Activity of the Orvinans.

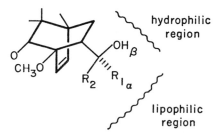

β, 20   a, 210

S, 4   R, 190

S, 4   R, 780

bridge. The tertiary hydroxyl group is directed above the bicyclic ring system toward a hydrophilic site on the receptor as shown in Fig. 1. It is the synergism and competition of binding at these 2 regions that determines the activity of the bridged-oripavine analgesics. If both a hydrophilic and a lipophilic interaction

Fig. 1. Proposed orvinol conformer of greatest agonist activity. The pendant alcohol is oriented for maximum interaction with the hydrophilic (H) and lipophilic (L) regions.

cannot occur, the compound will have poor activity. If both sites are occupied the analgesic response will be significantly magnified. The lipophilic side-chain is needed for high activity but the formation of an intermolecular hydrogen bond is a necessary supplement to achieve the extremely potent activity of etorphine and similar derivatives. This model for the side-chain locale provides a rationale for understanding the activity of the various ethenotetrahydro-oripavines prepared in this work and of other opiates, and should have predictive application to the enkephalins.

REFERENCES

Dixon, W. J. (1965) *Am. Stat. Assoc. J.* 967.
Fulmor, W., Lancaster, J. E., Morton, G. O., Brown, J. J., Howell, C. F., Nora, C. T. & Hardy, R. A. (1967) *J. Am. Chem. Soc.* 89, 3322.
Janssen, P. A. J., Neimegeers, C. J. E. & Dony, J. G. H. (1963) *Arzneim-Forsch.* 13, 502.
Loew, G. H. & Berkowitz, D. S. (1979) *J. Med. Chem.* 22, 603.
Michne, W. F. (1978) *J. Med. Chem.* 21, 1322.
Reich, H. J., Reich, I. L. & Wollowitz (1978) *J. Am. Chem. Soc.* 100, 5981.
Shanklin, J. R., Johnson, C. R., Ollinger, J. & Coates, R. M. (1973) *J. Am. Chem. Soc.* 95, 3429.

DISCUSSION

PORTOGHESE: Do you believe the 19-hydroxy group to be a hydrogen bonding donor or an acceptor?

RAPOPORT: I think it is a donor, but I have no data since it is not possible to make an ether without increasing the size.

NAKANISHI: Is there a possibility that the hydroxy group could hydrogen bond rather comfortably with the π-cloud of the double bond, which would give you a conformation different from that suggested by you?

RAPOPORT: This possibility has been excluded by NMR spectroscopy.

RAZDAN: Analogues, in which the double bond has been removed still have activity, so it is not really interacting and taking part in the activity. We have carried out the Diels-Alder reaction on morphinans, in which the oxide ring was eliminated, and have observed an attack of the dienophile from the opposite side. These compounds show very little analgesic activity.

KROGSGAARD-LARSEN: Do your data provide evidence that you are dealing with the same type of opioid receptors or is it possible that you are shifting between different types of receptors?

RAPOPORT: That is certainly possible. However, we are in the process of having these compounds evaluated by much more sophisticated pharmacological tests.

RAZDAN: Up till now all the peptides have shown activity with the δ-receptors, and no opioid compounds have shown some δ-receptor activity. We now have a compound, which seems to have interaction with the δ-receptors.

DJERASSI was inspired to the following comments:

I sit in Copenhagen
Under the heavy crystal chandeliers
Of the Royal Danish Academy.
The lecturer talks of opiates,

Of molecular improvements of morphine
Hundreds of times more powerful.

Feeling no pain,
Having been tranquilized
By Professor Henry Rapoport,
The audience barely breathes.
I write furiously
On my pad.
I am not copying formulae.
I am writing verse.

It is a known fact
That morphine does not sedate
Everyone. Most, but not all.

I am disappointed:
Rapoport's synthetic opiates
Are equally imperfect.

The Dibenzo[a,d]cycloalkenimines: Redesign of the Pavinan Skeleton to Obtain Useful Biological Activity

P. S. Anderson, B. V. Clineschmidt, M. E. Christy, B. E. Evans & G. G. Yarbrough

INTRODUCTION

Natural products have played a major role in drug therapy as well as serving as a rich source of leads for the medicinal chemist to explore in the pursuit of new and improved therapeutic agents. An interesting example of this can be found in use of the hydrocarbon backbone (dibenzo[a,d]cycloheptene) of isopavine as a building block to which various amine-containing appendages are attached as side chains (Fig. 1). Among the drugs derived, in principle, by this operation are the tricyclic antidepressants related to amitriptyline (Kaiser & Zirkle 1970), butaclamol type neuroleptics (Bruderlein *et al.* 1975), and a large number of cyproheptadine analogs having a spectrum of antihistaminic, anticholinergic, antiserotonin and antidopamine activities (Randall *et al.* 1979, Ogren *et al.* 1978). While this approach to drug design has been highly productive, attempts to derive therapeutic agents through modifications of pavinan or isopavinan skeletons in which the nitrogen bridge is retained have been less successful (Stermitz 1973, Brossi *et al.* 1980). These attempts have focused primarily on deletion of oxygen substituents from the aromatic rings (Walker *et al.* 1971, Dobson *et al.* 1968, Davis *et al.* 1969), and rearrangement of non-benzenoid skeletal atoms (Gootjes *et al.* 1972, Blaser *et al.* 1969). Transformations of this type have led to discovery of compounds with modest anticonvulsant activity, but these agents generally have lacked potency and other potentially useful biological properties.

The success of the dibenzo[a,d]cycloalkene approach to drug design may be related to binding requirements for amines attached to this ring system at pharmacologically relevant sites in the brain. Structure-activity relationship for

Merck Sharp & Dohme Research Laboratories West Point, Pennsylvania, 19486 U.S.A.

NATURAL PRODUCTS AND DRUG DEVELOPMENT, Alfred Benzon Symposium 20.
Editors: P. Krogsgaard-Larsen, S. Brøgger Christensen, H. Kofod, Munksgaard, Copenhagen 1984.

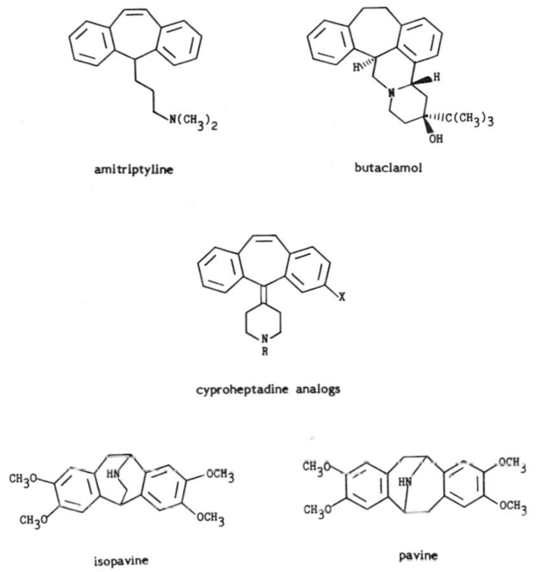

Fig. 1. Compounds of pharmacological interest that contain the hydrocarbon backbone of isopavine as a substructure, isopavine and pavine.

blockade of neurotransmitter receptors and/or uptake sites suggest that the preferred locus for nitrogen in structures of this type is near the plane of one of the aromatic rings and at some fixed distance from it (Humber *et al.* 1979, Snyder & Feinberg 1975). This spatial orientation of nitrogen is prohibited by the geometrical constraints of intact pavinan and isopavinan skeletons. Described here, are structural changes in deoxygenated pavinan and isopavinan skeletons that do not alter the gross three-dimensional shape of these molecules nor the approximate location of nitrogen but do influence biological activity in useful ways. Further, the placement of a single methyl group on these frameworks but not on the deoxygenated isopavinan skeleton is shown to be effective in enhancing biological potency.

THE 9,10-DIHYDROANTHRACEN-9,10-IMINES

Several years ago, a research program was initiated in our laboratories to investigate biological properties of 1,4-dihydronaphthalen-1,4-imines (Anderson *et al.* 1977). These nitrogen-bridged compounds proved to have modest anticonvulsant activity. In the course of this study, several of the related 9,10-

dihydroanthracen-9,10-imines were synthesized (Anderson *et al.* 1979). They also were found to possess modest anticonvulsant activity. In pursuing variation of this activity with further minor structural change, the fortuitious discovery was made that placement of alkyl substituents on the benzhydryl carbon atoms of anthracenimines resulted in a dramatic increase in anticonvulsant activity as well as appearance of central sympathomimetic and apparent anxiolytic activity. The maximal effect on these activities was achieved when a methyl group was placed on each benzhydryl carbon atom. While the efficaciousness of ethyl groups was nearly that of the methyl, bridgehead propyl substituents clearly had a deleterious effect on potency. The level and spectrum of biological activities appeared to be relatively insensitive to the electronic influence of substituents on the aromatic rings and the size of those attached to the nitrogen atom. Thus, it was apparent that methyl groups on the benzhydryl carbon atoms were key to the biological activity profile and potency of the 9,10-dihydro-anthracen-9,10-imines.

Inspection of Dreiding models demonstrated that the benzhydryl methyl groups were conformationally fixed on the face of the rigid hydrocarbon framework that contained the nitrogen bridge. Therefore, it was of interest to test the biological importance of this conformational relationship. Scission of a bond joining nitrogen to a bridgehead carbon atom relaxed the rigidity of the system and placed the C-methyl groups on the hydrocarbon face opposite to that with the nitrogen substituent. The biological consequence of this change was a decrease in anticonvulsant potency and loss of central sympathomimetic activity. Thus, the structural arrangement of nitrogen bridge and benzhydryl alkyl substituents on the same side of the hydrocarbon backbone appeared to be critically related to pharmacological profile.

To test whether or not the availability of the electron pair on nitrogen was biologically important, the N-oxide and methiodide derivatives of anthracenimine 3 were prepared. Both were inactive. During the synthesis of the N-oxide, it became apparent that 9,10-dihydroanthracen-9,10-imines were subject to oxidative deamination by a cheleotropic elimination mechanism (Gribble & Anderson *et al.* 1976). Treatment of 3 with hydrogen peroxide in methanol gave, in addition to the desired N-oxide, 9,10-dimethylanthracene. In view of the known mutagenic activity of this and related anthracenes, it became desirable to determine whether or not 9,10-dimethylanthracene was a metabolite of 3 in mammals. Subsequent demonstration that anthracenes were, in fact, metabolites of anthracenimines in rats and dogs precluded further interest in developing a member of this family for human pharmacology studies (Hucker *et al.* 1978). However, the role of ring-system geometry in expression of biological activity suggested that ring expansion of the hydrocarbon framework should be explored in a search for active compounds of this type that could not be metabolized to anthracenes.

THE DIBENZO[a,d]CYCLOALKENIMINES

Comparative superimposition of anthracenimines and certain dibenzo[a,d] cycloalkenimines having 7- and 8-membered cycloalkene rings with the aid of a molecular graphics system highlighted the common structural features of these molecules. Each contained a benzhydryl carbon (2 in the case of the anthracenimine) to which the nitrogen bridge is attached. Superimposition of the benzhydryl carbons and attached nitrogen bridges allowed significant overlap of the aromatic rings and benzhydryl substituents in these structures. This exercise demonstrated that the structural elements key to the biological activity of the anthracenimines were present in dibenzo[a,d]cyclohepten-5,10-imines and dibenzo[a,d]cycloocten-5,12- and 6,12-imines. Initially, these compounds were seen as ring-expanded analogs of the anthracenimines with added carbon atom(s) strategically positioned to prevent loss of nitrogen by oxidatively mediated cheleotropic elimination. Alternatively, dibenzo[a,d]cyclooocten-5,12- and 6,12-imines can be viewed as being constructed by changing the position of a methylene group in the hydrocarbon backbone of the pavinan skeleton (Fig. 2).

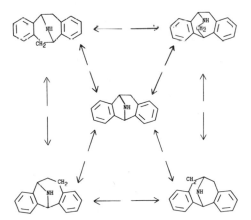

Fig. 2. Methylene group placement and deletion relationships among the dibenzo[a,d]cyclo-alkenimine, pavine and isopavine skeletons.

The pavinan, isopavinan and dibenzo[a,d]cyclooctenimine skeletons are all interrelated by shifts of a single methylene group, either within the framework of the hydrocarbon backbone or between the bridge and the backbone as shown in Fig. 2. Deletion of this methylene group from any of these structures produces the dibenzo[a,d]cyclohepten-5,10-imine ring system. Whether viewed as ring-expanded anthracenimines or pavinan analogs in which the framework has been reorganized, these molecules all have a similar three-dimensional shape as shown by models and graphics (Fig. 3). In each construction, bridgehead substituents and the nitrogen-bridge are fixed conformationally on one face of the hydrocarbon backbone as was the case with the anthracenimines. These molecules offered an opportunity to test the influence of molecular size, symmetry, and, to a degree, shape on the ability of a bridgehead methyl group to enhance biological activity in dibenzo[a,d]cycloalkenimines and related structures. Therefore, a strategy was devised for the synthesis of dibenzo[a,d]

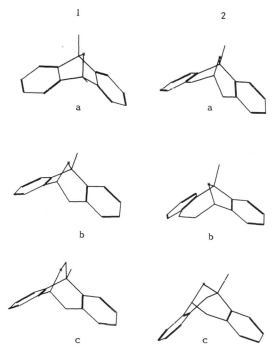

Fig. 3. Structures modeled by computer graphics for the minimum energy conformation of: (Column 1) (a) 9,10-dimethylanthracen-9,10-imine (b) 5-methyl-5H-dibenzo[a,d]cyclohepten-5,10-imine (c) Isopavinan skeleton; (Column 2) (a) 12-methyl-5H-dibenzo[a,d]cycloocten-6,12-imine (b) 12-methyl-5H-dibenzo[a,d]cycloocten-5,12-imine (c) Pavinan skeleton.

cyclohepten-5,10-imines and dibenzo[a,d]cycloocten-6,12- and 5,12-imines with and without methyl substituents at the benzhydryl bridgehead position.

CHEMISTRY

The 9,10-dihydroanthracenimines described here were synthesized by cyclo-addition of benzene to the appropriate isoindoles (Anderson *et al.* 1979). In the homologous dibenzo[a,d]cycloalkenimines, the 7- and 8-membered cycloalkene rings precluded use of a Diels-Alder cyclo-addition approach to these structures. Isopavinan and pavinan alkaloids have been prepared by oxidative cyclization of 1-benzyl-1,2,3,4-tetrahydroisoquinolines (Rice *et al.* 1980). While dibenzo [a,d]cycloocten-6,12-imine could, in principle, be derived by oxidative cycliza-tion of 3-benzyl-1,2,3,4-tetrahydroisoquinolines, interest in deoxygenated anal-ogs and in a general method for synthesizing all of the target dibenzo[a,d] cycloalkenimines suggested that an alternative approach should be pursued.

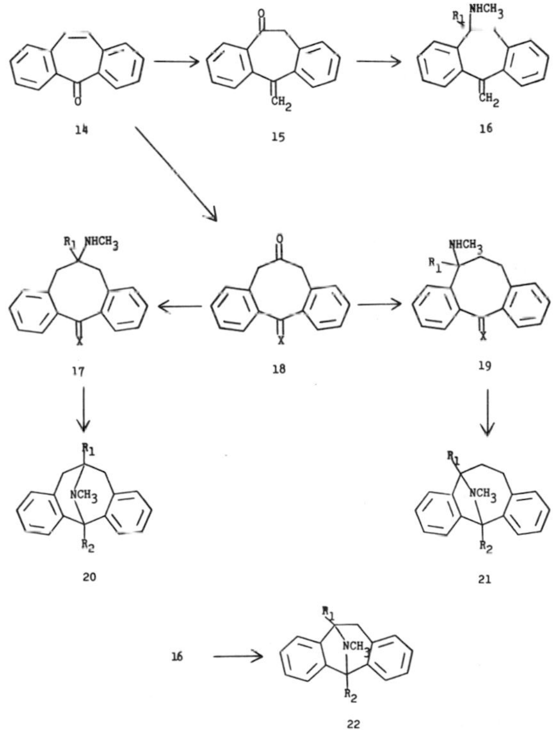

Scheme 1

The facilitating role of entropy in transannular reactions of appropriately substituted 7- and 8-membered cycloalkenes suggested that syntheses might be designed to make use of this principle. Thus, a strategy (Scheme 1) was evolved to construct the required hydrocarbon frameworks containing appropriate function for subsequent transannular nitrogen ring closure (Christy *et al.* 1979, Evans *et al.* 1979). The design further encompassed a common starting material, ketone **14**, for all of the target structures, and a pathway free from stereochemical complications. The latter point was achieved by holding the benzhydryl carbon in an sp^2 hybridized state until the ring closure step. In the case of aminoketones **17** and **19** (X=O), cyclization to ring-tautomer carbinolamines **20** and **21** (R_2=OH) was spontaneous. The amines having a methylene group at the benzhydryl position, **16**, **17** and **19** (X=CH₂), cyclized on accepting an electron from an electron donor in what appeared to be a radical mediated process (Evans & Anderson 1981). All of the dibenzocycloalkenimines described here were conveniently synthesized as briefly outlined in Scheme 1.

BIOLOGICAL RESULTS

Biological results obtained for compounds in this report are given in Table I. The data are presented as ED_{50} values for protection against electroshock convulsions [EST], protection against metrazol-induced convulsion [M], blockade of the convulsant effect of bicuculline [B], and induction of ipsilateral postural asymmetries in caudate-lesioned mice [T]. The latter test reflected the stimulant properties of these compounds. Data were obtained in female mice from Carworth Farms (5 mice/dose level). Each compound was administered i.p. at dose levels of 6, 30 and 150 mg/kg, or one-tenth of these values. The influence on biological activity of methyl group(s) placed at benzhydral bridgehead positions (compounds **2**, **3**, **5**, **8** and **11**) can be seen on inspection of these data. In each ring system, this substituent enhanced anticonvulsant activity and introduced measurable stimulant activity. In the anthracenimines, methyl groups at both benzhydryl bridgehead positions were required for the maximal effect. A second methyl substituent at the non-benzhydryl bridgehead position in dibenzocycloalkenimines **6** and **9** had a modestly adverse impact on potency. In addition to having the activities illustrated here, selected members of this family of nitrogen-bridged cycloalkenes were active in tests for anxiolytic activity (restoration of shock-suppressed behavior in rodents and "taming" in monkeys). The structure-activity relationship for this activity generally paral-

Table I

Summary of the anticonvulsant and turning activity for the dibenzo[a,d]cycloalkenimines and related compounds.

Structure Type	R₁	R₂	Number	ED₅₀ (mg/kg) [B]	[M]	[EST]	[T]
	H	H	1	10	15	>150	>150
	H	CH₃	2	4.2	7.6	7.6	>150
	CH₃	CH₃	3	1.0	0.03	4.1	7.6
	H	H	4	5.8	15	5.1	>150
	H	CH₃	5	0.24	0.16	1.7	1.2
	CH₃	CH₃	6	4.0	3.3	5.1	4.5
	H	H	7	17	27	22	>150
	H	CH₃	8	0.7	0.6	1.7	2.7
	CH₃	CH₃	9	9.2	3.3	5.7	10.5
	H	H	10	14	92	35	>150
	H	CH₃	11	16	9	13	128
	H	H	12	–	2.5	3.5	>150
	H	CH₃	13	–	6.7	6.7	>150

The ED₅₀ (mg/kg) values for protection against bicuculline [B], metrazol [M], and electroshock-induced [EST] convulsions and induction of ipsilateral postural asymmetries in caudate-lesioned mice [T] were estimated from data obtained in Carworth Farm's mice in which each compound was injected i.p., at doses of 150, 30 and 6 mg/kg or one tenth of these values (5 mice/dose level).

leled those shown for anticonvulsant action in Table I. As was the case with the anthracenimines, biological activity was relatively insensitive to substituents on nitrogen and/or the aromatic rings (data not shown).

DISCUSSION

The 9,10-dihydroanthracen-9,10-imines and dibenzo[a,d]cycloalkenimines are related by a common benzhydryl carbon atom and similar molecular shape. They are distinguished by differences in molecular volume, conformational flexibility and symmetry properties. Molecular volume and conformational mobility are minimized in the ring-strained anthracenimines. In the dibenzo [a,d]cyclohepten-5,10-imines, molecular volume is expanded with minimal increase in conformational flexibility. Volume is expanded again to obtain the dibenzo[a,d]-cyclooctenimines which have the highest degree of conformational flexibility in this family of compounds. Maximal flexibility is achieved with the dibenzo[a,d]cycloocten-5,12-imines. Two conformations of this ring system are permitted. In the lower energy conformation, the aromatic rings are placed in positions similar to those seen with the other dibenzocycloalkenimines described here. The higher energy conformation produced a more skewed arrangement of these rings. In the anthracenimines and dibenzocycloocten-6,12-imines, the nitrogen bridge is symmetrically placed with respect to the aromatic rings. In the former, but not the latter case, identical views of the molecular framework are obtained from either end of the bridge. The dibenzo[a,d]cycloheptenimines and dibenzo[a,d]cycloocten-5,12-imines are bridged by nitrogen in a dissymmetrical manner which preserves the dihydroisoindole substructure of the anthracenimines. In all of these compounds, the conformational space occupied by the benzhydryl methyl substituent is similar, but not identical (Fig. 3). The space occupied by this group is defined by a bond angle directed approximately 20° above the plane of one of the aromatic rings. The volume of this region must be limited since analogs in which this substituent was larger than ethyl were not biologically active. Since a methyl group at the benzhydryl carbon had a similar biological effect in each of the structural types described here, this would appear to be the critical geometrical relationship needed for potency enhancement. The less pronounced effect of this substituent seen with dibenzo[a,d]cycloocten-5,12-imines may be related to significant population of the higher energy conformation where this angle approaches zero degrees. A similar situation was encountered with the isopavinan skeleton (Brooks *et al.* 1973). In this conformationally rigid system, a methyl group added to the benzhydryl carbon (compound 13) was found to be in the plane of one aromatic ring and this substituent did not have a potency enhancing effect. The significance of this observation, of course, is tempered by the fact that nitrogen is not directly attached to the benzhydryl carbon in this system. The isomeric 5,10-(iminomethano)-5H-dibenzo[a,d]cycloheptene needed to clarify this point has been synthesized and its ED_{50} (63 mg/kg) determined for prevention of electroshock-induced convulsions (Gootjes *et al.* 1972). The analog with the bridgehead methyl substituent is yet to be prepared.

CONCLUSION

As the anthracenimines and dibenzo[a,d]cycloalkenimines discussed here share a common structure-activity pattern, they would appear to form a homologous pharmacological family. It is defined by a tricyclic hydrocarbon framework with a nitrogen-bridged central ring flanked by 2 aromatic rings to form at least one benzhydryl bridgehead carbon. The family can be generated by successive additions of methylene groups to the hydrocarbon backbone of its simplest member, 9,10-dihydroanthracen-9,10-imine. Alternatively, transposition of a methylene group in the pavine skeleton to a new position in the hydrocarbon moiety so that a benzhydryl carbon is formed can be viewed as defining the larger members of this group. Placement of a methyl substituent on this carbon in each of these structures enhanced anticonvulsant activity and introduced apparent central stimulant and anxiolytic activities. One of these analogs (+)-5-methyl-10,11-dihydro-5H-dibenzo[a,d]cyclohepten-5,10-imine (Clineschmidt *et al.* 1982a, 1982b) is being evaluated clinically for these activities.

REFERENCES

Anderson, P. S., Christy, M. E., Colton, C. D., Halczenko, W., Ponticello, G. S. & Shepard, K. L. (1979) Synthesis of 9,10-dihydroanthracen-9,10-imines. *J. Org. Chem.* 44, 1519–1533.
Anderson, P. S., Christy, M. E., Engelhardt, E. L., Lundell, G. F. & Ponticello, G. S. (1977) N-Trimethylsilylpyrroles as dienes in the synthesis of 1,4-dihydronaphthalen-1,4-imines and isoindoles. *J. Heterocycl. Chem.* 14, 213–218.
Blaser, R., Imfeld, P. & Schindler, O. (1969) Über derivate von 9,10-methaniminomethano-9,10-dihydroanthracen. *Helv. Chim. Acta 52,* 2197–2200.
Brooks, J. R., Harcourt, D. N. & Waigh, R. D. (1973) Cyclisation of N-(prop-2-ynyl)-benzylamines. Part II. Synthesis of 1,2-dihydro-3-phenylisoquinolines and an isopavine derivative. *J. Chem. Soc. (Perkin I),* 2588–2591.
Brossi, A., Rice, K. C., Mak, C.-P., Reden, J., Jacobson, A. E., Nimitkitpaisan, Y., Skolnick, P. & Daly, J. (1980) Mammalian alkaloids. 8. Synthesis and biological effects of tetrahydropapaveroline related 1-benzyltetrahydroisoquinolines. *J. Med. Chem.* 23, 648–652.
Bruderlein, F. T., Humber, L. G. & Voith, K. (1975) Neuroleptic agents of the benzocyclo-heptapyridoisoquinoline series. 1. Synthesis and stereochemical and structural requirements for activity of Butaclamol and related compounds. *J. Med. Chem.* 18, 185–189.
Christy, M. E., Anderson, P. S., Britcher, S. F., Colton, C. D., Evans, B. E., Remy, D. C. & Engelhardt, E. L. (1979) Transannular reactions of dibenzo[a,d]cyclo alkenes. 1. Synthesis of dibenzo[a,d]cycloocten-6,12-imines and dibenzo[a,d]cyclohepten-5,10-imines. *J. Org. Chem.* 44, 3117–3127.
Clineschmidt, B. V., Martin, G. E. & Bunting, P. R. (1982a) Anticonvulsant activity of (+)-5-methyl-10,11-dihydro-5H-dibenzo[a,d]-cyclohepten-5,10-imine (MK-801), a substance with potent anticonvulsant, central sympathomimetic and apparent anxiolytic properties, *Drug Dev. Res. 2,* 123–134.
Clineschmidt, B. V., Williams, M., Witoslawski, J. J., Bunting, P. R., Risley, E. A. & Totaro, J. A. (1982b) Restoration of shock-suppressed behavior by treatment with (+)-5-methyl-10,11-

dihydro-5H-dibenzo[a,d]cyclohepten-5,10-imine (MK-801), a substance with potent anticonvulsant, central sympathomimetic and apparent anxiolytic properties. *Drug Dev. Res. 2,* 147–163.

Cordell, G. H. (1981) Pavine and isopavine alkaloids. In: *Introduction to Alkaloids. A Biogenetic Approach,* pp. 372–379, Wiley-Interscience, New York.

Davis, M. A., Dobson, T. A. & Jordan, J. M. (1969) Transannular reactions in the dibenzo [a,d]cycloheptene series. IV. 10,5-ketone-amide interactions. *Can. J. Chem. 47,* 2827–2835.

Dobson, T. A., Davis, M. A. & Hartung, A. M. (1968) Transannular reactions in the dibenzo [a,d]cycloheptene series. III. Preparation of 11-substituted-10,11-dihydro-10,5-(iminomethano)-5H-dibenzo[a,d]cycloheptines. *Can. J. Chem. 46,* 3391–3397.

Evans, B. E. & Anderson, P. S. (1981) Transannular reactions of dibenzo[a,d]cycloalkenes. 3. Nature of the amine to olefin ring closure. *J. Org. Chem. 46,* 140–143.

Evans, B. E., Anderson, P. S., Christy, M. E., Colton, C. D., Remy, D. C., Rittle, K. E. & Engelhardt, E. L. (1979) Transannular reactions of dibenzo[a,d]cycloalkenes. 2. Synthesis of bridgehead substituted dibenzo[a,d]cycloalkenimines by a regiospecific transannular amine to olefin addition. *J. Org. Chem. 44,* 3127–3135.

Gootjes, J., Funcke, A. B. H. & Timmerman, H. (1972) Experiments in the 5H-dibenzo-[a,d]cycloheptene series. *Arzneim.-Forsch. 22,* 632–635.

Gribble, G. W., Allen, R. W., Anderson, P. S., Christy, M. E. & Colton. C. D. (1976). Oxidative deamination of aromatic 1,4-imines, a new synthesis of polynuclear aromatic hydrocarbons. *Tetrahedron Lett.,* 3673–3676.

Hucker, H. B., Balletto, A. J., Christy, M. E. & Anderson, P. S. (1978) A novel deamination reaction: Metabolism of 9,10-dihydro-9,10,11-trimethylanthracen-9,10-imine to 9,10-dimethylanthracene. In: *Biological Oxidation of Nitrogen,* ed. Gerrod, J. W., pp. 483–488. Elsevier/North Holland Biomedical Press, New York.

Humber, L. G., Bruderlein, F. T., Philipp, A. H., Gotz, M. & Voith, K. (1979) Mapping the dopamine receptor. 1. Features derived from modifications in ring E of the neuroleptic butaclamol. *J. Med. Chem. 22,* 761–767.

Kaiser, C. & Zirkle, C. L. (1970) Antidepressant drugs. In: *Medicinal Chemistry, 3rd, ed.,* ed. Burger, A., pp. 1470–1480. Wiley-Interscience, New York.

Ogren, S.-O., Hall, H. & Kohler, C. (1978) Studies on the stereoselective dopamine receptor blockade in the rat brain by rigid spiro amines. *Life Sci. 23,* 1769–1773.

Randall, W. C., Anderson, P. S., Cresson, E. L., Hunt, C. A., Lyon, T. F., Rittle, K. E., Remy, D. C., Springer, J. P., Hirshfield, J. M., Hoogsteen, K., Williams, M., Risley, E. A. & Totaro, J. A. (1979) Synthesis, assignment of absolute configuration, and receptor binding studies relevant to the neuroleptic activities of a series of chiral 3-substituted cyproheptadine atropisomers. *J. Med. Chem. 22,* 1222–1230.

Rice, K. C., Ripka, W. C., Reden, J. & Brossi, A. (1980) Pavinan and isopavinan alkaloids. Synthesis of racemic and natural thalidine, bisnorargemonine, and congeners from N-nor-reticuline. *J. Org. Chem. 45,* 601–607.

Snyder, S. H. & Feinberg, A. P. (1975) Phenothiazine drugs: structure-activity relationships explained by a conformation that mimics dopamine. *Proc. Nat. Acad. Sci. 72,* 1899–1903.

Stermitz, F. R. & Williams, D. K. (1973) The synthesis of N-methylhomopavine[(±)-homo-argemonine]. *J. Org. Chem. 38,* 2099–2100.

Walker, G. N., Alkalay, D., Engle, A. R., Kempton, R. J. (1971) Synthesis of 5-oxo-10,11-dihydro-5H-dibenzo[a,d]cycloheptene-10-carboxylic acids, corresponding nitriles, and related bridged lactones, hemiketals, lactams, amines, amidoximes, and amidines (5,10-epoxymethano and 5,10-iminomethano compounds). *J. Org. Chem. 36,* 466–478.

DISCUSSION

RAZDAN: Can your testing system indicate the possibility of using these compounds, in grand mal or petit mal type of epilepsy?

ANDERSON: The target is an anti-convulsant agent that can be used in children, since a serious problem is that many children, who are treated with present anti-convulsant agents for long periods of time, as adults never overcome the side-effects associated with that treatment. We don't absolutely know whether our compound works specifically in grand mal or petit mal.

ANAND: Have you some more detailed information about the mode of action of these compounds?

ANDERSON: We have done extensive neurochemical studies on (+)-5-methyl-10,11-dihydro-5H-dibenzo(a,d)cyclohepten-5,10,imine, but obtained few results. The only thing we can say is that all the pharmacological activity is in fact blocked by the α-1 adrenergic blocker prazosin. We have done radio-ligand displacement studies for all of the known neurotransmitters and benzo-diazepine-type drugs. This compound does not bind in concentrations lower than micromolar to any of those receptors.

ATTA-UR-RAHMAN: Reactions analogous to the radical-mediated cyclization of **16, 17** and **19** have been described.

ANDERSON: That's right, but not in such a good yield.

KUTNEY: An alternative way of eliminating the N-oxide group of the dibenzo-cycloalkenes is the classical Cope-elimination. Alkylation of the angular carbons might simply retard the N-oxide elimination.

ANDERSON: The N-oxides of all the new compounds are stable under ordinary conditions, and the N-oxide group appears not to be eliminated metabolically. All these compounds are negative in the Ames test, and in other tests for mutagenic and carcinogenic potential.

BAKER: Did you try to introduce a double bond in the 8-membered ring of compound **21**?

ANDERSON: Yes. This double bond has a rather dramatic effect on the conformation of these molecules and they are considerably less active.

RAPOPORT: Did you put any substituents on the aromatic nuclei?

ANDERSON: Yes, substituents on the aromatic rings have little influence on the biological activity of these compounds.

RAZDAN: As far as I am aware all the anticonvulsants show tolerance over a period.

ANDERSON: We have looked very carefully at these compounds both in terms of tolerance and to see if they are self-administered. They are not self-administered by animals, and the animals do not develop tolerance.

Ergot Alkaloids and Their Derivatives in Medicinal Chemistry and Therapy

P. A. Stadler† & R. K. A. Giger

Ergot alkaloids have a fascinating history. Their role and significance have undergone a radical change over the centuries. What was widely feared as a terrifying poison during the Middle Ages has been gradually converted into many valuable agents for medicinal use.

The ergot drug is primarily found in the dark violet sclerotia of the fungus *Claviceps purpurea,* commonly found on rye. As some of the various names of the drug indicate its application in gynaecology, for example the German name Mutterkorn, there are good reasons to assume that the knowledge of such usage dates back to very early times. In spite of this, ergots appeared in the medical literature relatively late: in 1582, Adam Lonitzer, the author of a book on medicinal herbs, described for the first time the use of raw extracts of ergot sclerotia for inducing child birth and for stopping post-partum bleeding.

ERGOTAMINE AND ERGOMETRINE (ERGONOVINE, ERGOBASINE)

The beginning of scientific research on ergot dates back to 1918, when the first chemically pure alkaloid of the cyclol type, ergotamine 1, was isolated and which exhibited the entire pharmacological spectrum of action of the raw drug extract (Stoll 1918). In 1935, 4 different research groups independently isolated ergometrine 2 (Dudley & Moir 1935, Stoll & Burckhard 1935, Kharash & Legault 1935, Thompson 1935). In comparison to ergotamine 1, the new alkaloid 2 was shown to have a much simpler chemical constitution, consisting

† The vacuum created by the untimely demise of Dr. P. Stadler will be acutely felt by his colleagues and friends for a long time to come.

Preclinical Research, Pharma Department, Sandoz Ltd., CH-4002 Basle, Switzerland.

NATURAL PRODUCTS AND DRUG DEVELOPMENT, Alfred Benzon Symposium 20.
Editors: P. Krogsgaard-Larsen, S. Brøgger Christensen, H. Kofod, Munksgaard, Copenhagen 1984.

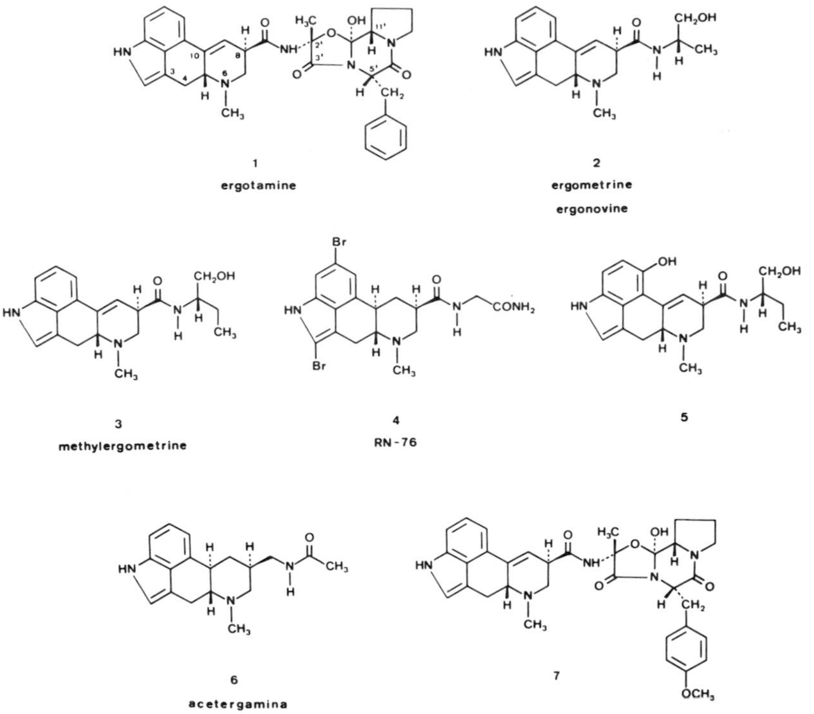

Fig. 1. Genuine ergot alkaloids and synthetic ergolines with high oxytocic activity.

of the 2 moieties d-lysergic acid and l-alaninol. A few years later, the structure of ergometrine could be demonstrated by partial synthesis (Stoll & Hoffmann 1938). This opened the way for its industrial production, and new modifications of this natural ergot derivative could be undertaken. Ergometrine proved to be a highly active and reliable uterotonic, which could be introduced as a therapeutic agent. Because of its greater specificity, better oral absorption, more rapid onset of action and lack of cumulation it gradually replaced ergotamine in the already mentioned obstetric indications and became the standard drug for stopping post-partum bleeding.

To complete the picture of this historical account on ergot research, some supplementary information has to be added. Ergometrine contains 3 asymmetric carbon atoms, which implies the existence of 8 stereoisomers. All of these were prepared and it could be shown that only ergometrine itself exhibited a high oxytocic activity (Stoll & Hofmann 1943a).

SYNTHETIC OXYTOCIC AGENTS

Among the synthetic homologues of ergometrine the next highest, methyl-ergometrine **3**, was found to be superior in its pharmacological properties and about twice as active as the parent compound **2**. Methylergometrine is presently used worldwide with the brand name Methergin® in obstetric and post-partum hemorrhage.

Nevertheless, the search for new oxytocic agents continued, leading to 2,13-dibromo-dihydrolysergic acid glycine amide **4**, which possessed extremely high oxytocic activity in rabbit uterus *in situ*. However, disappointing results in the clinic led to its demise as a therapeutic agent (Rutschmann & Schreier 1965). Probably similar circumstances were experienced with acetergamina **6**, reported to have a specific oxytocic activity comparable with that of ergometrine **2** (Fregnan & Glaesser 1968). Nevertheless, other more potent compounds than methylergometrine would be produced: an example is 12-hydroxy-methyl-ergometrine **5**, which is about 8-times more active than **3**, but its low chemical stability prevented its introduction as a therapeutic drug (Stadler *et al.* 1964a). Later the 5'-p-methoxy-ergotamine derivative **7** was found to be about 6-times more active than the parent compound, but at that time medical interest for drugs with this profile of action in obstetrics had declined and **7** was not developed any further (Stadler & Stuetz 1973).

POSSIBLE PHARMACOPHORES OF THE ERGOLINE RING-SYSTEM

The tetracyclic ergoline ring-system is rather special because of its unique ability to directly interact with various neurotransmitter systems, like the serotonin-ergic-, noradrenergic- and dopaminergic-systems. Fig. 2 shows the possible structural relationships between the ergoline ring-system and the neurotrans-mitter serotonin **8**, noradrenaline **9** and dopamine **10** (Lindberg *et al.* 1982). Knowledge of the ergoline pharmacophore fragments is important for a better understanding of the structure-activity relashionships, and as an instrument for the rational design of more selective derivatives. At the moment it is not definitively established which of the indicated alternatives A and B (or both) are the relevant interactions. For DA-receptor stimulation the pyrrole ethylamine moiety (alternative **10B** in Fig. 2) seems to be the correct one (Nichols 1976, Bach *et al.* 1980).

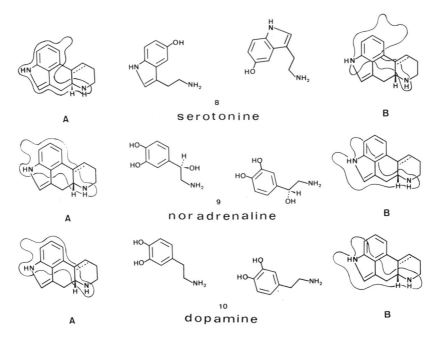

8
serotonine

9
noradrenaline

10
dopamine

A   B

Fig. 2. Possible 5-HT-, NA- and DA-pharmacophores of the ergoline ring system.

Binding studies in vitro

In any case, convincing evidence has been accumulated that ergolines can interfere with many receptor sites. To illustrate this, the IC50 values of several important ergot compounds at 8 different binding sites are given in Table I (Closse *et al.* 1983).

A typical representative of the genuine ergot peptide akaloids, ergotamine **1**, shows high affinity to serotonin—1 and —2, α-2 and α-1, dopamine-1 and -2 binding sites, whilst there is almost no affinity to the histamine-1 and the muscarinic-cholinergic binding sites.

In contrast to the complex binding profile of ergotamine, a more selective one is observed with nicergoline **27**, which shows a very high affinity to the α-1 binding sites, while binding to serotonin-1 and -2 is medium or poor to all other sites.

Although the values given in Table I should be interpreted with caution, it follows that ergot compounds can show quite different binding profiles and remarkably high affinity towards various binding sites and, hence, probably, to different types of receptors.

Table I

IC50 values of 8 ergot compounds at 8 different binding sites.

receptor-type	serotonine-1	serotonine-2	alpha-2	alpha-1	dopamine-1	dopamine-2	histamine-1	muscarinic cholinergic
membrane preparation from	whole rat brain	rat frontal cortex	rat brain minus cerebellus	whole rat brain	calf caudate	calf caudate	rat brain minus cerebellum	rat brain minus cerebellum
ligand	^3H-serotonine	^3H-spiperone	^3H-clonidine	^3H-WB-4101	^3H-dopamine	^3H-spiperone	^3H-pyrilamine	^3H-QNB
ergotamine 1	9 ± 1	4 ± 1	3 ± 1	22 ± 4	56 ± 10	7 ± 2	> 10'000	> 10'000
DHE 11	8 ± 1	13 ± 5	5 ± 1	15 ± 1	33 ± 7	9 ± 1	> 10'000	> 10'000
DH-ergocornine 23	85 ± 15	25 ± 3	5 ± 1	10 ± 3	50 ± 5	5 ± 1	> 10'000	> 10'000
LSD 32	44 ± 3	14 ± 3	65 ± 16	531 ± 6	30 ± 6	65 ± 5	1300 ± 150	inactive
nicergoline 27	175 ± 5	90 ± 3	825 ± 150	3 ± 1	2500 ± 250	1000 ± 100	6300 ± 750	550 ± 500
bromocriptine 35	225 ± 15	76 ± 15	29 ± 5	33 ± 7	84 ± 4	13 ± 3	inactive	> 10'000
CQ 32-084 48	5000	26 ± 4	480 ± 50	3300	120 ± 35	25 ± 5	1500 ± 200	inactive
mesulergine 49	< 10'000	15 ± 2	710 ± 250	4250	1400 ± 300	140 ± 15	6250 ± 750	inactive

The pluripotent biological action of the ergot alkaloids

In fact ergot alkaloids exhibit an astonishingly wide spectrum of biological actions, which is rarely found in any other group of natural products: α-adrenoreceptor blockade, serotonin antagonism, blood-pressure increasing or lowering activity, the already mentioned uterotonic activity, action on the central nervous system such as induction of hyperthermia, emesis, dopaminergic and neuroleptic activity and, finally, the newly discovered action on the secretion of pituitary hormones. In the last column of Table II (Berde & Stürmer 1978) a ratio between the highest and lowest activity of the listed compounds is given. These ratios range between 25 to more than 5000. Consequently, one of the tasks of the medicinal chemist working in the ergot field is to try to obtain compounds with a more selective rather than a higher biological activity. The relative predominance of these main effects varies from compound to compound. One or more activities may be completely absent and other effects may even be enhanced. Based on these biological effects, the search for substances of clinical value has yielded drugs against migraine and other vascular headaches, orthostatic circulatory disturbancies, senile cerebral insufficiency, hypertension in the elderly, infertility due to hyperprolactinemia, acromegaly, parkinsonism, tumor of hypophysis and last but not least uterine atonia.

30*

Table II

Activity profiles of some ergot compounds. The relative activities of 7 compounds on 10 biological parmameters are listed. The potency of the most active compound in each test beeing arbitrarily set at 1000.

Substance / Parameter	Ergot-amine	Bromo-criptine	Dihydro-ergotamine	Dihydro-ergotoxine mesylate[a]	Methyl-ergometrine	Methyser-gide	LSD	Max. Min.
α-Adrenoceptor blockade isol. guinea pig seminal vessel	50	230	350	1000	<0.4	<0.4	1	>2500
5HT-receptor blockade isol. rat uterus	10	3	40	10	250	1000	250	330
Pressor activity spinal cat, i.v.	1000	<10	120	30	<10	30	10	>100
Uterotonic activity rabbit in situ, i.v.	500	Inhibition of Me-ergo-metrine	Inhibition of Me-ergo-metrine	Inhibition of Me-ergo-metrine	1000	40	670	>1000
Inhibition of fertility in rats, s.c.	50	1000	<40	70	<80	<40	<40	>25
Influence on body temperature, rabbit, i.v.	+ 3	+ 2.5	−	−	+ 14	+ 0.2	+ 1000	>5000
Emetic activity in the dog, i.v.	1000	410	85	540	210	<1	<3	>1000
Dopaminergic stereotyped behaviour in rats, i.p.	<1	630	<1	<1	310	<1	1000	>1000
Contralateral turning behaviour in rats, 6-OHDA leasioned, s.c.	<1	1000	<1	10	400	<1	730	>1000
Inhibition of NA-stimulated cAMP-synthesis in rat cerebral cortex slices in vitro	400	190	240	1000	2.5	5	60	400

ANTIMIGRAINE ERGOT COMPOUNDS

For the treatment of migraine attack, ergotamine 1, was introduced into therapy in 1928 (Tzanck 1928, Trautmann 1928) on the assumption that its curative effect was due to its sympathicolytic action. Even today the underlying mechanism of action is not well understood, however, the vasoconstrictor activity of 1 appears to be at least partly responsible for it. To abort the beginning of a migraine attack, ergotamine had to be injected i.v. because of its slow onset of action after oral administration. This disadvantage was partly overcome by a combination of 1 with caffein: Cafergot® is effective by the oral route.

A favorable change in the spectrum of activity occurred when the double bond at position 9, 10 in the lysergic acid moiety of ergotamine 1 was hydrogenated: the symphathicolytic-adrenolytic effects were specifically enhanced, whereas vasoconstriction and stimulation of central sympathetic structures were attenuated. Consequently dihydroergotamine 11, DHE, was introduced as prophylactic agent for the treatment of migraine. DHE shows beneficial effects in the treatment of other forms of vascular headache also.

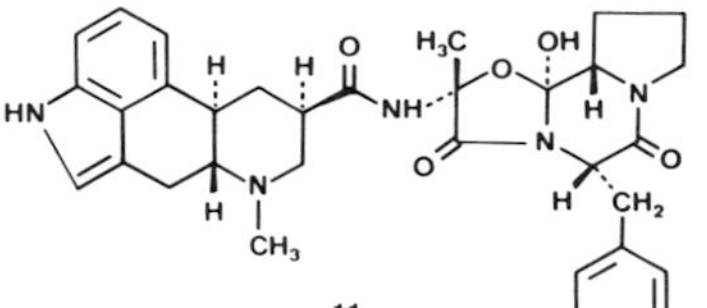

11

dihydroergotamine . DHE

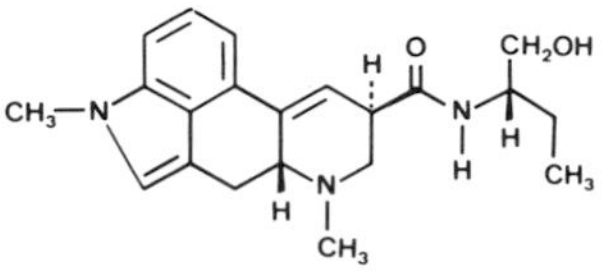

12

methysergide

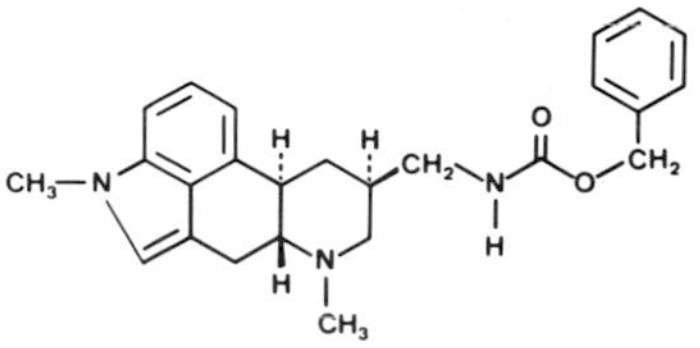

13

methergoline , MCE

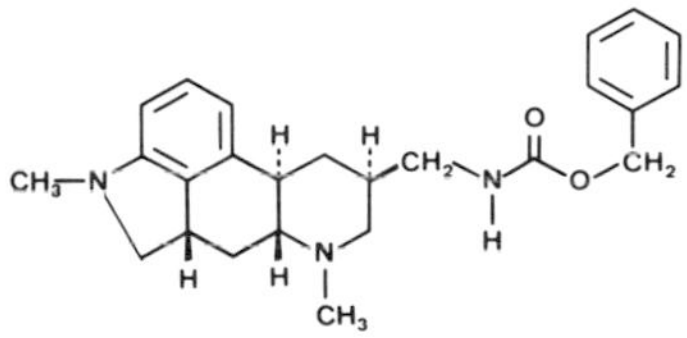

14

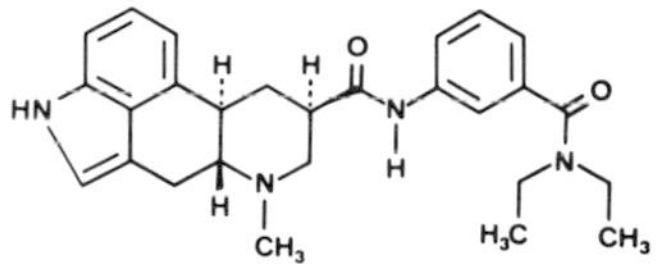

15

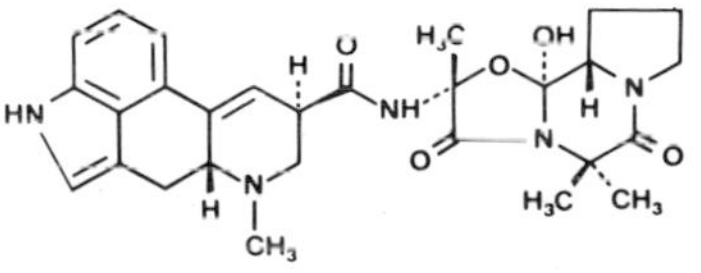

16

Fig. 3. Ergot drugs for the treatment of migraine, vascular headache and other compounds, which have been developed.

In 1957, a procedure for the selective methylation of N-1 in the ergoline ring system using liquid ammonia followed by methyliodide was developed (Bernardi *et al.* 1964). Among many derivatives prepared by this method methysergide **12**, the 1-methyl-derivative of methylergometrine **3**, attracted the interest because of its very strong and selective serotonin antagonistic effect. The hydrogen maleinate of methysergide **12**, Deseril®, was succesfully introduced into therapy for the treatment of carcinoid syndrome and, later, it turned out to be the most effective substance for the prevention of migraine attacks.

Methergoline **13**, easily obtained from 1,6-dimethyl-8-β-amino methyl-ergoline (Bernardi *et al.* 1964), was developed because of its high antiserotonin activity on the rat uterus (Beretta *et al.* 1965), and, later, for its favorable spectrum of activity in man, was introduced to the market under the trade name of Liserdol®* for the treatment of migraine and vascular headaches. In the corresponding 2,3-dihydro-derivative **14**, another potent serotonin antagonist was found (Arcamone & Franceschi 1973).

However, already in the early 1960's a way to the systematic variation of ergotamine was opened (Stadler *et al.* 1964b, Hofmann *et al.* 1963). A result of this work was, for example, the ergopeptine-derivative **16**, called 5'-methyl-ergoalanine (Stadler *et al.* 1971). Under the code name MD-121 this compound was found to be the most active vasoconstrictor of the ergopeptine series in man, about 6-times more active than ergotamine. Nevertheless, because of its very strong side effects MD-121 had to be dropped.

The same fate was shared by the N-dihydrolysergoyl-m-amino-benzoic acid diethylamide **15**, which showed a selective action on veins. Its development was stopped because of toxicity problems (Stadler 1978).

Coming back to DHE **11**, it has to be emphasized that its clinical indication is not restricted to migraine prophylaxis. Due to its action on α-adrenoceptors, **11** is able to constrict hypotonous veins rather selectively. This venotonic effect has proved beneficial for the treatment of orthostatic disorders (trade name: Dihydergot®). Furthermore, in combination with heparine, **11** has found broad application in post-operative prophylaxis of thrombosis and embolism, where the DHE component reduces venous stasis.

ERGOT ALKALOIDS OF THE DIHYDRO-ERGOTOXINE GROUP

Besides DHE, other dihydro-derivatives of natural ergot peptide alkaloids show interesting profiles of activity. The most important ones are listed in Fig. 4.

Dihydroergocristine **23**, enlarges arterioles and precapillary segments, but has a tonic action on veins. Its indications are therefore edemas, varicose illnesses and chronic venous insufficiency. In the form of the mesylate **23**, it constitutes a component of the antihypertensive Brinerdine® and of the venotonic Sandovene®.

---

* Registered trade mark of Farmitalia.

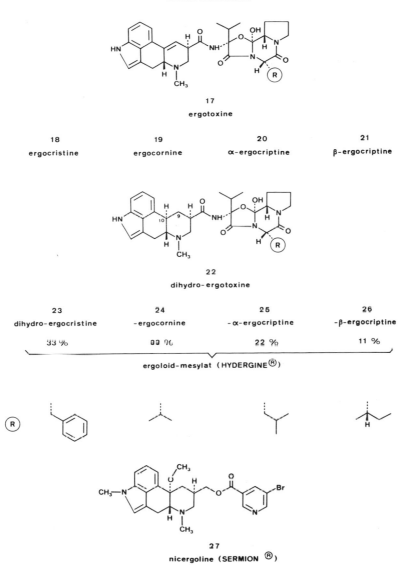

17

ergotoxine

18   19   20   21

ergocristine   ergocornine   α-ergocriptine   β-ergocriptine

22

dihydro-ergotoxine

23   24   25   26

dihydro-ergocristine -ergocornine   -α-ergocriptine   -β-ergocriptine

33 %   99 %   22 %   11 %

ergoloid-mesylat (HYDERGINE®)

27

nicergoline (SERMION ®)

Fig. 4. The genuine ergot alkaloids of the ergotoxine group, dihydroergotoxine and nicergoline.

Catalytic hydrogenation of ergotoxine **17**, which is a mixture from natural sources of the 4 genuine ergot peptide alkaloids ergocristine **18**, ergocornine **19**, α- and β-ergocriptine **20** and **21**, yielded a valuable new medicament in 1943 (Stoll & Hofmann 1943b). The drug consists of one third dihydroergocristine **23**, one third dihydroergocornine **24** and one third of a 2:1 mixture of dihydro-α and β-ergocriptine **25** and **26**, all in the form of the mesylate. The generic is ergoloid-mesylate, the trade name Hydergine®. This drug was introduced into therapy as a mild antihypertensive agent, especially for the elderly; then clinical investigations revealed another important indication: Hydergine® improves many symptoms of cerebral insufficiency, related to age, by stimulating intellectual capabilities, ameliorating social behavior and promoting mood elevation. In addition, Hydergine® improves cerebral metabolism, especially of oxygen, and stabilizes the tonus of intra- and extracranial blood vessels. More recently, it could be demonstrated that it stimulates dopamine and serotonin receptors, blocks particularly presynaptic α-adrenoceptors, thus, enhancing the liberation of endogenous noradrenaline in the brain. Its mechanism of action is complex and still under further investigation (Ermini & Markstein 1982). However, its beneficial action in elderly people is well documented.

In consideration of the eminent importance of the discussed indications of Hydergine®, it is somehow strange that up to now, only one other ergot derivative, nicergoline **27** (Sermion®*), which is a potent blocking agent for α-1 adrenoceptors, has found use in the CNS-field (Bernardi *et al.* 1966, Arcari *et al.* 1972).

ERGOT DERIVATIVES WITH HYPOTENSIVE ACTION

Now and then, unwanted side effects like hypotension are observed with ergot compounds. An example for this is the natural clavine alcaloid lysergol **28** (Yamatodani 1960, Abe *et al.* 1961), which is easily obtainable by reduction of d-lysergic acid methylester (Stoll *et al.* 1949). Being a strong central dopaminergic agent lysergol is not selective enough. Beside hypotension, cardiovascular disturbances also appear as a side effect. To give an example of the efforts of many years ago in this field, the parmacochemistry of lysergol as a lead substance will be discussed in some detail.

The goal was to find an ergot derivative with more potent antihypertensive activity than that of lysergol, and devoid of the undesired side effects mentioned above. The method was, of course, variations of the lead molecule by partial synthesis.

---

* Registered trade mark of Farmitalia.

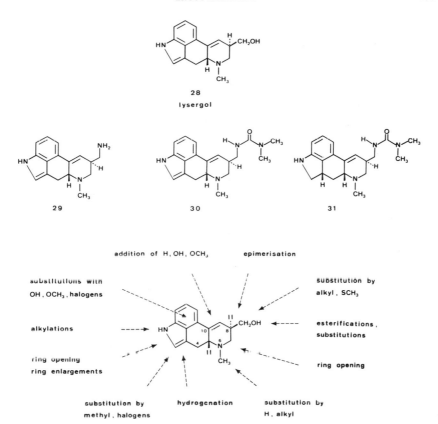

Fig. 5. Ergot derivatives with preponderant hypotensive activity and other chemical modifications performed on lysergol.

Initially, lysergol **28** was converted into the amino-derivative **29**, which proved to be a good starting point for further modifications. For example the corresponding N-formyl derivative exhibited a much higher antihypertensive activity than the lead **28**. Among a series of amido-, urethan- and urea-derivatives of **29**, compound **30** showed a very high, long-lasting and fairly specific antihypertensive activity, and an acceptable acute toxicity in mice and rats (Fehr *et al.* 1974). A single dose of 0.05 mg/kg remarkably lowered the blood pressure in Grollmann-rats (Grollmann 1944), the effect lasting for more than a day. Consequently, **30** was chosen for further development. In the clinic, low doses of 2 to 4 mg lowered blood-pressure considerably, but at higher doses vomiting occurred occasionally. So **30** was abandoned.

In the 2,3-dihydro derivative **31** the next candidate for development was found (Gull *et al.* 1978). But, in clinical trials, **31** showed no advantage in comparison to **30** and, therefore, was also discarded. The most important chemical modifications performed on lysergol are indicated at the foot of Fig. 5. At the moment the aim to find a selective antihypertensive agent on the basis of a simple ergoline derivative has not been reached and the hunt is still continuing.

ERGOT DERIVATIVES ACTING MAINLY ON THE CNS

Another challenging aspect of ergot pharmacochemistry which has not yielded substantial new results either, except for the action on basal ganglia and the hypothalamic tract (*vide infra*) is the selection of derivatives acting specifically on the central nervous system. The reason for this may be the notorious hallucinogenic properties of LSD **32** (Hofmann 1979), which led the scientists involved to step back from this project. However, it has to be noted that LSD, applied at subhallucinogenic doses in man, still shows anxiolytic and anti-depressive activities. It is regrettable that the separation of these highly valuable effects from the hallucinogenic ones by a systematic variation of the LSD molecule has not been attempted.

Compound **33**, easily accessible by reaction of lysergol-mesylate with azabicyclo[3,2,2]nonane (Stadler & Stuetz 1974), produced sedative effects in mice, an inhibition of conditioned avoidance behaviour in rats, was ineffective

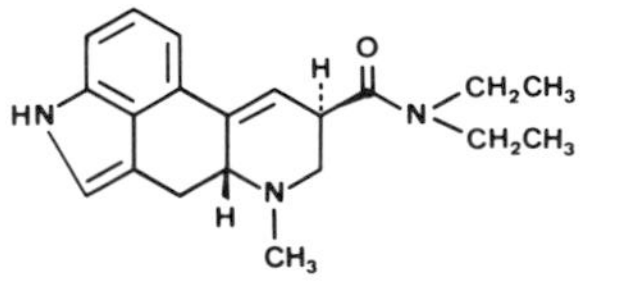

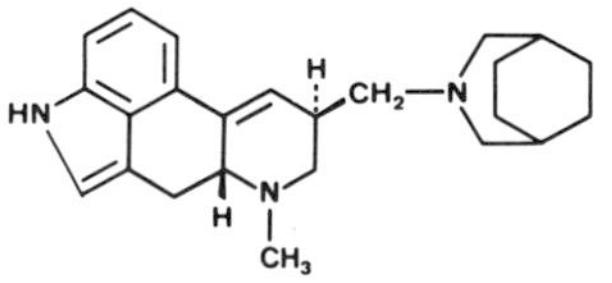

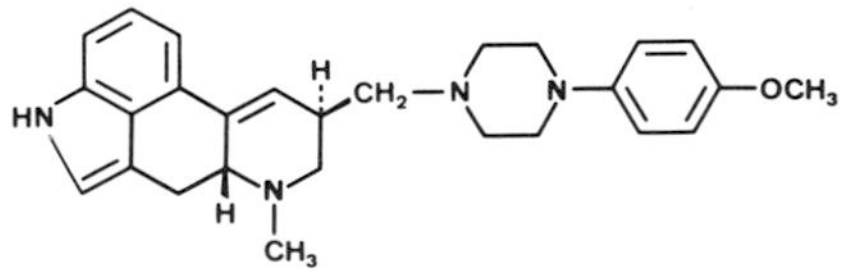

Fig. 6. Ergot compounds with preponderant activities on the central nervous system.

in peripheral circulation tests and, because of this unique pattern of activity, was selected from a series of dialkylated lysergylamines, for development. Its high sedative potency was confirmed in other animal species, but at higher doses leucocytopenia occurred occasionally and this compound had to be dropped.

Of a series of about 100 compounds with similar structure, PTR 17-402 **34**, attracted attention by its high psychostimulant effects on the CNS of rats and mice (Troxler & Hofmann 1971). Although fears that **34** might be hallucinogenic were disproved by administration to volunteers, it was, nevertheless, abandoned because clear-cut therapeutic efficacy in depressed and geriatric patients could not be found.

The discussed failures in ergot pharmacochemistry indicate that although many of the prepared compounds showed the desired activities in preliminary pharmacological tests, to obtain a valuable drug, even starting from a good lead, is still a difficult task. In fact selectivity rather than high biological activity is the main problem that has to be solved. This appears to be particularly difficult in the ergot field, as the deduction of structure-activity relationships seems to be practicable only within a narrowly restricted series of homologues.

DOPAMINERGIC ERGOT COMPOUNDS

The year 1954 saw the opening of a new and exciting chapter in the medicinal chemistry and pharmacology of ergot. Shelesnyak reported his finding that ergotoxine **17** (Fig. 4), prevented deciduoma formation in pseudopregnant rats, which led him to conclude that ergotoxine **17** acts via the hypothalamus and pituitary by inhibiting prolactin secretion (Shelesnyak 1954). This was the first observation of the agonistic action of ergot alkaloids on dopamine receptors. For about 10 years, this discovery remained without further consequences. However, after it was realized that ergocriptine, hitherto considered to be a single entity, was actually a mixture of the 2 alkaloids α- and β-ergocriptine, **20** and **21** respectively (Schlientz *et al.* 1967, 1968), the α-form beeing the most active genuine alkaloid of the peptide type in the Shelesnyak test, a great number of new ergopeptide alkaloids were prepared and tested, with the aim of retaining specific prolactin-inhibiting activity and eliminating the oxytocic and vasoconstrictor side effects of the parent compound **20**. This objective was finally reached with 2-bromo-α-ergocriptine-mesylate **35**, later named bromocriptine (Schneider *et al.* 1977). In comparison to α-ergocriptine, bromocriptine showed a higher antiprolactin activity (Flueckiger & Wagner 1968). Clinical results with

35 indicating for the first time the suppression of prolactin secretion in man, were published in 1971 (Lutterbeck *et al.* 1971). Soon afterwards, evidence for a stimulation of central dopamine neurons by bromocriptine was found (Corrodi *et al.* 1973). Finally, about 6 years ago, bromocriptine was registered with the brand the name Parlodel®, Pravidel® in the indications: prolactin-dependent diseases like galactorrhea, infertility, growth hormone-dependent acromegaly, prolactinomas and Parkinsonism. Last, but not least, it has to be mentioned that bromocriptine was shown to possess antidepressive properties comparable to the classic tricyclic antidepressants (Theohar *et al.* 1981, 1982).

In Fig. 7, some structure-activity relationships of bromocriptine derivatives are given. As a screening test, the inhibition of implantation in inseminated rats was used (Flueckiger *et al.* 1978), the potency of bromocriptine being arbitrarily set at 100. Even minor molecular changes led to substantial losses of biological activity, for example: methylation in position 1, epimerisation in 8 or 5' and hydrogenation of the 9, 10 double bond. The structures of the alkyl substituents in position 2' and 5' are critical for the activity: at 2' maximum activity is obtained with isopropyl and in 5' with isobutyl. Knowing that the peptide part alone, is devoid of any pharmacological action, the fact that even minor structural variations of this moiety leads to remarkable changes is quite surprising.

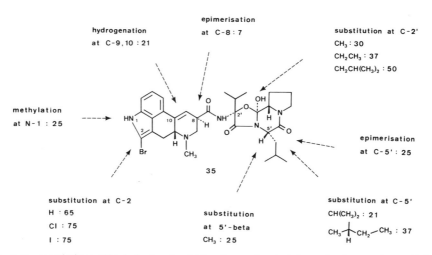

Fig. 7. Bromocriptine and its derivatives in which only one chemical change has been performed. The values given represent the relative activities in % in comparison to the activity of bromocriptine 35 in the inhibition of the implantation in rats.

Simple ergoline derivatives

Already 15 years ago, parallel to the efforts in the ergopeptide alkaloids field, the search for compounds with high and specific central dopaminergic activity was focussed on simple ergolines. Some natural ergolines such as agroclavine **36**, elymoclavine **37**, lysergol **28** and dihydrolysergol **38**, which exhibit high, albeit unspecific, dopaminergic activity (Edwardson 1968, Mantle 1968) were selected as starting material for chemical modifications.

At that time, the Ungerstedt model was proposed as a screening test for central dopaminergic activity (Ungerstedt 1971, Ungerstedt & Arbuthnott 1970). Extensive chemical work led to a large group of development compounds, which are listed in Fig. 9.

The homolysergic acid nitril **39** was prepared in 1966 (Troxler & Stadler 1968a, 1968b). Four close derivatives of this substance, all with hydrogenated D-ring were developed by different companies and reached the clinics. The most potent one was CM 29-712, **41**. However, all had to be dropped because other compounds were found to be more interesting.

In 1946, it was found that 8-α' and 8-β-amino-ergolenes and -ergolines can easily be prepared by Curtius degradation of the corresponding hydrazides of lysergic- and dihydrolysergic acid (Hofmann 1946). In this, as well as among the group of substances mentioned above, the highest activities are obtained with the α-orientation of the substituent at C-8. The best-known compound is probably lisuride **44** (Zikan & Semonsky 1960). Its hydrogen maleinate has been introduced into therapy as antiprolactin agent in 1982, under the trade name Dopergin®*.

While **44** is a strong dopamine agonist, dihydrolisuride **45** is a mixed agonist-antagonist (Wachtel & Dorow 1983), and 2-bromo-lisuride **46** is a dopamine

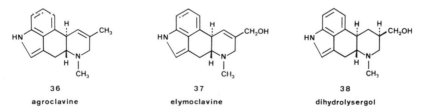

| 36 | 37 | 38 |
| agroclavine | elymoclavine | dihydrolysergol |

Fig. 8. Natural ergot alkaloids choosen for chemical modification on the search of central dopaminergic agents.

---

* Registered trade mark of Schering AG.

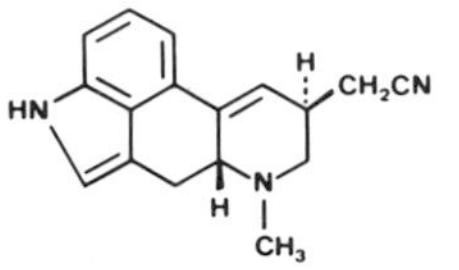

Fig. 9. Ergot derivatives developed as central dopaminergic agents.

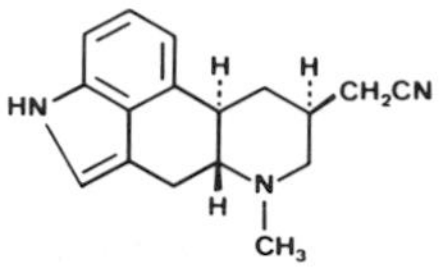

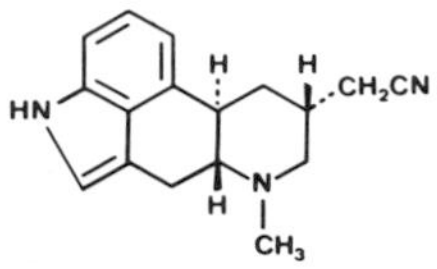

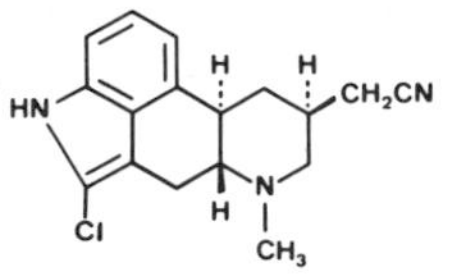

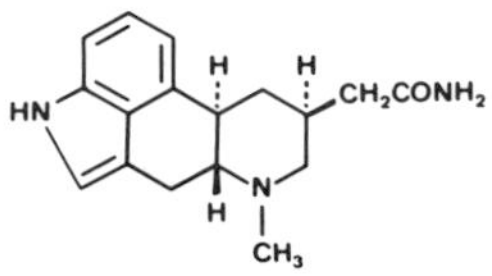

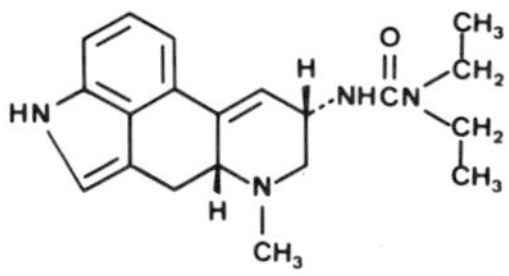

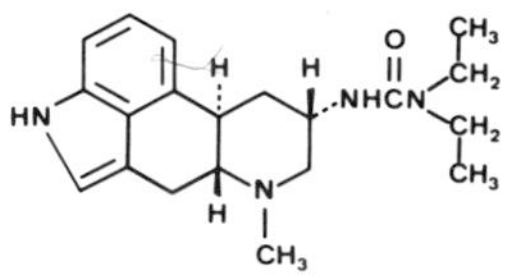

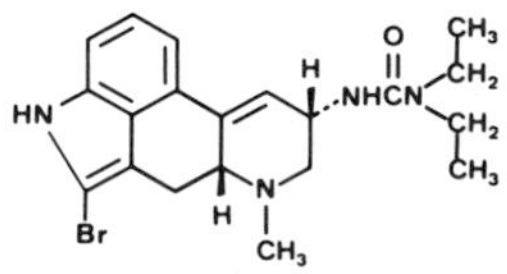

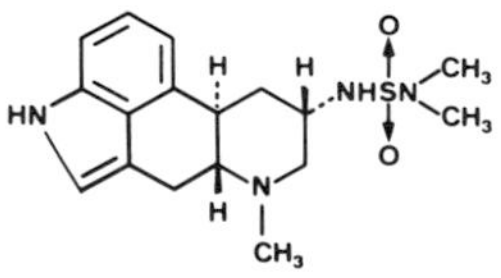

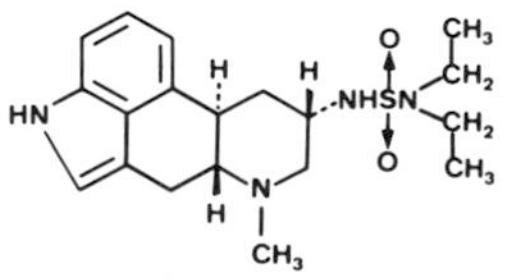

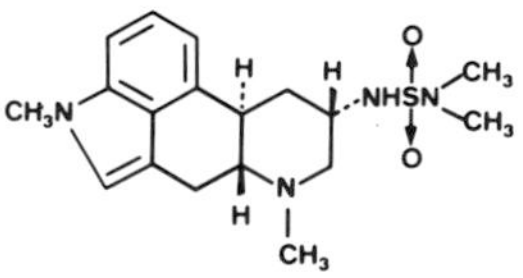

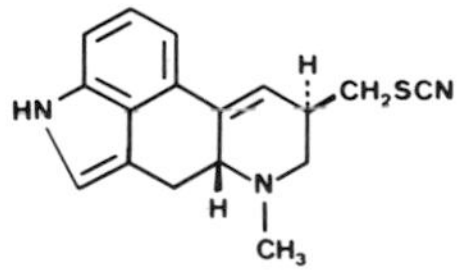

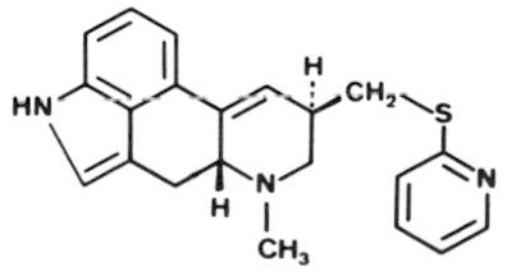

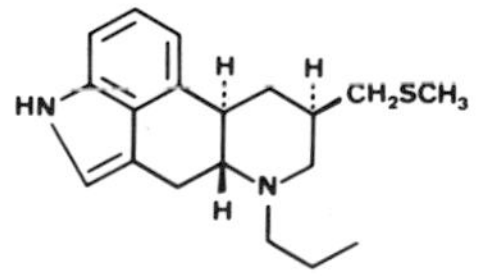

antagonist (Wachtel 1983), and might be useful as a neuroleptic agent. From the lower row of compound CU 32-085, **49** (Stuetz *et al.* 1982) looks most promising as anti-Parkinson agent in clinical trials (Flueckiger *et al.* 1983).

A simple derivative of thiolysergol, the rhodanide **50**, was one of the first compounds selected for development as anti-Parkinson agent. It was later abandoned in favour of CF 25-397 **51**, which showed a unique pharmacological profile (Stuetz *et al.* 1978), being selectively active in the Ungerstedt-test. In clinic, **51** was not convincing as anti-Parkinson agent, it was further investigated in geriatric conditions, but was not satisfactory in other respects and was discarded. It has been more common with ergot than other drugs that clinical results imposed a shift to different or new medical uses.

Finally, pergolide **52**, a very highly active central dopaminergic agent, is undergoing clinical trials and most probably will be commercialized in the near future (Fuller *et al.* 1979).

NEW COMPOUNDS BASED ON THE ERGOLINE PARTIAL STRUCTURE
In recent years, increasing interest was shown for compounds whose structure contains only portions of the ergoline skeleton. The pyrazoles **53** and **54**, both related to pergolide **52**, belong to this group and showed high and more selective

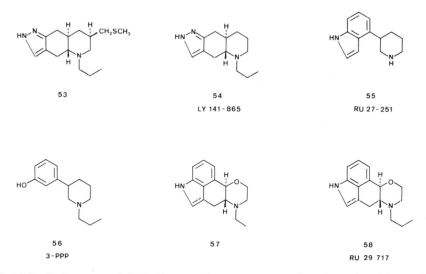

Fig. 10. Synthetic compounds in development whose structure contains only portion of the ergoline skeleton and close derivatives of them.

action, particularly a very selective D2-dopaminergic activity, but a shorter half life than the corresponding ergolines (Kornfeld *et al.* 1982). **54** exhibited besides bradycardia, dilation of blood vessels and, hence, antihypertensive activity (Hahn *et al.* 1983). The underlying mechanisms of action being peripheral presynaptic dopamine agonism.

RU 27-251 **55** was reported to act in animals selectively on the pituitary, decreasing prolactin levels: confirmation of this highly interesting finding in man has not yet been obtained (Boissier *et al.* 1982).

With 3-PPP **56** it has been shown that a reduction of the ergoline ring system to a bicyclic structure is possible without loss of the dopaminergic activity (Hjort *et al.* 1981, Nilsson *et al.* 1982).

The 9-oxa-ergolines **57** (Jones 1980) and **58** (Nedelec *et al.* 1983) developed almost simultaneously by 2 different laboratories, show that for high dopaminergic activity a substituent at C-8 is not essential, and that an oxygen at C-9 rather strengthens potency, since **58** is reported to be equipotent with pergolide.

The high number of compounds under development with dopaminergic activity presented in this review gives an idea of the potential of pharmaco-chemical research stimulated by the forerunner bromocriptine. There are good reasons to assume that clinical applications of these drugs are far from being exhausted yet. Besides the established action of the ergot on the secretion of prolactin and growth hormone, effects on other hormones like the gonado-tropins (LH) could be found in animal experiments.

It is, therefore, reasonable to expect that new indications for the ergot compounds will be discovered in the near future. Ergot was and still is a real treasure house for valuable drugs!

REFERENCES

Abe, M., Yamatodani, S., Yamano, T. & Kusumoto, M. (1961) Isolation of lysergol, lysergene and lysergine from saprophytic cultures of ergot fungi. *Agric. Biol. Chem. (Tokio) 25,* 594–595.

Arcamone, F. & Franceschi, G. (1973) *Ger. Auslegeschrift 1'695'752.*

Arcari, G., Bernardi, L., Bosisio, G., Coda, S., Fregnan, G. B. & Glaesser, A. H. (1972) 10-Methoxyergoline derivatives as alpha-adrenergic blocking agents. *Experientia 28,* 819–820.

Bach, N. J., Kornfeld, E. C., Jones, N. D., Chaney, M. O., Dorman, D. E., Paschal, J. W., Clemens, J. A. & Smalstig, E. B. (1980) Bicyclic and tricyclic ergoline partial structures. Rigid 3-(2-aminoethyl)pyrroles and 3- and 4-(2-aminoethyl)pyrazoles as dopamine agonists. *J. Med. Chem. 23,* 481–491.

Berde, B., Stürmer, E. (1978) in B. Berde & H. O. Schild, *Ergot Alkaloids and Related Compounds,* Springer Berlin, page 4.

Beretta, C., Ferrini, R. & Glaesser, A. (1965) 1-Methyl-8-beta-carbobenzyloxy-aminomethyl-10-

alpha-ergoline, a potent and long-lasting 5-hydroxytryptamine antagonist. *Nature 207,* 421–422.

Bernardi, L., Camerino, B., Patelli, P. & Redaelli, S. (1964) Ergolines. I. Derivatives of D-6-methyl-8-beta-aminomethyl-10-alpha-ergoline. *Gazz. Chim. Ital. 94,* 936–946.

Bernardi, L., Bosisio, G. & Goffredo, O. (1966) U.S. Patent 3'228'943.

Boissier, J. R., Nedelec, C., Oberlander, C. & Labrie, F. (1982) Simplified ergolines as new dopamine agonists. *Acta Pharmaceutica Suecica, Suppl. 1983:2,* 120–131.

Closse, A., Frick, W., Dravid, A., Bolliger, G., Hauser, D., Sauter, A. & Tobler, H. J. (1983) Classification of drugs according to receptor binding profiles, (in preparation).

Corrodi, H., Fuxe, K., Hoeckfeld, T., Lidbrink, P. & Ungersted, U. (1973) Effect of ergot drugs on central catechol amine neurons. Evidence for a stimulation of central dopamine neurons. *J. Pharm. Pharmacol. 25,* 409–412.

Dudley, H. W. & Moir, C. (1935) The substance responsible for the traditional clinical effect of ergot. *Br. Med. J. I,* 520–523.

Edwardson, J. A. (1968) The effects of agroclavine, an ergot alkaloid, on pregnancy and lactation in the rat. *Br. J. Pharmacol. 33,* 215–216.

Ermini, M. & Markstein, R. (1982) Hydergine therapy: mechanism of action. *Br. J. Clin. Pract. Symp. Suppl. 16,* 27–31.

Fehr, T., Stuetz, P., Stadler, P. A., Hummel, R. & Salzmann, R. (1974) Antihypertensiv wirksame Harnstoffderivate des 8-beta-Aminomethyl-6-methyl-ergolens. *Eur. J. Med. Chem. 9,* 597–601.

Flueckiger, E. & Wagner, H. R. (1968) 2-Br-alpha-Ergokryptin: Beeinflussung von Fertilitaet und Laktation bei der Ratte. *Experientia 24,* 1130–1131.

Flueckiger, E., Briner, U., Doepfner, W., Kovacs, E., Marbach, P. & Wagner, H. R. (1978) Prolactin secretion inhibition by a new 8-alpha-amino-ergoline, CH 29-717. *Experientia 34,* 1330–1332.

Flueckiger, E., Briner, U., Enz, A., Markstein, R. & Vigouret, J. M. (1983) *Dopaminergic Ergot Compounds:* an overwiev. Lisuride and other dopamine agonists. Ed. by D. B. Calne *et al.,* pp 1–9. Raven Press, New York.

Fregnan, G. B. & Glaesser, A. (1968) Structure-activity relationship of various acyl derivatives of 6-methyl-8-beta-aminomethyl-10-α-ergoline (dihydrolysergamine). *Experientia 24,* 150–151.

Fuller, R. W., Clemens, J. A., Kornfeld, E. C., Snoddy, H. D., Smalstig, E. B. & Bach, N. J. (1979) Effects of (8-beta)-8-[(methylthio)methyl]-6-propylergoline on dopaminergic function and brain dopamine turnover in rats. *Life Sci. 24,* 375–382.

Grollman, A. (1944) A simplified procedure for inducing chronic renal hypertension in the mammal. *Proc. Soc. Exp. Biol. Med. 57,* 102–104.

Gull, P., Haut, H. & Pfaeffli, P. (1978) *Ger. Offen.* 2'810'774.

Hahn, R. H., Macdonald, B. R. & Martin, M. A. (1983) Antihypertensive activity of LY141865, a selective presynaptic dopamine receptor agonist, *J. Pharmacol. Exp. Ther. 224,* 206–214.

Hjort, S., Carlsson, A., Wikstroem, H., Lindberg, P., Sanchez, D., Hacksell, U., Arvidsson, L.-E., Svensson, U. & Nilsson, J. L. G. (1981) 3-PPP, a new centrally acting DA-receptor agonist with selectivity for autoreceptors. *Life Sci. 28,* 1225–1238.

Hofmann, A. (1946) Uber den Curtius'schen Abbau der isomeren Lysergsaeuren und Dihydrolysergsaeuren. *Helv. Chim. Acta 30,* 44–51.

Hofmann, A., Ott, H., Griot, R., Stadler, P. A. & Frey, A. J. (1963) Die Synthese und Stereochemie des Ergotamins. *Helv. Chim. Acta 46,* 2306–2328.

Hofmann, A. (1979) *LSD-Mein Sorgenkind,* Verlag: Klett-Cotta.

Jones, J. H. (1980) U.S. Pat. 4'238'486.

Kharash, M. S. & Legault, R. R. (1935) New active principles of ergot. *Science 81,* 388, 614–615.

Kornfeld, E. C., Bach, N. J., Titus, R. D., Nichols, C. L. & Clements, J. A. (1982) Ergoline and apomorphine partial structures and hybrids. *Acta Pharm. Suecica Suppl. 1983, 2,* 83–97.

Lindberg, P., Wikstroem, H., Sanchez, D., Arvidson, L.-E., Hacksell, U., Nilsson, J. L. G., Hjorth, S. & Carlsson, A. (1982) A structural comparison between dopamine- and serotonine-receptor agonist. *Acta Pharm. Suecica, Suppl. 1983, 2,* 48–55.

Lutterbeck, P. M., Pryor, J. S., Varga, L. & Wenner, R. (1971) Treatment of non-puerperal galactorrhoea with an ergot alkaloid. *Br. Med. J. 3,* 228–229.

Mantle, P. G. (1968) Inhibition of lactation in mice following feeding with ergot sclerotia (*Claviceps fusiformis*) from the bulrush millet (*Pennisetum typhoides*) and an alkaloid component. *Proc. R. Soc. Ser. B. 170,* 423–434.

Nedelec, L., Pierdet, A., Faveau, P., Euvrard, C., Proulx-Ferland, L., Dumont, C., Labrie, F. & Boissier, J. R. (1983) Synthesis and central dopaminergic activities of racemic hexahydro-7H-indolo[3,4-gh]-[1,4]benzoxazine derivatives (racemic 9-oxaergolines). *J. Med. Chem. 26,* 522–527.

Nichols, D. E. (1976) Structural correlation between apomorphine and LSD. Involvement of dopamine as well as serotonine in the action hallucinogens. *J. Theor. Biol. 59,* 167–177.

Nilsson, J. L. G., Ardvidsson, L. E., Hacksell, U., Johansson, A., Svenson, U., Carlson, A., Hjoerth, S., Lindberg, P., Sanchez, D. & Wikstroem, H. (1982) Design of new agonists for dopamine- and serotonine receptors. *Acta Pharm. Suecica, Suppl. 1983,2,* 37–47.

Rutschmann, J. & Schreier, E. (1965) Swiss Pat. Nr. 394225.

Shelesnyak, M. C. (1954) Ergotoxine inhibition of deciduoma formation and its reversal by progesterone. *Am. J. Physiol. 179,* 301–304.

Schlientz, W., Brunner, R., Ruegger, A., Berde, B., Stuermer, E. & Hofmann, A. (1967) Beta-Ergokryptine, a new alcaloid of the ergotoxinc group. *Experientia 23,* 991–992.

Schlientz, W., Brunner, R., Ruegger, A., Berde, B., Stuermer, E. & Hofmann, A. (1968) Beta-Ergokryptin, ein neues Alkaloid der Ergotoxin-Gruppe. *Pharm. Acta Helv. 43,* 497–509.

Schneider, H. R., Stadler, P. A., Stuetz, P., Troxler, F. & Seres, J. (1977) Synthese und Eigenschaften von Bromokryptin. *Experientia 33,* 1412–1413.

Stadler, P. A., Frei, A. J., Troxler, F. & Hofmann, A. (1964a) Selektive Reduktions- und Oxydationsreaktionen an Lysersaure-Derivaten. 2,3-Dihydro und 12-Hydroxy-Lysergsaure-amide. *Helv. Chim. Acta 47,* 756–769.

Stadler, P. A., Frei, A. J., Ott, H. & Hofmann, A. (1964b) Die Synthese des Ergosins und des Valin-Analogen der Ergotamin-Gruppe. *Helv. Chim. Acta 47,* 1911–1921.

Stadler, P. A., Hofmann, A. & Troxler, F. (1971) Swiss Pat. 503'031.

Stadler, P. A. & Stuetz, P. (1973) Swiss Pat. Nr. 534683.

Stadler, P. A. & Stuetz, P. (1974) US-Patent 3'833'585.

Stadler, P. A. (1978) *Ger. Offenlegung* 2'802'023.

Stoll, A. (1918) Swiss Pat. 79879.

Stoll, A. & Burckhardt, E. (1935) Ergobasine, a new water-soluble alkaloid from Seigel ergot. *C. R. Acad. Sci Paris 200,* 1680–1682.

Stoll, A. & Hofmann, A. (1938) Partialsynthese des Ergobasins, eines natuerlichen Mutterkorn-alkaloids sowie seines optischen Antipoden. *Hoppe-Seyler's Z. Physiol. Chem. 251,* 155–163.

Stoll, A. & Hofmann, A. (1943a) Partialsynthese von Alkaloiden vom Typus des Ergobasins. *Helv. Chim. Acta 26,* 944–965.

Stoll, A. & Hofmann, A. (1943b) Die Dihydroderivate der natuerlichen linksdrehenden Mutter-kornalkaloide. *Helv. Chim. Acta 26,* 2070–2081.

Stoll, A., Hofmann, A. & Schlientz, W. (1949) Die stereoisomeren Lysergole und Dihydro-lysergole. *Helv. Chim. Acta 32,* 1947–1956.

Stuetz, P. L., Stadler, P. A., Vigouret, J. M. & Jaton, A. (1978) Ergot alkaloids. New ergolines as selective dopaminergic stimulants. *J. Med. Chem. 21,* 754–757.

Stuetz, P. L., Stadler, P. A., Vigouret, J. M. & Jaton, A. (1982) Derivate von (5R, 8S, 10R)-8-Amino-6-methylergolin als zentral wirksame dopaminerge Stimulantien. *Eur. J. Med. Chem. 17,* 537–541.

Theohar, C., Fischer-Cornelssen, K., Akesson, H. O., Ansari, J., Gerlach, J., Harper, P., Ohman, R., Ose, E. & Stegink, A. J. (1981) Bromocriptine as antidepressant. *Curr. Ther. Res. 30,* 830–842.

Theohar, C., Fischer-Cornelssen, K., Brosch, H., Fischer, E. K. & Petrovic, D. (1982) A comparative, multicenter trial between bromocriptine and amitriptyline in the treatment of endogenous depression. *Drug Res. 32 (II), 7,* 783–787.

Thompson, M. R. (1935) Active principles of ergot. *Science 81,* 636–639.

Trautmann, E. (1928) Die Beeinflussung migraeneartiger Zustaende durch ein sympathikus-hemmendes Mittel (Gynergen). *Muench. Med. Wochenschr. 75,* 513.

Troxler, F. & Stadler, P. A. (1968a) French Patent 1'439'953.

Troxler, F. & Stadler, P. A. (1968b) Ergot alkaloide. LXVIII. Partial synthesis of 6 methyl 8-ergolene-8-beta-acetic acid and some of its derivatives. *Helv. Chim. Acta 51,* 1060–1068.

Troxler, F. & Hofmann, A. (1971) Swiss Pat. 505'828.

Tzanck, A. (1928) Le traitement des migraines par le tartrate d'ergotamine. *Bull. Mem. Soc. Med. Hop. Paris 44,* 1057–1061.

Ungerstedt, U. & Arbuthnott, G. W. (1970) Quantitative recording of rotational behavior in rats after 6-hydroxy-dopamine lesions of the nigrostriatal dopamine system. *Brain Res. 24,* 485–493.

Ungerstedt, U. (1971) Postsynaptic supersensitivity after 6-hydroxy-dopamine-induced degeneration of the nigro-striatal dopamine system. *Acta Physiol. Scand. Suppl. 367,* 69–93.

Wachtel, H. (1983) 2-Bromolisuride: an ergot derivative with potential neuroleptic activity. *Kongressband der Fruehtagung der Deutschen Pharmakologischen Gesellschaft, Mainz, Nr. 360,* page R90.

Wachtel, H. & Dorow, R. (1983) Dual action on central dopamine function of trans-dihydro-lisuride, a 9,10-dihydrogenated analogue of the ergot dopamine agonist lisuride. *Life Sci. 32,* 421–432.

Yamatodani, S. (1960) Ergot fungus. XLII. Some derivatives of the clavine series ergot akaloids. *Takeda Kenkyusho Nempo 19,* 15–24.

Zikan, V. & Semonsky, M. (1960) Mutterkornalkaloide XVI. Einige N-(D-6-Methylisoergolenyl-8)-, N-(D-6-Methylergolenyl-8)- und N-(D-6-Methylergolin(I)-yl-8)-N'-substituierte Harnstoffe. *Collect. Czech. Chem. Commun. 25,* 1922–1928.

DISCUSSION

ANDERSON: In our work on the 9-oxa-ergolines we also prepared isomers with the unnatural absolute configuration. During this work we made the interesting discovery that at least in the oxa-ergolines concerned, the a-adrenergic agonist activity resides only in one of the optical antipodes. Have you made similar observations in connection with you work on the ergolines? Have you looked at any of the unnatural isomers.

GIGER: Yes, we did, and we found the same thing in the ergolene series.

KROGSGAARD-LARSEN: You mentioned that the sub-hallucinogenic doses, LSD had anxiolytic effects. Does the structure-activity analysis of your compounds allow you to suggest which profile of LSD is responsible for the anxiolytic effect?

GIGER: This is very difficult. Actually, you can only sort this out from studies in man, and we did not test many compounds in this study.

ARCAMONE: We have always been curious to know why Sandoz has always preferred to work on the unsaturated derivatives, although, as you have already shown, the 9,10-dihydro-compounds maintain all the activities of the alkaloids and also are more stable. My second question is: what is known about the metabolism of bromocriptine and related compounds?

GIGER: We actually do prefer to work on the dihyro-derivatives because, as you said, they are more stable and they are better tolerated. One of the problems of ergot in terms of therapeutic application is to reduce toxicity. About the metabolism of bromocriptine and related compounds in man we did not know very much until recently (1,2). The reason for this is that we apply very low doses, only a few mg, and, therefore, it is not easy to map out the metabolism. I can give you the following pieces of information: the peptide part appears to prevent metabolism of the lysergic acid part. With bromocriptine we don't find metabolites of the lysergic acid moiety. In fact, we can detect 2 major pathways. The first one involves metabolism in the proline ring. This is the principle metabolism attack. Then we have a minor pathway: the hydrolytic cleavage of the amide bridge, which cuts the 2 molecules into 2 pieces. We still don't know if these metabolites are active or not.

RAPOPORT: I assume you are making your dihydro-derivatives by catalytic hydrogenation?

GIGER: Right.

RAPOPORT: Do these reactions proceed stereo-specifically?

GIGER: Yes.

WITKOP: Those who have read Albert Hoffmann's book "LSD – My Problem Child" may still wonder about the uniqueness of this molecule. Axelrod and I, a long time ago, studied its metabolism, and one of the effects of the hydroxylases is to attack the 2 position which you have protected by bromine. Are you able to shed more light on the unusual and unique properties of LSD?

GIGER: No, I don't think so. The work that was done on LSD is pretty old, and the company has not been interested in pursuing this work. A main difference between the ergot peptides and small molecules like LSD, appears to be that the small molecules give rise to metabolites originating in the lysergic acid moiety, as you pointed out in the case of LSD, and sometimes these metabolites are highly active. These metabolites should contribute to the spectrum of activity *in vivo*.

(1) Maurer, G., Schreier, E., Delaborde, S.,Loosli, H. R., Nufer, R. & Shula, A. P. (1982) *Eur. J. Drug. Met. & Pharmacokin 7,* 281–292.
(2) Maurer, G., Schreier, E., Delaborde, S., Nufer, R., Shukla, A. P. (1983) *Eur. J. Drug Met. & Pharmacokin 8,* 51–62.

Structure-Activity Studies and Development of Drugs from Cannabinoids

Raj K. Razdan

For generations man has treated diseases with a mixture of herbs and natural products known to possess pharmacological properties. It is only since the turn of the century that our scientific knowledge has led to the introduction of novel synthetic drugs for the treatment of disease. The inspiration for the design of such new drugs can invariably be traced back to structure modification of biologically active natural products. Marijuana is an excellent example of a natural product that has immense therapeutic potential. In spite of its fascinating pharmacological and toxicological profile, this fertile lead has not been exploited most likely because of a reluctance to develop a therapeutic agent from a drug of abuse. In recent years, however, there has been a dramatic change in the acceptance of marijuana and its active constituent Δ^9-THC as a drug, since it has been found serendipitously to be more effective than presently available drugs for controlling nausea in cancer chemotherapy and in the treatment of glaucoma.

Voluminous literature has appeared on the chemistry of marijuana and Δ^9-THC (family of compounds known as cannabinoids), their pharmacology, biochemistry and toxicology. Extensive Structure-Activity Relationships (SAR) have been developed in THC's and numerous carbocyclic and heterocyclic analogs have been synthesized. The first cannabinoid drug, nabilone, has recently been marketed as an anti-emetic in Canada while others are under development in Europe and the U.S.A. The potential of cannabinoids as clinically useful drugs is now beginning to emerge (Razdan & Howes 1983).

With this background, a brief survey of SAR in THC's and the development of therapeutic agents particularly in the field of analgesics and glaucoma will be presented.

Sisa Incorporated, Cambridge, Massachusetts, 02138 U.S.A.

NATURAL PRODUCTS AND DRUG DEVELOPMENT, Alfred Benzon Symposium 20.
Editors: P. Krogsgaard-Larsen, S. Brøgger Christensen, H. Kofod, Munksgaard, Copenhagen 1984.

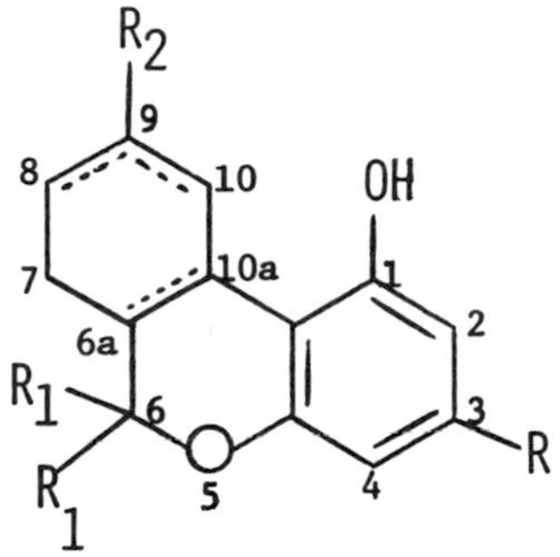

Fig. 1. Dibenzopyran numbering system of THC's.

SAR IN THC's

Based on CNS pharmacological profiles in laboratory animals the SAR in cannabinoids can be summarized as follows:

1. Essentially a benzopyran structure with an aromatic hydroxyl group at 1-position and an alkyl or alkoxyl group on the 3-position are a requirement for activity.

2. The position and the environment around the aromatic hydroxyl group are very important for activity, viz.:
   a. The OH at position C-1 is in itself necessary for CNS activity;
   b. esterification of the phenol retains, whereas etherification eliminates activity. Replacement of the OH by NH_2 retains while SH eliminates activity;
   c. methyl substituents at C-10 in the alicyclic ring can significantly influence the CNS activity.

3. Substitution in the aromatic ring by electronegative groups such as COOH, acetyl eliminates activity, whereas alkyl and OH retain activity.

4. A minimum length of the aromatic side chain is a requirement for activity. Branching of the side chain, increases potency.

5. The gem-dimethyl group in the pyran-ring is optimum for activity. Replacement of one of the gem-dimethyl group by a hydroxyl methyl group retains activity. Replacement of pyran O by N and ring expansion by one carbon can retain activity.

6. In the alicyclic ring the position of the double bond in Δ^9-, Δ^8-, or $\Delta^{6a,10a}$ retains activity. A 6a,10a-*trans* junction increases and a *cis* junction decreases activity. The natural THC's are active in the 10aR, 6aR series only. A methyl

at C-9 increases activity but metabolism to the 9-hydroxymethyl is not a prerequisite for THC activity.

7. The alicyclic ring can be substituted by a variety of nitrogen and sulfur-containing rings without loss of CNS activity. With the nitrogen and sulfur analogs the optimum CNS activity is obtained when the heteroatom is in a phenethyl orientation, i.e., inserted in place of C-9 or C-7.

8. Planarity of the alicyclic ring is not a necessary criterion for activity.

9. In both carbocyclic and heterocyclic analogs, opening the pyran ring generally decreases activity.

ANALGESICS

Some 20 years ago, we started the development of therapeutic agents from this field. Our initial focus was on analgesics, as anecdotal data pointed to the relief of pain associated with migraine headaches, menstrual cramps and toothache. The possibility of developing novel analgesics from a class of compounds which have (i) a non-opiate chemical structure and mechanism of action, (ii) no physical dependence liability, and (iii) an extraordinarily low toxicity with little or no respiratory depression, seemed very attractive to us. At the time Δ^9-THC, the active constituent of marijuana, was just becoming available and was reported to be active in the hot-plate and tail-flick tests (Grunfield & Edery 1969), (Buxbaum et al. 1969). It should be noted, however, that under stringent test procedures as used for narcotic analgesics (Harris & Pierson 1964), Δ^9-THC showed only minimal activity (Dewey et al. 1972). In the writing test Δ^9-THC was found to be inactive at lower doses, but at higher doses it did display activity. More importantly, unlike the narcotic-antagonist analgesics, it did not produce physical dependence, but a tolerance to most of the CNS effects of Δ^9-THC was observed with no cross-tolerance to morphine (McMillan et al. 1970). In the last 9 years there have been 4 relatively well-controlled studies of the analgesic activity of Δ^9-THC in man (Hill et al. 1974, Noyes et al. 1975, Regelson et al. 1976, Raft et al. 1977). The results have been inconclusive and it is generally accepted that Δ^9-THC is not a useful analgesic.

In our own work, on the basis of some structural relationships between THC's and morphine, we synthesized several heterocyclic analogs as potential analgesics. They showed good antinociceptive activity in laboratory animals (Table I) and were active in the tail-flick test but only when less stringent methodology in terms of control-reaction time and cut-off times were used. There is, however,

Table I

Analgesic activity of selected nitrogen and sulfur analogs

STRUCTURE	ED$_{50}$ - MG/KG, PO		
	HOT PLATE (MOUSE)	ANTI WRITHING (MOUSE)	TAIL FLICK (RAT)
CH$_2$C≡CH (SP-1) ... C_9H_{19}	7.7	4.3	13.8
CH$_2$C≡CH (SP-106) OC(CH$_2$)$_3$N ... C_9H_{19}	4.2	12.0	12.5
... OH ... C_9H_{19}	4.3	10.3	2/.7
... OH ... C_9H_{19}	5.7	8.6	2.7
... CH$_3$ OH ... C_9H_{19}	1.4	4.7	1.4

no question that these analogs showed greater analgesic activity than Δ^9-THC (Pars *et al.* 1977).

A comparison of the nitrogen analog SP-1 with morphine and pentazocine was carried out in the morphine-dependent monkey. It was found that SP-1, unlike morphine, exacerbates abstinence in the single-dose suppression test in withdrawn monkeys. In addition, in a non-withdrawn monkey it produced signs of withdrawal similar to those seen on administration of pentazocine. A more complete explanation of the SAR of this series of compounds is discussed in a review (Pars *et al.* 1977). One of these compounds, nabitan (SP-106) (Razdan *et al.* 1976), has been evaluated clinically for analgesic activity.

Other researchers have also been interested in the analgesic potential of the cannabinoids. May and his colleagues (Wilson & May 1974, 1975, Wilson *et al.* 1976) synthesized a number of 9-nor-9β-hydroxy-THC analogs which had good

Table II

Analgesic activity of SP-1 and its esters

$$CH_2C\equiv CH$$

(chemical structure: OR, O, C_9H_{19})

Compound	R	ED50 MG/KG Hot Plate (Mouse)[A]		ED50 MG/KG Writhing (Mouse)[B]		ED50 MG/KG Tail Flick (Rat)
		P.O.	I.V.	P.O.	I.V.	P.O.
SP-1	H	7.7 (4.2-12.7)	0.58 (0.3-1.12)	4.3 (3.2-5.9)	0.08 (0.02-0.28)	13.8 (4.5-23.9)
SP-106	C-CH₂CH₂CH₂N⟨⟩ .HCL	4.2 (2.0-6.8)	2.1 (1.0-4.1)	12.0 (9.3-16.9)	0.26 (0.14-0.49)	12.7 (9.4-15.7)
SP-178	C-CHCH₂CH₂N⟨⟩ .2HCL CH₃	4.6 (1.5-14.2)	1.6 (0.8-3.2)	12.2 (7.7-33.2)	0.35 (0.2-0.6)	9.8 (6.6-13.6)
SP-204	C-CHCH₂CH₂N⟨⟩ .2HCL CH₃ CH₃	3.8 (1.6-8.9)	1.2 (0.7-2.2)	7.3 (2.7-20.3)	0.43 (0.15-1.22)	10.7 (6.7-13.0)
Morphine		19.5 (8.2-46.2)	4.3 (2.7-7.0)	N.T.	0.26 (0.085-0.79)	N.T.

(A) Carried out at $58°C$
(B) 0.5% Acetic Acid Administered I.P. (0.4 ML)

analgesic activity in laboratory animals. The 9-nor-9β- hydroxyhexahydro-cannabinol (Fig. 2) had potent analgesic actions which were partially antagonized by naloxone (Bloom *et al.* 1977).

This prompted Milne and Johnson (1981) to combine our concept of nitrogen analogs with those of May to produce a series of potential analgesics. One of these compounds, levonantradol (Fig. 2) showed potent antinociceptive activity in animals. This was not antagonized by naloxone although, like morphine, levonantradol blocks abstinence signs in morphine-dependent dogs and rats. Cross tolerance between morphine and levonantradol does suggest some common pathway in their mechanism of action, but not an action at opiate receptors. Clinically, levonantradol demonstrated analgesic activity against post-operative pain (Jain *et al.* 1981) when compared to placebo. Even though doses of 1.5 to 3.0 mg were used, no dose-response relationship was observed.

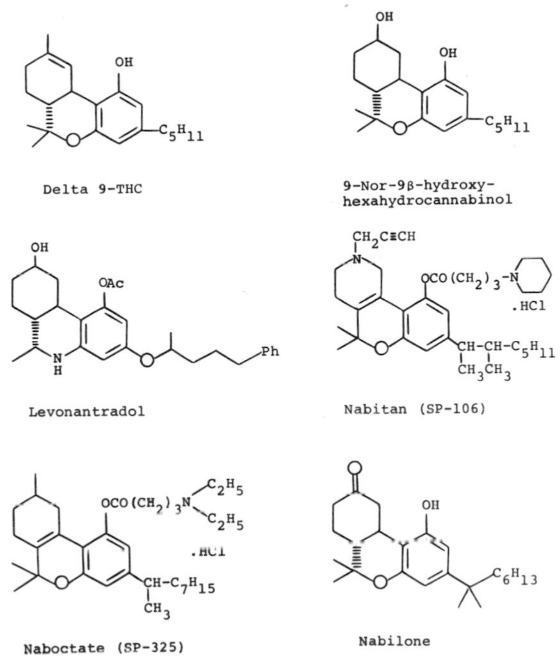

Fig. 2. Various cannabinoids discussed in this article

Duration of action was at least 6 h. The side effects observed in this study were characteristic of cannabinoids in general.

As mentioned before, the nitrogen analogs showed good antinociceptive activity in laboratory animals. From SP-1, the parent compound, a series of water-soluble analogs was prepared and SP-106 (nabitan) was selected for initial clinical work. It shares many of the pharmacological properties of SP-1, but without the potent tachycardia. Nabitan has been studied extensively in animals and is free of dependence liability and is not self-administered in monkeys. It has been evaluated in 3 laboratories for analgesic activity in man. In the first study (Staquet et al. 1978), it was shown that nabitan (4 mg) and codeine (50 mg) were indistinguishable from each other and both were more effective than a placebo in relieving pain.

A second study in patients with post-operative cancer pain was carried out by Houde and Wallenstein (Houde et al. 1978, Harris 1979, Houde & Wallenstein 1982). They determined that nabitan was approximately 6 times as potent as codeine in the relief of chronic pain. A high incidence of disturbing side effects was experienced by this population of subjects, especially at the 8.0 mg dose, in spite of the fact that in studies for glaucoma and emesis, higher doses were used with few, if any, serious side effects. The stressed condition of the patients from this study, or the use of strong narcotics at times close to the administration of nabitan, may account for the observed effects. In a third study, Jochimsen *et al.* (1978) failed to demonstrate analgesia with nabitan at 2 mg and 4 mg in cancer patients.

In summary, it is clear from Houde's study that nabitan is an orally active analgesic with codeine-like efficacy but at doses where the incidence of side effects is high. To achieve better selectivity of analgesic activity, we are presently developing 2 other compounds SP-178 and SP-204 (Table II) which are very closely related to nabitan and have shown better separation between analgesia and other side effects in CNS profiling.

GLAUCOMA

Glaucoma is one of the major causes of blindness in the world. It is a condition of the eye where higher than normal intraocular pressure (IOP) progressively affects the field of vision resulting in irreversible blindness. Early observations by Hepler and Frank (1971) demonstrated that smoking marijuana resulted in a decrease of IOP in normal subjects. Several reports have since appeared confirming the IOP-lowering effects of marijuana or Δ^9-THC in both normal subjects (Hepler *et al.* 1972, Shapiro 1974, Perez-Reyes *et al.* 1976, Cooler & Gregg 1977), and glaucoma patients (Hepler *et al.* 1976, Lockhart *et al.* 1977), and are reviewed elsewhere (Razdan & Howes 1980). Although Δ^9-THC has been reported to lower IOP in animals when administered topically, these results have not been confirmed in glaucoma patients (Merritt *et al.* 1981, Green & Roth 1982).

As part of an ongoing program in our laboratories (Meltzer *et al.* 1981, Pars *et al.* 1977), we have developed 2 compounds (Fig. 2) nabitan (SP-106) and naboctate (SP-325), which reduce IOP in animals and in man, and are potential anti-glaucoma drugs.

Drugs from the cannabinoid class produce a number of side effects such as tachycardia, orthostasis and subjective CNS effects which could limit their therapeutic use. The object of our development program has been to prepare a compound in which a good separation of therapeutic and side effects exists. To achieve these goals, we have looked for lowering of intraocular pressure in animals, combined with a low incidence of tachycardia. Identified candidates were then evaluated clinically.

Mean IOP 8mg Nabitan (20 eyes)

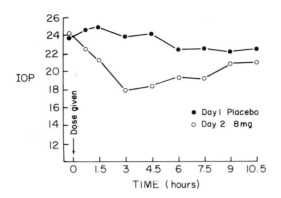

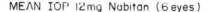

Fig. 3.

Our earliest evaluations were with nabitan (Razdan *et al.* 1976). This has been studied by Weber *et al.* (1981) and Tiedeman *et al.* (1981). It showed a decrease in IOP in normotensive human volunteers (Weber *et al.* 1981). The falls in IOP were small, but none of the subjects in this study had a starting IOP of greater than 18.0 mmHg. At high doses, nabitan caused a mild tachycardia (Weber *et al.* 1981). Subjects receiving 10 mg or more, reported marijuana-like side effects. In a further clinical study on ocular hypertensives (Tiedeman *et al.* 1981), nabitan showed a lowering of IOP (Figs. 3, 4). This was a double-masked study carried out over a period of 2 days. On the first day, the subject received

MEAN IOP 12mg Nabitan (6 eyes)

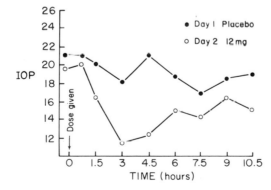

Fig. 4.

only placebo; on the second day either a placebo or the test drug. The results show that nabitan caused a dose-related fall of IOP. Mild tachycardia was observed and some incidents of orthostasis occurred. In an effort to reduce the cardiovascular side effects, a different compound, naboctate (SP-325), was developed (Razdan & Howes 1981).

Naboctate (SP-325) lowered the IOP of normotensive rabbits at doses of 5, 10 and 20 mg/kg orally. The peak effect was observed after 3 h, at which time a dose-related response was observed. The duration of action in these experiments was about 6 h. SP-325 caused a slight increase in heart rate in conscious rats given doses of 5, 10 and 20 mg/kg orally. A small non-dose-related hypotension was observed at $3\frac{1}{2}$ to $5\frac{1}{2}$ h in these animals. In the anesthetized animal, no significant cardiovascular effects were observed. SP-325 did not affect respiratory parameters in any of these experiments. When challenges of neurotransmitters were used, SP-325 exerted a weak anticholinergic effect. In the rat, the incidence of tachycardia with naboctate was much less than that seen with Δ^9-THC or nabitan.

The acute LD_{50} (p.o.) in the rat and the rabbit was >1500 and >1000 mg/kg respectively. In a 30-day subchronic study using rats and rabbits, SP-325 caused behavioral effects, which disappeared by the end of the first week. These included ataxia and sedation. No gross pathology was observed and microscopic analysis of tissues revealed no drug-related pathological changes.

In a Phase I study (Weber & Howes 1981) in 20 healthy normal volunteers, 5 subjects received 1.75 mg; 11, 3.50 mg, and 4, 5.0 mg of naboctate by the oral route. Their starting IOP varied from 10 to 20 mmHg. The IOP data for each dose group is shown in Fig. 5. The falls in IOP in the 3.5 mg and 5.0 mg groups were significantly larger than that observed in the 1.75 mg group. Previous experience indicates that clinical changes of 2 or 3 mm are all that are usually observed in normotensive subjects. The data indicates a significant ocular hypotensive effect of naboctate, which was long lasting with pressures still reduced 9 h after administration. No evidence of orthostasis was seen at 1.75 mg or 3.5 mg, but at 5 mg dose orthostasis was observed in 2 of 4 subjects. An increased pulse rate was observed in all subjects at the 5.0 mg level. At the lower doses, insignificant changes were noticed which were not dose related.

From the clinical data obtained so far, naboctate given orally appears to be potent with a long duration of action in normotensive subjects with no major side effects and is superior to nabitan.

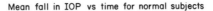

Mean fall in IOP vs time for normal subjects

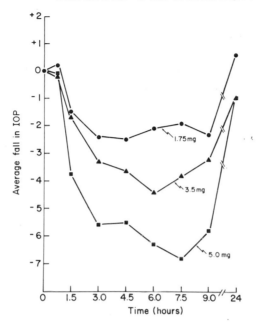

Fig. 5.

Topical activity

In the normotensive rabbit, naboctate administered topically gave a weak ocular hypotensive response. However, by temporarily elevating the IOP of the rabbit using the water-loading procedure described by Vareilles *et al.* (1977), we have been able to demonstrate an ocular hypotensive action to topically administered naboctate. In this model naboctate at 0.2%, 0.5% and 1% shows a dose-related response on the IOP as shown in Figs. 6, 7, 8. The results obtained in our laboratory with timolol (0.25%) confirm the data reported by Vareilles *et al.* (1977). In this model naboctate at 0.2% appears to be superior to timolol.

In summary, the 2 cannabinoids we have examined lower IOP in humans. The best route of administration, oral or topical, is yet to be determined, and is presently under active investigation. We conclude that marijuana and synthetic cannabinoids appear to have a place in the therapy of glaucoma.

It is obvious that cannabinoids display a wide range of biological activity. The future development of drugs from this area will undoubtedly depend on the success achieved by structural changes to provide selectivity of pharmacological

Effect of Naboctate (0.2% topically) on the IOP of water loaded rabbits

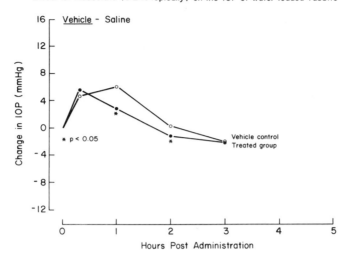

Fig. 6.

action (Razdan & Howes 1983). Because of remarkably low toxicity, and no, or very low, physical dependence liability, the concept of drug development from cannabinoids is based on very sound foundations. Indeed, it is surprising that such development did not take place sooner.

Effect of Naboctate (0.5% topically) on the IOP of water loaded rabbits

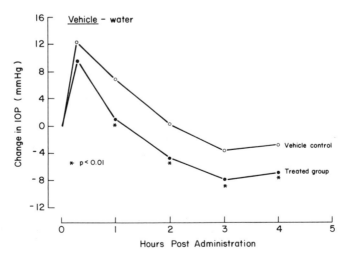

Fig. 7.

Effect of Naboctate (1.0% topically) on the IOP of water loaded rabbits

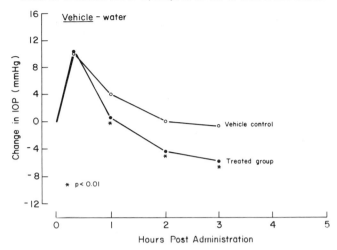

Fig. 8.

REFERENCES

Bloom, A. S., Dewey, W. L., Harris, L. S. & Brosius, K. K. (1977) 9-Nor-9β-hydroxyhexa-hydrocannabinol a cannabinoid with potent antinociceptive activity; comparison with morphine, *J. Pharmacol. Exp. Ther. 200*, 263 70.

Buxbaum, D., Sanders-Bush, E. & Efron, D. (1969) Analgesic activity of tetrahydrocannabinol (THC) in the rat and mouse. *Fed. Proc. 28*, 735.

Cooler, R. & Gregg, J. M. (1977) Effect of delta-9-tetrahydrocannabinol on intraocular pressure in humans. *South Med. J. 70*, 951–54.

Dewey, W. L., Harris, L. S. & Kennedy, J. A. (1972) Some pharmacological and toxicological effects of *1*-trans Δ^8 and *1*-trans-Δ^9-tetrahydrocannabinol in laboratory rodents. *Arch. Int. Pharmacodyn. Ther. 196*, 133–45.

Green, K. & Roth, M. (1982) Ocular effects of topical administration of Δ^9-tetrahydrocannabinol in man. *Arch. Opthalmol. 100*, 265–67.

Grunfield, Y. & Edery, H. (1969) Psychopharmacological activity of the active constituents of hashish and some related cannabinoids. *Psychopharmacologia, 14*, 200–10.

Harris, L. S. & Pierson, A. K. (1964) Narcotic antagonists in the Benzomorphan series. *J. Pharmacol. Exp. Ther. 143*, 141–48.

Harris, L. S. (1979) Cannabinoids as analgesics. In: *Mechanisms of Pain and Analgesic Compounds*, eds. Beers, R. F. & Bassett, E. G., pp. 467–474. Raven Press, New York.

Hepler, R. S. & Frank, I. M. (1971) Marihuana smoking and intraocular pressure. *J. Am. Med. Assoc. 217*, 1392.

Hepler, R. S., Frank, I. M. & Ungerleider, J. T. (1972) Pupillary constriction after marihuana smoking. *Am. J. Opthalmol. 74*, 1185–90.

Hepler, R. S., Frank, I. M. & Petrus, R. (1976) Ocular effects of marihuana smoking. In: *The Pharmacology of Marihuana*, eds. Braude, M. C. & Szara, S., pp. 815–824. Raven Press, New York.

Hill, S. Y., Schwin, R., Goodwin, D. W. & Powell, B. J. (1974) Marihuana and pain, *J. Pharmacol. Exp. Ther. 188,* 415–18.

Houde, R. W., Wallenstein, S. L., Rogers, A. & Kaiko, R. F. (1978) Annual Report of the analgesic studies section of the Sloan-Kettering Cancer Center. *Report to the Committee on Problems of Drug Dependence.* pp. 149–168. National Academy of Sciences, Washington, D.C.

Houde, R. W. & Wallenstein, S. L. (1982) Personal communication.

Jain, A. K., Ryan, J. R. McMahon, F. G. & Smith, G. (1981) Evaluation of intramuscular Levonantradol and placebo in acute post-operative pain. *J. Clin. Pharmacol. 21,* 320–26S.

Jochimsen, P. R., Lawton, R. L., Ven Steeg, K. & Noyes, R. L. (1978) Effect of benzopyrano-pyridine, a Δ^9-THC congener on pain. *Clin. Pharmacol. Ther. 24,* 223–27.

Lockhart, A. B., West, M. E. & Lowe, H. I. C. (1977) *West Indian Med. J. 26,* 66–70.

McMillan, D. E., Harris, L. S., Frakenheim, J. M. & Kennedy, J. S. (1970) *1*-trans-Δ^9-tetrahydrocannabinol in pigeons: Tolerance to the behavioral effects. *Science 169,* 611–12.

Meltzer, P. C., Dalzell, H. C. & Razdan, R. K. (1981) Drugs derived from Cannabinoids. Part 8. The synthesis of side-chain analogues of $\Delta^{6a,10a}$ tetrahydrocannabinol. *J. Chem. Soc. Perkin I.,* 2825–29; and previous papers in the series.

Merritt, J.C., Perry, D. D., Russell, D. N. & Jones, B. F. (1981) Topical Δ^9-tetrahydrocannabinol and aqueous dynamics in glaucoma. *J. Clin. Pharmacol. 21,* 467–71S.

Milne, G. M. & Johnson, M. R. (1981) Levonantradol: a role for central prostanoid mechanisms. *J. Clin. Pharmacol. 21,* 367–74S.

Noyes, R., Jr., Brunk, S. F., Baram, D. A. & Canter, A. (1975) Analgesic effects of Δ^9-tetrahydrocannabinol. *J. Clin. Pharmacol. 15,* 139–43.

Pars, H. G., Razdan, R. K. & Howes, J. F. (1977) Potential therapeutic agents derived from the cannabinoid nucleus. In: *Advances in Drug Research, Vol. 11,* eds. Harper, N. J. & Simmonds, A. B., pp. 97–189. Academic Press, New York.

Perez-Reyes, M., Wagner, D., Wall, M. E. & Davis, K. H. (1976) Intravenous administration of cannabinoids and intraocular pressure. In: *The Pharmacology of Marihuana,* eds. Braude, M. C. & Szara, S., pp. 829–832. Raven Press, New York.

Raft, D., Gregg, J., Ghia, J. & Harris, L. S. (1977) Effects of intravenous tetrahydrocannabinol on experimental and surgical pain. *Clin. Pharmacol. Ther. 121,* 26–33.

Razdan, R. K., Zitko-Terris, B., Pars, H. G., Plotnikoff, N. P., Dodge, P. W., Dren, A. T., Kyncl, J. & Somani, P. (1976) Drugs derived from cannabinoids. 2. Basic esters of nitrogen and carbocyclic analogs. *J. Med. Chem. 19,* 454–61.

Razdan, R. K. & Howes, J. F. (1980) Recent advances in the pharmacological treatment of glaucoma. *Rev. Pure Appl. Pharmacol. Sc. 1,* 183–213.

Razdan, R. K. & Howes, J. F. (1981) Naboctate, a novel cannabinoid with antiglaucoma activity. *Fed. Proc. 40,* 278.

Razdan, R. K. & Howes, J. F. (1983) Drugs related to tetrahydrocannabinol. *Med. Res. Rev. 3,* 119–46.

Regelson, W., Butler, J. R., Schulz, J., Kirk, T., Peek, L., Green, M. L. & Zalis, M. O. (1976) Δ^9-THC as an effective anti-depressant and appetite stimulating agent in advanced cancer patients. In: *Pharmacology of Marihuana. Vol. 2,* eds. Braude, M. C. & Szara, S. pp. 763–776. Raven Press, New York.

Shapiro, D. (1974) The ocular manifestation of the cannabinols. *Opthalmologica 168,* 366–69.

Staquet, M., Gnatt, C. & Machin, D. (1978) Effect of a nitrogen analog of tetrahydrocannabinol on cancer pain. *Clin. Pharmacol. Ther. 23,* 397–401.

Tiedeman, J. S., Shields, M. B., Weber, P. A., Crow, J.A., Cochetto, D. M., Harris, W. A. & Howes, J. F. (1981) Effects of synthetis cannabinoids on elevated intraocular pressure. *Opthalmology 88,* 270–77.

Vareilles, P., Silverstone, D., Plazonnet, B., LeDonarec, J. C., Seens, M. L. & Stone, C. A. (1977) Comparison of the effects of timolol and other adrenergic agents on intraocular pressure in the rabbit. *Invest. Ophthalmol. Visual Sc. 16,* 987–96.

Weber, P. A. & Howes, J. F. (1981) Lowering of intraocular Pressure in normotensive human volunteers by naboctate. ARVO Abstracts, p. 196, Abstract # 3 (Supplement to *Invest. Opthalmol. Visual Sc. 20,* No. 3, March, 1981).

Weber, P., Bianchine, J. & Howes, J. F. (1981) Nabitan Hydrochloride: Ocular hypotensive effect in normal human volunteers. *Glaucoma 3,* 163–66.

Wilson, R. S. & May, E. L. (1974) 9-Nor-Δ^8-tetrahydrocannabinol, a cannabinoid of metabolic interest. *J. Med. Chem. 17,* 475–76.

Wilson, R. S. & May, E. L. (1975) Analgesic properties of the tetrahydrocannabinoids, their metabolites and analogs. *J. Med. Chem. 18,* 700–3.

Wilson, R. S., May, E. L., Martin, B. R. & Dewey, W. L. (1976) 9-Nor-9-hydroxy-hexahydro-cannabinols synthesis, some behavioral and analgesic properties and comparison with the tetrahydrocannabinols. *J. Med. Chem. 19,* 1165–67.

DISCUSSION

DJERASSI: Suppose one gave naboctate (SP-325) to a group of ordinary people, would they have any marijuana-type effect?

RAZDAN: If you give sufficiently high doses, yes. After doses of 5 mg people said that they noticed effects similar to those of a glass of beer.

DJERASSI: Yes, but my point is, do you think that it is at all possible from a legal-political standpoint that such a drug would ever be approved in the Western countries which follow typical FDA regulations?

RAZDAN: Nabilone is marketed and used in Canada and the USA. Any drug has to stand on its own. If naboctate can help patients with glaucoma more effectively than other drugs, then why not use it.

DJERASSI: The history of mankind is full of the use of recreational drugs, including alcohol and the cannabinoids. This, actually may suggest that we do need a "harmless" recreational drug. Could, in fact, the medicinal chemist and the pharmacologist design a "harmless" recreational drug, which could substitute for the existing ones, all of which are really undesirable?

RAZDAN: In that sense, cocaine comes pretty close to it. But all such compounds may inherently have undesired effects.

ANDERSON: How much is known about the mechanism of action of naboctate?

RAZDAN: I did not have time to touch on this. I should state that we have not done the mechanistic study on naboctate, but mechanistic studies have been done on other cannabinoids, such as Δ^9-THC. Green & Pederson (1) reported that when Δ^9-THC was applied *in vitro* to a ciliary body iris tissue preparation of albino rabbit, the aqueous secretion was reduced and membrane permeability was increased. They also found with *in vivo* experiments in rabbits that the IOP decreased by 25–30% and total outflow facility of the eye increased by 60–70% following intravenous administration of Δ^9-THC. On the basis of these experiments, they concluded that Δ^9-THC appears to vasoconstrict the different blood vessels to the ciliary epithelium, causing a fall in both blood pressure and flow to the region of aqueous humor formation. Thus, the mechanism of IOP reduction may be due to decreased secretion and increased outflow of aqueous secretion and, thus, appears to be different from those of β-blockers and other antiglaucoma agents.

ANDERSON: Do you know what the rate of penetration of the epithelial layer of the cornea is?

RAZDAN: No, at the present time we are working on the formulation. As naboctate is an ester, we have some problems with hydrolysis. But we have found that you can keep it for one month in solution without much loss of activity.

ANDERSON: I assume that you do have a soluble formulation.

RAZDAN: These are water soluble compounds. Actually, they have detergent properties.

KROGSGAARD-LARSEN: It was my impression from your talk that the mechanism of action of these compounds is rather complex and that they also affect the cholinergic system? If so, then you would possibly be able to explain most of the effects on the basis of the cholinergic profile, for example, the analgesic effect and the effects on blood pressure.

RAZDAN: There is no complete answer to this question. We have hypothesized on the basis of work we did in the 1970s, that inhibition of prostaglandin biosynthesis may be important. Right now the picture is quite complicated, and I think that inhibition of prostaglandins biosynthesis, stimulation of PGE_2-synthesis, and blockade of the receptor, may all be involved and may be relevant for the different effects of different cannabinoids. For a detailed discussion see (2).

ALBUQUERQUE: I am surprised that these cannabinoids have not yet been thoroughly studied in the sensory systems. Such studies and also studies on the central GABA system should be performed in order to achieve a better understanding of the mechanism of action of the compounds concerned.

RAZDAN: I do not know whether the studies you mentioned have been done or not. One problem in relation to the development of this class of compound is that there are no good animal models. In this situation, it has been very difficult to establish studies in the human clinic.

WALL: A major problem in relation to the glaucoma patients is that most of them are elderly, and here tachycardia is a very dangerous situation. For this reason, the ophthalmologist that you referred to has almost given up his work with THC on the glaucoma patient he brought with him to North Carolina.

RAZDAN: As I pointed out, this is a very important side-effect, which we are trying to eliminate.

WALL: The use of many valuable cancer drugs is frequently inhibited because of intractable nausea. In recent years, there have been several symposia on the use of THC and certain analogues against this. I was wondering whether any of your compounds have shown promising effects in these conditions?

RAZDAN: I did not touch on that because of lack of time. I just mentioned that nabilone is already on the market as an anti-nauseant, and other compounds are under development in this field.

WALL: Nabilone was removed for a while, I think.

RAZDAN: That was 3–4 years ago. The toxicologists at Eli Lilly carried out the toxicology in dogs, and a metabolite of nabilone proved to be very toxic in this species. This was a specific effect in dogs, but in monkeys there were no toxicological problems.

WALL: I would think that the ketone group of nabilone would be reduced, and in fact I thought that the corresponding alcohol was the active metabolite.

RAZDAN: The ketone group of nabilone is reduced. Eli Lilly has done all the kinetic work on this compound.

WALL: Which one of the epimeric alcohols is the active one?

RAZDAN: The β-form is active, the α-form is inactive. I did not have time to go into these SAR studies.

(1) Green, K. & Pederson, J. E. (1973) *Exp. Eye Res. 15,* 449–507.
(2) Razdan, R. K. & Howes, J. F. (1983) *Med. Res. Rev. 3,* 119–146.

Amanita muscaria in Medicinal Chemistry. I. Muscimol and Related GABA Agonists with Anticonvulsant and Central Non-Opioid Analgesic Effects

Erik Falch, Vibeke Christensen,* Poul Jacobsen, Jette Byberg & Povl Krogsgaard-Larsen

The amino acid, 4-aminobutyric acid (GABA) (Fig. 1) is the major inhibitory neurotransmitter in the mammalian central nervous system (CNS) (Curtis & Johnston 1974). GABA is known to be involved in the central regulation of a variety of physiological functions including cardiovascular mechanisms (DeFeudis 1981), the sensation of pain (Hill *et al.* 1981, Kendall *et al.* 1982, DeFeudis 1982, Christensen *et al.* 1982), and anxiety (Hoehn-Saric 1983). Furthermore, accumulating evidence strongly suggests that the symptoms associated with epilepsy and Huntington's chorea are caused by impaired transmission at GABA-operated synapses (Roberts *et al.* 1976, Krogsgaard-Larsen *et al.* 1979b, Morselli *et al.* 1981, Meldrum 1982). These findings have brought agents with GABA stimulating effects into focus as potential therapeutic agents.

In diseases with advanced neuronal degeneration only the postsynaptic receptors are potential pharmacological sites of attack (Krogsgaard-Larsen 1981), and, consequently, GABA-agonist therapies appear to be of primary interest (Krogsgaard-Larsen & Falch 1981).

As the antinociceptive effects of GABA-mimetics are not mediated by the opiate receptors (Hill *et al.* 1981, Christensen *et al.* 1982, Kendall *et al.* 1982), it might be possible to develop GABA-ergic strong analgesics devoid of the undesired side-effects of the opiates.

The Royal Danish School of Pharmacy, Department of Chemistry BC, DK-2100 Copenhagen.
* H. Lundbeck & Co, A/S, Department of Pharmacology, DK-2500 Valby, Copenhagen, Denmark.

NATURAL PRODUCTS AND DRUG DEVELOPMENT, Alfred Benzon Symposium 20.
Editors: P. Krogsgaard-Larsen, S. Brøgger Christensen, H. Kofod, Munksgaard, Copenhagen 1984.

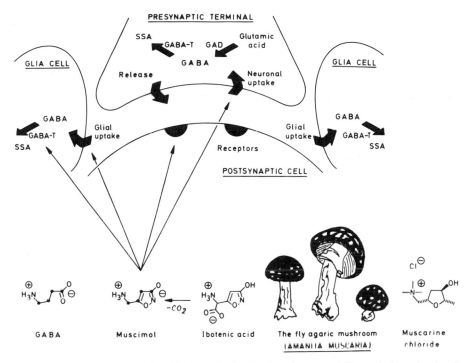

Fig. 1. The structures of ibotenic acid, biosynthesized by *Amanita muscaria* Fr., and of muscimol and GABA. The structural similarity between muscimol and GABA is indicated.

MUSCIMOL, A PSYCHOACTIVE CONSTITUENT OF *AMANITA MUSCARIA*

The mushroom *Amanita muscaria* Fr. (Fig. 1), the fly agaric, has psychotropic effects, which manifest themselves after consumption of the fresh or dried mushrooms (Waser 1979). The use of the fly agaric as an inebriant among certain Siberian tribes may represent a degeneration of traditions, which played a part in ancient Indo-European religious ceremonies (Wasson 1979). The plant Soma, which was deified and consumed by Indo-European priests, probably is identical with *Amanita muscaria* Fr. (Wasson 1968).

In 1954 muscarine (Fig. 1) was isolated in a pure state and its structure unequivocally established (Eugster & Waser 1954). Muscarine has cholinergic effects in the peripheral nervous system (Waser 1979), but the quaternary ammonium group prevents muscarine from entering the CNS after systemic administration, and, consequently, muscarine cannot be responsible for the central effects of the fly agaric.

Two decades ago, the isolation and structure determination of the centrally active constituents of *Amanita muscaria* Fr. were reported (Takemoto *et al.* 1964, Eugster *et al.* 1965, Bowden & Drysdale 1965). The compounds proved to be zwitterionic 3-isoxazolol derivatives, a new type of naturally occurring compound. Ibotenic acid [(*RS*)-α-amino-3-hydroxy-5-isoxazoleacetic acid],

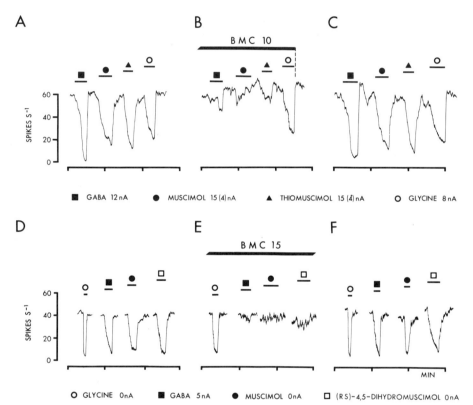

Fig. 2. A, B, C. The effect of BMC on the inhibition of the firing of a cat-spinal interneurone by glycine (○, 8 nA, 0.5 M); GABA (■, 12 nA, 0.2 M); muscimol (●, 15 nA), and thiomuscimol (▲, 15 nA), all ejected micro-electrophoretically for the times indicated by the symbols and horizontal bars. The muscimol and thiomuscimol solutions were 0.05 M in 0.165 M-NaCl; the figures in brackets indicate the approximate currents ejecting these heterocycles. The neurone was fired by the continuous ejection of DL-homocysteate (10 nA, 0.2 M). A, before; B, during BMC (10 nA) terminated at the vertical broken line; C, 4 min after B.

D, E, F. The effect of BMC on the inhibition of the firing of another cat-spinal interneurone by glycine (○, 0 nA, 0.5 M); GABA (■, 5 nA, 0.2 M); muscimol (●, 0 nA, 0.1 M), and (*RS*)-4,5-dihydromuscimol (□, 0 nA, 0.2 M) ejected as above. D, before; E, during BMC (15 nA), terminated at the vertical broken line; F, 1–8 min after terminating the administration of BMC. (From Krogsgaard-Larsen *et al.* 1979a).

which is an analogue of glutamic acid (see subsequent chapter), is synthesized by the mushroom, whereas muscimol (5-aminomethyl-3-isoxazolol), which is not present in the fresh mushrooms, is formed in the dried plant material by decarboxylation of ibotenic acid (Fig. 1), a process which is not catalyzed by enzymes (Eugster 1969).

MUSCIMOL AS A LEAD FOR THE DEVELOPMENT OF SPECIFIC GABA AGONISTS

As illustrated in Fig. 1 muscimol is a heterocyclic analogue of GABA. Muscimol is a powerful agonist at the post-synaptic GABA-receptor complex sensitive to the antagonists bicuculline (BIC) and bicuculline methochloride (BMC) (Fig. 6) (Curtis et al. 1971, Krogsgaard-Larsen et al. 1979a). The depressant effect of muscimol on the firing of 2 different cat spinal neurones and the blockade of this effect by BMC is illustrated in Fig. 2. The effective receptor interaction of muscimol can also be detected in vitro, muscimol being an inhibitor of the receptor binding of GABA at concentrations in the low nanomolar range (Krogsgaard-Larsen et al. 1979a).

Muscimol is, however, not a specific GABA agonist (Fig. 1). It also interacts with the GABA-transport (uptake) systems, although the ratio between the receptor and uptake affinities of muscimol is substantially higher than in the case of GABA (Fig. 3) (Krogsgaard-Larsen et al. 1979a, Schousboe et al. 1979), and muscimol is a substrate for the GABA-metabolizing enzyme GABA:2-oxoglutarate aminotransferase (GABA-T) (Fowler et al. 1983). Muscimol actually is transported by the neuronal GABA-uptake system (Johnston et al. 1978), and metabolites formed within the GABA-nerve terminals may contribute to the toxicity of muscimol after systemic administration to animals and man. In contrast to GABA, and in spite of its zwitterionic structure, muscimol is capable of penetrating the blood-brain barrier (BBB) (Moroni et al. 1982). This characteristic and its potency as a GABA agonist has made muscimol a useful lead structure for the design of specific GABA agonists with favourable pharmacokinetic properties (Krogsgaard-Larsen & Falch 1981, Krogsgaard-Larsen et al. 1981a).

Conversion of muscimol into the bicyclic compounds 4,5,6,7-tetrahydro-isoxazolo[5,4-c]pyridin-3-ol (THIP) (Gaboxadol) and 4,5,6,7-tetrahydroiso-xazolo[4,5-c]pyridin-3-ol (THPO) (Fig. 3) resulted in a "separation" of the GABA receptor and uptake affinities of muscimol. Thus, THIP is a specific

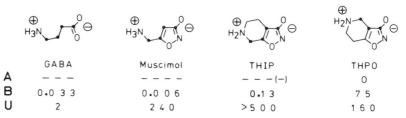

	GABA	Muscimol	THIP	THPO
A	– – –	– – – –	– – –(–)	0
B	0.0 3 3	0.0 0 6	0.1 3	7 5
U	2	2 4 0	>5 0 0	1 6 0

Fig. 3. Structures and biological effects of GABA, mucimol, and the bicyclic muscimol analogues THIP and THPO. *A:* The GABA agonist activity relative to that of GABA (---) as determined micro-electrophoretically (Curtis *et al.* 1971); *B:* Inhibition of GABA receptor binding *in vitro* (IC$_{50}$, μM) using rat-brain membranes (Falch & Krogsgaard-Larsen 1982); *U:* Inhibition of neuronal GABA uptake *in vitro* (IC$_{50}$, μM) using a crude synaptosomal fraction isolated from rat brain (Jacobsen *et al.* 1982).

GABA agonist (Krogsgaard-Larsen *et al.* 1977, 1979a) whereas THPO is an inhibitor of GABA uptake with selective effect on glial GABA uptake, but without significant receptor affinity (Krogsgaard-Larsen 1980).

The conformationally rigid structure of THIP compared with its potency and specificity as a GABA agonist (Krogsgaard-Larsen *et al.* 1977, Alger & Nicoll 1982) indicates that THIP essentially reflects the receptor-active conformations of muscimol and GABA. In order to map-out in detail the structural requirements for activation of the post-synaptic GABA receptor, the relationship between structure and GABA-agonist activity of a variety of muscimol analogues has been studied (Krogsgaard-Larsen *et al.* 1979a, Krogsgaard-Larsen & Falch 1981, Krogsgaard-Larsen *et al.* 1983a). While (RS)-dihydromuscimol and thiomuscimol are almost equipotent with muscimol (Fig. 2), analogues containing other heterocyclic rings are very weak or inactive (Fig. 4). This reflects that the degree of delocalization of the negative charges of (RS)-dihydromuscimol and thiomuscimol are comparable with that of GABA, whereas the electronic structures of the rings of isomuscimol and **3** are distinctly different. Unfortunately, lack of specificity limits the value of (RS)-dihydromuscimol as well as thiomuscimol, both compounds being substrates for GABA-T (L. J. Fowler, unpublished), and while thiomuscimol does not affect GABA uptake *in vitro,* (RS)-dihydromuscimol is comparable with muscimol as an inhibitor of neuronal and glial GABA uptake (Schousboe *et al.* 1979, Krogsgaard-Larsen *et al.* 1979a).

As exemplified in Fig. 4, homologation of the side chain of muscimol and/or introduction of alkyl groups into various positions of the molecules reduce the

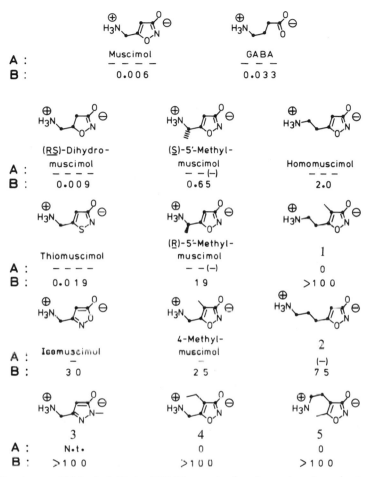

Fig. 4. Structures and biological effects of GABA, muscimol, and a number of muscimol analogues. *A* and *B:* see legend for Fig. 3.

effects on the GABA receptors. Only (*S*)-5'-methylmuscimol and homo-muscimol are potent GABA agonists. It is worth noting that whereas the *S*-isomer of 5'-methylmuscimol is some 30-times more potent than the *R*-isomer in inhibiting the receptor binding of GABA, these isomers are virtually equi-potent as GABA agonists on cat spinal neurones (Falch & Krogsgaard-Larsen 1982, Krogsgaard-Larsen *et al.* 1983a). This observation suggests that the ion channel-coupled post-synaptic GABA receptors (Fig. 6) and the GABA-receptor recognition sites, as measured in binding experiments, exhibit different

510FALCH ET AL.

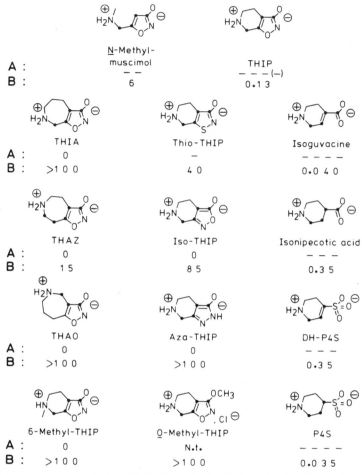

Fig. 5. Structures and biological effects of THIP, *N*-methylmuscimol, and a number of mono- and bicyclic GABA analogues derived from THIP. *A* and *B:* see legend for Fig. 3.

degrees of stereoselectivity, emphasizing the limitations of binding studies in investigations of GABA-receptor mechanisms.

While THIP is a specific and very active GABA agonist, *N*-methylmuscimol is only moderately potent (Fig. 5) (Krogsgaard-Larsen *et al.* 1977, 1982a), indicating that the presence of secondary amino groups in muscimol analogues does not, *per se,* prevent effective activation of the GABA receptors, and that THIP is locked in a shape easily recognized and bound by the receptors.

As exemplified in Fig. 5, alterations of the structure of THIP along certain lines result in substantial or complete loss of GABA-agonist activity. Thus, 6-methyl-THIP, 5,6,7,8-tetrahydro-4*H*-isoxazolo[5,4-*c*]azepin-3-ol (THIA), and 5,6,7,8-tetrahydro-4*H*-isoxazolo[4,5-*d*]azepin-3-ol (THAZ) have little or no effect on the GABA receptors. These compounds are, however, antagonists at the glycine receptors on cat spinal neurones (Krogsgaard-Larsen *et al.* 1982a). Similarly, structural modifications of the heterocyclic anionic moiety of THIP have dramatic effects (Fig. 5). Only 4,5,6,7-tetrahydroisothiazolo[5,4-*c*]pyridin-3-ol (thio-THIP) has significant GABA-agonist activity (Krogsgaard-Larsen *et al.* 1983b) emphasizing the pronounced structural specificity of the GABA receptors.

Replacement of the 3-isoxazolol anion of THIP by carboxylate or sulphonate groups did, on the other hand, lead to a series of potent and specific BMC-sensitive GABA agonists (Krogsgaard-Larsen *et al.* 1977, 1980, E. Falch, unpublished). It is, however, interesting to note that introductions of a double bond into the molecules of isonipecotic acid and piperidine-4-sulphonic acid (P4S) have opposite effects. While isoguvacine is an order of magnitude more

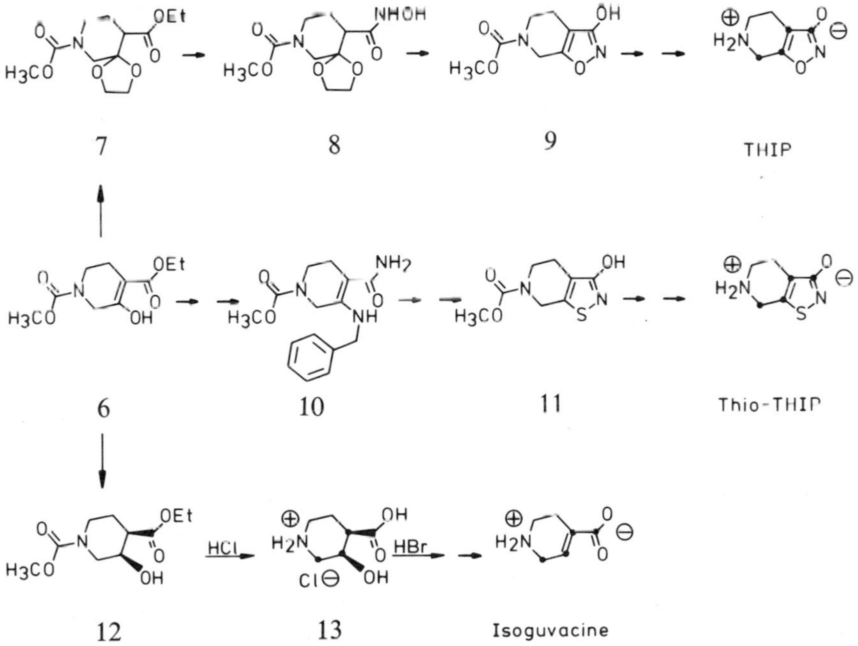

Scheme 1

potent than isonipecotic acid as an inhibitor of GABA-receptor binding, the unsaturated analogue of P4S, 1,2,3,6-tetrahydropyridine-4-sulphonic acid (DH-P4S) is proportionally weaker than P4S, and micro-electrophoretic studies have disclosed the same relative order of potency of these compounds as BMC-sensitive GABA agonists *in vivo*. These observations seem to suggest that the replacement of the carboxylate group of this class of GABA agonists by a sulphonate group affects the mechanism of interaction of the compounds concerned with the GABA receptors (see later section of this chapter).

SYNTHESES OF SOME HETEROCYCLIC GABA AGONISTS
In Scheme 1, the last steps of the multi-step sequences for the syntheses of THIP (Krogsgaard-Larsen 1977), and thio-THIP (Krogsgaard-Larsen *et al.* 1983b), and for one of the syntheses of isoguvacine (Krogsgaard-Larsen & Christiansen 1979) are outlined. The key intermediate **6** was converted into the ketalized hydroxamic acid **8**, which was partially deprotected and cyclized under strong acid conditions to give **9**. After deprotection of **9**, THIP was isolated in the zwitterionic form.

The enamino amide **10**, derived from **6**, was treated with hydrogen sulphide, and oxidation of the crude intermediate of unknown structure with bromine gave **11** in rather poor yields. Acid deprotection of **11** followed by an ion-exchange purification step gave thio-THIP, which was isolated as the chloride.

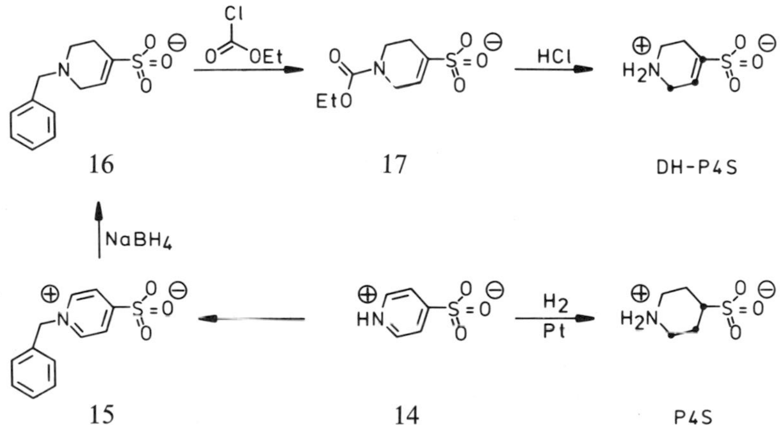

Scheme 2

The hydroxy amino acid **13** was obtained from **6** *via* catalytic hydrogenation followed by relatively mild hydrolysis of **12**. Prolonged treatment with hydrobromic acid converted **13** into isoguvacine.

Scheme 2 summarizes the syntheses of P4S and DH-P4S (Krogsgaard-Larsen *et al.* 1980, E. Falch, unpublished). The quaternary derivative **15** of pyridine-4-sulphonic acid **14** was converted into protected DH-P4S **17** *via* a hydride reduction step followed by a modified von Braun reaction. Upon acid deprotection of **17** zwitterionic DH-P4S crystallized from the reaction medium.

MOLECULAR PHARMACOLOGY OF THE POST-SYNAPTIC GABA-RECEPTOR COMPLEX

In Fig. 6, our present knowledge of the structure of the post-synaptic GABA-receptor complex is summarized (Olsen 1981, Skolnick & Paul 1981, Krogsgaard-Larsen 1981). The chloride channel is regulated by the GABA receptor consisting of 2 (Olsen *et al.* 1981), or possibly 3 GABA-binding sites (Falch &

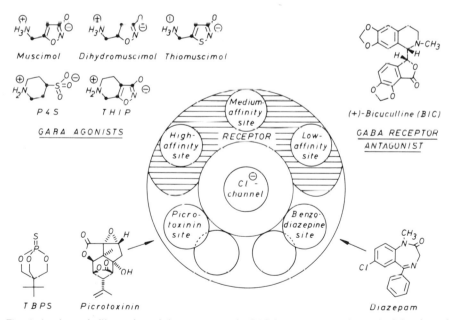

Fig. 6. A schematic illustration of the post-synaptic GABA-receptor complex and of the sites of action of some GABA agonists, the receptor antagonist bicuculline, and various other compounds. (From Krogsgaard-Larsen 1983).

Krogsgaard-Larsen 1982). The receptor function appears to be subject to modulation by various additional units, which can be detected *in vitro* as distinct binding sites for the benzodiazepines (Squires & Braestrup 1977), and picrotoxinin (Olsen 1981). A number of cage convulsants including *t*-butylbicyclophosphorothionate (TBPS) interact potently with the latter binding site (Squires *et al.* 1983). As indicated in Fig. 6, there is some evidence of heterogeneity of both the benzodiazepine and the picrotoxinin binding sites (Olsen 1981).

The physiological relevance of the mulitiple GABA-receptor sites and of these additional sites of the GABA-receptor complex is unknown, but the intimate contact and allosteric interactions between these sites as detectable *in vitro,* may reflect certain aspects of the dynamic properties of the GABA receptors (Olsen 1981, Squires *et al.* 1983).

The interaction of GABA agonists with the GABA-receptor complex *in vitro* has been extensively studied (Braestrup *et al.* 1979, Krogsgaard-Larsen & Falch 1981). These studies have disclosed striking differences between the effects on benzodiazepine binding of different "structural classes" of GABA agonists and pronounced effects of temperature and chloride ions on the degree of GABA agonist-induced stimulation of benzodiazepine binding (Supavilai & Karobath 1980). GABA and the GABA agonists muscimol, (*RS*)-dihydromuscimol, and thiomuscimol (Fig. 4), all of which have a certain degree of conformational mobility, quite effectively activate benzodiazepine binding (Fig. 7) (Braestrup *et al.* 1979). GABA agonists with more rigid structures or containing sulphonic acid groups have less effect in this test system (Krogsgaard-Larsen & Falch 1981, Krogsgaard-Larsen 1983, P. Jacobsen, E. Falch, C. Braestrup & P. Krogsgaard-Larsen, unpublished).

In Fig. 7, the effects of muscimol, THIP, and P4S on benzodiazepine binding at 30°C and in the presence or absence of chloride ions are illustrated. The presence of chloride substantially enhances the ability of these GABA agonists to stimulate benzodiazepine binding, probably reflecting the intimate contact between the receptor sites concerned and the chloride-ion channel (Fig. 6). The addition of chloride actually converts P4S from a deactivator to an activator of benzodiazepine binding, and similar effects of chloride were observed for DH-P4S (Fig. 5) (E. Falch, D. R. Curtis, P. Jacobsen & P. Krogsgaard-Larsen, unpublished).

The pharmacological relevance of these dissimilar effects of different types of potent GABA agonists on benzodiazepine binding *in vitro* is unknown. The results illustrated in Fig. 7 are reminiscent of partial GABA-agonist effects of

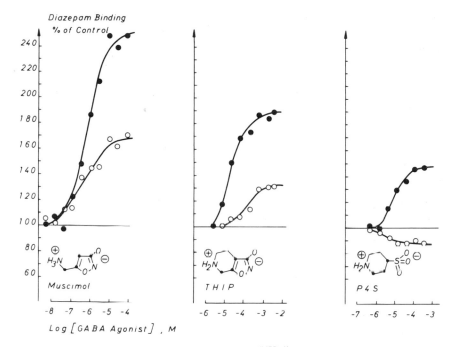

Fig. 7. Effects of some GABA agonists on the binding of ³H-diazepam at 30°C in the *presence* ● or *absence* ○ of 0.15 M-NaCl. Experiments were performed in analogy with published procedures (Braestrup *et al.* 1979, E. Falch, D. R. Curtis, P. Jacobsen & P. Krogsgaard-Larsen, unpublished).

THIP and P4S, but an interpretation of these *in vitro* observations must await the results of detailed electrophysiological studies in progress.

Our studies on the molecular pharmacology of GABA agonists have embraced labelling of THIP and P4S (Krogsgaard-Larsen *et al.* 1982b), and comparative studies on the binding of radioactive GABA, THIP and P4S (Falch & Krogsgaard-Larsen 1982, Krogsgaard-Larsen *et al.* 1983a). While the K_D values for these ligands are comparable, considerable differences between the corresponding binding capacities (B_M values) were measured (Table I). The density of the high-affinity binding sites for THIP was particularly low. While there is no obvious correlation between these data and the different effects of the GABA agonists concerned on benzodiazepine binding, the characteristics of the binding of ³H-THIP strongly suggest that the potent effects of THIP in animals and man are mediated by the medium-affinity GABA-receptor site (Krogsgaard-Larsen *et al.* 1983a).

PHARMACOKINETIC ASPECTS OF GABA AGONISTS

All compounds so far known with specific GABA-agonist actions have zwitterionic structures. Small, and frequently negligible, fractions of amino acids exist as unionized molecules in solution, the ratio between the concentrations of ionized and non-ionized molecules (I/U ratio or zwitterion constant) being a function of the difference between the pKA-I and -II values (Krogsgaard-Larsen & Falch 1981, Krogsgaard-Larsen *et al.* 1983b). A great difference between the 2 pKA values of neutral amino acids is tantamount to high I/U ratios for the compounds.

As amino acids are likely to penetrate the blood-brain barrier (BBB) in the non-ionized form, it is of pharmacological interest to develop analogues of GABA with small differences in the pKA values, and, thus, low I/U ratios, compared to GABA. Neither GABA (pKA 4.0, 10.7; I/U 800,000), isoguvacine (pKA 3.6, 9.8; I/U 200,000), nor P4S (pKA<1, 10.3; I/U>1,000,000) are capable of penetrating the BBB. On the other hand, approximately 0.1% of doses of THIP (pKA 4.4, 8.5; I/U 1,500) and muscimol (pKA 4.8, 8.4; I/U 900) exist as non-ionized molecules in aqueous solution, and this value can explain why THIP and muscimol enter the brain after peripheral administration in animals and man (Schultz *et al.* 1981, Moroni *et al.* 1982, Christensen *et al.* 1982). The very low I/U ratios for thiomuscimol (pKA 6.1, 8.9; I/U 13) and thio-THIP (pKA 6.1, 8.5; I/U 16) suggest that these compounds are capable of penetrating the BBB very easily (Krogsgaard-Larsen 1981, Krogsgaard-Larsen *et al.* 1983b).

Table I

Binding data and kinetic constants for radioactive GABA, THIP, and P4S[a]

Binding and kinetic parameters	Radioactive ligand		
	^{3}H-GABA	^{3}H-THIP	^{3}H-P4S
K_{D1} (nM)	6±3	4±2	6±2
B_{M1} (pmol/mg)	0.31±0.1	0.05±0.03	0.55±0.15
K_{D2} (nM)	175±35	80±23	56±15
B_{M2} (pmol/mg)	1.7±0.4	0.5±0.1	0.96±0.35
K_{D3} (nM)	>5,000	>10,000	>1,500
k_{on} ($M^{-1}min^{-1}$)	$2 \cdot 10^7$	–	$7 \cdot 10^7$
k_{off} (min^{-1})	0.2	–	0.8

a The receptor-binding studies (Falch & Krogsgaard-Larsen 1982) and the measurement of the kinetic constants for the high-affinity sites (Krogsgaard-Larsen *et al.* 1981b) were performed as described elsewhere in detail.

As discussed in an earlier section of this chapter, muscimol is a non-specific GABA agonist (Figs. 1, 3), and the toxicity and metabolism of muscimol (Moroni *et al.* 1982, Christensen *et al.* 1982) further reduce the pharmacological importance of this compound. So far, the metabolites of muscimol have not been identified. THIP, on the other hand, is well tolerated by various animal species (Christensen *et al.* 1982). It is active after oral administration and excreted unchanged and, to some extent, in a conjugated form in the urine of animals and humans (Schultz *et al.* 1981). The conjugate of THIP has not been isolated in a pure form, but it has chromatographic properties identical with those of synthetic THIP-*N*-glucoronide (B. Schultz, H. Mikkelsen & P. Krogsgaard-Larsen, unpublished). In the rat THIP is active for up to 3 h, and in the rhesus monkey for 4–5 h in analgesia tests (Christensen *et al.* 1982). In an attempt to obtain prolonged pharmacological actions and to avoid undesired effects at peak concentrations, a sustained release preparation of THIP is now under development.

PHARMACOLOGICAL AND CLINICAL STUDIES ON GABA AGONISTS

Among various pharmacological effects of THIP, its anticonvulsant properties in animals (Meldrum & Horton 1980, Christensen & Larsen 1982, Löscher 1982), its analgesic effects in a variety of animal models (Hill *et al.* 1981, Christensen & Larsen 1982, Kendall *et al.* 1982, Grognet *et al.* 1983), its inhibition of food intake in the rat (Blavet *et al.* 1982), and the decreases in blood pressure observed after injection of THIP into the brain ventricles of cats (Gillis *et al.* 1982) may have therapeutic interest.

In Table II, the GABA-agonist actions of muscimol, THIP, and a number of related compounds are compared with their anticonvulsant and analgesic effects in the indicated test systems. In general, there is a positive correlation between the GABA-agonist actions of these compounds and their effects in the animal-behavioural models concerned in agreement with these effects being mediated by the GABA receptors.

So far, the analgesic effects of THIP in animals and man have been most extensively studied (Christensen *et al.* 1982). The inability of naloxone to reverse THIP-induced analgesia in animals (Hill *et al.* 1981, Kendall *et al.* 1982) indicates that THIP does not interact directly with the opiate receptors. The lack of effect of BIC on THIP analgesia may suggest that a distinct subtype of GABA receptors mediates this effect of THIP, which in most animal models and in man

Table II

GABA agonist, anticonvulsant and analgesic activities of muscimol and various analogues[a]

COMPOUND	STRUCTURE	BIOLOGICAL ACTIONS		
		GABA AGONISM ON CAT SPINAL NEURONES (Rel. Potency)	ANTAGONISM OF ISONIAZIDE CONVULSIONS	ANALGESIA GRID SHOCK TEST
			(ED_{50}, μmol/kg, i.p.)	
Muscimol		– – – –	2	3
N-Methyl-muscimol		– –	>200	>200
(S)-5'-Methyl-muscimol		– – (–)	23	77
THIP		– – – (–)	9	16
6-Methyl-THIP		0	>200	>200
O-Methyl-THIP		N.t.	>200	>200
THPO		0	>200	>200
THIA		0	N.t.	>200
THAO		0	N.t.	>200

[a] The GABA-agonist activities, determined micro-electrophoretically (Curtis *et al.* 1971, Krogs-gaard-Larsen *et al.* 1979a), the effects on isoniazide-induced convulsions (Christensen *et al.* 1982), and the analgesic effects (Christensen & Larsen 1982) were measured as described elsewhere in detail.

is comparable in potency with that of morphine (Christensen *et al.* 1982, Grognet *et al.* 1983). THIP has been reported to have positive effects in chronic anxiety patients (Hoehn-Saric 1983). This combination of anxiolytic and analgesic effects combined with the observation that THIP, in contrast to morphine, does not cause respiratory depression (Christensen *et al.* 1982) has stimulated the interest in THIP, and in GABA agonists in general, as analgesic drugs.

ACKNOWLEDGEMENTS

This work was supported by grants from the Danish Medical Research Council. The collaboration with Professor D. R. Curtis, Canberra, Australia, and Drs. L. Brehm and H. Hjeds, Copenhagen, is gratefully acknowledged. The secretarial assistance of B. Hare and the technical assistance of U. Geneser, J. S. Johansen, J. B. Pedersen and S. Stilling are gratefully acknowledged.

REFERENCES

Alger, B. E. & Nicoll, R. A. (1982) Pharmacological evidence for two kinds of GABA receptors on rat hippocampal pyramidal cells studied in vitro. *J. Physiol. (London) 328,* 125–141.

Blavet, N., DeFeudis, F. V. & Clostre, F. (1982) THIP inhibits feeding behaviour in fasted rats. *Psychopharmacology 76,* 75–78.

Bowden, K. & Drysdale, A. C. (1965) A novel constituent of *Amanita muscaria. Tetrahedron Lett.* 727–728.

Braestrup, C., Nielsen, M., Krogsgaard-Larsen, P. & Falch, E. (1979) Partial agonists for brain GABA-benzodiazepine receptor complex. *Nature 280,* 331–333.

Christensen, A. V. & Larsen, J.-J. (1982) Antinociceptive and anticonvulsive effect of THIP, a pure GABA agonist. *Pol. J. Pharmacol. Pharm. 34,* 127–134.

Christensen, A. V., Svendsen, O. & Krogsgaard-Larsen, P. (1982) Pharmacodynamic effects and possible therapeutic uses of THIP, a specific GABA agonist *Pharm. Weekbl. Sci. Ed. 4,* 145–153.

Curtis, D. R., Duggan, A. W., Felix, D. & Johnston, G. A. R. (1971) Bicuculline, an antagonist of GABA and synaptic inhibition in the spinal cord of the cat. *Brain Res. 32,* 69–96.

Curtis, D. R. & Johnston, G. A. R. (1974) Amino acid transmitters in the mammalian central nervous system. *Ergebn. Physiol. 69,* 97–188.

DeFeudis, F. V. (1981) GABA and "neuro-cardiovascular" mechanisms. *Neurochem. Int. 3,* 113–122.

DeFeudis, F. V. (1982) 4-Aminobutyric acid and analgesia. *Trends Pharmacol. Sci. 3,* 444–446.

Eugster, C. H. (1969) Chemie der Wirkstoffe aus dem Fliegenpilz. *Fortschr. Chem. Org. Naturst. 27,* 261–321.

Eugster, C. H., Müller, G. F. R. & Good, R. (1965) Wirkstoffe aus *Amanita muscaria:* Ibotensaeure und Muscazon. *Tetrahedron Lett.* 1813–1815.

Eugster, C. H. & Waser, P. G. (1954) Zur Kenntnis des Muscarins. *Experientia 10,* 298–300.

Falch, E. & Krogsgaard-Larsen, P. (1982) The binding of the GABA agonist [^{3}H]THIP to rat brain synaptic membranes. *J. Neurochem. 38,* 1123–1129.

Fowler, L. J., Lovell, D. H. & John, R. A. (1983) The reaction of muscimol with 4-aminobutyrate aminotransferase. *J. Neurochem. 41,* 1751–1754.

Gillis, R. A., Williford, D. J., Souza, J. D. & Quest, J. A. (1982) Central cardiovascular effects produced by the GABA receptor agonist drug, THIP. *Neuropharmacology 21,* 545–547.

Grognet, A., Hertz, F. & DeFeudis, F. V. (1983) Comparison of the analgesic actions of THIP and morphine. *Gen. Pharmacol. 14,* 585–590.

Hill, R. C., Maurer, R., Buescher, H. H. & Roemer, D. (1981) Analgesic properties of the GABA-mimetic THIP. *Eur. J. Pharmacol. 69,* 221–224.

Hoehn-Saric, R. (1983) Effects of the GABA agonist THIP on chronic anxiety patients. *Psychopharmacol. Bull. 19,* 114–115.

Jacobsen, P., Labouta, I. M., Schaumburg, K., Falch, E. & Krogsgaard-Larsen, P. (1982) Hydroxy- and amino-substituted piperidinecarboxylic acids as 4-aminobutyric acid agonists and uptake inhibitors. *J. Med. Chem. 25,* 1157–1162.

Johnston, G. A. R., Kennedy, S. M. E. & Lodge, D. (1978) Muscimol uptake, release and binding in rat brain slices. *J. Neurochem. 31,* 1519–1523.

Kendall, D. A., Browner, M. & Enna, S. J. (1982) Comparison of the antinociceptive effect of GABA agonists: evidence for a cholinergic involvement. *J. Pharmacol. Exp. Ther. 220,* 482–487.

Krogsgaard-Larsen, P. (1977) Muscimol analogues. II. Synthesis of some bicyclic 3-isoxazolol zwitterions. *Acta Chem. Scand. B31,* 584–588.

Krogsgaard-Larsen, P. (1980) Inhibitors of the GABA uptake systems. *Mol. Cell Biochem. 31,* 105–121.

Krogsgaard-Larsen, P. (1981) 4-Aminobutyric acid agonists, antagonists, and uptake inhibitors. Design and therapeutic aspects. *J. Med. Chem. 24,* 1377–1383.

Krogsgaard-Larsen, P. (1983) GABA agonists: Structural, pharmacological and clinical aspects. In: *Metabolic Relationship between Glutamine, Glutamate and GABA in the CNS,* eds. Hertz, L., Kvamme, E., McGeer, E. & Schousboe, A., pp. 537–557 Alan R. Liss, Inc., New York.

Krogsgaard-Larsen, P., Brehm, L. & Schaumburg, K. (1981a) Muscimol, a psychoactive constituent of *Amanita muscaria,* as a medicinal chemical model structure. *Acta Chem. Scand. B35,* 311–324.

Krogsgaard-Larsen, P. & Christiansen, T. R. (1979) GABA agonists. Synthesis and structure-activity studies on analogues of isoguvacine and THIP. *Eur. J. Med. Chem. 14,* 157–164.

Krogsgaard-Larsen, P. & Falch, E. (1981) GABA agonists. Development and interactions with the GABA receptor complex. *Mol. Cell. Biochem. 38,* 129–146.

Krogsgaard-Larsen, P., Falch, E., Peet, M. J., Leah, J. D. & Curtis, D. R. (1983a) Molecular pharmacology of the GABA receptors and GABA agonists. In: *CNS Receptors – From Molecular Pharmacology to Behaviour,* eds. Mandel, P. & DeFeudis, F. V., pp. 1–13. Raven Press, New York

Krogsgaard-Larsen, P., Falch, E., Schousboe, A., Curtis, D. R. & Lodge, D. (1980) Piperidine-4-sulphonic acid, a new specific GABA agonist. *J. Neurochem. 34,* 756–759.

Krogsgaard-Larsen, P., Hjeds, H., Curtis, D. R., Leah, J. D. & Peet, M. J. (1982a) Glycine antagonists structurally related to muscimol, THIP, or isoguvacine. *J. Neurochem. 39,* 1319–1324.

Krogsgaard-Larsen, P., Hjeds, H., Curtis, D. R., Lodge, D. & Johnston, G. A. R. (1979a) Dihydromuscimol, thiomuscimol, and related heterocyclic compounds as GABA analogues. *J. Neurochem. 32,* 1717–1724.

Krogsgaard-Larsen, P., Johansen, J. S. & Falch, E. (1982b) Deuterium labelling of the GABA agonists THIP, piperidine-4-sulphonic acid and the GABA uptake inhibitor THPO. *J. Labelled Compd. 19,* 689–701.

Krogsgaard-Larsen, P., Johnston, G. A. R., Lodge, D. & Curtis, D. R. (1977) A new class of GABA agonist. *Nature 268*, 53–55.

Krogsgaard-Larsen, P., Mikkelsen, H., Jacobsen, P., Falch, E., Curtis, D. R., Peet, M. J. & Leah, J. D. (1983b) 4,5,6,7-Tetrahydroisothiazolo[5,4-*c*]pyridin-3-ol and related analogues of THIP. Synthesis and biological activity. *J. Med. Chem. 26*, 895–900.

Krogsgaard-Larsen, P., Scheel-Krüger, J. & Kofod, H. eds. (1979b) *GABA-Neurotransmitters. Pharmacochemical, Biochemical and Pharmacological Aspects*, Munksgaard, Copenhagen.

Krogsgaard-Larsen, P., Snowman, A., Lummis, S. C. & Olsen, R. W. (1981b) Characterization of the binding of the GABA agonist [^{3}H]piperidine-4-sulphonic acid to bovine brain synaptic membranes. *J. Neurochem. 37*, 401–409.

Löscher, W. (1982) Comparative assay of anticonvulsant and toxic potencies of sixteen GABA-mimetic drugs. *Neuropharmacology 21*, 803–810.

Meldrum, B. (1982) Pharmacology of GABA. *Clin. Neuropharmacol. 5*, 293–316.

Meldrum, B. & Horton, R. (1980) Effects of the bicyclic GABA agonist, THIP, on myoclonic and seizure responses in mice and baboons with reflex epilepsy. *Eur. J. Pharmacol. 61*, 231–237.

Moroni, F., Forchetti, M. C., Krogsgaard-Larsen, P. & Guidotti, A. (1982) Relative disposition of the GABA agonists THIP and muscimol in the brain of the rat. *J. Pharm. Pharmacol. 34*, 676–678.

Morselli, P. L., Löscher, W., Lloyd, K. G., Meldrum, B. & Reynolds, E. H. eds. (1981) *Neurotransmitters, Seizures, and Epilepsy*, Raven Press, New York.

Olsen, R. W. (1981) GABA-benzodiazepine-barbiturate receptor interactions. *J. Neurochem. 37*, 1–13.

Olsen, R. W., Bergman, M. O., Van Ness, P. C., Lummis, S. C., Watkins, A. E., Napias, C. & Greenlee, D. V. (1981) Gamma-aminobutyric acid receptor binding in mammalian brain: Heterogeneity of binding sites. *Mol. Pharmacol. 19*, 217–227.

Roberts, E., Chase, T. N. & Tower, D. B., eds. (1976) *GABA in Nervous System Function*, Raven Press, New York.

Schousboe, A., Thorbek, P., Hertz, L. & Krogsgaard-Larsen, P. (1979) Effects of GABA analogues of restricted conformation on GABA transport in astrocytes and brain cortex slices and on GABA receptor binding. *J. Neurochem. 33*, 181–189.

Schultz, B., Aaes-Jørgensen, T., Bøgesø, K. P. & Jørgensen, A. (1981) Preliminary studies on the absorption, distribution, metabolism, and excretion of THIP in animal and man using 14C-labelled compound. *Acta Pharmacol. Toxicol. 49*, 116–124.

Skolnick, P. & Paul, S. M. (1981) Benzodiazepine receptors. *Ann. Rep. Med. Chem. 16*, 21–29.

Squires, R. F. & Braestrup, C. (1977) Benzodiazepine receptors in rat brain. *Nature 266*, 732–734.

Squires, R. F., Casida, J.E., Richardson, M. & Saederup, E. (1983) 35S-*t*-Butyl-bicyclophos-phothionate binds with high affinity to brain specific sites coupled to GABA-A and ion recognition sites. *Mol. Pharmacol. 23*, 326–336.

Supavilai, P. & Karobath, M. (1980) The effect of temperature and chloride ions on the stimulation of [^{3}H]flunitrazepam binding by the muscimol analogues THIP and piperidine-4-sulphonic acid. *Neurosci. Lett. 19*, 337–341.

Takemoto, T., Nakajima, T. & Sakuma, R. (1964) Isolation of a flycidal constituent "ibotenic acid" from *Amanita muscaria* and *A. pantherina*. *J. Pharm. Soc. Jpn. 84*, 1233–1234.

Waser, R. G. (1979) The pharmacology of *Amanita muscaria*. In: *Ethnopharmacologic Search for Psychoactive Drugs*, eds. Efron, D. H., Holmstedt, B. & Kline, N. S., pp. 419–439. Raven Press, New York.

Wasson, R. G. (1968) *Soma. Divine Mushroom of Immortality,* Harcourt Brace Jovanovich, New York.

Wasson, R. G. (1979) Fly agaric and man. In: *Ethnopharmacologic Search for Psychoactive Drugs,* eds. Efron, D. H., Holmstedt, B. & Kline, N. S., pp. 405–414. Raven Press, New York.

DISCUSSION

RAZDAN: What is the activity range for analgesia of THIP?

FALCH: THIP has been tested in a variety of animal models and in patients. The relative potency of THIP and morphine depends somewhat on the species used, but in most models and in humans THIP is approximately equipotent with morphine.

BRØGGER CHRISTENSEN: You mentioned in your talk that muscimol might be toxic because it is metabolized. Do you have any idea of the structure of the toxic metabolites, or of the mechanism underlying the metabolism of muscimol?

FALCH: Muscimol is a substrate for the transaminating enzyme GABA-T, but the structures of the metabolites are not known.

LAZDUNSKI: Is there any effect of benzodiazepines on the binding of radioactive THIP to the medium – or on low-affinity GABA receptor sites?

FALCH: It has not been studied yet, but investigations along these lines have a high priority in our laboratories. Other groups have studied the benzodiazepines' influence on the binding of GABA, but the technique required for such studies is not fully developed.

LAZDUNSKI: I was asking about THIP which appears to recognize rather selectively, low-affinity GABA receptor sites.

FALCH: While the effects of a variety of GABA agonists on benzodiazepine binding have been studied in great detail, the "reverse effects" have only been studied using GABA itself as a ligand.

NAKANISHI: Has anyone made the bicyclic isoxazole N-oxide related to THIP? This might be an interesting model compound for studies of the agonist specificity of the GABA receptors. What is the pK_a-value for the 3-hydroxy-isoxazole?

FALCH: Such analogues have not been synthesized yet, but it would be relevant to consider this type of compound. The pK_a-values for 3-hydroxyisoxazoles are about 5.

PORTOGHESE: you showed a receptor model containing 3 binding sites. Do your binding studies exclude the existence of only 2 GABA receptor sites?

FALCH: We have analyzed our binding data for radioactive GABA, THIP, and P4S very throughly using computer programmes. The data are consistent with 3 binding sites, and attempts to fit the data to a 2-sided model almost always give less satisfactory results. I wish to emphasize that the K_d-value for the low-affinity site really is too high for satisfactory characterization.

Amanita muscaria in Medicinal Chemistry. II. Ibotenic Acid Analogues as Specific Agonists at Central Glutamate Receptors

*Povl Krogsgaard-Larsen, Elsebet Ø. Nielsen, Anne Engesgaard, Jørn Lauridsen, Lotte Brehm & Jan J. Hansen**

Certain amino acids play a key role in the function of the mammalian central nervous system (CNS) (Curtis & Johnston 1974). While 4-aminobutyric acid (GABA) is the major inhibitory neurotransmitter in the brain, glutamic acid (GLU), and possibly also aspartic acid (ASP), are assumed to be the major excitatory neurotransmitters.

Extensive electrophysiological and neurochemical studies during the past 3 decades have shed some light on the extremely complex functions of GABA in the CNS, although our knowledge of the mechanisms underlying the GABA neurotransmission is still incomplete (Roberts *et al.* 1976, Krogsgaard-Larsen *et al.* 1979). As a result of the development of GABA mimetics with potent and specific actions, the pharmacology of GABA is now in a stage of rapid development (Krogsgaard-Larsen 1981).

Compared with GABA, studies of the excitatory neurotransmission processes are at a very early stage. GLU, as well as ASP, are capable of exciting virtually all neurones in the CNS, and the ubiquity of GLU in the CNS, its involvement in protein synthesis and nitrogen metabolism, and its role as a precursor for GABA make specific studies of GLU neurotransmission processes difficult (Roberts *et al.* 1981). A prerequisite for progress in this field, is the development of agents by which the GLU receptors and other synaptic mechanisms can be specifically manipulated.

The Royal Danish School of Pharmacy, Department of Chemistry BC, DK-2100 Copenhagen, and *The Technical University of Denmark, Department of Applied Biochemistry, DK-2800 Lyngby, Denmark

NATURAL PRODUCTS AND DRUG DEVELOPMENT, Alfred Benzon Symposium 20.
Editors: P. Krogsgaard-Larsen, S. Brøgger Christensen, H. Kofod, Munksgaard, Copenhagen 1984.

NATURALLY OCCURRING ANALOGUES OF GLUTAMIC ACID

A number of heterocyclic analogues of GLU have been isolated from natural sources as exemplified in Fig. 1 (Davies *et al.* 1982). Ibotenic acid (IBO), which is biosynthesized by *Amanita muscaria,* and muscazon, formed by photochemical rearrangement of IBO, can be isolated from the dried mushroom (Eugster 1969). Quisqualic acid (QUIS) is a constituent of *Quisqualis fructus* (Takemoto *et al.* 1975), and willardiine has been isolated from *Acacia willardinia* (Evans *et al.* 1980). The pyrrolidine amino acids kainic acid and domoic acid are produced by *Digenea simplex* (Ueno *et al.* 1955) and *Chondria armata,* respectively (Takemoto *et al.* 1966).

With the exception of muscazon (Curtis *et al.* 1979), all of these amino acids are neuronal excitants, which are more potent than GLU after micro-electrophoretic administration near central neurones (Biscoe *et al.* 1976, Davies *et al.* 1982), and like GLU they cause degeneration of neurones after local

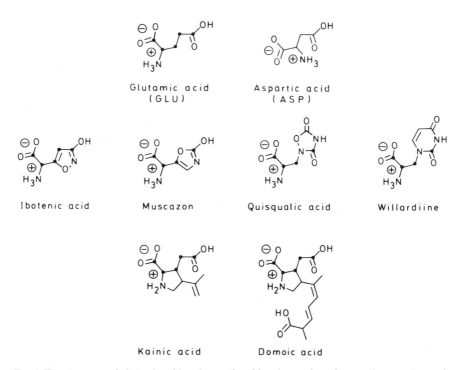

Fig. 1. The structure of glutamic acid and aspartic acid and a number of naturally occurring amino acids structurally related to glutamic acid.

injection into animal brains (Coyle *et al.* 1981). The pharmacological effects and patterns of neuronal degeneration observed after such injections have been shown to mimic the symptoms and alterations of neuronal pathways observed in patients suffering from epilepsy or Huntington's chorea (Coyle *et al.* 1981). As most, if not all, of these effects, apparently, are the results of hyperactivation of central excitatory amino acid receptors, these receptors have been brought into focus as potential pharmacological sites of attack. Antagonists at these receptors obviously have therapeutic interest, and the availability of such compounds and specific agonists is a necessary condition for satisfactory receptor characterization (Watkins 1981, Krogsgaard-Larsen & Honoré 1983).

CLASSIFICATION OF CENTRAL, EXCITATORY AMINO ACID RECEPTORS
Although all of the excitatory heterocyclic amino acids depicted in Fig. 1 are structural analogues of GLU, these compounds do not interact with a homogeneous population of receptors. Based on the relative sensitivity of these GLU analogues and the GLU agonist (*R*)-N-methylaspartic acid (N-Me-*D*-ASP, NMDA) to different antagonists the excitatory amino acid receptors are at present most conveniently subdivided into 3 classes (Fig. 2) (Watkins 1981, Davies *et al.* 1982, Krogsgaard-Larsen & Honoré 1983):

1. "QUIS receptors", at which (*S*)-glutamic acid diethyl ester (GDEE) acts as a relatively selective, but weak, antagonist (Hall *et al.* 1979),
2. "NMDA receptors", which can be blocked by a number of compounds including 2-amino-5-phosphonovaleric (2APV) and α-amino-adipic acid (α-AA), of which 2APV is the most potent antagonist so far known (Watkins 1981), and,
3. "kainic acid receptors", at which certain lactonized derivatives of kainic acid, notably **1** and **2** (Fig. 2), show selective antagonistic properties (Goldberg *et al.* 1981).

This receptor classification obviously is artificial, and the physiological relevance of these subclasses of receptors is not clear. Kainic acid binds with high affinity to a distinct class of receptor sites (Simon *et al.* 1976), assumed to represent pre-synaptic GLU receptors which stimulate the release of GLU and ASP from pre-synaptic terminals (Ferkany *et al.* 1982). Domoic acid (Fig. 1) appears to be the most potent agonist known at the "kainic acid receptors" (Watkins 1981). Very little is known about the location and physiological function of the "NMDA receptors" (Watkins 1981, Coyle *et al.* 1981).

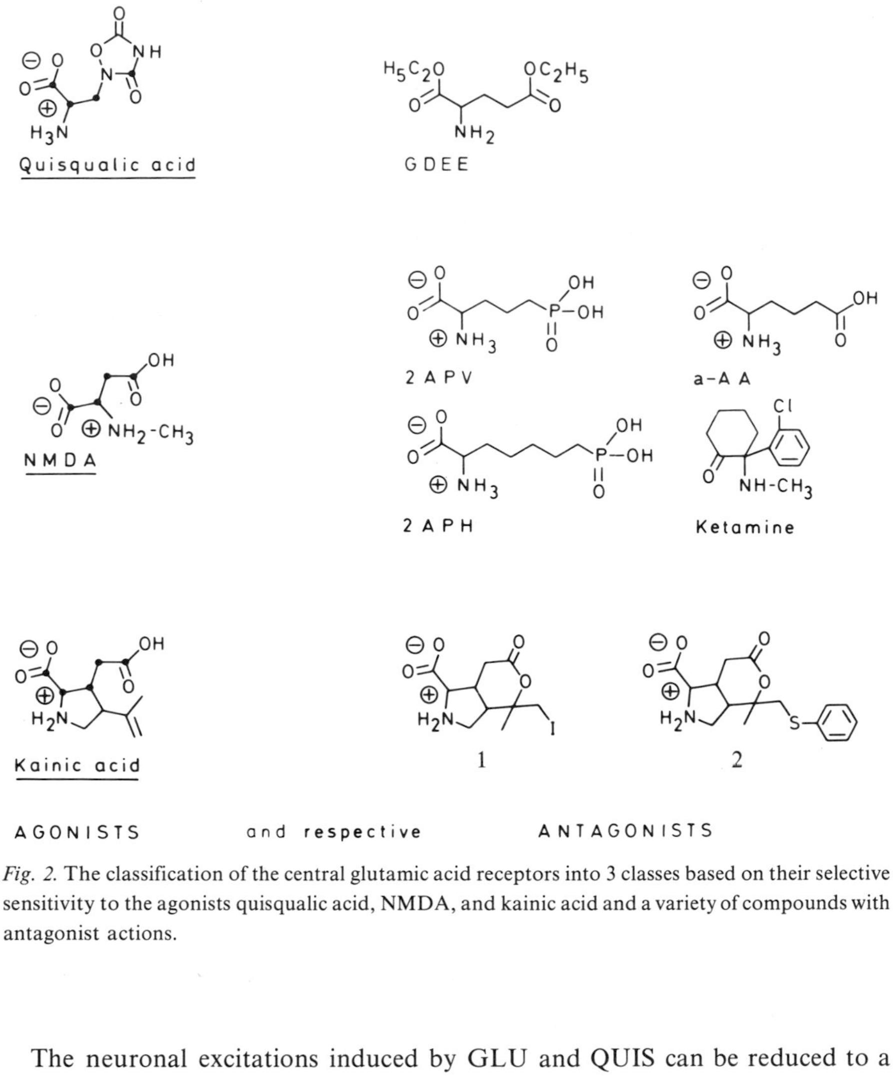

Fig. 2. The classification of the central glutamic acid receptors into 3 classes based on their selective sensitivity to the agonists quisqualic acid, NMDA, and kainic acid and a variety of compounds with antagonist actions.

The neuronal excitations induced by GLU and QUIS can be reduced to a similar extent by GDEE, and both amino acids are relatively insensitive to NMDA and kainic acid antagonists (Fig. 2) (Watkins 1981, Goldberg *et al.* 1981). These observations suggest that the "QUIS receptors" primarily represent the class of receptors associated with the excitation of central neurones by GLU. Consequently, there is a considerable interest in specific agonists and antagonists for the GDEE-sensitive "QUIS receptors". QUIS is, however, far from being an ideal tool for studies of these receptors. QUIS does for example bind tightly to the "kainic acid receptors" (Simon *et al.* 1976).

The primary objective of our studies on the central excitatory neurotransmission processes is the development of specific agonists at the GDEE-sensitive "QUIS receptors". In this phase of the project, IBO has proven to be a useful lead.

STRUCTURE ACTIVITY STUDIES ON IBOTENIC ACID AND
RELATED COMPOUNDS

During the past few years, the *in vivo* and *in vitro* effects of IBO on central neurotransmission processes have been quite extensively studied (Nistri & Constanti 1979, Curtis *et al.* 1979, Krogsgaard-Larsen *et al.* 1981). IBO is chemically unstable (Eugster 1969), and it appears to interact with all types of excitatory receptors, primarily the "NMDA receptors" (Curtis *et al.* 1979). In an attempt to distinguish these actions of IBO and with the aim of optimizing the effect on the "QUIS receptors", a number of analogues of IBO have been synthesized and tested (Hansen & Krogsgaard-Larsen 1980, Krogsgaard-Larsen *et al.* 1980, Honoré & Lauridsen, 1980, Honoré *et al.* 1982, Krogsgaard-Larsen *et al.* 1981).

A CNDO/2-molecular orbital study has shown that a conformation of the fully charged molecule of IBO similar to conformation II in Fig. 3 is energetically favourable in the conservative state (Borthwick & Steward 1976). Allowance for an aqueous medium, however, predicts a change in the conservative-molecule minimum-energy conformation from II into I (Fig. 3) (Borthwick & Steward 1976). In the bicyclic IBO analogue (*RS*)-3-hydroxy-4,5,6,7-tetrahydroisoxazolo[5,4-*c*]pyridine-7-carboxylic acid (7-IIPCA) the structural element equivalent to IBO has been locked in a conformation similar to conformation I (Fig. 3) (P. Krogsgaard-Larsen, E. Ø. Nielsen & D. R. Curtis, unpublished). Micro-electrophoretic studies disclosed that 7-HPCA is a powerful agonist at the GDEE-sensitive "QUIS receptors" having virtually no effect on "NMDA receptors" (Fig. 3), and binding studies have shown that 7-HPCA may reflect the conformation of IBO and GLU at the "QUIS receptors".

The pharmacological profile of (*RS*)-α-amino-3-hydroxy-4-methyl-5-isoxazoleacetic acid (4-methyl-IBO) at single cat spinal neurones is qualitatively similar to that of IBO, although the introduction of a methyl group on the ring of IBO gives a compound, which is essentially weaker. Similarly, homologation of the side chain of IBO results in a much weaker analogue, but in contrast to IBO and 4-methyl-IBO, (*RS*)-α-amino-3-hydroxy-5-isoxazolepropionic acid (homo-

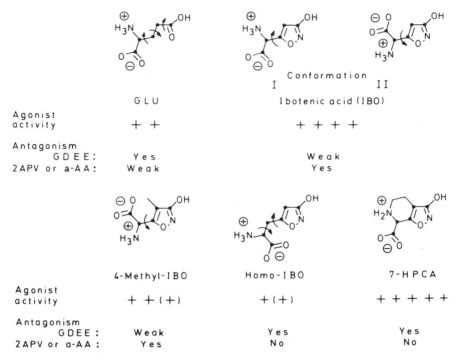

Fig. 3. Structure-activity studies on glutamic acid, ibotenic acid, and a number of ibotenic acid analogues. The conformational mobility around some carbon-carbon bonds is indicated by arrows.

IBO) selectively activates "QUIS receptors" though much weaker than 7-HPCA (Fig. 3) (Krogsgaard-Larsen et al. 1980).

The susceptibility of IBO to decarboxylation (Eugster 1969) prompted us to synthesize (RS)-α-amino-3-hydroxy-5-methyl-4-isoxazolepropionic acid (AMPA), which is a chemically stable analogue of IBO still containing a GLU-structure element (Fig. 4) (Hansen & Krogsgaard-Larsen 1980). Like 7-HPCA (Fig. 3), AMPA proved to be a very potent GDEE-sensitive GLU agonist, insensitive to the NMDA antagonists 2APV or α-AA (Fig. 4) and with no effect on "kainic acid receptor" sites in vitro (Krogsgaard-Larsen et al. 1980, 1982).

The assumption that steric effects of the methyl group of AMPA forces the GLU-structure element of the molecule to adopt a more or less folded conformation (Fig. 4) (Krogsgaard-Larsen et al. 1980), led us to propose that AMPA and GLU interact with the "QUIS receptors" in somewhat folded conformations. This hypothesis was supported by structure-activity studies

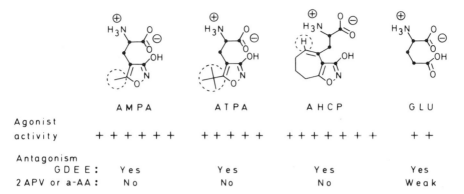

	AMPA	ATPA	AHCP	GLU
Agonist activity	+ + + + +	+ + + + +	+ + + + + + +	+ +
Antagonism				
GDEE:	Yes	Yes	Yes	Yes
2 APV or a-AA:	No	No	No	Weak

Fig. 4. Structure-activity studies on glutamic acid and a number of ibotenic acid analogues. The steric effects of certain groups are indicated.

on (*RS*)-a-amino-3-hydroxy-5-*tert*butyl-4-isoxazolepropionic acid (ATPA) (Krogsgaard-Larsen *et al.* 1982), and (*RS*)-α-amino-3-hydroxy-7,8-dihydro-6*H*-cycloheptatrieno[1,2-*d*]isoxazole-4-propionic acid (AHCP) (P. Krogsgaard-Larsen, E. Ø. Nielsen & D. R. Curtis, unpublished). Like AMPA, both ATPA and, in particular, AHCP, are very powerful agonists at GDEE-sensitive receptors with no significant effects on "NMDA receptors" (Fig. 4), or "kainic acid receptor" sites. It should be noted that the backbone of AHCP, which is assumed to bind to the receptors, unlike those of 7-HCPA (Fig. 3), AMPA, and ATPA, consists of 6 carbon atoms. In any case, the structure-activity studies on the compounds depicted in Fig. 3 and Fig. 4, emphasize that the agonist conformations recognized by the "QUIS, NMDA and kainic acid receptors" are different.

Fig. 5 illustrates the conformations of 7-HPCA (L. Brehm, unpublished), and AMPA (Honoré & Lauridsen 1980), in the crystalline states as established by X-ray analyses. In the 7-HPCA molecule the isoxazole ring is planar and the 6-membered ring is in a half-chair conformation with the carboxylate group in an equatorial position. The 7-HPCA and AMPA molecules are both highly selective agonists at the "QUIS receptors" (Figs. 3, 4). The conformations of the 2 molecules in the solid states are quite different (Fig. 5). Force-field calculation performed by use of the programme MM2 (Allinger 1977) on AMPA indicate energy barriers less than 29 kjoule/mol for rotation around the C(4)–C(7) bond. This indicates that the molecule is rather flexible and that conformations different from the one observed in the crystal are accessible. By alteration of the

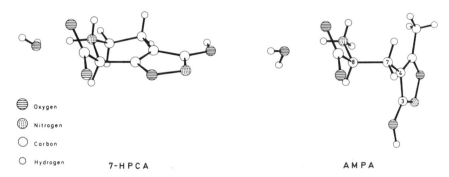

Oxygen
Nitrogen
Carbon
Hydrogen
7-HPCA
AMPA

Fig. 5. The conformations of 7-HPCA and of AMPA monohydrates in the crystalline states as established by X-ray analyses.

torsion angle C(3)-C(4)-C(7)-C(8) to *ca.* 180° the conformation of AMPA, found in the crystalline state, is changed into a conformation, which is comparable with that of 7-HPCA in the crystalline state. In the light of this similarity and the relatively small energy barriers between the different conformations of AMPA, the conformation of 7-HPCA observed in the solid state may represent the active conformations of IBO and AMPA at the "QUIS receptors".

3
5
6
4
7
9
8
7-HPCA
CH2N2
HNO2
BuLi,
HBr
IRA
400
, H2O

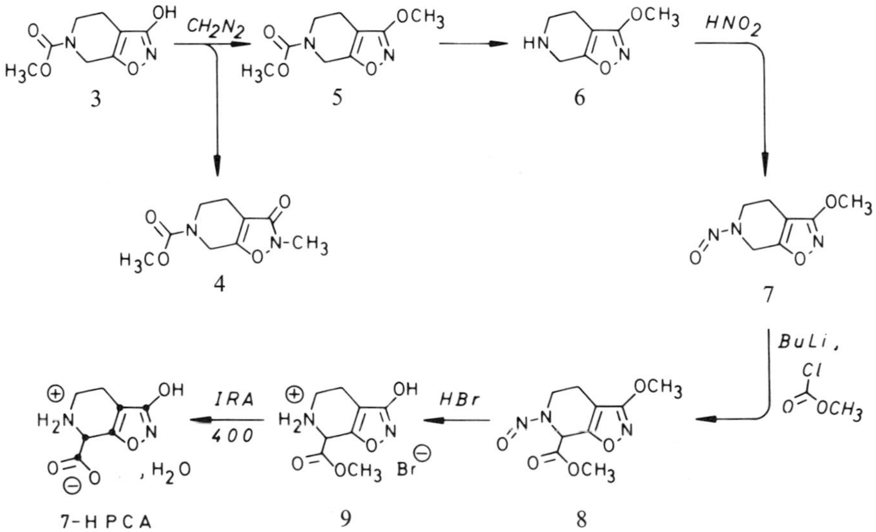

Scheme 1

SYNTHESES OF ANALOGUES OF IBOTENIC ACID

All of the IBO analogues so far discussed have been synthetized *via* multi-step sequences. In Scheme 1, the last steps of the reaction sequence for the preparation of 7-HPCA are outlined (P. Krogsgaard-Larsen, E. Ø. Nielsen & D. R. Curtis, unpublished). The bicyclic 3-isoxazole 3 (Krogsgaard-Larsen 1977) was converted into a separable mixture of 4 and 5. Treatment of 6, obtained by alkaline hydrolysis of 5, with nitrous acid transformed it into the *N*-nitroso derivative 7. As indicated, a methoxycarbonyl group was then introduced regiospecifically into position 7 of 7 to give 8, which was stepwise deprotected to give 7-HPCA. In order to avoid decarboxylation of the final product the last reaction step was an ester hydrolysis of 9, accomplished on a strongly basic ion exchange-resin without significant loss of the carboxylate group.

The last steps of the multi-step synthesis of AHCP are shown in Scheme 2 (P. Krogsgaard-Larsen, E. Ø. Nielsen & D. R. Curtis, unpublished). Oxidation of the 3-methoxyisoxazole 12 gave a mixture of the ketones 13 and 14, the latter compound being the major product. The allylic bromination of 15, obtained from 14 *via* a Grignard reaction, proceeded regiospecifically. Deprotection of 17 was accompanied by quite extensive decomposition, and AHCP could only be isolated in relatively poor yields.

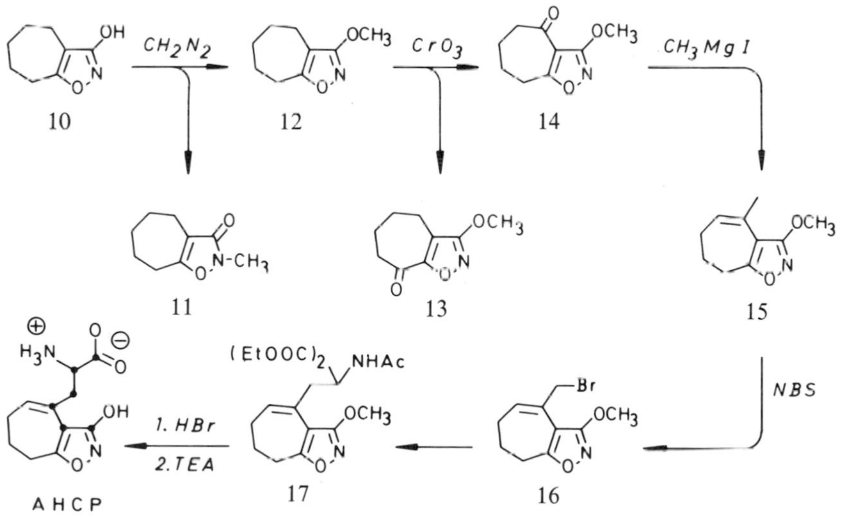

Scheme 2

STEREOSTRUCTURE-ACTIVITY STUDIES ON AMPA AND GLUTAMIC ACID

(*R*)- and (*S*)-GLU are approximately equipotent as excitants when administered micro-electrophoretically near neurones in the mammalian CNS (Curtis & Watkins 1960). As both of these isomers appear to be substrates for the low-affinity transport system, assumed to be responsible for the synaptic inactivation of GLU (Cox *et al.* 1977), the apparent equipotency of these optical antipodes cannot be explained by a more rapid removal from the synaptic environments of the more effective receptor agonist. The excitatory effect of (*R*)-GLU is, however, more sensitive to NMDA antagonists than that of (*S*)-GLU (Fig. 6) (Watkins 1981), indicating that (*R*)-GLU, more pronounced than the (*S*)-isomer, is an agonist at both "NMDA and QUIS receptors". These observations seem to indicate that (*S*)-GLU actually is the more effective agonist at the GDEE-sensitive "QUIS receptors" assumed to be the physiologically relevant post-synaptic GLU receptors (see earlier sections of this chapter). As AMPA appears to be a specific agonist at these receptors (Fig. 4) (Krogsgaard-Larsen *et al.* 1980), it was of interest to study the excitatory effects of the optical antipodes of AMPA.

Both (*R*)- and (*S*)-AMPA have recently been obtained by enzymatic resolution (Hansen *et al.* 1983), and shown to be GDEE-sensitive, 2APV-insensitive excitants of cat spinal neurones, (*S*)-AMPA being the more active isomer (Fig. 6) (Krogsgaard-Larsen *et al.* 1982). Thus, both (*S*)-GLU and (*S*)-AMPA are more effective in exciting the GDEE-sensitive "QUIS receptors" than the respective (*R*)-enantiomers.

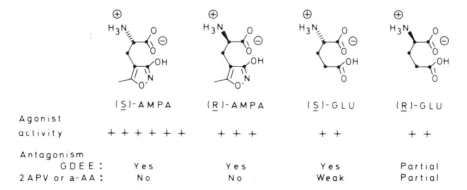

Fig. 6. Structure-activity studies on the optical antipodes of AMPA and glutamic acid.

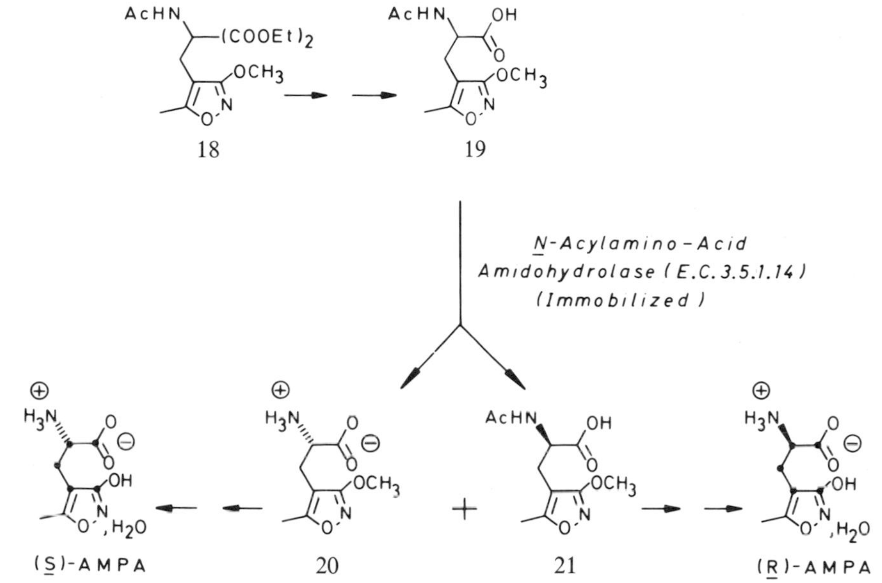

Scheme 3

The resolution of AMPA is illustrated in Scheme 3 (Hansen *et al.* 1983). Under appropriate conditions an immobilized form of the enzyme *N*-acylaminoacylase (E.C. 3.5.1.14) deacetylated the (*S*)-form of **19** in an apparently stereospecific manner. Deprotection of the corresponding amino acid **20** and of the acetylated (*R*)-form **21** to give (*S*)- and (*R*)-AMPA, respectively, proceeded without detectable racemization. The methoxylated compound **19** proved to be a better substrate for the enzyme than the corresponding 3-isoxazolol derivative, *N*-acetyl-AMPA, which has 2 acid moieties.

RADIOACTIVE AMPA AS A LIGAND FOR STUDIES OF CENTRAL GLUTAMIC ACID RECEPTORS

The apparent high degree of specificity of AMPA for post-synaptic GLU receptors, prompted the synthesis of radioactive AMPA (Scheme 4) for receptor binding and autoradiographic studies. In model experiments using deuterium gas, the bromomethyl group of **22** was converted almost quantitatively into a monodeuteriomethyl group in **23** (indicated by an asterisk in Scheme 4), and acid deprotection of **23** proceeded without significant loss of deuterium

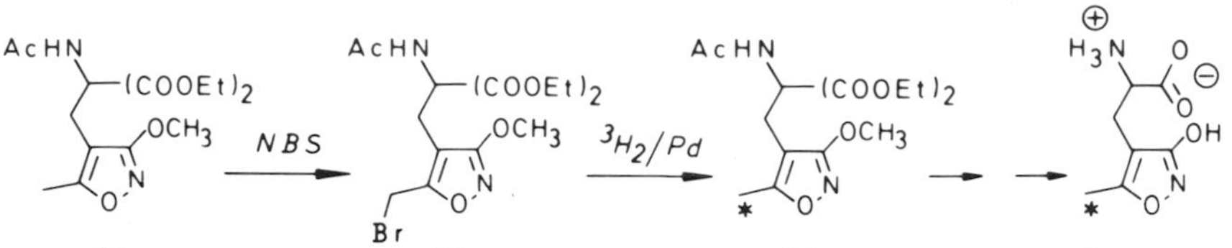

Scheme 4

(Lauridsen & Honoré 1981). This reaction sequence was used by New England Nuclear, Boston, U.S.A. to prepare ^{3}H-AMPA with a specific radioactivity of *ca.* 15 Ci/mmol.

The pharmacological characteristics of ^{3}H-AMPA binding were studied using a membrane preparation exhibiting a single binding site (K_D 300 nM, B_{max} 2.7 pmol·mg[−1] protein), and shown to be distinctly different from those of the binding sites for ^{3}H-GLU and ^{3}H-kainic acid (Honoré *et al.* 1981, 1982, Simon *et al.* 1976).

A comparison of the activity of a number of IBO analogues as agonists at the GDEE-sensitive "QUIS receptors" and as inhibitors of ^{3}H-GLU, ^{3}H-kainic acid, and ^{3}H-AMPA binding is illustrated in Table I. Within this group of compounds there obviously is no correlation between the *in vivo* effects and the ability to displace ^{3}H-GLU and ^{3}H-kainic acid from their receptor sites (Krogsgaard-Larsen *et al.* 1980, 1982, Honoré *et al.* 1981, Hansen *et al.* 1983). This lack of correlation between the GDEE-sensitive excitatory activities and the effects on ^{3}H-kainic acid binding is in agreement with the kainic acid receptor sites being distinctly different from the receptors associated with the neuronal excitation by GLU (Ferkany *et al.* 1982).

There is, on the other hand, no obvious explanation of the conspicuous discrepancy between the potencies of the compounds as GDEE-sensitive neuronal excitants and as inhibitors of ^{3}H-GLU binding. It is possible that the excitatory actions of the compounds are mediated by a subpopulation of GLU receptors (Krogsgaard-Larsen & Honoré 1983). The density of the ^{3}H-AMPA binding sites is only about 10% of that of the ^{3}H-GLU sites (Honoré *et al.* 1982). This observation and the correlation between the potencies of the compounds as GDEE-sensitive neuronal excitants and as inhibitors of ^{3}H-AMPA binding (Table I) suggest that the ^{3}H-AMPA binding sites represent the physiological post-synaptic GLU receptors (Krogsgaard-Larsen & Honoré 1983). According-

Table I

Structure-activity studies on glutamic acid and some ibotenic acid analogues

COMPOUND	AGONIST ACTIVITY ON CAT SPINAL NEURONES GDEE SENSITIVE (Rel. Potency)	INHIBITION OF THE BINDING OF RADIOACTIVE (IC_{50}, μM)		
		GLU	KAINIC ACID	AMPA
GLU	+ +	0.5	0.4	1
(S)-AMPA	+ + + + + +	>100	>100	0.6
(R)-AMPA	+ + +	>100	>100	5
Homo-IBO	+ (+)	7.5	>100	16
4-Me-homo-IBO	+ + +	45	>100	2
4-Br-homo-IBO	+ + + + +	110	>100	3

The effects of the compounds on single cat spinal neurones were measured micro-electrophoretically (Krogsgaard-Larsen *et al.* 1980, 1982). The binding studies using radioactive GLU (Honoré *et al.* 1981), kainic acid (Krogsgaard-Larsen *et al.* 1980), and AMPA (Honoré *et al.* 1982) were performed as described elsewhere.

ly, QUIS, (S)-GLU, (S)-AMPA, and AHCP are the most potent inhibitors of ^{3}H-AMPA binding so far tested (Honoré *et al.* 1982, Hansen *et al.* 1983, E. Ø. Nielsen & J. Lauridsen, unpublished).

The recent demonstration of specific binding of ^{3}H-AMPA to cultured mouse CNS neurones (Hösli *et al.* 1983), supports the view that this ligand is likely to be a useful tool for the mapping of central GLU neurones, as well as for the development of new agonists and antagonists for the post-synaptic GLU receptors.

IBOTENIC ACID HOMOLOGUES AS AGONISTS OR ANTAGONISTS AT
EXCITATORY AMINO ACID RECEPTORS

The observation that homologues of GLU and related phosphonoamino acids are antagonists at the "NMDA receptors" (Fig. 2) (Watkins 1981) prompted the syntheses of homologues of IBO (Hansen & Krogsgaard-Larsen 1980, T. Honoré & J. Lauridsen, unpublished). While homo-IBO is a weak, GDEE-sensitive GLU agonist (Figs. 3, 7) (Krogsgaard-Larsen *et al.* 1980), the higher homologues (*RS*)-α-amino-3-hydroxy-5-isoxazolebutyric acid ((2)homo-IBO) and (*RS*)-α-amino-3-hydroxy-5-isoxazolevaleric acid ((3)-homo-IBO) are moderately potent antagonists at "NMDA receptors" (Fig. 7) (Krogsgaard-Larsen *et al.* 1981). In the GLU homologues and the phosphonoamino acids (Fig. 2), the "NMDA antagonist" properties reside in the (*R*)-isomers (Watkins 1981). Enzymatic resolution of homologues of IBO, using processes analogous with those outlined in Scheme 3 are in progress.

The present structure-activity studies have shed light on the active conformations of agonists at the "QUIS receptors", assumed to represent the physiological post-synaptic GLU receptors. Onc of the objectives of the present project is to develop antagonists at these receptors, and, thus, the problem is to convert the described potent GDEE-sensitive GLU agonists such as 7-HPCA (Fig. 3), AMPA, and AHCP (Fig. 4), into analogues with high affinity for, and without intrinsic activity at, the receptors concerned. Pertinent model compounds are at present being synthesized in our attempt to reach this goal.

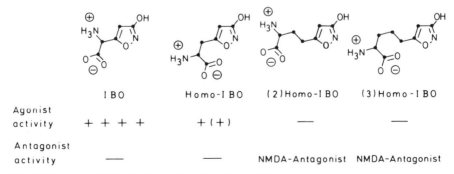

Fig. 7. Structure-activity studies on ibotenic acid and 3 homologues.

ACKNOWLEDGEMENTS

This work has been supported by grants from The Danish Medical Research Council and The Foundation for Technical Chemistry of The Technical University of Denmark. The collaboration with Professor D. R. Curtis, Canberra, Australia, and Dr. T. Honoré, Copenhagen, is gratefully acknowledged. Part of the synthetic work was performed by P. Krogsgaard-Larsen at the School of Pharmacy, University of Kansas, Lawrence, U.S.A., and fruitful discussions with Professors M. Mertes and L. A. Mitscher are gratefully acknowledged.

REFERENCES

Allinger, N. L. (1977) Conformational analysis. 130. MM2. A hydrocarbon force field utilizing V_1 and V_2 torsional terms. *J. Am. Chem. Soc. 99*, 8127–8134.

Biscoe, T. J., Evans, R. H., Headley, P. M., Martin, M. R. & Watkins, J. C. (1976) Structure-activity relations of excitatory amino acids on frog and rat spinal neurones. *Br. J. Pharmacol. 58*, 373–382.

Borthwick, P. W. & Steward, E. G. (1976) Ibotenic acid: further observations on its conformational modes. *J. Mol. Struct. 33*, 141–144.

Cox, D. W. G., Headley, P. M. & Watkins, J. C. (1977) Actions of L- and D-homocysteate in rat CNS: a correlation between low-affinity uptake and the time courses of excitation by microelectrophoretically applied L-glutamate analogues. *J. Neurochem. 29*, 579–588.

Coyle, J. T., Bird, S. J., Evans, R. H., Gulley, R. L., Nadler, J. V., Nicklas, W. J. & Olney, J. W. (1981) Excitatory amino acid neurotoxins: selectivity, specificity, and mechanisms of action. *Neurosci. Res. Prog. Bull. 19*, 333–427.

Curtis, D. R. & Johnston, G. A. R. (1974) Amino acid transmitters in the mammalian central nervous system. *Ergebn. Physiol. 69*, 97–188.

Curtis, D. R., Lodge, D. & McLennan, H. (1979) The excitation and depression of spinal neurones by ibotenic acid. *J. Physiol. (London) 291*, 19–28.

Curtis, D. R. & Watkins, J. C. (1960) The excitation and depression of spinal neurones by structurally related amino acids. *J. Neurochem. 6*, 117–141.

Davies, J., Evans, R. H., Jones, A. W., Smith, D. A. S. & Watkins, J. C. (1982) Differential activation and blockade of excitatory amino acid receptors in the mammalian and amphibian central nervous systems. *Comp. Biochem. Physiol. 72C*, 211–224.

Eugster, C. H. (1969) Chemie der Wirkstoffe aus dem Fliegenpilz. *Fortschr. Chem. Org. Naturst. 27*, 261–321.

Evans, R. H., Jones, A. W. & Watkins, J. C. (1980) Willardiine: a potent quisqualate-like excitant. *J. Physiol. (London) 308*, 71P–72P.

Ferkany, J. W., Zaczek, R. & Coyle, J. T. (1982) Kainic acid stimulates excitatory amino acid neurotransmitter release at presynaptic receptors. *Nature 298*, 757–759.

Goldberg, O., Luini, A. & Teichberg, V. I. (1981) Lactones derived from kainic acid: novel selective antagonists of amino acid-induced Na^+ fluxes in rat striatum slices. *Neurosci. Lett. 23*, 187–191.

Hall, J. G., Hicks, T. P., McLennan, H., Richardson, T. L. & Wheal, H. V. (1979) The excitation of mammalian central neurones by amino acids. *J. Physiol. (London) 286,* 29–39.

Hansen, J. J., Lauridsen, J., Nielsen, E. & Krogsgaard-Larsen, P. (1983) Enzymatic resolution and binding to rat brain membranes of the glutamic acid agonist, α-amino-3-hydroxy-5-methyl-4-isoxazolepropionic acid. *J. Med. Chem. 26,* 901–903.

Hansen, J. J. & Krogsgaard-Larsen, P. (1980) Isoxazole amino acids as glutamic acid agonists. Synthesis of some analogues and homologues of ibotenic acid. *J. Chem. Soc. Perkin Trans. I.* 1826–1833.

Honoré, T. & Lauridsen, J. (1980) Structural analogues of ibotenic acid. Syntheses of 4-methylhomoibotenic acid and AMPA, including the crystal structure of AMPA, monohydrate. *Acta Chem. Scand. B34,* 235–240.

Honoré, T., Lauridsen, J. & Krogsgaard-Larsen, P. (1981) Ibotenic acid analogues as inhibitors of [^{3}H]glutamic acid binding to cerebellar membranes. *J. Neurochem. 36,* 1302–1304.

Honoré, T., Lauridsen, J. & Krogsgaard-Larsen, P. (1982) The binding of [^{3}H]AMPA, a structural analogue of glutamic acid, to rat brain membranes. *J. Neurochem. 38,* 173–178.

Hösli, E., Krogsgaard-Larsen, P. & Hösli, L. (1983) Binding sites for the glutamate-analogue [^{3}H]AMPA in cultured rat brainstem and spinal cord. *Brain Res. 268,* 177–180.

Krogsgaard-Larsen, P. (1977) Muscimol analogues. II. Synthesis of some bicyclic 3-isoxazolol zwitterions. *Acta Chem. Scand. B31,* 584–588.

Krogsgaard-Larsen, P. (1981) 4-Aminobutyric acid agonists, antagonists, and uptake inhibitors. Design and therapeutic aspects. *J. Med. Chem. 24,* 1377–1383.

Krogsgaard-Larsen, P., Hansen, J. J., Lauridsen, J., Peet, M. J., Leah, J. D. & Curtis, D. R. (1982) Glutamic acid agonists. Stereochemical and conformational studies of DL-α-amino-3-hydroxy-5-methyl-4-isoxazolepropionic acid (AMPA) and related compounds. *Neurosci. Lett. 31,* 313–317.

Krogsgaard-Larsen, P. & Honoré, T. (1983) Glutamate receptors and new glutamate agonists. *Trends Pharmacol. Sci. 4,* 31–33.

Krogsgaard-Larsen, P., Honoré, T., Hansen, J. J., Curtis, D. R. & Lodge, D. (1980) New class of glutamate agonist structurally related to ibotenic acid. *Nature 284,* 64–66.

Krogsgaard-Larsen, P., Honoré, T., Hansen, J. J., Curtis, D. R. & Lodge, D. (1981) Structure-activity studies on ibotenic acid and related muscimol analogues. In: *Glutamate as a Neurotransmitter,* eds. Di Chiara, G. & Gessa, G. L., pp. 285–294. Raven Press, New York.

Krogsgaard-Larsen, P., Scheel-Krüger, J. & Kofod, H. eds. (1979) *GABA-Neurotransmitters. Pharmacochemical, Biochemical and Pharmacological Aspects,* Munksgaard, Copenhagen.

Lauridsen, J. & Honoré, T. (1981) Preparation of deuterium labelled α-amino-3-hydroxy-5-methyl-4-isoxazolepropionic acid (AMPA) *J. Labelled Compd. 18,* 1479–1484.

Nistri, A. & Constanti, A. (1979) Pharmacological characterization of different types of GABA and glutamate receptors in vertebrates and invertebrates. *Prog. Neurobiol. (Oxford) 13,* 117–235.

Roberts, E., Chase, T. N. & Tower, D. B. eds. (1976) *GABA in Nervous System Function,* Raven Press, New York.

Roberts, P. J., Storm-Mathisen, J. & Johnston, G. A. R. eds. (1981) *Glutamate: Transmitter in the Central Nervous System,* John Wiley & Sons, Chichester & New York.

Simon, J. R., Contrera, J. F. & Kuhar, M. J. (1976) Binding of [^{3}H]-kainic acid, an analogue of L-glutamate, to brain membranes. *J. Neurochem. 26,* 141–147.

Takemoto, T., Daigo, K., Kondo, Y. & Kondo, K. (1966) Studies on the constituents of *Chondria armata.* VIII. On the structure of domoic acid. *J. Pharm. Soc. Jpn. 86,* 874–877.

Takemoto, T., Nakajima, T., Arihara, S. & Koiki, K. (1975) Studies on the constituents of *Quisqualis fructus.* II. Structure of quisqualic acid. *J. Pharm. Soc. Jpn. 95,* 326–332.

Ueno, Y., Nawa, H., Ueganagi, J., Morimoto, H., Nakamori, R. & Matsuoka, T. (1955) Studies on the active compounds of *Digenea simplex:* Ag and related compounds. *J. Pharm. Soc. Jpn. 75,* 807–844.

Watkins, J. C. (1981) Pharmacology of excitatory amino acid receptors. In: *Glutamate: Transmitter in the Central Nervous System,* eds. Roberts, P. J., Storm-Mathisen, J. & Johnston, G. A. R., pp. 1–24. John Wiley & Sons, Chichester & New York.

DISCUSSION

ALBUQUERQUE: Did you calculate the density of the AMPA binding sites in the cultured spinal neurones?

KROGSGAARD-LARSEN: We did not calculate the density. I can inform you that the density of the binding sites for radioactive AMPA was about 10% of that for radioactive glutamic acid in binding studies using rat brain synaptic membranes, suggesting that the AMPA sites represent only a subpopulation of the total number of binding sites for glutamic acid.

ANDERSON: Many of the studies on receptor-active conformations that have been done with other neurotransmitter systems, including GABA, usually conclude that the active conformation is one of the minimum energy conformations, and those frequently turn out to be fully extended conformations. This apparently is not the case with glutamic acid agonists. I wonder if you could comment on that, and is this, in fact, the first example of an amino acid neurotransmitter that is active in a folded conformation?

KROGSGAARD-LARSEN: It seems to be the case for glutamic acid based on the described indirect studies. We see the same thing for GABA. In the GABA field we have some good model compounds including THIP. In the light of the specificity of THIP as a GABA agonist, it is fair to conclude that THIP represents the active conformation of muscimol and also GABA. But this particular conformation of muscimol is not the conformation of lowest energy.

BLUNDEN: A much more fundamental question: One would imagine that ibotenic acid would be present in the mushroom as a feeding deterrent agent. Yet, in fact, the fungus is quite readily eaten by a number of organisms. You indicated that ibotenic acid had an effect on the snail Helix. Is it known if there are any detoxification mechanisms in the lower forms of life, because you don't find a pile of dead organisms around these mushrooms, although many animals eat them?

KROGSGAARD-LARSEN: There are 2 aspects of your question which I think are important. On the surface of the mushroom you have a red colour, in which ibotenic acid is incorporated chemically. Below this coloured material, you find a yellow coloured layer containing the free ibotenic acid. So it is possible that the animals can eat the surface of the mushrooms without getting too much ibotenic acid. I am, however, not sure that ibotenic acid *per se* is the dangerous compound. Ibotenic acid possibly has to be converted into muscimol before it really kills them, because muscimol is extremely active on the central neurones of most lower animals. The rate of conversion of ibotenic acid into muscimol may be different in different animals.

NAKANISHI: Would it be relevant to try to develop photoaffinity labels for the glutamic acid receptors?

KROGSGAARD-LARSEN: The problem here is that the glutamic acid receptors are very difficult to study, because glutamic acid is involved in a variety of processes in the brain, not only in neurotransmission, but also in nitrogen metabolism, energy metabolism, and it acts as a precursor for GABA. It has multiple functions, and, consequently, there must be many different active sites for glutamic acid in the brain, besides the receptors. It is going to be extremely difficult to pick up specifically the receptors. But in this respect some of the compounds I have described might represent useful models.

NAKANISHI: My question actually is pertinent to domoic acid, which you showed on a slide. A number of analogues of domoic acid are being synthesized with the purpose of labelling the receptors to which it binds – does this approach make sense?

KROGSGAARD LARSEN: By definition, it would not be an unreasonable approach. I am glad to hear that the work on domoic acid is being continued. The problem with domoic acid is that the plant which is producing this unique amino acid is dying. We may not have a natural source for domoic acid anymore.

NAKANISHI: The natural source, which was thought to be extinct, has been rediscovered.

LAZDUNSKI: I will start with a comment on Dr. Nakanishi's question. In order to be successful in a photoaffinity experiment you must have the right combination of number of receptor sites and adequate receptor affinity. In the case of glutamic acid the affinity appears to be between 0.1 and 1 micromolar, and with the number of different binding sites that are known for glutamic acid you will probably have little change to be successful with an affinity label. You have to gain 2 orders of magnitude in the affinity, in order to start affinity labelling experiments in order to identify the receptor.

KROGSGAARD-LARSEN: May I comment further on this problem? The affinity of agonists for the quisqualic acid-preferring glutamate receptors is relatively low, in the micromolar range. In the case of the kainic acid receptor type, it is, however, much lower. It is in the nanomolar range, and domoic acid is the most potent agonist at this type of receptors.

NAKANISHI: The reason I mentioned domoic acid is because it has the extended side chain. It has been more easy to play around with.

LAZDUNSKI: Are your agonists active on the glutamate receptors of muscles of insects? Are these compounds very toxic for insects?

KROGSGAARD-LARSEN: We have not studied the effects of these compounds on the muscles of crustaceans or insects. Ibotenic acid is very toxic for some animals, but as I mentioned before, I think that ibotenic acid has to be converted, i.e. decarboxylated, into muscimol, before it acts. Ibotenic acid very effectively kills flies, whereas AMPA, which is resistant to decarboxylation, has no effect on flies. As AMPA is more potent than ibotenic acid as an agonist, the glutamic receptors apparently do not mediate the killing effects of ibotenic acid.

ATTA-UR-RAHMAN: Have any of the glutamic acid agonists been demonstrated to be very effective in the clinic?

KROGSGAARD-LARSEN: All glutamic-acid agonists so far known are neurotoxic. However, the patterns of neuronal degeneration of the different agonists are different. So, hopefully, it will be possible to separate neuroexitation and neurotoxicity. If this is possible, pharmacological or even clinical studies might be relevant in this field.

RAPOPORT: You might consider the possibility of synthesizing ibotenic acid.

KROGSGAARD-LARSEN: Ibotenic acid is very difficult to synthesize. The yields of published procedures are extremely low. We are trying to develop alternative syntheses, but we are faced with quite severe problems.

RAPOPORT: On the basis of addition to vinylglycine?

KROGSGAARD-LARSEN: No, we are trying to develop a completely different synthetic route.

Concluding Remarks

Bernhard Witkop

Professor Kofod, ladies and gentlemen. We have talked about recognition sites, I think, metaphorically speaking, this site and place is now approriate to give recognition to the success of the symposium and to the accomplishments and wisdom of the managing staff. We let a 100 topics, as it were a 100 flowers blossom, and by now some older topics, such as the ergot alkaloids, look like a Japanese *Bonsai.* We crossed, nationally and scientifically, boundaries with equal ease, and each participant is free to select his favourite impressions, carry them home, and let them grow and mature, a privilege of a pluralistic society. We used as a vehicle of communication the universal language of chemistry that, like music, is understandable without limitation throughout the world's scientific community. In addition, there was a special communication. As the Japanese say "*I-shin den-shin*", i.e., from heart to heart.

The Alfred Benzon Foundation's planning made possible this meeting between East and West, the New World and the Old World, thus, creating reservoirs of goodwill, and centres of crystallization for new ideas and types of collaboration. Those of us who were present in Strasbourg 3 years ago at the international congress with a similar topic "Natural Products as Medicinal Agents" cannot resist the temptation of comparison. In Strasbourg, more than 1,000 participants laboured for a week to produce a volume containing more multa than multum. Here, we addressed a truly interdisciplinary programme with 35 speakers in their double rôle as listeners, in only 4 days. We might perhaps have extended the opportunity for discussion by special round-table workshops with not more than 3–5 interdisciplinary topics. As we also think of suggestions for the printed proceedings of this symposium, the pedagogic, and possibly sales value, of such a book might be increased by having a glossary, in which the individual authors try to explain, in the simplest terms possible, the meaning of phenomena, such as fast and slow channels, receptor ionophores,

NATURAL PRODUCTS AND DRUG DEVELOPMENT, Alfred Benzon Symposium 20.
Editors: P. Krogsgaard-Larsen, S. Brøgger Christensen, H. Kofod, Munksgaard, Copenhagen 1984.

desensitization, or the properties of special toxins. For this suggestion, I found in Professor Kofod a willing receptor with positive co-operativity.

More and more, in the words of Arnold Toynbee, the history of mankind becomes a race between education and catastrophy. We touched ever so lightly on the problem of fertility control, fully aware of the great urgency of a speedy solution, as we do live in a "*MAD*" world, that is a world of *M*utually *A*ssured *D*estruction. We are aware of the gradation of information not all of which can be stored as knowledge, and not all knowledge contributes to experience, leave alone wisdom or *sapientia,* the increasingly questionable hallmark of *homo sapiens.* Information should have a negative entropy. Otherwise, it is equivalent to confusion. This interpretation of the character of information, we owe it to Claude Shannon, should be remembered in the preparation of legible slides.

Our conference has given old and new clues to the management of diseases and problems of public health, be they infectious diseases, control of cancer, or the most common disease, old age. In keeping, as a *basso ostinato*, the guiding theme of selective receptors as the basis for the mechanism of action of actual and potential therapeutic agents, we have kept the tenor of this symposium on a high level of molecular biology and have helped Professor Kofod to avoid the misleading and perilous stigma of the daily newspapers, expressed in a possible dreaded headline, "Danish Academy Embraces and Endorses Herbal Medicine".

As you now join me in a rousing vote of thanks to the ever active staff of the symposium and of the Alfred Benzon Foundation, the repetitiousness of this gesture may not tire Professor Kofod too much, so that he may not say, like the late John Jacob Astor at the height of the confusion of the sinking of the "Titanic": "I have been ringing for some ice, but this, this is too much".

The graceful setting for the symposium in the Royal Danish Academy of Sciences and Letters prompted Professor Carl Djerassi to draw certain parallels between men of science and men of letters.

The editors are happy to include the poem overleaf in the Proceedings, thus, to quote the author, "adding a touch of levity to an otherwise very serious collection of papers".

WHY ARE...

548

WHY ARE CHEMISTS NOT POETS?

Take the chemist.
By definition
The synthesizer of molecules;
The dissector of molecules;
The manipulator of molecules.

For molecules read words:
You have defined the poet.

Why then
Are chemists never poets?

Initially chemists always dilute.
Eventually they always concentrate,
Evaporate, distill
To reach their chemical goal.

While some poets dilute,
The best are thickeners.
(No wonder the German poet is a Dichter.*)*
They thicken, dichten, *concentrate,*
Distill,
Until the poem is compacted.

Why then
Are chemists not poets?

Chemists work in fume hoods,
Wearing safety glasses,
Behind explosion-proof shields,
In a partial vacuum,
Under some inert atmosphere.

Can you imagine a poet
Writing in such a laboratory?
Writing sterile,
Non-explosive,
Non-inflammable,
Vacuous poems?
Poems which, if they stink,
Are kept in a rarefied atmosphere
To hide the stench?

Now you know why
There is no future
For a careless chemist,
A cautious poet.

Carl Djerassi

Subject Index

A-23187, 411
Abdominis muscle, 285
Abeo-diene, 125
Abortifacient, 373
Acacia, 35, 526
Acanthaster, 171
Acetergamina, 464, 465
Acetylcholine, 301, 325
   analogues, cyclic, 322
Acetylcholinesterase, 287, 306
Acetyldigoxin, 19
Acetylpyridine methiodide, 287,
   305, 306
Achyrocline, 394
Aconitine, 325, 330
Aconitum, 394
Acosamine, 268
Acromegaly, 467, 476
Acronychia, 235
Acronycine, 234
Actinomadura, 195, 197, 198, 273
Actinomycetes, 217, 267
Actinoplanes, 195, 198
Action potentials, 315, 326
Actodigin, 340
Acylagmatine amidase, 244
Acylaminoacylase, N-, 535
Adaline, dihydro, 284
Addiction, 439
Adenosine analogues, 158
Adenosylmethionine bio-
   methylation, 166
Adoniside, 20
Adriamycin, 267, 277
Aescin, 19
Agardhiella, 186
Agglutinins, 184
Agmatine, 243
Agrimonia, 99
Agrimophol, 99
Agroclavine, 477
AHCP, 531, 533
Ajmalicine, 19, 51
Alamethicin, 291
Alanine, 284
Alantolactone, 414

Albomycin, 214, 226
Aldo-keto reductase,
   mammalian, 274
Alginic acids, 400
Alkaloid, quinolinium, 202
Alkaloids, 122, 253, 302
   phenanthroquinolizidine, 199
   production of, 70
   pyrrolizidine, 390
Allantoin, 19
Alpha-adrenergic, 461, 484
Alpinetin, 111
Alpinia, 107
Althaea, 394
Alzheimer's disease, 294
Amanita, 284, 289, 305, 504, 525
Amatoxins, 284
Ames test, 461
Amikacin, 71, 72
Amino-methylhex-ynoic acid, 41
Aminoadipic acid, 527
Aminobutyric acid (GABA),
   504, 525
   betaine, 181
Aminopeptidase, 244
Aminovaleric acid betaine, 182
Amitriptyline, 450
Amofrutin, 200
Amomum, 107
Amorpha, 200
Amorphane, 96
AMPA, 530, 534, 535
Amylase, 180
Anabaena, 285, 302
Anabasine, 20
Anaesthetic, 317
Analgesia, THIP, 523
Analgesic, 284, 439, 488, 504, 517
Analgeticum, 154
Anaphylatoxins, 411
Anatoxin, 322
   -A, 284, 302
   conformation, 299
Androctonus, 326, 329, 330
Andrographolide, 20
Androstene, 19-nor, 172

Anemonia, 326, 330
Angelica, 400
Angina pectoris, 103
Aniba, 115
Anicetus, 37
Anisodamine, 20
Ansamacrolides, 197
Ansamitocins, 197
Anthopleura, 330
Anthracen-imines, dihydro, 451
Anthracyclines, 267
Anthracyclinones, 267
Anthrone, 229
Anti-allergic, 155
Anti-amphetamine, 155
Anti-arhytmic agent, 332
Anti-arthritic, 152
Anti-cholinergic, 450
Anti-convulsant, 151, 332, 450,
   451, 452, 456, 504, 517
Anti-depressant, 153, 450
Anti-dopamine, 450
Anti-fertility, 355, 358
Anti-fungal, 152
Anti-hypertensive, 337
Anti-inflammatory, 154, 160
Anti-malaria, 34, 95
Anti-nociceptive, 488
Anti-serotonin, 450
Anti-snake venom, 39
Anti-tumor activity, 141, 394
Antibiotic resistance raising, 72
Antibiotics, 179, 193, 213
   aminocyclitols, 197, 205
   anthracyclines, 198
   from higher plants, 198, 207
   isoflavones, 198
   marine sources, 211
   polyether, 197
   production of, 70, 73
Antibodies, monoclonal, 300
Anticholinergic, 494
Antidepressive, 474, 476
Antigens, 67
Antiglaucoma agents, 500
Antihepatitis agents, 101

558

medicine, China, 94
medicine, Pakistan, 121
medicine, Thai, 107
systems of medicine, China, 79, 42
systems of medicine, India, 78, 79
Trans-bis-Q, 305
Tremors, 155
Tributyltin hydride, 271
Trichilia, 34
Trichillins, 34
Trichoderma, 284
Trichosanthin, 355
Trifluoroacetic acid, 410
Trilobolide, 407
Trimethylsilyl chloride, 38
Tripdiolide, 47, 57
Triphenylphosphonium, hydroxypropyl-, 117
Tripterygium, 46, 56
Triterpenes, 33, 99
Triterpenoid, 135, 124
Trypsin, 180
Tryptamine, 136
  NN-dimethyl, 51
Tryptanthrin, 201
Tubaic acid, 232
Tubercidin, deoxy-iodo, 158
Tubocurarine, 19, 24, 310

Tubulosine, 205
Tumors, 228, 467
Tylocebrine, 205
Tylophorine, 205

Ubiquinones, 393
Ulvaline, 183
Umbelliferone, 383
  methyl, 383
Umstimmungs-therapie, 394
Unani-Tibb system, 78, 79
Urotensin, 284
Utero-evacuant, 362
Uterotonic, 464, 467
Uzarigenin, 340, 342

Vaccine, 67
Vallesiachotamine, 51
Vasicine, 355
Veratraldehyde, 117
Veratridine, 325, 330
Veratrum alkaloids, 325
Victomycin, 239
Vinblastine, 47, 121, 130
  anhydro, 48, 53, 141
Vinca, 25
Vincadifformine, 128
Vincaleukoblastine, 19, 25
Vincamine, 20, 121, 136
Vincristine, 130

Vindoline, 47, 51, 127, 130
  epi-, 128
Viscum, 400
Vitamin E, 387
Walker Ca-256, 99
Warburganal, 33
Warburgia, 33, 34
Willardiine, 526
Wittig reaction, 117
Wuweizisu, 101, 385

Xanthone, 228, 237
Xanthotoxin, 19

YA56X, 239
YA56Y, 239
Yingzhaosu, 98, 106
Yohimbine, 20, 51
Yuanhuacine, 355

Zanthoxylum, 203
Zenks alkaloid medium, 50
Zingerone, 107
Zingiber, 107, 109, 110, 116
Zoapatanol analogues, 362
Zoapatanol, 355, 360, 373
Zoapatlin, 365
Zorbamycin, 239
Zorbonomycin, 239
Zymosan, 394